Partial Extraction Therapy in Implant Dentistry

Udatta Kher • Ali Tunkiwala
Editors

Partial Extraction Therapy in Implant Dentistry

Springer

Editors
Udatta Kher
Only Smiles Dental Centre
Mumbai
India

Ali Tunkiwala
Smiles by Design
Mumbai
India

ISBN 978-3-030-33609-7 ISBN 978-3-030-33610-3 (eBook)
https://doi.org/10.1007/978-3-030-33610-3

This Springer imprint is published by the registered company Springer Nature Switzerland AG
The registered company address is: Gewerbestrasse 11, 6330 Cham, Switzerland

Dear Meenakshi and Bhakti,
We wish to express our gratefulness for everything you remarkable women have done to enhance our lives.

Udatta & Ali

Foreword

As dentistry evolves, it takes pioneers and trendsetters to look into the future. Tooth replacement strategies are among the most critical of all dental procedures. Patients rely upon dental professionals to be able to minimize destruction and maximize the effect and esthetics of these artificial replacement teeth.

This book highlights a more minimally invasive approach developed over the past 2 decades and how "Partial Extraction Therapies" can be implemented into a modern dental practice. The authors have concisely adapted this technique as a routine protocol and have clarified the key factors of success in a systematic blueprint.

I hope that this book helps lead the next generation of dentists to look more closely at these modern-day tooth replacement procedures.

Maurice Salama, DDS
Team Atlanta Dental Clinic,
Atlanta, GA, USA
Scientific Editor Dentalxp.com

Foreword

The loss of a tooth sets off a cascade of events that ultimately lead to bone and soft tissue loss. Many techniques have been developed over the years to try and deal with this phenomenon. Most of these techniques have occasional success, and we are striving to find a technique that is more predictable and reproducible—predictable in that we can achieve the best result possible more often than not and reproducible in that it is not just a technique that is limited to highly skilled clinicians but one that can be achieved across the board. This book is an important milestone in helping practitioners with a step-by-step protocol in a technique that has slowly become a predictable and reproducible way to maintain the bone and soft tissue both in the short and long term.

I have no doubt that this book will help anyone wanting to get involved in these treatment protocols, thereby benefitting our patients and giving them the ideal treatment options they expect from us as practitioners.

These techniques are not easy and require a fair amount of surgical skill. Learning how to do them by reading up on the protocols will go a long way in giving you the necessary confidence to try this technique. Reading in itself is not enough, and I encourage everyone who wants to attempt this technique to get adequate training from an accredited institute or trainer and secondly to ensure that you have the correct instruments to carry out the procedure. Failure to follow these protocols may lead to increased failure and frustration.

These techniques will change the way you do implantology, and the improvement in the results you achieve will be staggering.

Howard Gluckman, BDS, MChD (OMP), PhD
Director, Implant and Aesthetic Academy,
Cape Town, South Africa

Preface

Leaving a part of the root behind intentionally when extracting a tooth prior to implant placement would seem unthinkable for most clinicians. When Narayan first introduced the concept of the socket shield technique to us in 2012, we instinctively dismissed it. The procedure sounded like a violation of the basic principles of implant dentistry.

Some cutting-edge work on Dental XP (one of the largest portal for online education) by Maurice Salama, Howard Gluckman, Snjezana Pohl and Jorge Campos Aliaga inspired us to warm up to the idea of placing an implant in close proximity to a partially extracted root.

The results we witnessed in the first few cases were spectacular and surpassed the outcomes of our earlier cases in every aspect. This motivated us to pursue the socket shield technique more frequently in our practices. Unfortunately, there was limited literature on the subject. We depended on the experience of the originators of partial extraction therapies (PET), Howard and Maurice, to guide us through the protocols.

In the past 5 years, PET procedures have gained immense popularity the world over. With the growing enthusiasm among clinicians, the time was ripe to introduce a set of guidelines for clinicians to follow in order to achieve consistently successful outcomes, minimize errors, and manage complications.

This guidebook on PET covers all aspects of treatment modality with an emphasis on case selection criteria and step-by-step demonstration of the technique. All three PET modalities—the socket shield procedure, pontic shield procedure, and root submergence technique—are described in the book. The restorative phase of the treatment involving the art of fabricating the interim and definitive restoration is described in great detail.

The contributors to the book, Sudhindra Kulkarni, Tarun Kumar, and Payal Kumar, have been early adopters of the PET procedure and bring their wealth of experience to the book. Fittingly, Narayan, who has been one of the earliest experts of the socket shield technique, has scripted the chapter on biological rationale for PET.

Any new technique needs several rounds of fine-tuning and establishing protocols. The newly developed technique should also be duplicable, in that any clinician anywhere in the world should be able to achieve comparable results if the methodology is followed. We acknowledge the contribution of the *PET Research Group* comprising selfless clinicians and researchers from all over the world who are teaching the right method of executing this technique and also contributing towards forming a consensus on certain contentious issues.

The introduction of any novel treatment protocol should be aimed at reducing morbidity, treatment duration, and overall cost, without any compromise to the final result. The PET is a patient-centric treatment approach, which apart from fulfilling all the above criteria also provides results that are superior to existing techniques. With evidence in favor of the technique increasing by the day, it is a matter of time before PET become part of mainstream implant practice. This book will provide a thorough understanding of all aspects of the technique while assisting clinicians in incorporating the procedure in their daily practices.

Mumbai, India — Udatta Kher
Mumbai, India — Ali Tunkiwala

Contents

Biologic Rationale for Partial Extraction Therapies

1

T. V. Narayan and Sudhindra Kulkarni

Abstract

Partial extraction therapies (PET) are a group of clinical procedures carried out wherein a part of the tooth is left behind in the alveolar socket at the time of extraction and the implant is placed either at the same time or later. This technique makes the body believe that the tooth is in the bone and makes it behave as such. The procedure relies on the concept that, the alveolar bone resorption is a consequence of loss of bundle bone and the only way to preserve the bundle bone is to retain the periodontal ligament attachment to it. This chapter will cover the biology of the periodontal tissues and the evolution of PET.

1.1 Introduction

Partial extraction therapies denote a collective term used to describe the maintenance of a root or a part of the root with the aim of preserving the natural contours of bone and soft tissue around implant-retained restorations. These include the root submergence technique [1], the socket-shield technique [2], the pontic-shield technique [3], and Glocker's technique [4] for ridge preservation. Details of each will be described in the further chapters of this book. The key to the rationale for partial extraction therapies lies in understanding alveolar bone development, bundle bone, and the dimensional changes associated with tooth loss, which will be discussed in the following sections.

T. V. Narayan (✉)
Private Practice, Bengaluru, Karnataka, India

S. Kulkarni
Department of Implantology, SDM Dental College, Sri Dharmasthala Manjunatheshwara University, Dharwad, Karnataka, India

Private Practice, Hubli, Karnataka, India

U. Kher, A. Tunkiwala (eds.), *Partial Extraction Therapy in Implant Dentistry*, https://doi.org/10.1007/978-3-030-33610-3_1

1.1.1 Alveolar Bone

Alveolar bone is one of the three supporting tissues of teeth. Along with periodontal ligament and cementum, they are collectively called the periodontium. Alveolar bone is composed of two structures—the alveolar process and the alveolar bone proper. Tooth buds of developing teeth are housed in the alveolar process during organogenesis and subsequently the roots of the teeth. The alveolar process of the jawbones is unique, since it develops for the teeth and along with the eruption of the teeth and is dependent on the presence of teeth for its maintenance, undergoing atrophy, once the teeth are lost. Alveolar bone consists of two plates of cortical bone separated by cancellous bone. In some areas the alveolar bone may be thin and have no cancellous bone (Figs. 1.1 and 1.2).

The spaces between the trabeculae of cancellous bone are filled with marrow (Fig. 1.2a), which is hematopoietic in early life and fatty later in life. The surface of the trabeculae of bone is lined by osteoblasts, which are responsible for bone formation. These osteoblasts get incorporated within the matrix of bone as it is laid down to form osteocytes, which lie in lacunae and communicate with each other via canaliculi to maintain the homeostasis of bone. Cells responsible for resorption of bone are the osteoclasts and are seen in resorption bays known as Howship's lacunae. Bone is a dynamic tissue and is continually forming and resorbing in response to

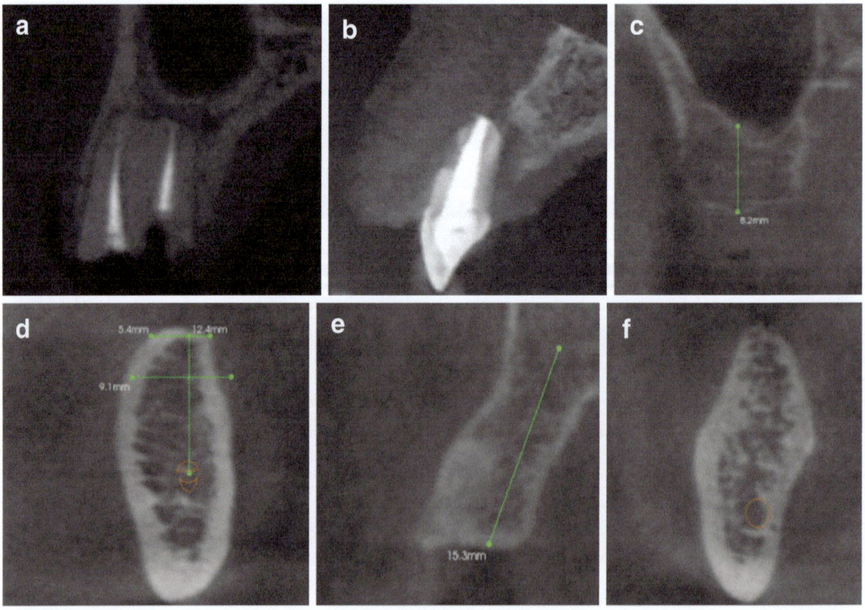

Fig. 1.1 (**a–f**) Different patterns of alveolar bone: (**a**) absence of cancellous bone between the cortical plates. (**b**) Loss of alveolar bone due to periodontal disease. (**c–f**) residual alveolar ridge with a cortical perimeter and a cancellous core in different areas of the maxilla and mandible

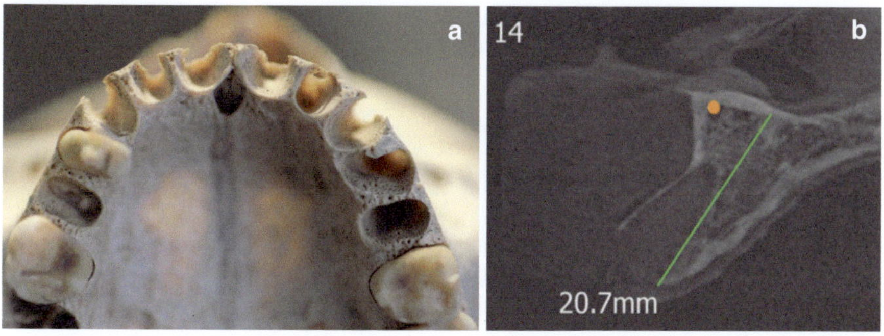

Fig. 1.2 (**a**) The alveolar bone proper can be visualized in the images. It is delicately thin and is easily destroyed by faulty extraction techniques. The marrow spaces appear as perforations giving the name cribriform plate. (**b**) The cone beam computed tomography (CBCT) section of a recently extracted tooth depicts the thinness of the labial plate

functional needs. While bone metabolism is under hormonal control, it is easily resorbed in response to inflammation, ischemia, and trauma.

Alveolar bone proper is that part of alveolar bone which actually lines the socket of the roots. It provides the attachment for the periodontal ligament fibers and is cortical in nature with perforations for nutrient channels, hence also known as cribriform plate. While the full length of the alveolar bone proper is available for periodontal ligament fiber attachment, in certain areas, the periodontal ligament fibers are embedded in the cementum and bone and undergo calcification. These are known as Sharpey's fibers, and this bone is known as bundle bone. The subsequent sections describe the bundle bone in greater detail.

1.1.2 Development of the Alveolar Bone

The alveolar bone development starts prenatally, concomitant with the membranous portions of the mandible and maxilla and strictly coordinated with the developing primary dentition and is based on molecular signaling as well as mechanical forces. The cells that participate in this event are the osteoblasts and osteoclasts. Interestingly, the osteoblasts that are responsible for the intramembranous ossification that produces the alveolar bone are derived from the ectomesenchymal cells that are present in the dental sac, also responsible for development of periodontal ligament and cememtum. This implies that ontogenically, the three structures of the periodontium have a common origin and that the alveolar bone belongs to the tooth. This is amply demonstrated by alveolar bone loss as a result of tooth loss.

The mandible develops in membrane around the Inferior alveolar nerve. This results in a bony trough in which the nerve lies, and the walls of which extend superiorly to form the alveolar process. This alveolar process will also house the developing tooth buds. While the development of the maxilla is more complex, the alveolar process, that will enclose the developing tooth buds, develops in much the same fashion as the mandible. Over time, these tooth buds will be separated by bony partitions, thereby creating sockets. This has been described in a very elegant paper by Kjaer and Bagheri [5].

1.1.3 Alveolar Bone Proper

The alveolar bone proper starts developing with the erupting tooth. After crown formation is complete, the complex interactions between the Hertwig's epithelial root sheath and the dental follicle, initiates cementogenesis with the differentiation of cementoblasts from the ectomesenchymal cells. Simultaneously, other ectomesenchymal cells differentiate into fibroblasts to form the periodontal ligament and another population differentiates into osteoblasts to give rise to alveolar bone proper, forming sockets for the roots. The fact that all these events occur synchronously allows for the embedding of PDL fibers into the cementum and alveolar bone proper.

As root formation progresses, the PDL continues to extend itself as does the alveolar bone proper continue to remodel. Bone is deposited apically and coronally, increasing the depth of the socket, remodeling and filling in around the root as the tooth erupts. It should be obvious now that the development of alveolar bone proper is purely a function of tooth formation and eruption and in cases of anodontia or lack of eruptive force, this will not develop.

1.1.4 Bundle Bone

Alveolar bone proper provides the attachment for Sharpey's fibers from the PDL. These are arranged in bundles and get calcified within the bone to provide a firm attachment. This part of the alveolar bone proper is referred to as bundle bone. Bundle bone merges with the adjacent lamellar bone which comprises the alveolar process. Bundle bone has an important role to play in tooth movement and periodontal disease progression. Understanding bundle bone is the key to understanding the rationale for partial extraction therapies, hence we will delve a little in-depth here.

Several papers have reported loss of bundle bone as the first event in the dimensional changes that take place after extraction and the explanation seems to lie in the fact that after tooth extraction, the bundle bone becomes non-functional through loss of its periodontal blood supply and undergoes complete resorption in the first few weeks [6–9]. Al Hezaimi and co-workers [9] analyzed the blood supply to buccal bone in monkeys and established that the blood supply to the buccal plate came mainly from the socket side of the alveolus i.e. via the periodontal ligament, the adjacent interdental bone, and supraperiosteal vessels emanating from the gingiva (Fig. 1.3). They also found that the buccal bone was composed of bundle bone and cortical bone, and that while the thickness of this bone was not uniform corono-apically, the thinnest area was at the coronal portion.

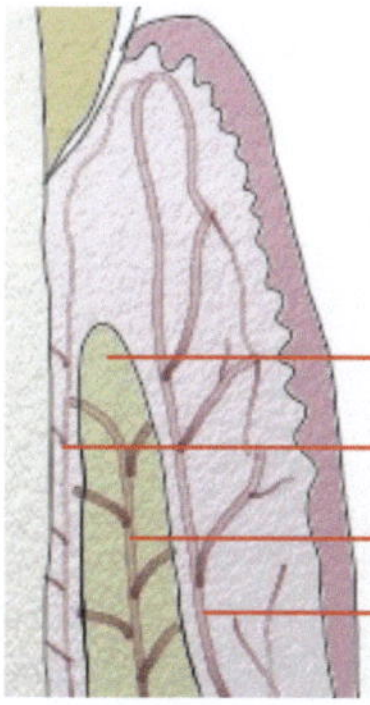

Fig. 1.3 Blood supply to the bundle bone

This implies that the periodontal ligament is a key player in maintaining the viability of the bundle bone as well as the outer cortex, and loss of a tooth will compromise this blood supply Fig. 1.3 and lead to a loss of bone.

One of the most cited pieces of published dental literature in the English language is the works of Araujo and Lindhe group [6–8, 10, 11], on the dimensional alterations of the alveolar ridge. Ridge alterations following tooth extractions in mongrel dogs described the phases of resorption after extraction as occurring in two phases: Phase one which occurred from within the socket and involved bundle bone. According to these authors, since most of the buccal crests of these sockets were made up of bundle bone, the dimensional loss was severe. In phase two, there was resorption from the surface of both bone walls.

The dimensions of bundle bone are reported to be 0.2–0.3 mm in width (apico-coronal) on the lingual plate, and at the buccal crest, 2 mm on the buccal crest, sometimes spanning the whole mesio-distal dimension of the crest. As a consequence, they found that following extraction, the buccal bone shows a vertical loss and the crest lies on an average 1.9 mm apical to the lingual crest. This may not be truly representative of what happens clinically in humans, but does offer a plausible explanation (Fig. 1.3).

In a 2009 systematic review, Van der Weijden and co-workers found only one article by Nevins et al. that corroborated these findings in humans. Their principal findings were a loss in width of 3.87 mm and a loss in height of 1.67–2.03 mm [12, 13].

In another systematic review from 2012, Niklaus Lang's group found that in human hard tissues, horizontal loss was 3.79 ± 0.23 mm and vertical reduction was 1.24 ± 0.11 mm on the buccal at the end of 6 months. Proximal bone loss was 0.84 ± 0.71 mm [14].

Chappuis [11] and co-workers, in an detailed CBCT based clinical study in humans, found that patients with a thin facial wall phenotype (<1 mm), showed a rapid vertical bone loss on the facial plate of (Median—7.5 mm), whereas those which had a facial plate thickness of greater than 1 mm, showed a median vertical

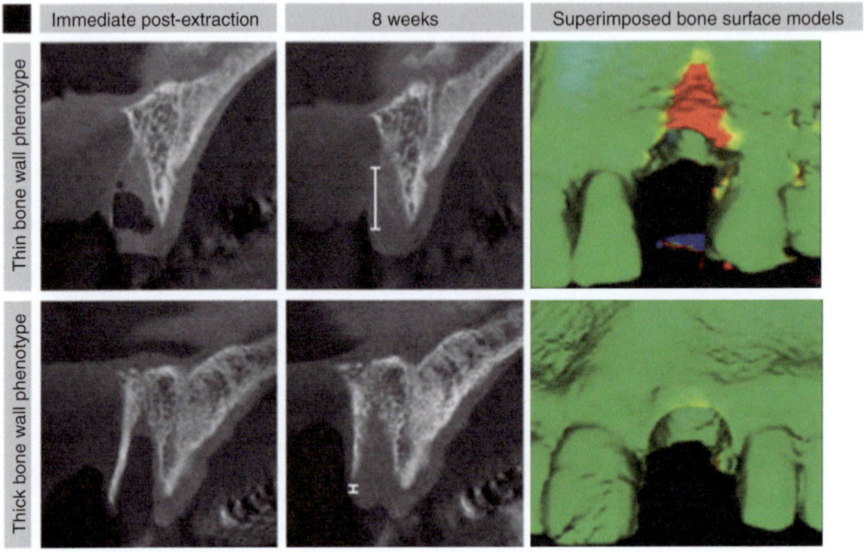

Fig. 1.4 Thin bone wall phenotypes with a facial bone wall thickness of 1 mm or less, revealed a progressive bone resorption pattern, leading to median vertical bone loss of 7.5 mm or 62% of the former facial bone height after 8 weeks of healing. This is in contrast to thick wall phenotypes, showing a facial bone wall thickness of more than 1 mm, displaying only a median vertical bone loss of 1.1 mm or 9%. The dimensional alteration pattern in single extraction sited with healthy neighboring dentition occurred mainly in the central area of the socket wall, whereas the proximal areas remained nearly unchanged after flapless tooth extraction at 8 weeks of healing [11] Printed with permission from Chappuis et al. [12]

bone loss of 1.1 mm. This implies that in facial plates that are greater than 1 mm thick, only part of it is bundle bone, and the loss of the tooth results in an early loss of this bundle bone on the socket side, without loss of the surface bone (Fig. 1.4).

With this background information, it is clear that the *bundle bone*, and the rest of the alveolar bone proper, *belongs to the tooth* and tooth loss will result in an obligatory loss of bone, starting with a rapid loss of bundle bone and continuing gradually to the rest of the alveolar bone over the long term.

The resorption of the alveolar ridge is more pronounced on the buccal than on the lingual aspect of the extraction socket [15, 16] and it is the loss of buccal tissues that is more prominent and compromises the outcomes in the esthetic areas [6, 7].

Howell et al. showed in 1970s that when endodontically treated submerged roots were left in the alveolar bone under complete dentures, hardly any resorption was seen at 10 years.

To prevent and/or minimize the resorption and mitigate the effects of bone loss after the removal of the teeth various treatment modalities such as immediate implants [10, 17, 18], use of graft materials to augment the socket [8, 19–22], and use of barrier membranes [18, 19] have been tried. Of the multitude of procedures tried above, none of them have been effective in achieving the said goal [7, 19–23] and thus complete preservation and/or entire regeneration of the extraction socket has not been achieved.

The loss of the periodontal ligament attachment to the buccal bone and loss of the bundle bone due to the extraction of the tooth/root has been determined as the principal factor in the loss of alveolar bone. This led to the emergence of the concept that, if a part of the root is retained, then it may be possible to retain the corresponding part of the bone.

With this background, Filippi et al. [24] showed that an ankylosed tooth retained bone, submerged roots allowed to form bone and cementum on top of them.

Salama et al. [1], in 2007, reintroduced root submergence in preserving alveolar bone width and height in the aesthetic zone under pontics between implants and teeth, for optimizing aesthetics.

Davarpanah and Szmukler-Moncler [25] published an alternative to extraction of deeply placed, impacted teeth that were not communicating with the oral cavity, clinically and radiographically healthy teeth that come in the pathway of implant placements. They suggested that, instead of removing the roots with invasive surgery it may be prudent to place the implants directly in contact with them. In small sample size of six patients with seven implants, they placed implants in contact with root fragments. They reported good success rates with some bone loss in one of the cases. Although the sample size was small, the paper was a positive step retaining healthy roots around implants and was an important milestone in the history of PET.

In 2010, Hurzeler et al. [3] conducted a beagle dog study to demonstrate that the retention of root helped in holding the alveolar volume. They used an enamel matrix derivative to fill the gap between the implant and the retained root. They reported, histologically, the formation and maintenance of supra-alveolar connective tissues, the formation of cementum along the root surface, but no-epithelial down migration between the root and the bone. The authors then depicted the first clinical case of the socket-shield technique, wherein the authors' placed the implant after preparing the shield in a manner depicted in the Fig. 1.5. The study showed that retaining the buccal aspect of the root did not interfere with osseointegration and that it may be beneficial in maintaining the buccal bone contour. This proof-of-principle study sets in motion the use of socket shield/PET as a treatment modality for the prevention of buccal tissue loss.

In 2013, Baumer et al. [26] published the first histological, clinical, and volumetric data of implants placed in beagle dogs after vertical separation of the buccal fragment. In their study, they removed the palatal portion of the root and then also split the buccal root into two parts. They placed the implants without any enamel matrix derivative and euthanized the animals at 4-months and conducted the histological evaluation. The implants had all integrated with new bone formation between the implant and the root fragment. They found that root fragment was well attached to the buccal bone with no signs of resorption. Clinically, too there were no visible signs of inflammation as all sites had healed well. Volumetrically, in one case that was reported, they showed good maintenance of buccal bone contours. Thus, this came to be a significant step in the evolution of PET techniques, as now it was proven that bone forms between the implant and the root fragment with no adverse effects on both, the implant as well as the root fragment.

In the same year, Kan et al. published the use of proximal shield to maintain interdental soft tissue in the aesthetic zone. Although it was just a case report, it did

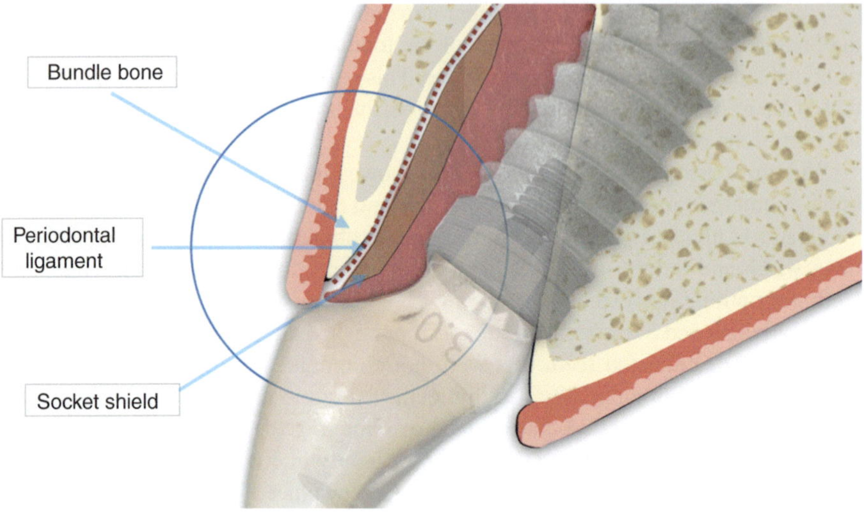

Fig. 1.5 Preservation of the bundle bone with a socket shield

open up newer possibilities in the management of the shield to harness the aesthetic potential of biologic entities around the implant with root fragments, intentionally prepared and left in the socket.

In 2014, Glocker et al. published a modified socket shield technique in three cases, in which they prepared the shield, but did not place an implant immediately in the alveolar socket. Implants were placed 6-months later. They concluded stating that the complete preservation of the buccal lamellar bone was observed intra-operatively in all three cases. This technique now became a viable alternative in cases where implant placement was not possible immediately after partial extraction.

In the same year, Siormpas et al. coined the term "root membrane technique" for cases in which there is an intentional retention of buccal root fragment to prevent buccal bone loss. The difference between the root membrane technique and the others was that, in this technique the implant deliberately touches the root fragment. They published clinical results and radiographic data of 46 patients followed up to 5 years post loading, with a success rate of 100% as far as implant integration was concerned and loss of one root to resorption that did not affect the implant.

In 2016, in a significant technique article, Gluckman et al. coined the term "Partial Extraction Therapy" that included various different terminologies under one name. Root submergence technique, socket shield technique, and pontic shield technique were collectively called partial extraction therapies. Figure 1.5 demonstrates the meaning of the various terms. Gluckman et al. then followed up with part 2 of the article in 2017 where they described the various procedures and technical aspects of partial extraction therapy.

At this point in literature it was well established that intentional retention of a part of the root on the labial side of the socket is indeed a good way to prevent buccal bone loss and thereby provide excellent tissue contours. It was also clear that the apex of the root should be totally removed and that no residual endodontic filling material must be retained behind on the shield.

In 2017, Gharpure and Bhatavadekar in a systematic review of the available literature on socket shield doubted the long-term outcomes of the procedure. It takes years, if not decades for a new technique to get refined in procedure and gain acceptance, and their review of the very limited literature at that point may have been premature. As clinicians we believe that the procedures under the umbrella of PET have very sound scientific basis as shown in animal and histological studies, as well as long-term case series. It is only a matter of time that the PET becomes a staple procedure in the surgical inventory for replacement of teeth with implants and we will start to see controlled clinical trials as well as histological studies happening in different part of the globe to substantiate the benefits of the same.

Sirompas et al., in 2018, published up to 10 years of retrospective data on clinical results of the root membrane technique for periodontal ligament-mediated immediate implant placements. A total of 182 patients received 250 immediate implants (230 maxilla, 20 mandible) after the root membrane concept and followed-up for a mean of 49.94 months. Overall, five implant failures were recorded. Ten-year cumulative implant survival rate of 97.3% (implant-based) and 96.5% (patient-based), respectively, was reported in this study. This by far is the most recent long-term data of the patients that have been treated with PET and is significant in its findings. Various other articles, mainly in form of case reports, have been published since 2018 till date.

As practitioners of this science and art, we the authors of this book feel that there is a very high amount of clinical evidence to support PET, and hence this book has been authored detailing every aspect of the PET procedure in a manner that is clinically relevant, technically reproducible, and evidence-based for the reader to incorporate it into their daily practice.

1.2 Partial Extraction Therapies

Root submergence technique (RST): A healthy root is left submerged below a fixed partial denture or an implant-supported fixed bridge (Fig. 1.6a).

Socket shield technique (SS): A part of the root is left attached to the labial bone, which aids in maintenance of the labial bone and soft tissue architecture. The labial root fragment is referred to as the 'shield' through all the chapters. An implant is placed in the palatal part of the socket in the same surgical appointment to support a restoration (Fig. 1.6b).

Pontic shield (PS): A part of the root fragment is left attached to the labial bone like the socket shield technique. Natural bone fill with or without a bone graft material is allowed to occur in the remainder of the socket. The purpose is to prevent the collapse of alveolar ridge below future pontic sites (Fig. 1.6c).

The timeline for the PET is described in a chart below (Fig. 1.6).

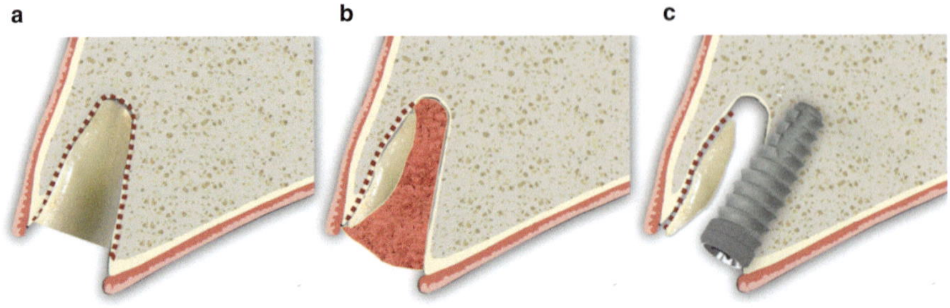

Fig. 1.6 Depiction of the various partial extraction therapies: (**a**) Root submergence. (**b**) Pontic shield. (**c**) Socket shield

1.3 Histological Evidence in PET Describing the Fate of the Root Fragment

Hürzeler et al. [3] in a proof-of-principle study done in animal models showed that, leaving behind the root and treating the dentine side of the root with enamel matrix protein derivative (Emdogain, Straumman, Basel, Switzerland) did not influence osseointegration. They found that there was no epithelial down growth, a 0.5 mm area coronal to the implant had connective tissue and a biological Junctional epithelium. Cementum had formed on the dentine surface, also visible were cemetoid, cementoblasts and there was absence of any osteoclasts. Even in those sites where the implants were placed close to the tooth there was presence of cementum and in gaps between the threads an amorphous mineralized tissue was observed.

Bäumer et al. [26] conducted a similar study in animals, but did not apply any EMD and found that new bone had formed in the gap between the implant and the dentine and the lingual side showed osseointegrated implant. The gaps between the threads showed bone fill, and in sites where the implant touched the tooth, no resorptive process was observed.

Zhang et al. [27], in a study done on dogs with four groups, extraction, extraction with socket graft with Bio-Oss collagen, SS only and SS with Bio-Oss collagen, found that in sites with SS in comparison to no SS shield sites, there was a good bone fill and better trabecular pattern.

Human histology for socket shield was found accidentally by three authors, Guarnieri et al. [28], Schwimer et al. [29] and Mitsias et al. [30].

Guarnieri et al. [28] found cellular cementum and cementocytes in an implant failure case where the implant was placed accidentally touching the fractured root and not the socket shield technique as we know it. They attributed the cementum formation to the inflammation and the extrusive action of the root fragment, possibly on account of it being luxated. This is not what we would expect around a socket shield, where only a stable fragment is left behind.

Schwimer et al. [29] found that there is bone fill in the gaps between the dentine and the implant for the full length of the implants.

Mitsias et al. [30], in a detailed histological analysis of an implant placed with the root membrane technique, which needed to be retrieved after 5 years in function, on account of a serious accident to the patient necessitating removal of a part of the maxilla, found the following:

1. Trabecular, mature bone at the interface of the implant. The bone was present between the implant and the root. The root membrane and the buccal bone plate appeared intact without any signs of resorption.
2. In the coronal portion, between the root and the implant, connective tissue without inflammatory infiltrate was present.
3. In the apical portion of the root, it was observed that the cementum migrated from the residual root to the implant surface.

Given the above evidence, it is easy to infer that the fate of the gap between the shield and the implant seems fairly consistent with the formation of bone and osseointegration, with varying degrees of non-inflamed connective tissue attachment in the crestal area of the implant and varying degrees of cellular cementum apically, particularly if the implant is in contact with the tooth fragment.

The current status of clinical and histological evidence of socket shield and PET has made it possible to apply this wonderful clinical application to practice (Fig. 1.7).

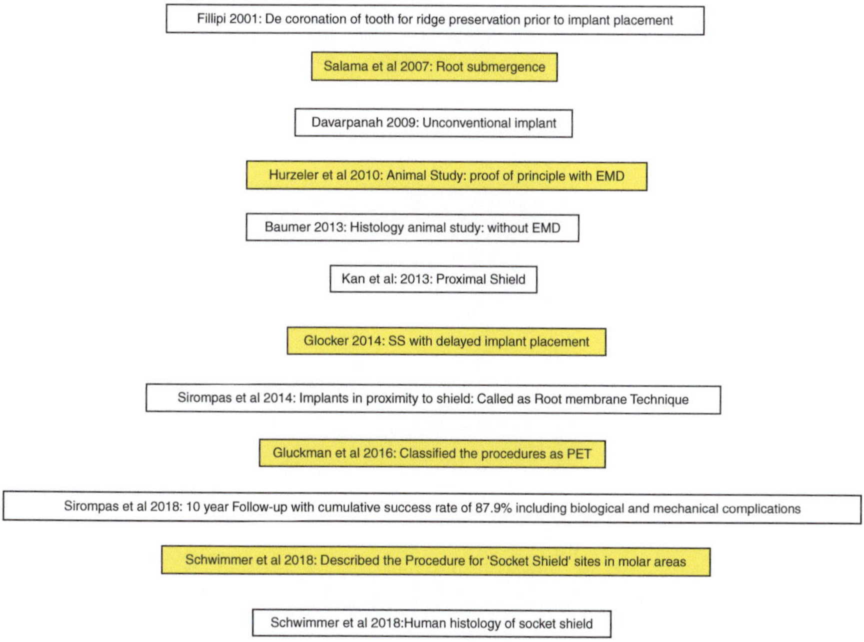

Fig. 1.7 The timeline describes the evolution of the Partial extraction therapies

By retaining a part of the root on the facial side, attached to its periodontal ligament, the body is tricked into believing that the root still exists, while the bundle bone as well as the marginal gingiva continues to get its blood supply from the periodontal ligament, thereby maintaining the hard and soft tissue contours, a phenomenon which could be referred to as "Biologic cheating". This forms the basis for the Socket shield technique [3] and its variants—the Pontic shield and Glocker's [4] technique for ridge preservation (Fig. 1.8).

The PET has made it possible to achieve outstanding esthetic and functional outcomes in challenging clinical situations. A comparison of the outcomes of PET and conventional implant is visibly appreciated in Fig. 1.9.

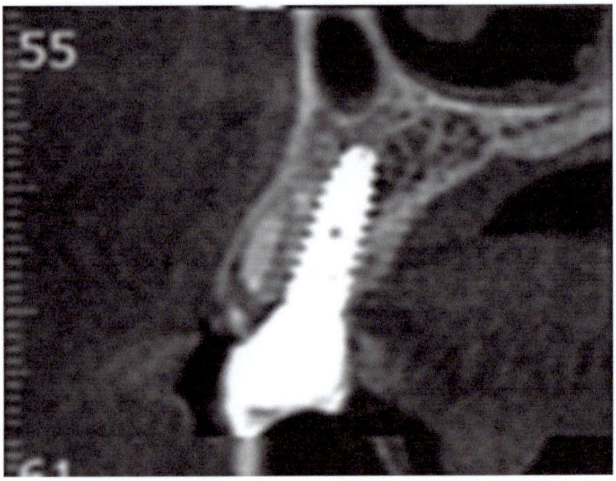

Fig. 1.8 One-year follow-up on a Socket shield showing bone fill between the shield and the implant, intact periodontal ligament between the buccal plate and the root sliver, as well as bone growth over the shield

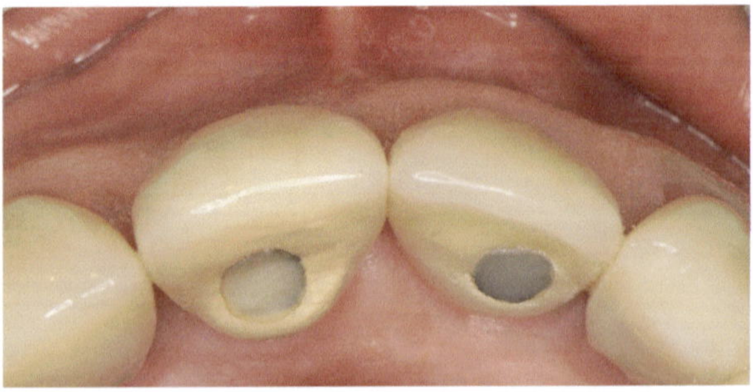

Fig. 1.9 Comparison of sites with PET (tooth21) and conventional implant therapy (tooth11). The stark difference in the contour is appreciable

1.4 Conclusion

Prof. Branemark introduced the concept of osseointergration more than five decades ago. Back then, clinicians were more focused on evaluating the ability of the human body to accept dental implants. Today, clinicians are seeking treatment options for their patients, wherein replacement of teeth with implants are virtually indistinguishable from what was given by Mother Nature. Partial extraction therapies are just getting started and are already making it possible to achieve near-natural outcomes with dental implants. The sound biological basis for the concept and the clinical and histological studies published so far is reassuring for clinicians to adopt these procedures in their practices. The following chapters will discuss in detail about PET techniques, outcomes, and possibilities in different areas of the jaw and also the errors, complications, and their management.

Acknowledgement Illustrations by: Udatta Kher.

References

1. Salama M, Ishikawa T, Salama H, Funato A, Garber D. Advantages of the root submergence technique for pontic site development in esthetic implant therapy. Int J Periodontics Restorative Dent. 2007;27(6):521–7.
2. Hürzeler MB, Zuhr O, Schupbach P, Rebele SF, Emmanouilidis N, Fickl S. The socket-shield technique: a proof-of-principle report. J Clin Periodontol. 2010;37(9):855–62.
3. Gluckman H, Du Toit J, Salama M. The pontic-shield: partial extraction therapy for ridge preservation and pontic site development. Int J Periodontics Restorative Dent. 2016;36(3):417–23.
4. Glocker M. Ridge preservation with modified "socket-shield" technique: a methodological case series. Dent J. 2014;2:11–21.
5. Kjaer I, Bagheri A. Prenatal development of the alveolar bone of human deciduous incisors and canines. J Dent Res. 1999;78(2):667–72.
6. Araújo MG, Lindhe J. Dimensional ridge alterations following tooth extraction. An experimental study in the dog. J Clin Periodontol. 2005;32(2):212–8.
7. Araújo MG, Lindhe J. Ridge preservation with the use of Bio-Oss collagen: a 6-month study in the dog. Clin Oral Implants Res. 2009;20(5):433–40.
8. Misawa M, Lindhe J, Araújo MG. The alveolar process following single-tooth extraction: a study of maxillary incisor and premolar sites in man. Clin Oral Implants Res. 2016;27(7):884–9.
9. Al-Hezaimi K, Levi P, Rudy R, Al-Jandan B, Al-Rasheed A. An extraction socket classification developed using analysis of bone type and blood supply to the buccal bone in monkeys. Int J Periodontics Restorative Dent. 2011;31(4):421–7.
10. Cardaropoli G, Araújo M, Lindhe J. Dynamics of bone tissue formation in tooth extraction sites. An experimental study in dogs. J Clin Periodontol. 2003;30(9):809–18.
11. Chappuis V, Araújo MG, Buser D. Clinical relevance of dimensional bone and soft tissue alterations post-extraction in esthetic sites. Periodontol 2000. 2017;73(1):73–83.
12. Chappuis V, Engel O, Shahim K, Reyes M, Katsaros C, Buser D. Soft tissue alterations in esthetic postextraction sites: a 3-dimensional analysis. J Dent Res. 2015;94(9 Suppl):187S–93S. https://doi.org/10.1177/0022034515592869.
13. Van der Weijden F, Dell'Acqua F, Slot DE. Alveolar bone dimensional changes of post-extraction sockets in humans: a systematic review. J Clin Periodontol. 2009;36(12):1048–58.

14. Tan WL, Wong TL, Wong MC, Lang NP. A systematic review of post-extractional alveolar hard and soft tissue dimensional changes in humans. Clin Oral Implants Res. 2012;23(Suppl 5):1–21.
15. Pietrokovski J, Massler M. Alveolar ridge resorption following tooth extraction. J Prosthet Dent. 1967;17(1):21–7.
16. Pietrokovski J, Massler M. Ridge remodeling after tooth extraction in rats. J Dent Res. 1967;46(1):222–31.
17. Cardaropoli G, Araújo M, Hayacibara R, Sukekava F, Lindhe J. Healing of extraction sockets and surgically produced – augmented and non-augmented – defects in the alveolar ridge. An experimental study in the dog. J Clin Periodontol. 2005;32(5):435–40.
18. Botticelli D, Berglundh T, Lindhe J. Hard-tissue alterations following immediate implant placement in extraction sites. J Clin Periodontol. 2004;31(10):820–8.
19. Araújo MG, Sukekava F, Wennström JL, Lindhe J. Ridge alterations following implant placement in fresh extraction sockets: an experimental study in the dog. J Clin Periodontol. 2005;32(6):645–52.
20. Lekovic V, Camargo PM, Klokkevold PR, Weinlaender M, Kenney EB, Dimitrijevic B, Nedic M. Preservation of alveolar bone in extraction sockets using bioabsorbable membranes. J Periodontol. 1998;69(9):1044–9.
21. Fickl S, Zuhr O, Wachtel H, Stappert CF, Stein JM, Hürzeler MB. Dimensional changes of the alveolar ridge contour after different socket preservation techniques. J Clin Periodontol. 2008;35(10):906–13.
22. Fickl S, Schneider D, Zuhr O, Hinze M, Ender A, Jung RE, Hürzeler MB. Dimensional changes of the ridge contour after socket preservation and buccal over building: an animal study. J Clin Periodontol. 2009;36(5):442–8.
23. Lekovic V, Kenney EB, Weinlaender M, Han T, Klokkevold P, Nedic M, Orsini M. A bone regenerative approach to alveolar ridge maintenance following tooth extraction. Report of 10 cases. J Periodontol. 1997;68(6):563–70.
24. Filippi A, Pohl Y, von Arx T. Decoronation of an ankylosed tooth for preservation of alveolar bone prior to implant placement. Dent Traumatol. 2001;17(2):93–5.
25. Davarpanah M, Szmukler-Moncler S. Unconventional implant treatment: I. Implant placement in contact with ankylosed root fragments. A series of five case reports. Clin Oral Implants Res. 2009;20(8):851–6.
26. Bäumer D, Zuhr O, Rebele S, Schneider D, Schupbach P, Hürzeler M. The socket-shield technique: first histological, clinical, and volumetrical observations after separation of the buccal tooth segment – a pilot study. Clin Implant Dent Relat Res. 2015;17(1):71–82.
27. Zhang Z, Dong Y, Yang J, Xu R, Deng Q. Effect of socket shield technique on alveolar ridge soft and hard tissues in dogs. J Clin Periodontol. https://doi.org/10.1111/jcpe.13073.
28. Guarnieri R, Giardino L, Crespi R, Romagnoli R. Cementum formation around a titanium implant: a case report. Int J Oral Maxillofac Implants. 2002;17(5):729–32.
29. Schwimer C, Pette GA, Gluckman H, Salama M, Du Toit J. Human histologic evidence of new bone formation and osseointegration between root dentin (unplanned socket-shield) and dental implant: case report. Int J Oral Maxillofac Implants. 2018;33(1):19–e23.
30. Mitsias ME, Siormpas KD, Kotsakis GA, Ganz SD, Mangano C, Iezzi G. The root membrane technique: human histologic evidence after five years of function. Biomed Res Int. 2017;2017:7269467.

Suggested Reading

Gluckman H, Salama M, Du Toit J. A retrospective evaluation of 128 socket-shield cases in the esthetic zone and posterior sites: partial extraction therapy with up to 4 years follow-up. Clin Implant Dent Relat Res. 2018;20(2):122–9.

Kan JY, Rungcharassaeng K. Proximal socket shield for interimplant papilla preservation in the esthetic zone. Int J Periodontics Restorative Dent. 2013;33(1):24–31.

Siormpas KD, Mitsias ME, Kontsiotou-Siormpa E, Garber D, Kotsakis GA. Immediate implant placement in the esthetic zone utilizing the "root-membrane" technique: clinical results up to 5 years postloading. Int J Oral Maxillofac Implants. 2014;29(6):1397–405.

Gluckman H, Salama M, Du Toit J. Partial extraction therapies (PET) part 1: maintaining alveolar ridge contour at pontic and immediate implant sites. Int J Periodontics Restorative Dent. 2016;36(5):681–7.

Gluckman H, Salama M, Du Toit J. Partial extraction therapies (PET) part 2: procedures and technical aspects. Int J Periodontics Restorative Dent. 2017;37:376–85.

Gharpure A, Bhatavadekar N. Current evidence on the socket-shield technique: a systematic review. J Oral Implantol. 2017;43(5):395–403.

Siormpas KD, Mitsias ME, Kotsakis GA, Tawil I, Pikos MA, Mangano FG. The root membrane technique: a retrospective clinical study with up to 10 years of follow-up. Implant Dent. 2018;27(5):564–74.

Schwimer CW, Gluckman H, Salama M, Nagy K, Du Toit J. The socket-shield technique at molar sites: a proof-of-principle technique report. J Prosthet Dent. 2019;121(2):229–33. https://doi.org/10.1016/j.prosdent.2018.05.006.

Surgical Technique for Socket Shield Procedure

2

Udatta Kher

Abstract

The socket shield procedure is a novel technique for post-extraction implant placement. Several modifications of the socket shield procedure and simultaneous implant placement have been presented since its inception. This chapter explains the most contemporary step-by-step surgical technique of the socket shield procedure with detailed illustrations and representative cases. The armamentarium necessary for the procedure is enlisted. Troubleshooting and tips to minimize errors are presented at the end of the chapter.

2.1 Introduction

Few procedures in modern-day implant dentistry have generated more interest and curiosity among clinicians than the socket shield technique. From the time of its introduction to the dental world in 2010, the original technique by Hurzeler et al. has seen a few modifications [1]. The partial extraction therapy (PET) procedures include the socket shield technique of post-extraction immediate implant placement. The PET technique is a deviation from the original socket shield technique and will be discussed in great detail in this chapter. The PET entails preparation of a shield by performing a partial extraction of the root. This is followed by a specific protocol of shaping the shield to enable ease of implant placement and fabrication of a provisional restoration. The goal of treatment is to achieve a satisfactory restoration that meets the esthetic and functional requirements of the patient. The procedure is technique-sensitive and should be ideally practiced by clinicians who are

U. Kher (✉)
Only Smiles Dental Centre, Mumbai, India

U. Kher, A. Tunkiwala (eds.), *Partial Extraction Therapy in Implant Dentistry*,
https://doi.org/10.1007/978-3-030-33610-3_2

trained in various aspects of implant dentistry such as minimally traumatic extractions of teeth, immediate implant placement, fabrication of chairside provisional restorations, and management of soft tissues around implant sites. Clinicians should also have a thorough understanding of the usage of various biomaterials like bone substitute materials and collagen membranes for the management of unexpected complications during the PET procedures.

Teeth selected for the socket shield technique are those that are indicated for extraction and simultaneous implant placement. Criteria for case selection and contraindications are discussed in great details in Chap. 3.

2.2 Diagnostic Tools

A good intraoral periapical radiograph and a cone beam CT scan showing cross-sectional views are mandatory. These views will allow the clinicians to detect any pathology associated with the root that is indicated for extraction. It will also allow the clinician to measure the root length and study the morphology of the surrounding alveolar bone. Mounted study casts are essential for analyzing the patient's occlusal scheme and will assist in planning for the final restoration.

2.3 Guidelines for Shield Preparation

Preparation of the shield in partial extraction therapy is an exacting procedure that needs great attention to detail. Errors in shield preparation can be detrimental to the long-term survival of the implants and surrounding alveolar bone. An ideal shield design should follow certain guidelines (Figs. 2.1 and 2.2). Minor variations in the shield preparation are described in the subsequent chapters.

An ideal shield preparation should exhibit the following:

1. No apical area of the tooth must remain. The shield preparation must ensure total removal and debridement of the apex of the tooth [1].
2. The shield must remain stable and should be completely immobile at the end of the preparation. Any movement will eventually lead to an infection, extrusion, resorption, and eventual loss of shield [2].
3. The shield should be thin enough to avoid any contact between shield and the implant [3]. A very thin shield, however, will be prone to mobility or migration.
4. The shield should be optimally thick enough to resist detachment from the labial bone, but should not be too thick so as to interfere with the implant placement [4]. A very thick shield will have a greater tendency to contact the implant after placement.

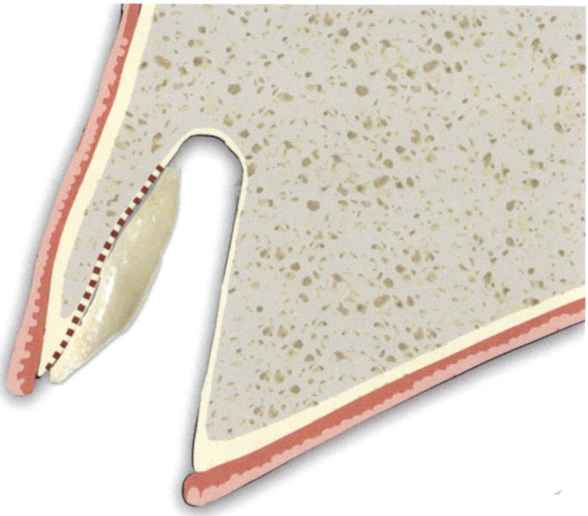

Fig. 2.1 Cross-sectional view showing ideal shield design

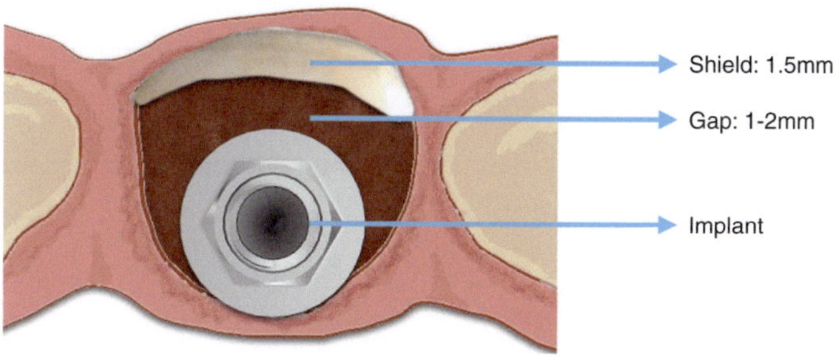

Fig. 2.2 Occlusal view showing ideal shield design, implant position and gap between implant and shield

Keeping these requirements in mind, the ideal shield design and dimension should be as follows (Figs. 2.1 and 2.2):

1. No palatal or apical portion of the root should be present.
2. The shield must be about two/third the length of the original root or at least 8 mm long, whichever is more [5].
3. The shield should be at least 1.5 mm in width, or one/fourth the buccolingual dimension of the root, whichever is lesser. Another guideline to follow is half the distance between the labial bone and the root canal space of the root to be sectioned [6].
4. It should follow curvature of labial bone from mesial to distal line angle.
5. It should be trimmed down to the level of labial bone crest [7].
6. It should have a bevel or S-shaped curve on the internal aspect [8].

Following these guidelines will go a long way in preventing complications (Chap. 10) [8].

2.3.1 Armamentarium

The following instruments are necessary for the shield preparation (Figs. 2.3 and 2.4):

1. Long shank carbide bur on high-speed air turbine drill.
2. Long shank round diamond bur of various diameters.
3. Football-shaped diamond bur.
4. Zekrya gingival retractor.
5. Fine-tipped elevators.
6. Curved artery forceps.
7. Bone curettes.

Customized kits that have a selection of various burs and diamonds for ease of shield preparation are available from different companies (Fig. 2.5).

1. PET kit (Brassler).
2. Root membrane kit (Megagen) [3].
3. Socket shield kit (Komet) [9].
4. PET kit (Megagen).

Rest of the armamentarium is the same as for any routine implant placement and the fabrication of a provisional restoration.

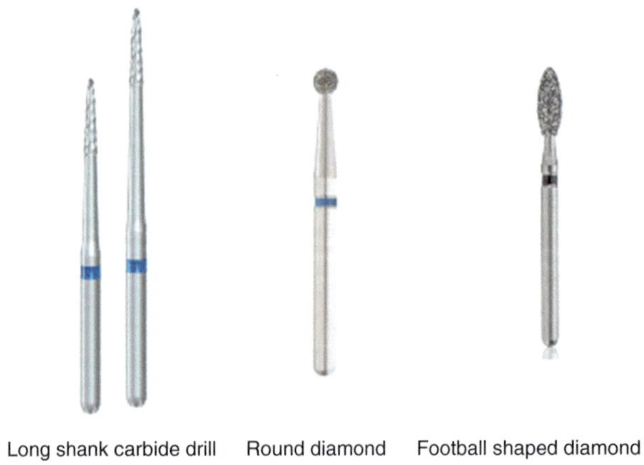

Fig. 2.3 Burs for shield preparation

Fig. 2.4 Zekrya Gingival protector

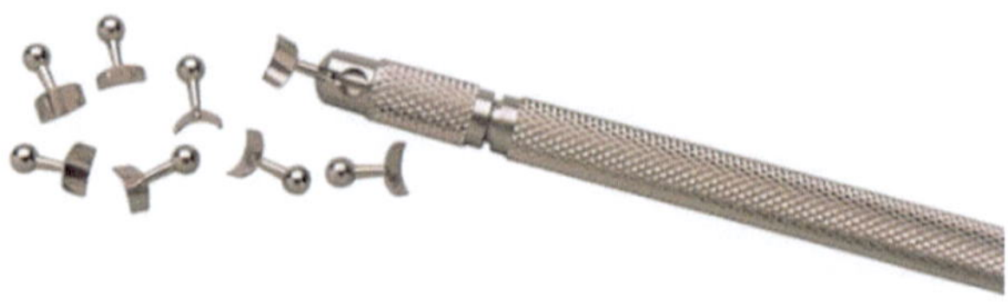

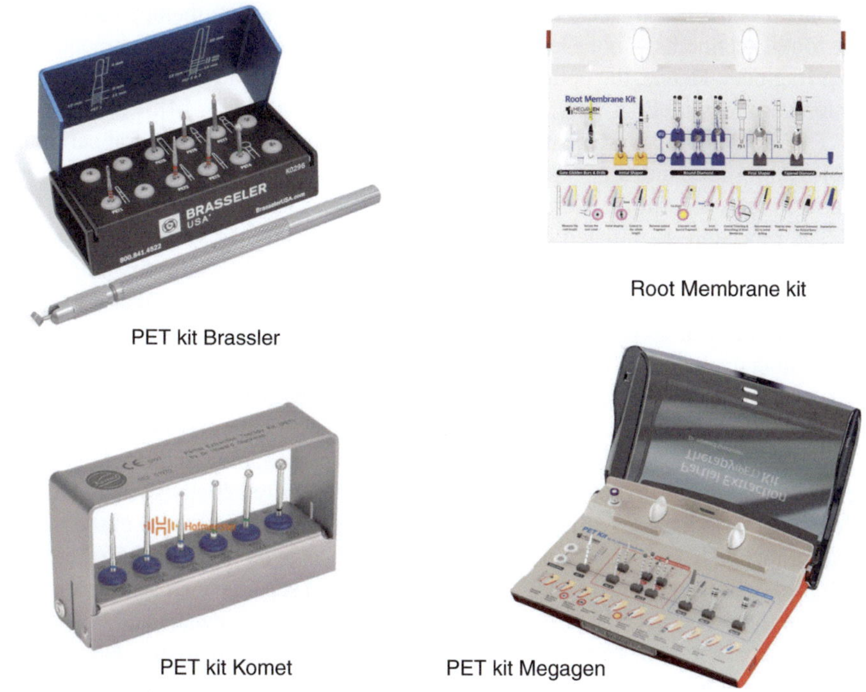

Fig. 2.5 Kits for shield preparation

2.3.2 The Step by Step Procedure

The surgical technique described in this chapter explains the procedure for a maxillary central incisor. The procedure for the maxillary lateral incisor would be similar. Minor changes in the technique are required for canines, mandibular teeth, and multi-rooted teeth, which are described in Chaps. 5 and 6. The procedure entails five principal steps:

- Sectioning of the root (partial extraction).
- Shield preparation.
- Implant placement.
- Management of the gap.
- Closure.

Step 1: Sectioning of the Root

The socket shield procedure is performed under local anesthesia.

The procedure may be performed flapless or with a conventional flap approach. If the socket dimension is large enough to allow access for tooth sectioning and extraction of the root apex, a flapless approach is preferred. Literature has enough evidence to show that when a flap is raised, the separation of the periosteum from the underlying bone may lead to resorption of the labial plate due to loss of periosteal blood supply [10–12]. In cases where access is difficult, when multiple teeth have to be prepared, or when the operator is inexperienced, raising a flap is preferred for better visualization. In traditional implant dentistry, raising a flap may lead to minor loss of the labial bone. But in socket shield or other partial extraction therapy cases, since the root is retained, the bone level will still be maintained due to its attachment to the root fragment. Hence, the option of raising the flap does not affect the final outcome as long as the guidelines for shield preparation are followed [13, 14].

The root length is first measured on the CBCT or an accurate intraoral periapical radiograph shot using a positioning device. In teeth with no prior endodontic treatment, an apex locator maybe used to measure the root length.

The procedure is initiated by sectioning of the coronal part of the tooth using a short shank carbide bur on a water-cooled high-speed drill. Using this long shank carbide drill, the root is sectioned in the coronal plane to separate the labial part of the root from the palatal part. The section is made through the root canal space almost throughout the length of the root. Endodontic rotary files can also be used to extirpate the canal contents and reach the apex of the root, prior to sectioning. An assessment of the root length can be accurately made by using an apex locator device. This step will ensure inadvertent damage to periapical bone during sectioning and shield preparation. As it approaches the apex, the drill is directed slightly labially so as to create a clean-cut mesiodistally. Gentle sweeping motions of the drill are made in the mesiodistal direction to separate the buccal and palatal halves of the root (Figs. 2.6 and 2.7). The mesiodistal sectioning should be complete so as to separate the palatal portion of the root from the buccal. The objective is to extract the entire palatal and apical portion of the root and keep the labial section firmly attached to the labial bone. Occasionally the palatal fragment may get extracted devoid of the apex. In such a scenario, the apex is drilled off carefully using the same long shank drill or a round bur on a straight surgical handpiece. Care is taken not to perforate the labial bone and create an inadvertent fenestration. Since single-rooted teeth are triangular in cross section, a wide sectioning will lead to damage of the adjacent teeth or bone. Periapical radiographs at this juncture of the procedure will assist the operator in ensuring that a correct path and depth of cut is being followed.

Once the section is made, the palatal fragment is carefully mobilized with a fine-tipped elevator. The tip of the elevator should rest between palatal bone and the palatal fragment of the root. It should never be positioned between the labial and palatal part of the tooth, as it may lead to an inadvertent fracture of the labial bone and mobility of the labial portion of the sectioned tooth. Gentle force is exerted to mobilize the fragment (Fig. 2.8). If the initial separation between labial and palatal fragment is

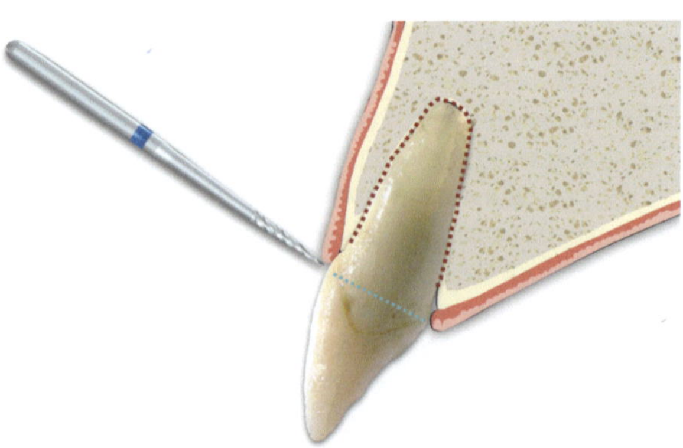

Fig. 2.6 Sectioning of the tooth

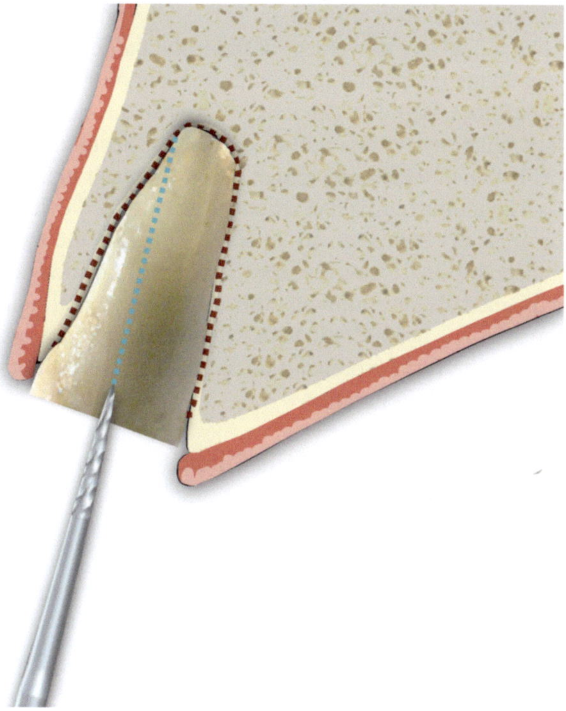

Fig. 2.7 Sectioning of the root

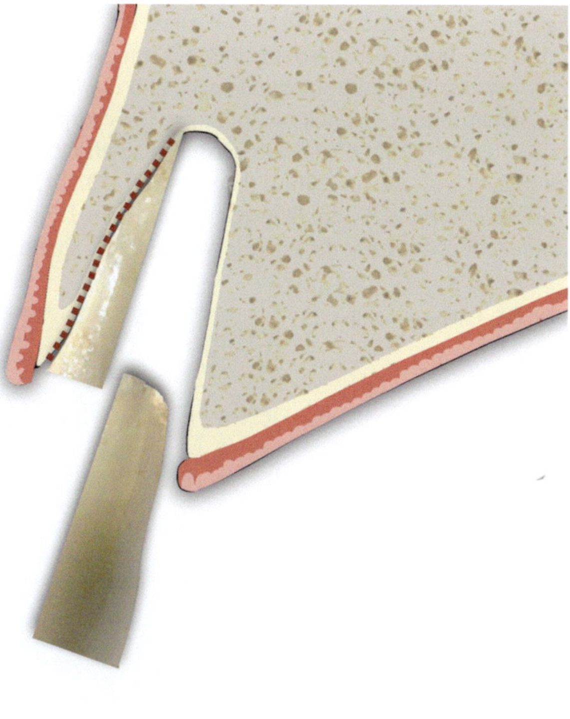

Fig. 2.8 Extraction of the palatal root fragment

complete, the palatal fragment gets easily mobilized. A finger is placed on the labial bone to feel any movement of the labial part of the root. In case there is difficulty in mobilizing the palatal fragment, the sectioning of the tooth should be revisited. The palatal root should be extracted only when the mesio-distal sectioning is complete. An incomplete sectioning will lead to an accidental movement of the labial fragment or extraction of the complete root. This will result in failure of the procedure.

The mobilized palatal fragment is extracted using fine-tipped extraction forceps or a curved hemostat. In an ideal situation, the extracted fragment has the apex attached to it. If not, the apex is carefully drilled with the long shank carbide as explained above. Following this step, a periapical radiograph is taken to ensure that the apex has been eliminated. Any visibility of radiopaque root filling material will necessitate further preparation so that the entire root canal contents are extirpated during shield preparation.

Step 2: Preparation of the Shield

Armamentarium:

1. Gingival retractors.
2. Long shank round diamond burs of various diameters.
3. Football-shaped diamond.

After the extraction of the palatal fragment, a small gingival retractor or similar instrument is used to protect the soft tissue from the drill (Fig. 2.9). A large round diamond bur is used at 200,000 rpm to trim the shield to the level of the bone. The same large diamond is used to thin down the shield in the coronal aspect. The ideal thickness should be approximately 1.5 mm. Another guideline for the thickness is halfway between the root canal space and the labial extent of the root. In essence, the shield should be thick enough to resist resorption and thin enough to leave sufficient space within the socket perimeter to allow for an optimally sized implant to be placed without contacting the shield [3, 13, 14]. For a lower incisor, the shield will have to be very thin, sometimes less than 1.5 mm to leave space for a narrow diameter implant. For the maxillary canine, the shield dimension can be kept thicker

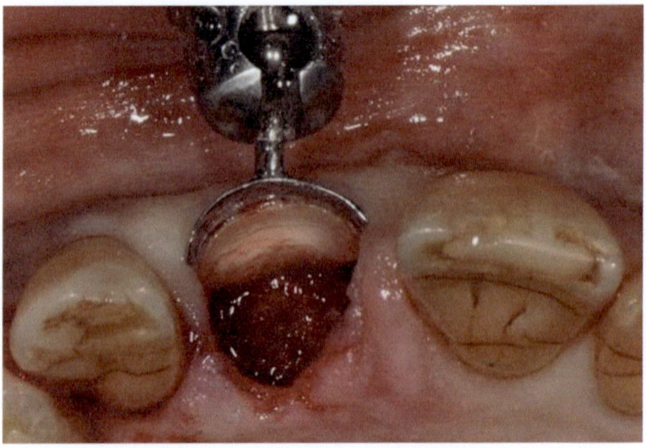

Fig. 2.9 Protection of the soft tissue

so as to accommodate an implant and have an optimum gap between the implant and the shield.

The shield should extend from mesio-labial to disto-labial line angle and follow the curvature of the labial bone contour [5]. The midfacial part of the shield should be made thin so that a contact with the implant is avoided. Schwimmer et al. have shown in their case report, a histological evidence of integration between root shield and the implant with presence of vital bone between them [15]. However, the authors believe in intentionally leaving a gap between the shield and the implant, so as to prevent inadvertent pressure of the implant against the shield. In spite of all efforts, a mild contact between the implant in the apical half of the shield maybe unavoidable.

The next step is to make an S-shaped preparation to bevel the shield on its internal aspect using a football-shaped diamond bur (Fig. 2.10). This preparation provides restorative space to accommodate the abutment and provides good emergence for the provisional crown. The objective is to ensure that there is no contact between the abutment and the provisional crown with the shield. The space will allow soft tissue to form over the shield and insulate it from the oral environment. This helps in forming a collar of healthy soft tissue around the neck of the implant (Figs. 2.10 and 2.11).

Once the shield preparation is complete, the socket is thoroughly irrigated with normal saline to flush out any remnants of tooth structure or gutta percha. A small-sized bone curette is used to clean the apical portion of the socket. A periapical radiograph is taken at this juncture to ensure that all the remnants of the gutta percha and the apex of the root are eliminated.

The site is now ready for the osteotomy and implant placement.

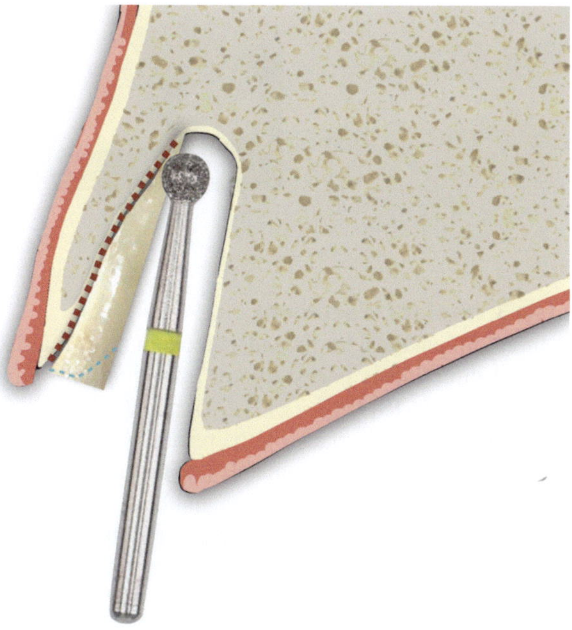

Fig. 2.10 Thinning the shield with a large round bur. Trimming the apical portion of the shield

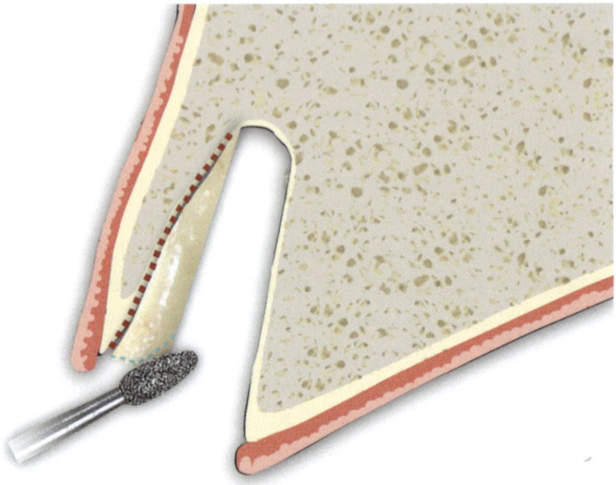

Fig. 2.11 Beveling of internal aspect of shield

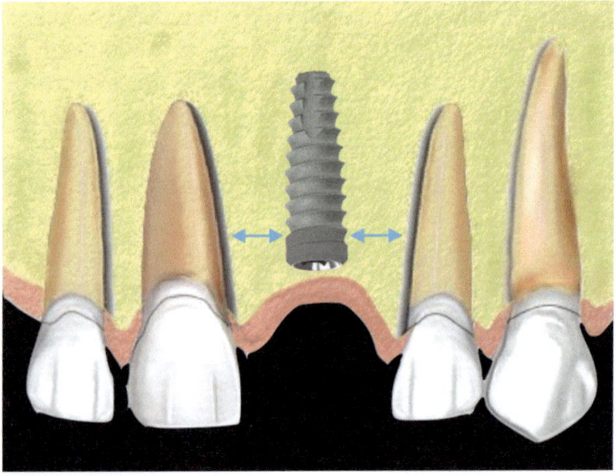

Fig. 2.12 Mesiodistal position

Step 3: Implant Placement

A three-dimensional implant placement in the mesiodistal, buccolingual, and apico-coronal direction is necessary for achieving an optimum emergence of the final restoration [16–18] (Figs. 2.12, 2.13, and 2.14).

The osteotomy is made on the palatal wall of the socket. The entry point of the osteotomy should be 3–4 mm apical to the palatal crest of bone when adequate palatal bone is available. When the palatal bone is reduced in thickness, the entry point should be shifted apically. Gluckman et al. have suggested guidelines for choosing

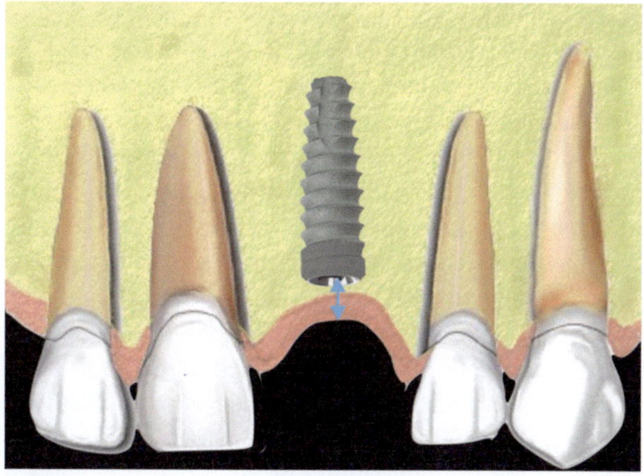

Fig. 2.13 Apicocoronal position

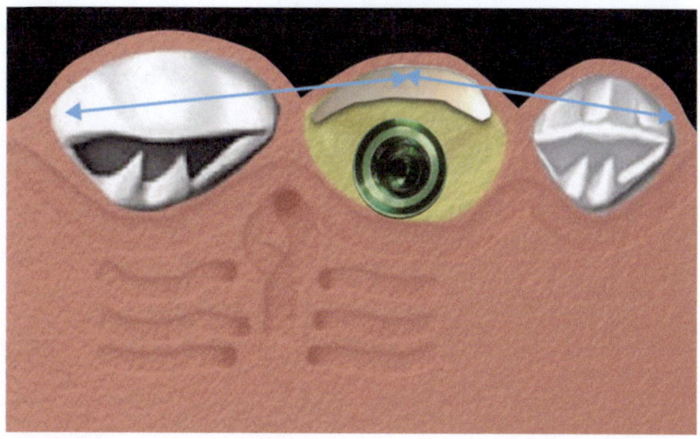

Fig. 2.14 Bucco-lingual position

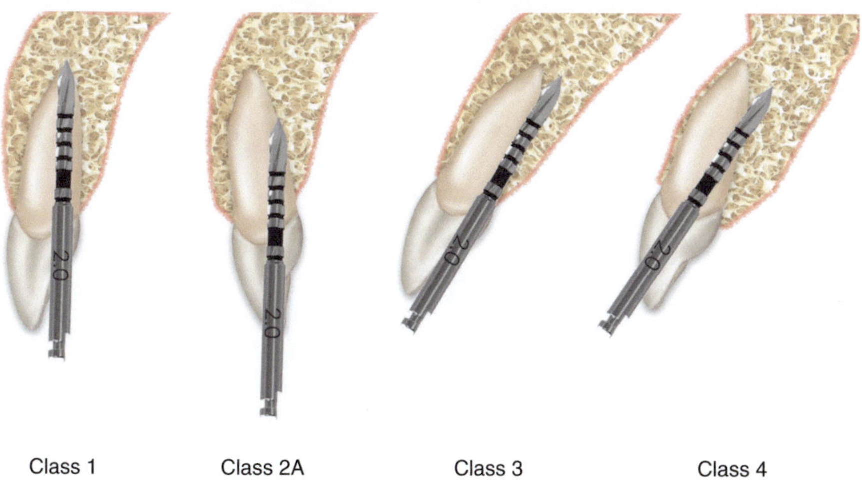

Fig. 2.15 Trajectories for implant placement based on radial plane position of the tooth in the socket

an entry point within the socket for immediate post-extraction implant placement [19]. Based on their classification for radial plane position of the tooth (ref. to Chap. 3), the implant trajectory can be planned (Fig. 2.15).

In most maxillary anterior sockets, the osteotomy commences from the palatal wall of the socket. The osteotomy should never commence from the apex of the socket if the tooth is facially positioned and the labial bone is thin. This will create a fenestration on the labial side and will get the implant too close to the shield. Not paying attention to this aspect of the osteotomy preparation can seriously impact the outcome of the treatment. Care should be taken to prevent any contact of the drill with the shield during osteotomy preparation. Sequential enlargement of the osteotomy must be performed based on the density of the bone. The diameter of the implant should be chosen so as to ideally leave a space of 1 to 1.5 mm between the shield and the labial part of the implant in the coronal aspect. The length of the implant should be such that it extends 2-3 mm beyond the apex of the root so as to achieve good primary stabilty from the periapical bone. Hence, the preparation is made 2–3 mm deeper than the apex of the socket on the palatal wall to accomodate the implant (Figs. 2.16, 2.17, and 2.18).

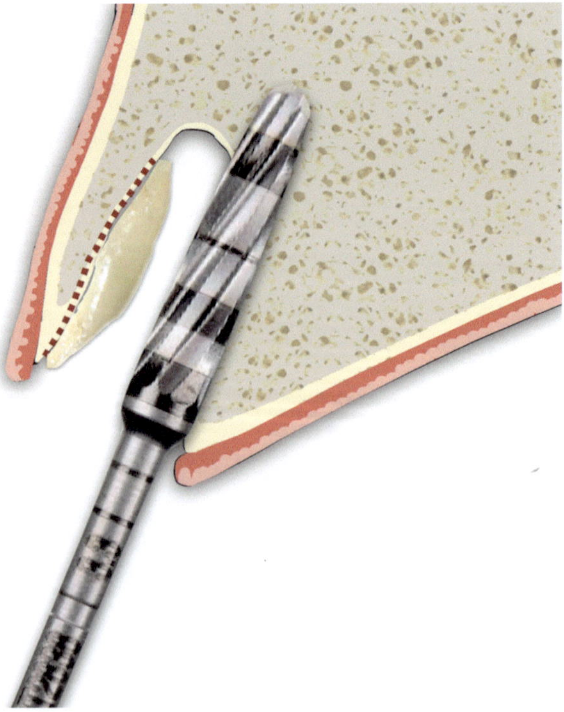

Fig. 2.16 Implant site preparation

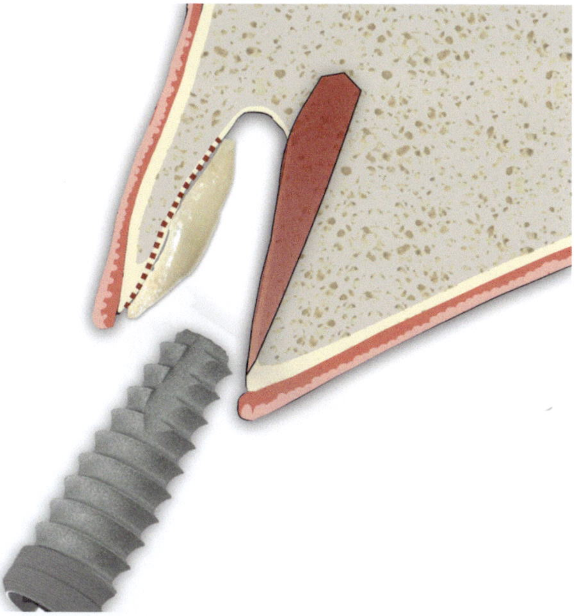

Fig. 2.17 Implant placement

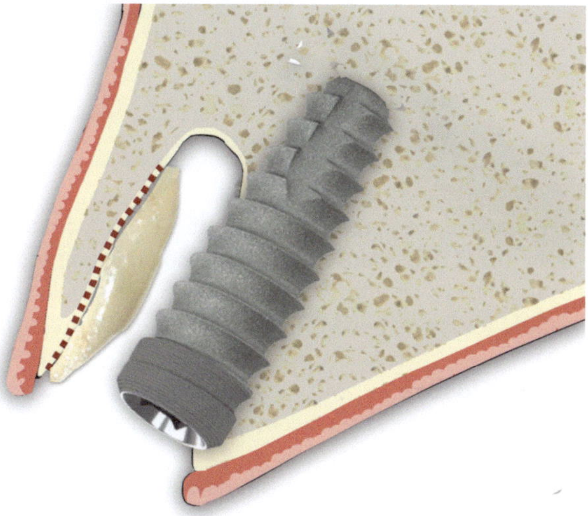

Fig. 2.18 Implant in final position

Step 4: Management of the Gap

So far there is no consensus on whether a biomaterial is required to fill the gap between the shield and the implant (Fig. 2.19). The retention of the blood clot in the gap is the key to bone formation between the shield and the implant. A prosthetic seal created with a well-contoured provisional restoration or a customized healing abutment prevents soft tissue ingress into the gap [3, 4]. The authors have not used a biomaterial in the gap for all their cases performed over a 5-year time frame and

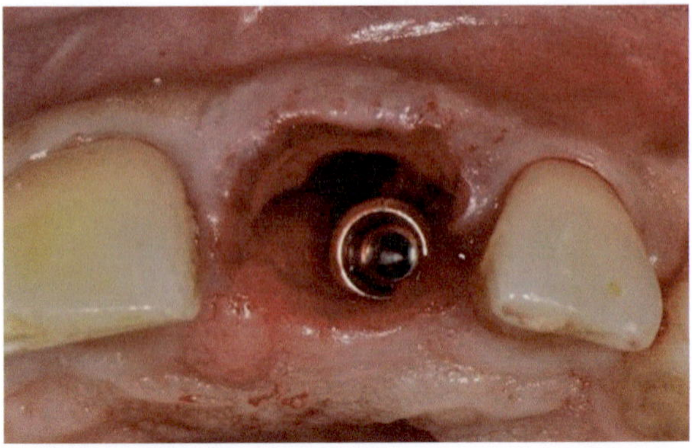

Fig. 2.19 Gap between implant and shield

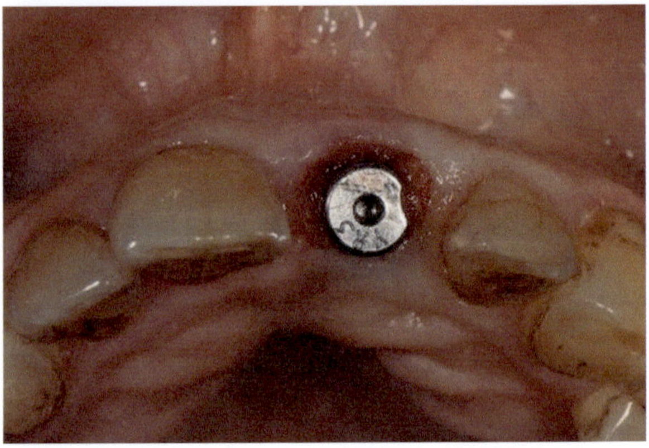

Fig. 2.20 Healing abutment

have found no compromise in the esthetic or functional outcome [5]. However, gaps larger than 3 mm, more commonly encountered in premolar and molar sockets, may be filled using an allograft or alloplastic material which would help in creating a scaffold for future bone formation and prevent the ingress of soft tissue [9, 21, 22].

Step 5: Closure

Closure of the socket is necessary to protect the underlying implant and seal the periphery of the socket.

There are four ways of closing the site.

1. Placement of a healing abutment: This is a simple and rapid way of closure [1, 3, 9, 22–24]. This is done when a tooth borne provisional restoration is planned. However, the soft tissue contour formed after healing may need some modification prior to impression making (Fig. 2.20). The gingival former can be placed directly or utilizing platelet-rich fibrin wrapped around it (poncho technique) [3].
2. Customizing a healing abutment to seal the socket: This option is chosen when the clinician chooses *not* to make an immediate fixed provisional crown on the implant (Figs. 2.21 and 2.22). Customization of the healing abutment will allow

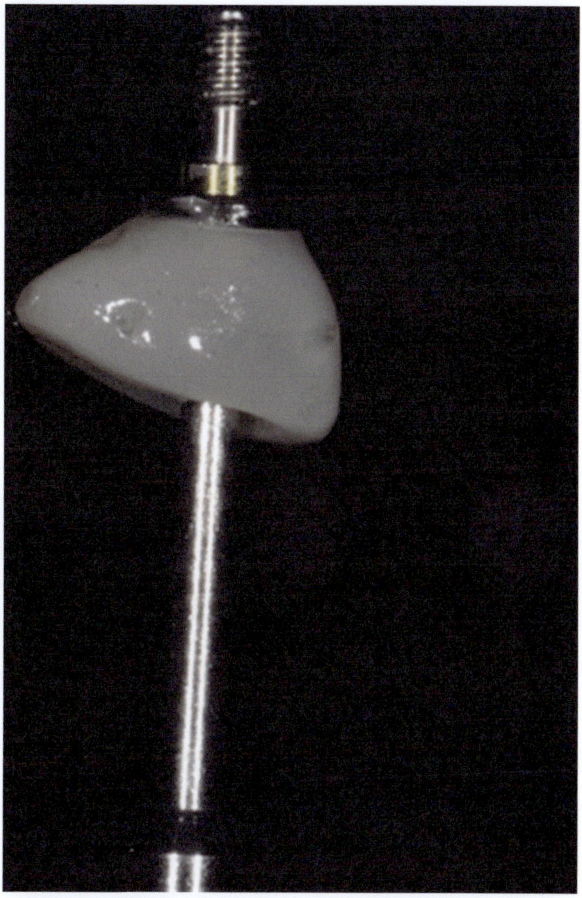

Fig. 2.21 Customized healing abutment

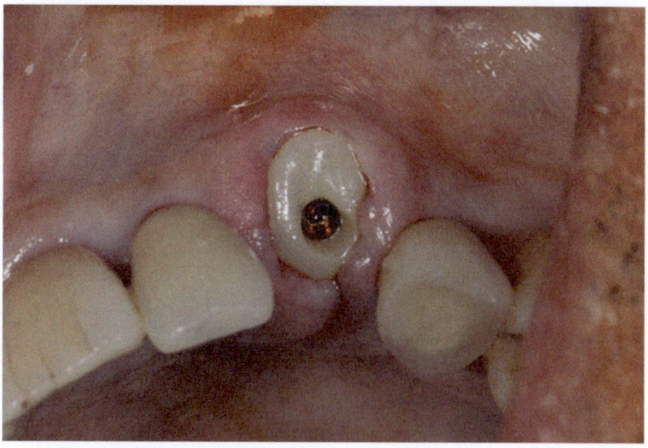

Fig. 2.22 Customized healing abutment

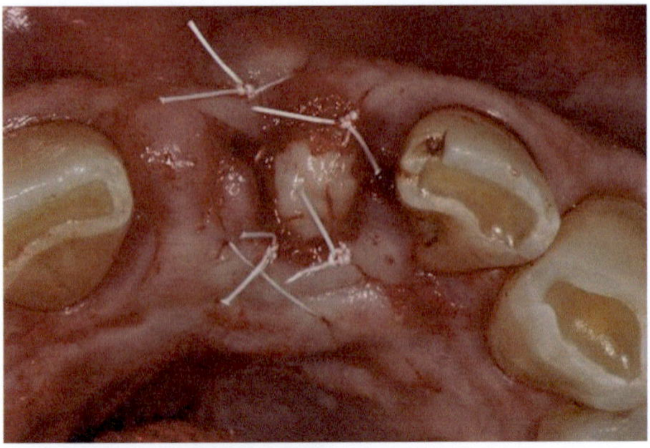

Fig. 2.23 Socket seal with palatal free gingival graft sutured with PTFE sutures

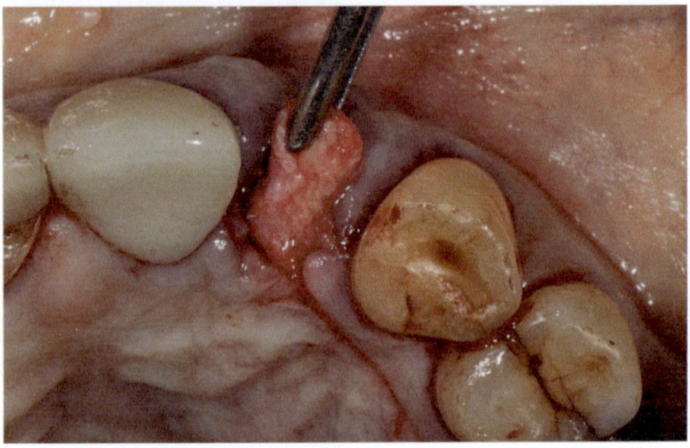

Fig. 2.24 Rotated palatal pedicled flap

effective development of tissue contours and help in maintaining the soft tissue architecture [7, 14, 25].

3. Placing a cover screw followed by a socket seal procedure: In the event of poor primary stability of the implant, the operator may prefer to submerge the implant [26]. A seal is achieved with a piece of free gingival graft from the palate or tuberosity which is sutured around the periphery of the socket (Fig. 2.23). Alternately, a rotated pedicled connective tissue graft from the palate maybe used to cover the socket (Fig. 2.24).
4. Making a screw retained provisional crown: This is the most preferred option when there is good primary stability of the implant and the occlusion is suitable for making a fixed restoration on the implant (Fig. 2.25). This will allow the patient to have an esthetic provisional restoration during the healing phase and help in maintaining the soft tissue contours for the definitive restoration [4–6, 27–30].

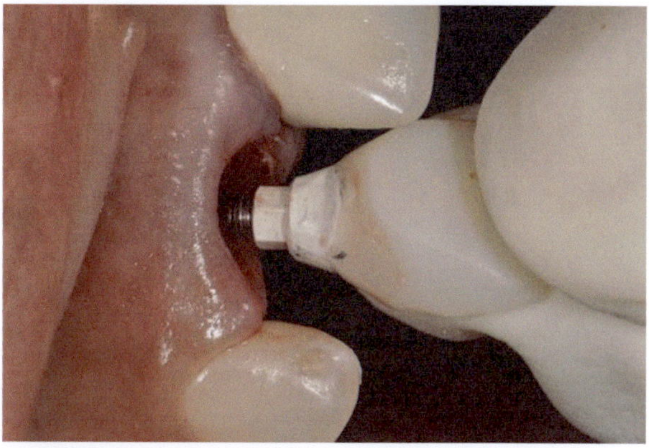

Fig. 2.25 Provisional crown over the implant

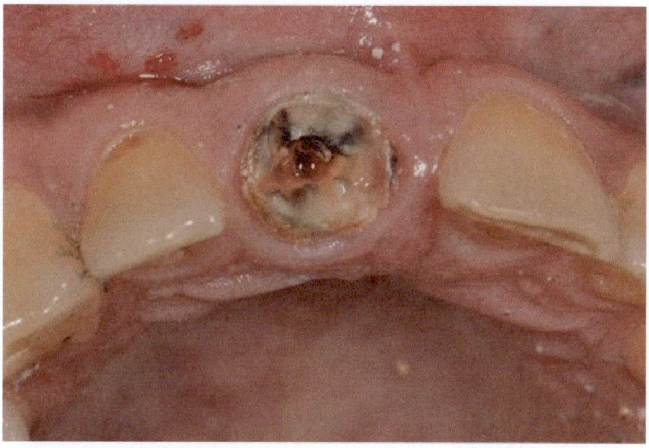

Fig. 2.26 Preoperative situation of a fractured tooth 11

2.3.3 Step by Step Protocol

The following is a case report of a 44-year-old man who reported with an unrestorable tooth 11. A socket shield procedure followed by implant placement and an immediate provisional crown was performed. The provisional crown was replaced with a lithium disilicate crown on a zirconia abutment after 3 months (Figs. 2.26, 2.27, 2.28, 2.29, 2.30, 2.31, 2.32, 2.33, 2.34, 2.35, 2.36, 2.37, 2.38, and 2.39).

2.4 Troubleshooting

1. Improper sectioning: Occasionally the sectioning of the root maybe inaccurate in direction and may not deliver the root fragment with the apex. Instead only a small palatal fragment may get extracted.

   In such a scenario, the apical portion can be further trimmed using the long shank carbide drill on a high-speed handpiece by accessing it through the socket (Fig. 2.40). In case the root is long and adequate access is not achievable through

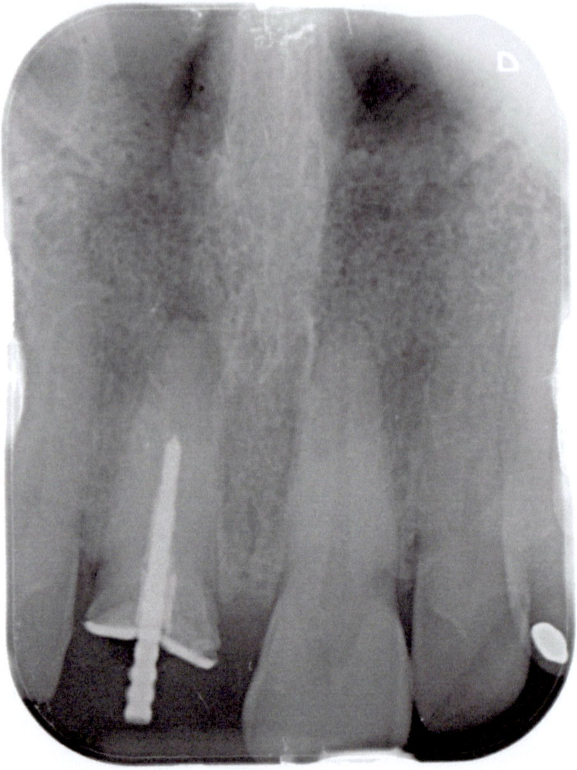

Fig. 2.27 Fractured tooth 11 on the X-ray

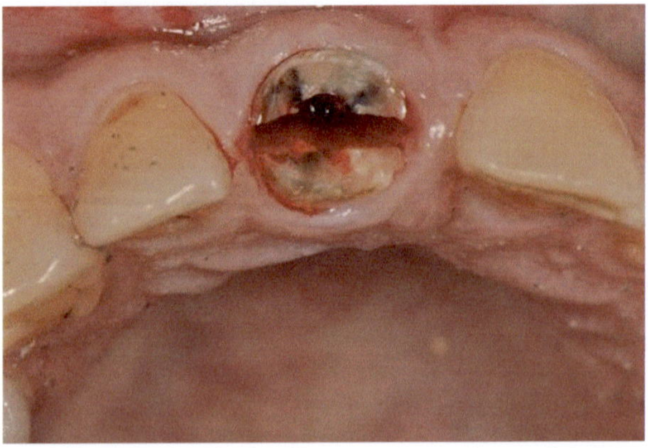

Fig. 2.28 Sectioning of the tooth with a long shank carbide bur

the socket, the apex can be accessed and trimmed away by making a labial incision and reflecting a flap (Chap. 6).

2. Mobility of the labial shield: There is always a possibility of inadvertent mobility of the labial fragment of the root while extracting. In such cases, the labial fragment should be carefully extracted and the case should be treated like a conventional immediate implant placement with a dual-zone grafting technique [31].

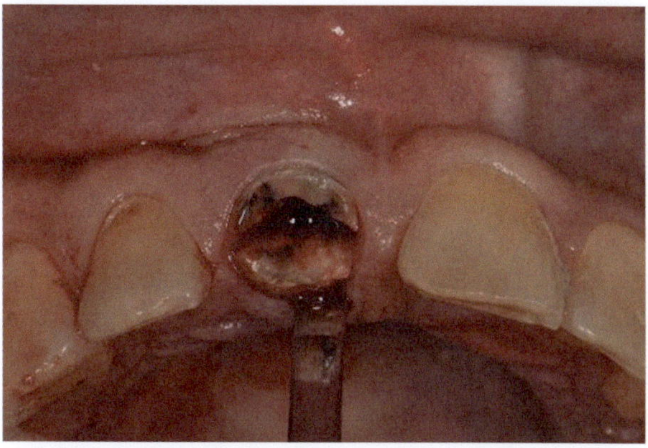

Fig. 2.29 Mobilization of the palatal fragment

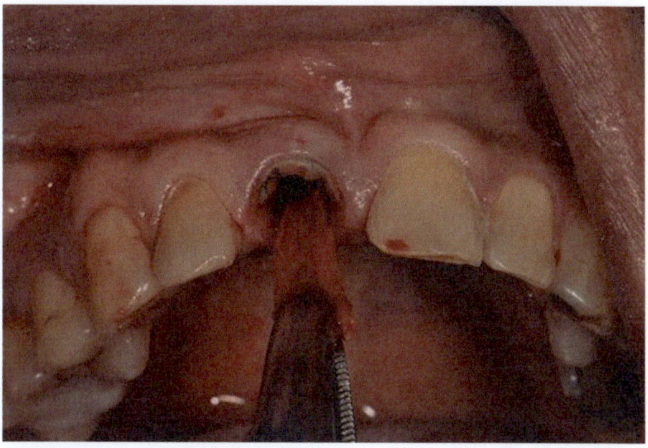

Fig. 2.30 Extraction of the palatal fragment

3. Labial fenestration: During the sectioning of the root there is a possibility of creating a labial fenestration near the apex of the root (Fig. 2.41). These fenestrations can be accessed and grafted using an esthetic buccal flap approach (Chap. 6).
4. Inadequate stability for the implant: If low insertion torque values are recorded while placing the implant, it is advisable not to make an immediate provisional restoration over the implant. In such a scenario the implant is submerged and a socket seal is created using a small piece of a free gingival graft or a palatal pedicle graft (Fig. 2.42).
5. Spinning implant: In case the implant stability is very low and if the implant is spinning internally after reaching its final position, it is advisable to remove the implant and do a staged implant placement as described by Glocker et al. [32] (Chap. 6). The resulting socket and defect created by the osteotomy should be grafted with a biomaterial and closed with a free gingival graft, pedicle flap, or a barrier membrane (Figs. 2.43 and 2.44).

Fig. 2.31 The extracted palatal fragment

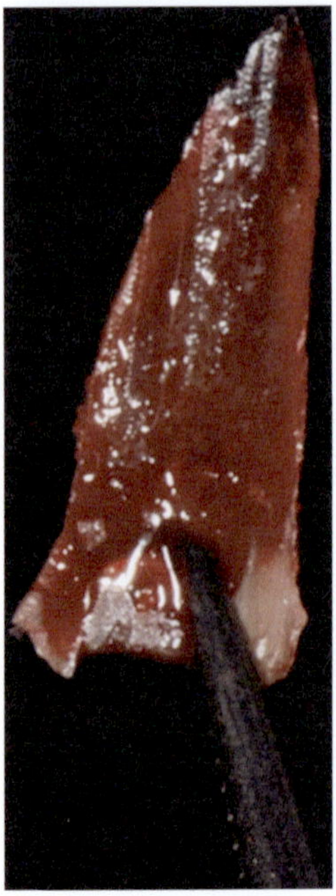

Fig. 2.32 Verification of the partial extraction and removal of apical root portion

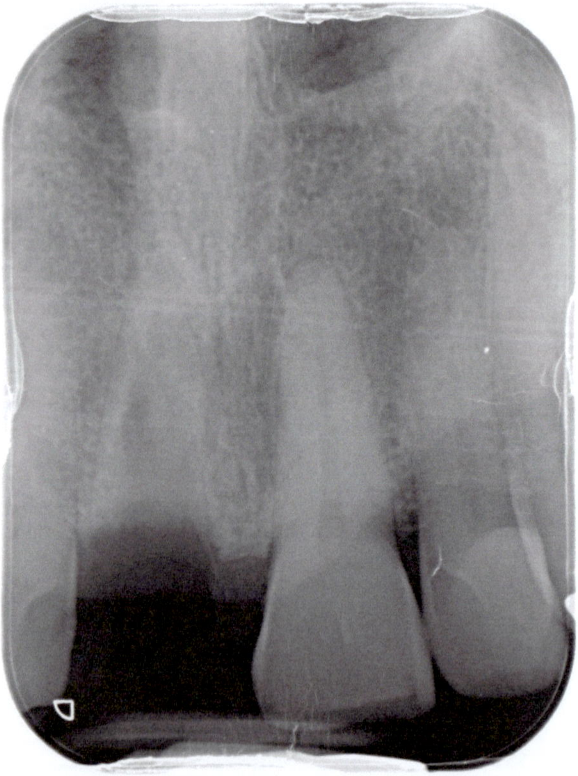

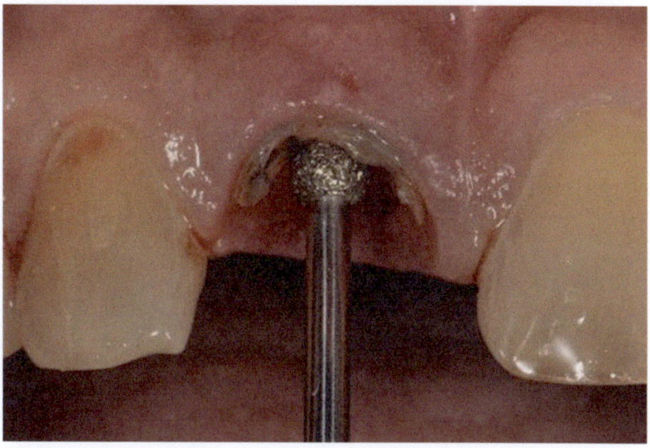

Fig. 2.33 Shield preparation

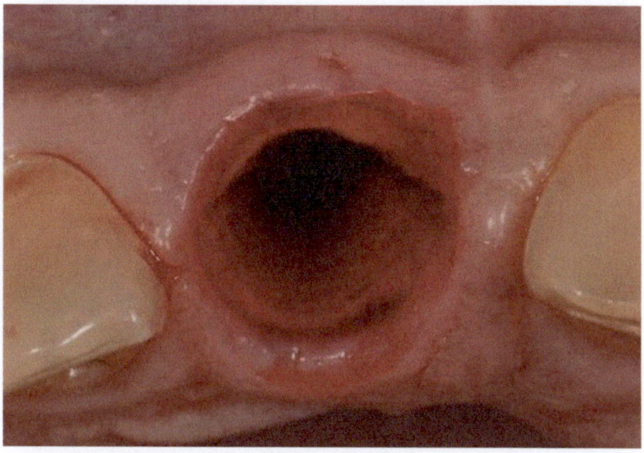

Fig. 2.34 Prepared shield

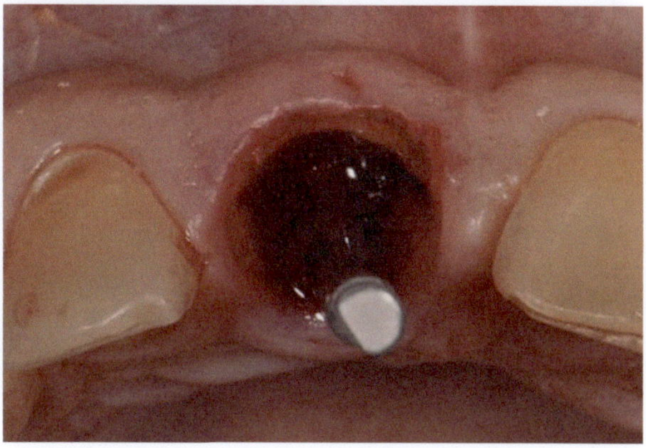

Fig. 2.35 Initiation of the osteotomy for implant placement

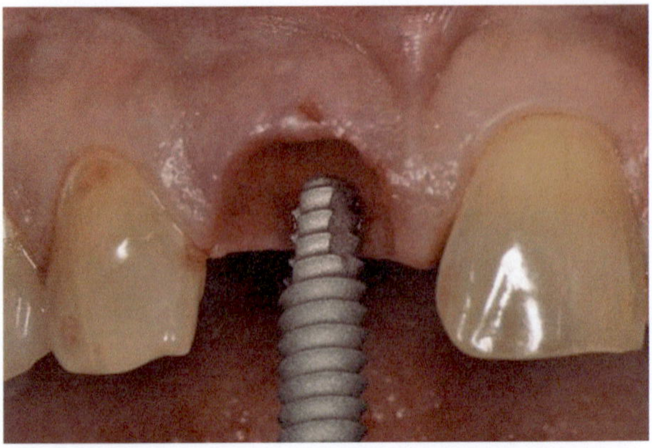

Fig. 2.36 Implant placement

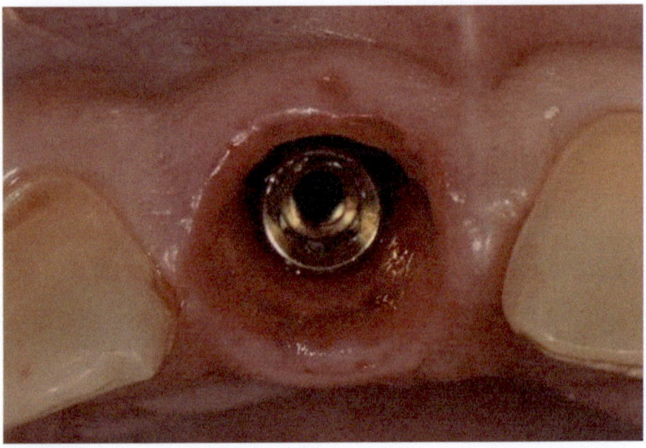

Fig. 2.37 Implant in final position

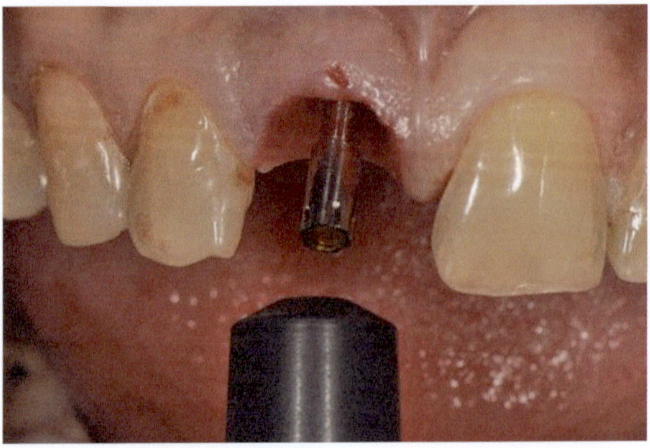

Fig. 2.38 Verification of primary stability by measuring ISQ value

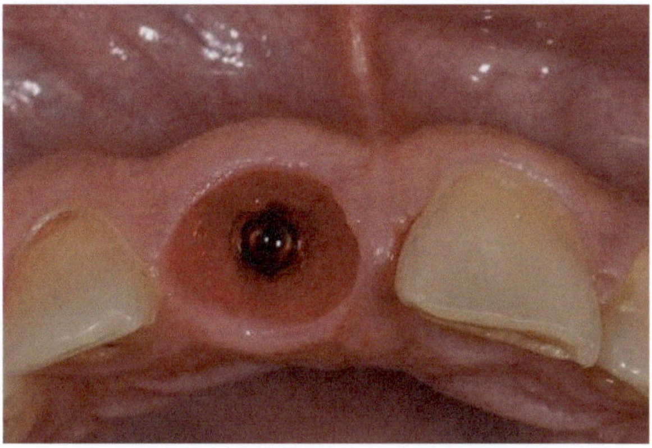

Fig. 2.39 Excellent tissue contours after removal of the screw retained provisional restoration 4 months after implant placement

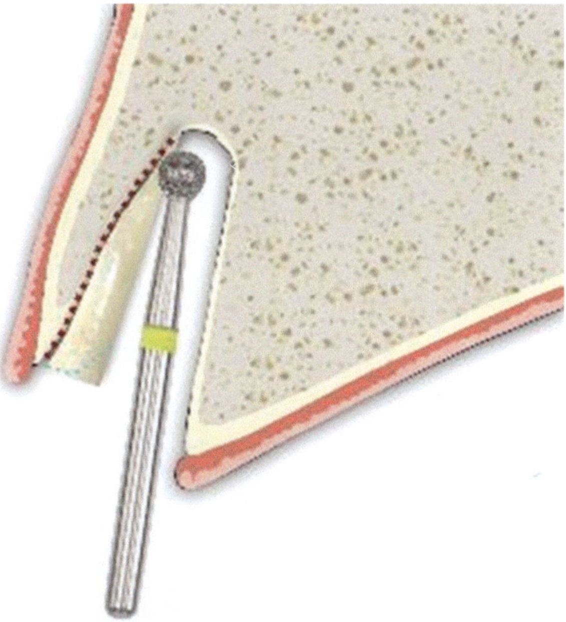

Fig. 2.40 Round bur on a straight handpiece to access apex of the root

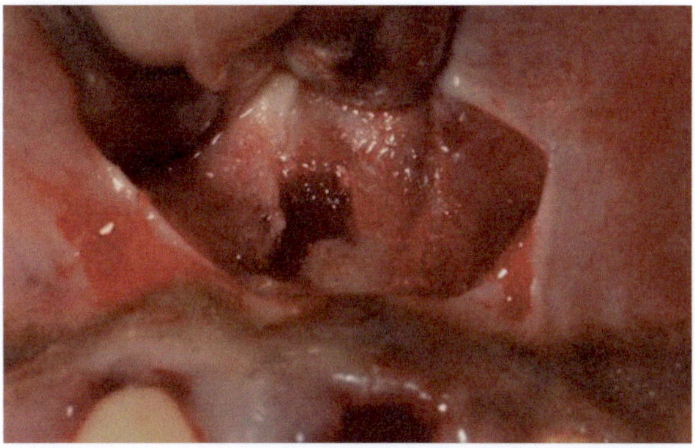

Fig. 2.41 Esthetic labial flap for access to apical fenestration

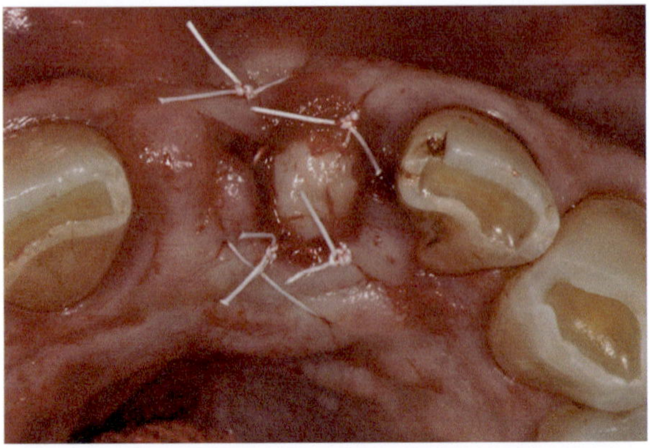

Fig. 2.42 Socket seal procedure done using a free gingival graft from the palate

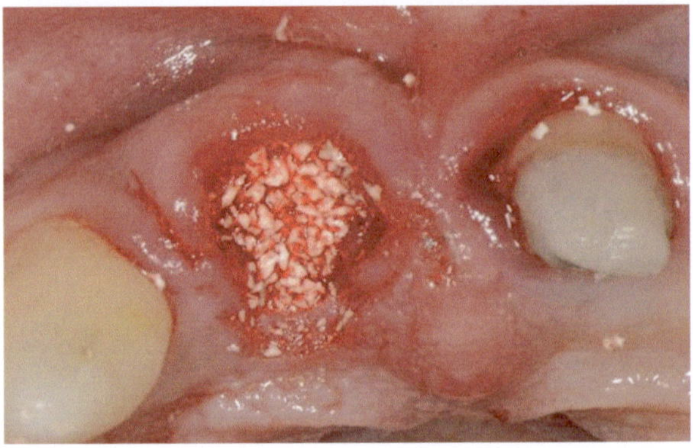

Fig. 2.43 Socket grafting after removal of a spinning implant

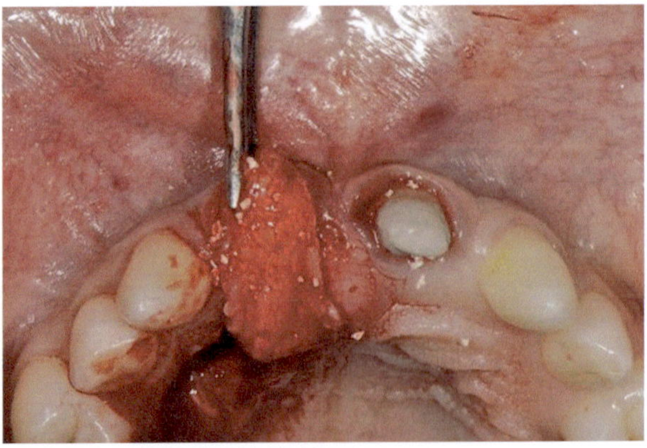

Fig. 2.44 Palatal pedicle flap

2.5 Conclusion

The socket shield procedure is a highly technique sensitive procedure. High level of expertise in post-extraction immediate placement and fabrication of a well-contoured chairside provisional restoration are essential for achieving a predictable outcome. Careful assessment of the root morphology with preoperative diagnostic aids is essential. Using the correct instrumentation and following surgical protocols for partial extraction of the root and shield preparation are mandatory for achieving successful outcomes. When executed correctly, the postoperative morbidity and complication rates are low and can be managed easily by conventional procedures (Chap. 10).

Acknowledgement Illustrations by: Udatta Kher.

References

1. Gluckman H, Salama M, Du Toit J. Partial extraction therapies (PET). Part 1: maintaining alveolar ridge contour at pontic and immediate implant sites. Int J Periodontics Restorative Dent. 2016;36:681–7.
2. Gluckman H, Du Toit J, Salama M. The socket-shield technique to support buccofacial tissues at immediate implant placement: A case report and review of the literature. Int Dent Africa Ed. 2015;5:1–7.
3. Mitsias ME. The root membrane concept: in the zone with the "triangle of bone". Dent Today. 2017;36(10):80.
4. Siormpas KD, Mitsias ME, Kontsiotou-Siormpa E, Garber D, Kotsakis GA. Immediate implant placement in the esthetic zone utilizing the "root-membrane" technique: clinical results up to 5 years post loading. Int J Oral Maxillofac Implants. 2014;29:1397–405.
5. Kumar PR, Kher U. Shield the socket: procedure, case report and classification. J Indian Soc Periodontol. 2018;22(3):266–72.
6. Mitsias ME, Siormpas KD, Prasad H, Garber D, Kotsakis GA. A step-by-step description of PDL-mediated ridge preservation for immediate implant rehabilitation in the esthetic region. Int J Periodontics Restorative Dent. 2015;35:835–41.
7. Gluckman H, Nagy K, Du Toit J. Prosthetic management of implants placed with the socket-shield technique. J Prosthet Dent. 2019;121(4):581–5.
8. Gluckman H, Salama M, Du Toit J. A retrospective evaluation of 128 socket shield cases in the esthetic zone and posterior sites: partial extraction therapy with up to 4 years follow-up. Clin Implant Dent Relat Res. 2017;20:122–9.
9. Gluckman H, Du Toit J, Salama M. The pontic shield: partial extraction therapy for ridge preservation and pontic site development. Int J Periodontics Restorative Dent. 2016;36:417–23.
10. Araujo MG, Lindhe J. Ridge alterations following tooth extraction with and without flap elevation: an experimental study in the dog. Clin Oral Implants Res. 2009;20:545–9.
11. Fickl S, Zuhr O, Wachtel H, Bolz W, Huerzeler M. Tissue alterations after tooth extraction with and without surgical trauma: a volumetric study in the beagle dog. J Clin Periodontol. 2008a;35:356–63.
12. Campelo LD, Camara JR. Flapless implant surgery: A 10-year clinical retrospective analysis. Int J Oral Maxillofac Implants. 2002;17:271–6.
13. Gluckman H, Salama M, Du Toit J. Partial extraction therapies (PET). Part 2: procedures and technical aspects. Int J Periodontics Restorative Dent. 2017;37(3):377–85.

14. Gluckman H, du Toit J, Salama M. Guided bone regeneration of a fenestration complication at immediate implant placement simultaneous to the socket-shield technique. Int Dent. 2015;5:58–66.
15. Schwimer C, Pette GA, Gluckman H, Salama M, Du Toit J. Human histologic evidence of new bone formation and osseointegration between root dentin (unplanned socket-shield) and dental implant: case report. Int J Oral Maxillofac Implants. 2018;33:e19–23.
16. Chen ST, Buser D. ITI treatment guide vol 3: implants in extraction sockets. In: Buser D, Belser U, Wismeijer D, editors. Implants in post-extraction sites: a literature update. Berlin: Quintessence Publishing Co, Ltd; 2008. p. 9–16.
17. Buser D, Martin W, Belser UC. Optimizing esthetics for implant restorations in the anterior maxilla: anatomic and surgical considerations. Int J Oral Maxillofac Implants. 2004;19(Suppl):43–61.
18. Kois JC. Predictable single tooth peri-implant esthetics: five diagnostic keys. Compend Contin Educ Dent. 2001;22:199–206.
19. Gluckman H, Pontes CC, Du Toit J. Radial plane tooth position and bone wall dimensions in the anterior maxilla: a CBCT classification for immediate implant placement. J Prosthet Dent. 2018;120:50–6.
20. Huwais S, Meyer EG. A novel osseous densification approach in implant osteotomy preparation to increase biomechanical primary stability, bone mineral density, and bone-to-implant contact. Int J Oral Maxillofac Implants. 2017;32:27–36.
21. Zhang Z, Dong Y, Yang J, Xu R, Deng F. Effect of socket-shield technique on alveolar ridge soft and hard tissue in dogs. J Clin Periodontol. 2019;46:256–63.
22. Schwimer CW, et al. The socket-shield technique at molar sites: A proof-of-principle technique report. J Prosthet Dent. 2018;121(2):229–33.
23. Esteve-Pardo G, Esteve-Colomina L. Clinical application of the socket-shield concept in multiple anterior teeth. Case Rep Dent. 2018;2018:Article ID 9014372.
24. Baumer D, Zuhr O, Rebele S, Hürzeler M. Socket shield technique for immediate implant placement—clinical, radiographic and volumetric data after 5 years. Clin Oral Implants Res. 2017;28:1450–8.
25. Machado A, Goncalves R, Pinheiro AD, Cordeiro Filho C, Rangel BC, Alto RM, Casado PL. Immediate implant and customized abutments: Esthetic peri-implant preservation alternative without immediate loading esthetic customized abutment. Int J Growth Factors Stem Cells Dent. 2019;2(1):8.
26. Chen C, Pan Y. Socket shield technique for ridge preservation: a case report. J Prosthodont Implantol. 2013;2:16–21.
27. Cherel F, Etienne D. Papilla preservation between two implants: a modified socket-shield technique to maintain the scalloped anatomy? A case report. Quintessence Int. 2014;45:23–30.
28. Hurzeler MB, Zuhr O, Schupbach P, Rebele SF, Emmanouilidis N, Fickl S. The socketshield technique: a proof-of-principle report. J Clin Periodontol. 2010;37:855–62.
29. Kan JY, Rungcharassaeng K. Proximal socket shield for interimplant papilla preservation in the esthetic zone. Int J Periodontics Restorative Dent. 2013;33:e24–31.
30. Aslan S. Improved volume and contour stability with thin socket-shield preparation in immediate implant placement and provisionalization in the esthetic zone. Int J Esthetic Dent. 2018;13:172–83.
31. Chu S, Salama M, Salama H, David AG, Saito H, Guido OS, Tarnow D. The dual-zone therapeutic concept of managing immediate implant placement and provisional restoration in anterior extraction sockets. Comp Contin Edu Dent (Jamesburg, NJ, 1995). 2012;33:524–34.
32. Glocker M, Attin T, Schmidlin PR. Ridge preservation with modified "socket-shield" technique: a methodological case series. Dent J. 2014;2:11–21.

Case Selection and Risk Assessment for PET

3

Udatta Kher, Ali Tunkiwala, and Payal Rajender Kumar

Abstract

Surgical procedures require a thorough understanding of the risks involved and possibility of complications that may occur following the surgery. This is more so important for newer techniques. Diagnosis and selection of the right case is the first step toward achieving a successful outcome. This chapter will help the reader understand the limitations of the PET procedure and evaluate the risk factors involved in performing the case. The indications for the socket shield procedure along with absolute and relative contraindications are listed along with clinical examples.

3.1 Introduction

The socket shield technique is a new addition to the myriad surgical procedures in implant dentistry. Clinicians new to this science ought to educate themselves, to understand the ideal indications while selecting cases. More importantly, clinicians need to understand which cases should not be undertaken for PET procedures. After having understood the step-by-step technique of the socket shield procedure in Chap. 2, it is prudent to follow guidelines for choosing the right cases in order to avoid intraoperative and postoperative complications.

U. Kher (✉)
Only Smiles Dental Centre, Mumbai, India

A. Tunkiwala
Smiles by Design, Mumbai, India

P. Rajender Kumar
Private Practice, New Delhi, India

U. Kher, A. Tunkiwala (eds.), *Partial Extraction Therapy in Implant Dentistry*,
https://doi.org/10.1007/978-3-030-33610-3_3

3.2 Case Selection

The first step in minimizing failures of surgical procedures is choosing cases appropriately. Emphasis should be on correct diagnosis of the clinical condition and assessment of risks involved in the procedure [1]. A systematic approach toward identifying the risks involved in the case should be practiced. A combination of clinical and radiographic data should be collected to analyze the suitability of the case for a socket shield procedure.

3.2.1 Clinical Assessment

Parameters for assessment of the possible risks involved during teeth replacement in the esthetic zone are described below. These are risk factors for any implant-based treatment options in the esthetic zone. They are also relevant for PET procedures.

Lip Line

Lip lines are classified as high, average, or low. The higher the lip line, higher will be the effort required to achieve a satisfactory esthetic result. The higher the lip line, greater is the tooth and gingival display and greater the risk of an unforgiving esthetic outcome in implant dentistry; should something not go as per plan (Figs. 3.1, 3.2, and 3.3). A low lip line is generally more forgiving since the teeth and soft tissue interface is not visible during speech or while smiling [2].

Tooth Position and Free Gingival Margin

If the free gingival margin of the tooth to be extracted is more coronal, the risk is lower, as minor mucosal recession will not lead to an esthetic compromise [3]. More apical level of the gingival margins will necessitate the use of adjunct surgical or orthodontic procedures prior to implant placement [4, 5] (Figs. 3.4 and 3.5).

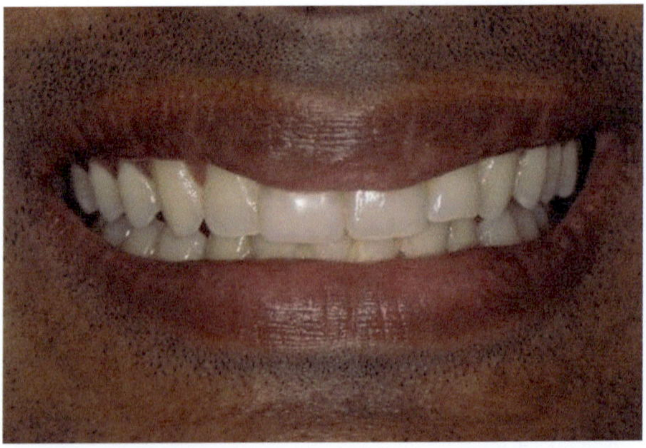

Fig. 3.1 Low lip line

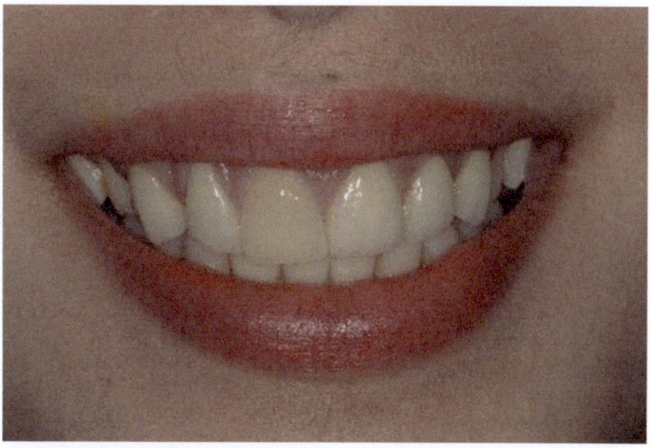

Fig. 3.2 Medium lip line

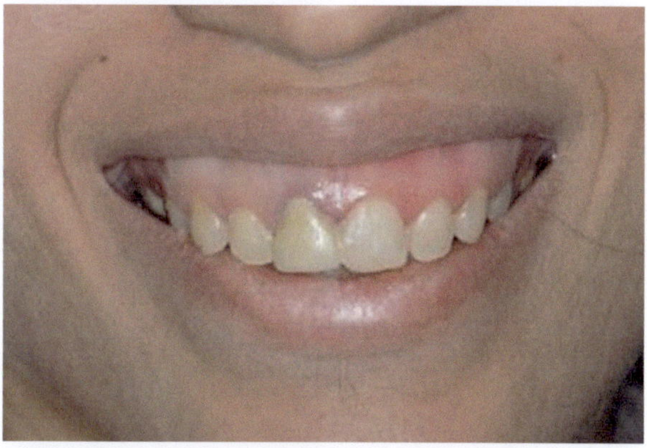

Fig. 3.3 High lip line

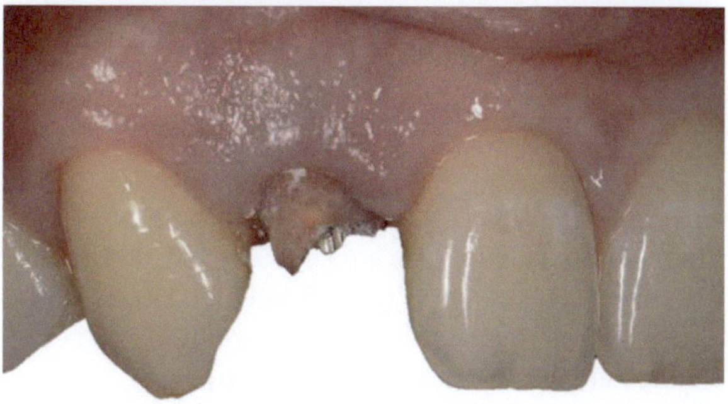

Fig. 3.4 Tooth position and free gingival margin (FGM) more coronal to adjacent teeth is an ideal starting point

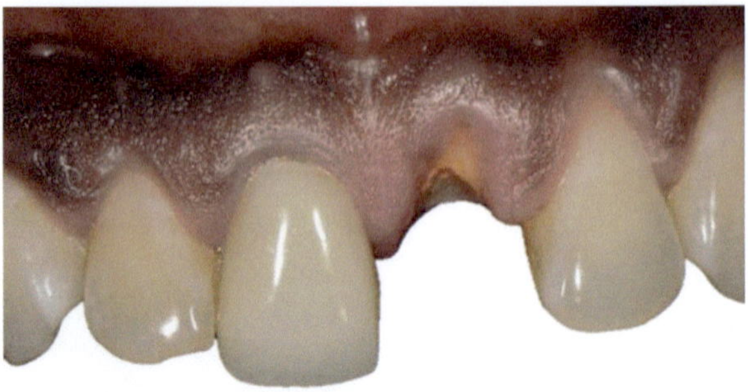

Fig. 3.5 Tooth position and FGM more apical to adjacent teeth will increase the risk of an esthetic compromise

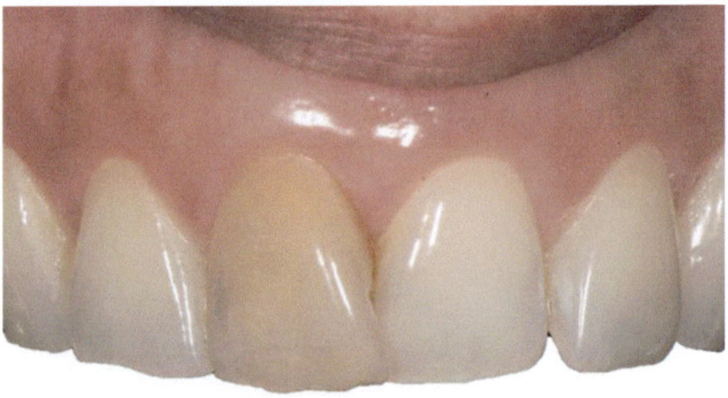

Fig. 3.6 Thin gingival biotype

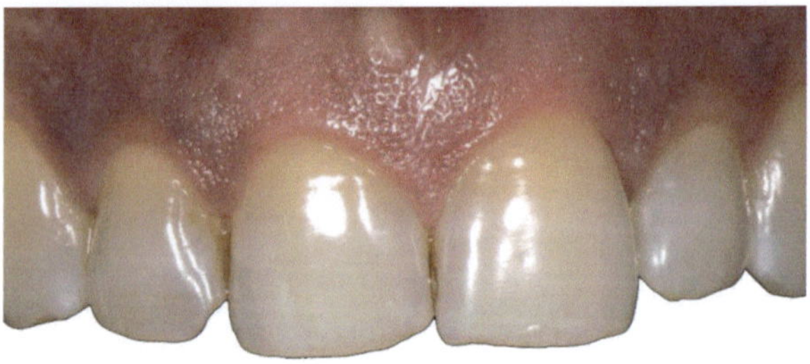

Fig. 3.7 Thick gingival biotype

Gingival Biotype

Thinner gingival biotypes are known to have a greater tendency toward post-extraction mucosal recession (Figs. 3.6 and 3.7). However, this tendency is greatly reduced in the socket shield procedure since the labial bone and surrounding soft tissue architecture are better maintained [4, 6].

Scallop of Gingival Margin and Tooth Shape

Teeth with high scallop and a triangular tooth form are more prone to recession and loss of interdental papilla compared to square- or oval-shaped teeth in conventional immediate post extraction cases. However in PET procedures this risk is lower as the labial bone and soft tissues are relatively undisturbed during the surgical procedure (Figs. 3.8, 3.9, and 3.10) [7, 8].

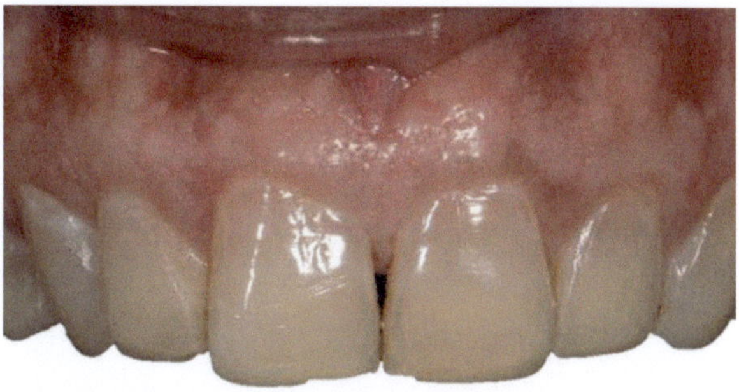

Fig. 3.8 Square teeth. Flat scallop

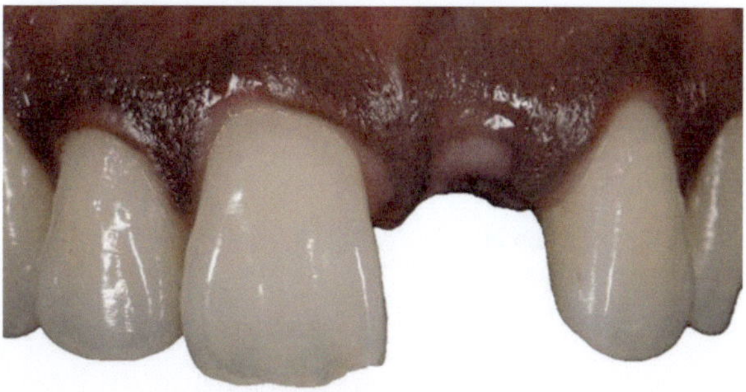

Fig. 3.9 Ovoid teeth. Medium scallop

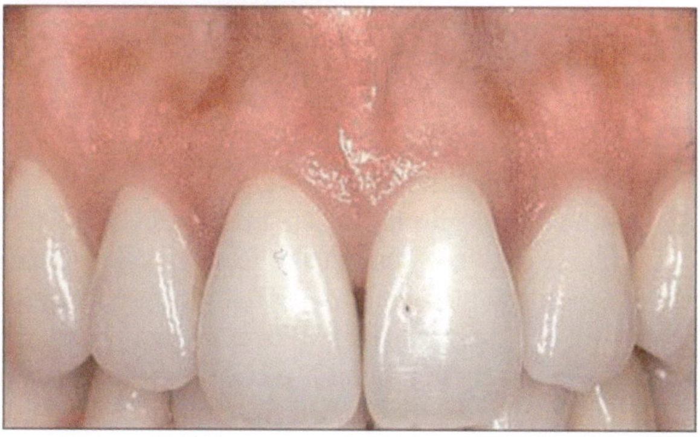

Fig. 3.10 Triangular teeth. High scallop

Interproximal Height of Bone

The height of interproximal bone will determine the possibility of attaining an intact interdental papilla (Fig. 3.11). Reduction in the height of interdental bone will lead to loss of interdental soft tissues resulting in a dark triangular space between the restored implant and the adjacent tooth. This will occur even in socket shield cases. Hence, proximal bone loss on the adjacent tooth should be considered as a risk factor for achieving optimal results even with the socket shield procedure [9, 10].

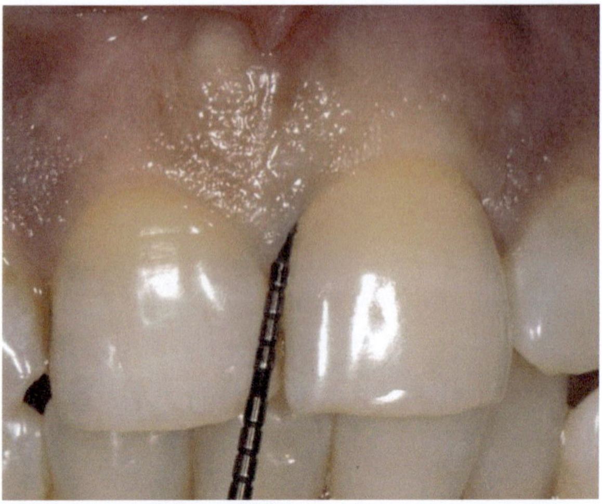

Fig. 3.11 The interproximal height of bone is an important parameter in achieving complete interdental fill after an implant is done

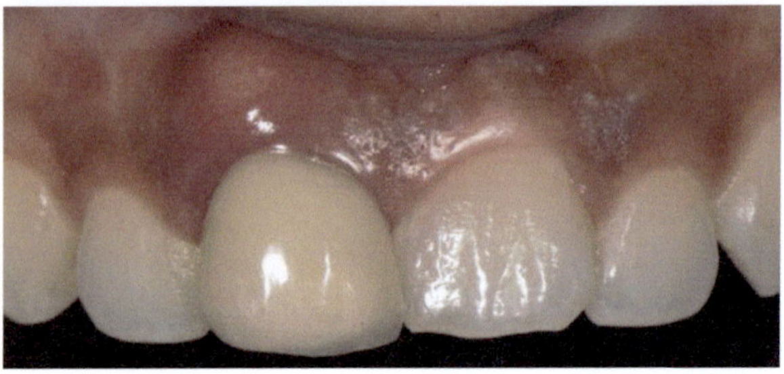

Fig. 3.12 Infection in connection with tooth 11

Infection at Implant Site

Any source of infection at the surgical site is likely to lead to a postoperative complication. Small-sized periapical infections can be successfully managed during the socket shield surgery (Chap. 6). Attempts at eliminating larger lesions may not be successful while performing partial extractions (Fig. 3.12). This may lead to a recurrence of the infection, progressive bone loss, soft tissue defects, and mobility or loss of shield. Hence periapical lesions should be considered to be a risk factor [11].

Available Restorative Space

A minimum of 5 mm restorative space is necessary inciso-gingivally for a screw-retained restoration and 8 mm is necessary for a cement-retained one. Careful evaluation of restorative space is necessary for the fabrication of a good provisional and definitive restoration (Figs. 3.13 and 3.14).

3.2.2 Radiological Assessment

Teeth positions with respect to its inclinations within the bone and the thickness of labial and palatal bone need to be considered while preparing the osteotomies in extraction sockets. For these reasons, it is mandatory to have a CBCT of the

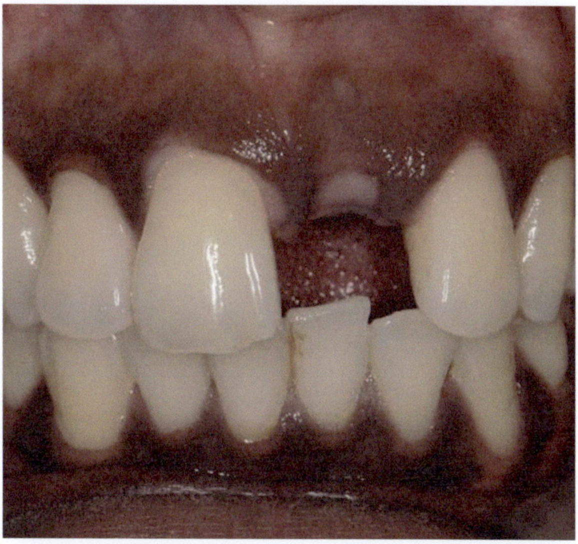

Fig. 3.13 Adequate restorative space

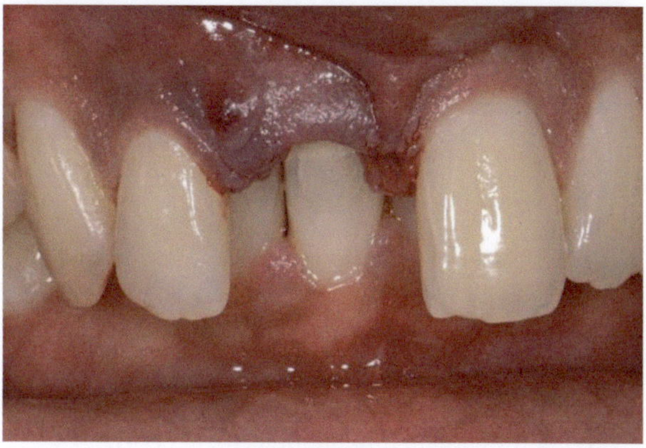

Fig. 3.14 Inadequate restorative space

preoperative condition before attempting socket/pontic shield procedures. Timings for implant placements, either staged or immediate, can be planned based on the anatomy of the alveolar bone. Osteotomy positions and trajectories of implants can be planned based on CBCT findings [12, 13]. The choice between cement- or screw-retained restorations can be made before implant placement on the basis of evaluating the cross-sectional images of the teeth indicated for a socket shield procedure.

Gluckman et al. introduced a new classification system for anterior maxillary tooth position with guidelines for immediate implant placement (Fig. 3.15). They classified the radial plane positions that helped in case selection and making decisions in immediate implant placements. The presence of adequate palatal bone is essential for preparing an osteotomy for immediate implant placement [13, 14].

Fig. 3.15 Classification of radial plane tooth position as described by Gluckman et al. [14]

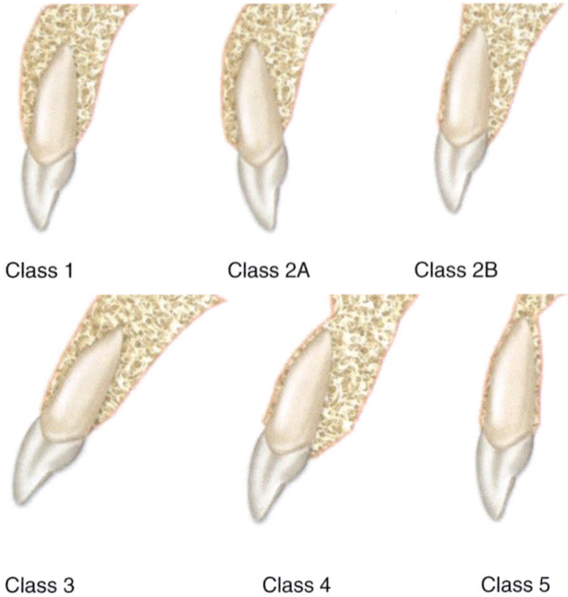

Class 1	Tooth positioned centrally within the ridge
Class 2A	Tooth retroclined with thick labial bone
Class 2B	Tooth retroclined with thin labial bone
Class 3	Proclined tooth with thick palatal and thin labial bone
Class 4	Tooth facially positioned
Class 5	Tooth with thin facial and palatal walls

According to his classification Class 5 which represents 0.7% of the total cases have bone neither facially, palatally, nor apically to provide primary stability. Hence Class 5 tooth root position is considered as a contraindication to PET procedures involving immediate implant placements [14].

Presence of complete buccal plate, as in Type 1 extraction sockets [15], with intact buccal bone, is advocated for immediate implant placements and an immediate provisional restoration. The presence or absence of the buccal plate of bone can be determined by preoperative CBCT. Maintaining this buccal plate is clinically significant to avoid midfacial recession [16].

3.3 Indications

The following points should be considered while choosing cases for a socket shield procedure:

1. *Firm but non-restorable tooth*: Teeth indicated for extraction which are broken down due to caries or trauma and cannot be restored effectively are ideally suited for PET procedures. Roots that lack adequate ferrule for supporting a post, core and crown are chosen for PET procedures. Both vital and endodontically treated

teeth can be selected for PET procedures. In case of endodontically treated teeth, the gutta percha in the canal helps in guiding the clinician to section the root along the correct axis. Teeth which have a metallic post may complicate the process since the procedure would entail removal of the post carefully prior to sectioning the root. Teeth which have metallic posts or any other rigid posts are prone to vertical root fractures and will complicate the process of partial extraction and shield preparation [17, 18].

Cone beam computed tomography should be used for the early detection of fractures in teeth. This will help the clinician to assess the risk involved in atraumatic preparation of the shield and preventing the accidental luxation of the shield (Figs. 3.16, 3.17, and 3.18).

2. *Periodontal status*: Teeth with healthy periodontal status i.e. with no gingival inflammation or bone loss are indicated and determine successful long-term outcome [19] (Fig. 3.19).
3. *Periapical lesions*: Since the apical tip of the root gets eliminated during the preparation of the shield, small periapical lesions can be managed through the socket. Teeth with larger periapical infections should be avoided for an immediate placement protocol, since achieveing primary stability for the implant can be extremely challenging. In teeth with longer roots such as canines, the apical pathology can be curetted through a remote semilunar vestibular incision similar to the one for apical surgeries (Chap. 6) (Fig. 3.20).

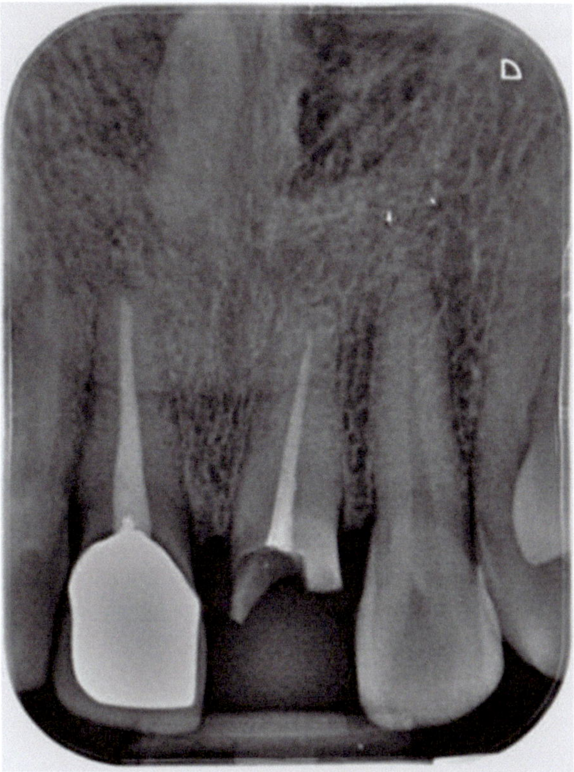

Fig. 3.16 Pre-operative intraoral periapical x-ray aids in evaluating mesiodistal inclination of the root, detecting periapical pathology and assessing the interproximal height of bone

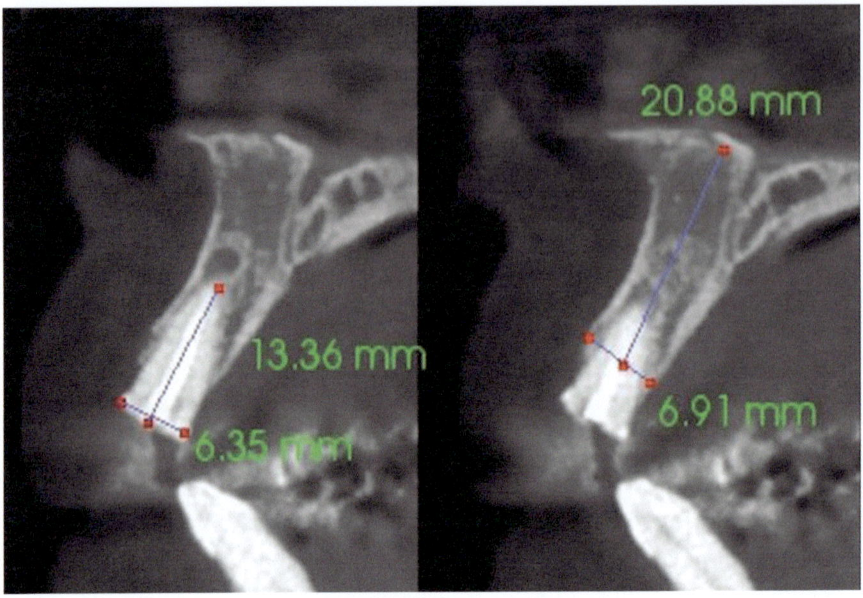

Fig. 3.17 Cone bean CT scans help in assessing presence of labial bone and the root position in the radial plane

Fig. 3.18 An ideal clinical situation for a socket shield procedure

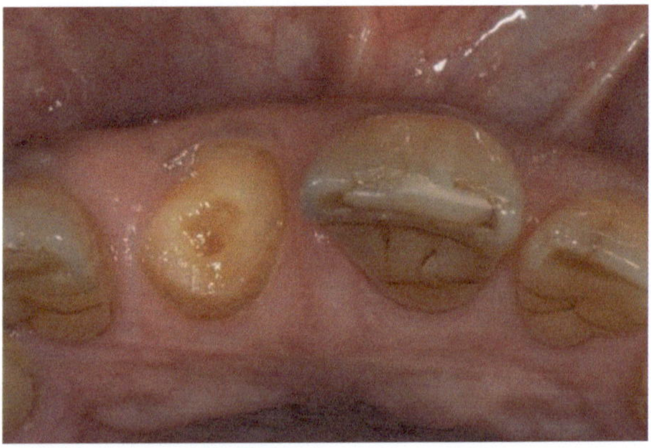

It is mandatory to confirm that the site is free of any active lesion and an active purulent infection is absent. Placing an implant in such a site is contraindicated due to the increased risk of failure [20]. Partial extraction therapy with immediate implant placement in sites exhibiting chronic periapical lesions can be considered, as long as thorough debridement of the infected socket is possible. Immediate implant placement in completely debrided sockets has been reported in the literature as a successful treatment modality with no disadvantages clinically, radiographically, or esthetically when compared to immediate implants in healthy sites [21, 22].

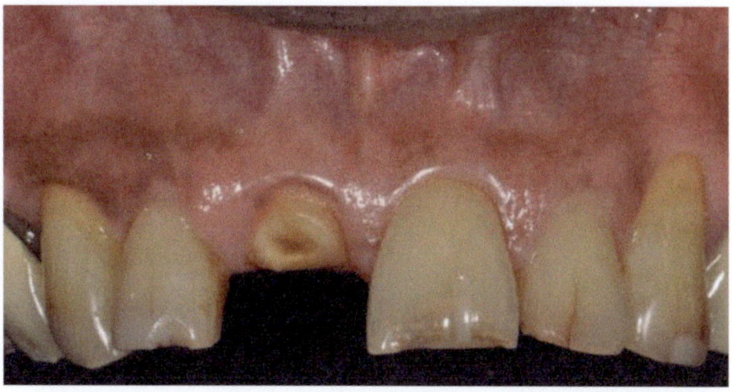

Fig. 3.19 Root with healthy periodontal condition

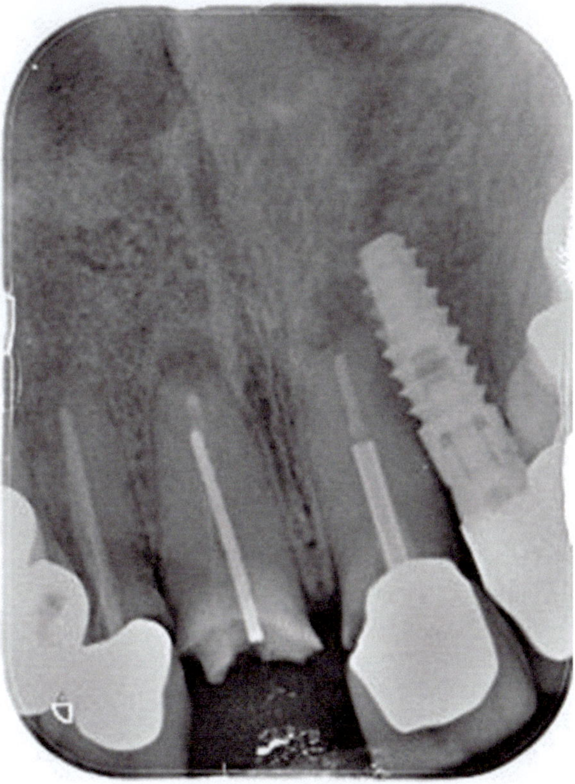

Fig. 3.20 Mild periapical lesion in relation to tooth 11. Also a small lesion in the adjacent tooth is a risk factor

4. *Adequate palatal/lingual and apical bone*: Achieving primary stability for the implant in postextraction immediate placements is mandatory [23–25]. Hence, even for the socket shield procedure it is a pre-requisite to have adequate apical and palatal/lingual bone. The bone configuration should allow proper implant placement so as to maintain a small gap between the labial part of the implant and the shield. In the event that the implant comes too close to the shield while being torqued in, the implant may exert pressure leading to dislodgement of the shield (Fig. 3.21).

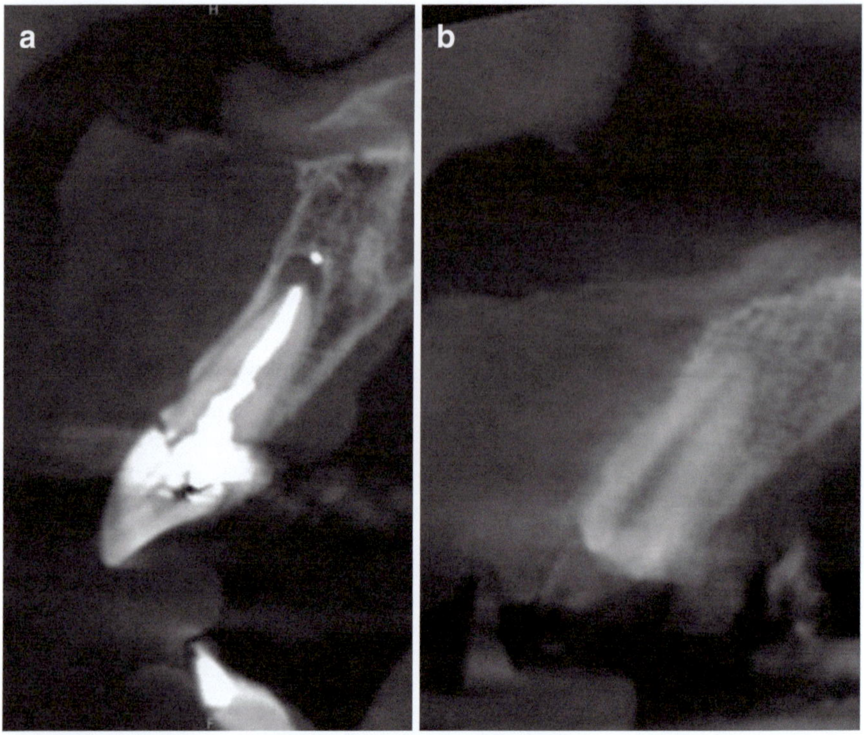

Fig. 3.21 (**a**) Limited amount of palatal bone. (**b**) Adequate amount of palatal bone

The amount of bone beyond the apex required to gain the initial stability is 3–5 mm [12]. However, the proximity to any vital structure such as the nasopalatine canal, the nasal floor can be a limiting factor that precludes immediate implant placement [26].

The sagittal root position should be assessed from CBCT and when the available bone around the failing tooth is deficient, a early/delayed approach for implant placement is preferred [27].

5. *Favorable occlusal scheme for immediate provisional and definitive restoration.*

   In a healthy mouth with no occlusal issues, restorative materials have a better chance of survival. In case of mutilated dentition, a comprehensive approach must be adopted to improve the occlusal scheme (Fig. 3.22).
6. *For multirooted teeth, having larger interradicular bone is beneficial* for achieving good primary stability for the implants (Fig. 3.23). Molars with fused roots and minimal or no inter radicular bone can pose a huge challenge for implant placement [28, 29].

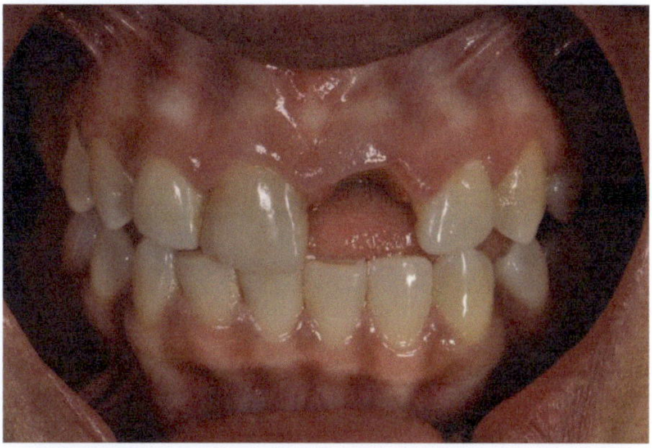

Fig. 3.22 Fractured tooth 21. Favorable occlusal scheme with adequate restorative space

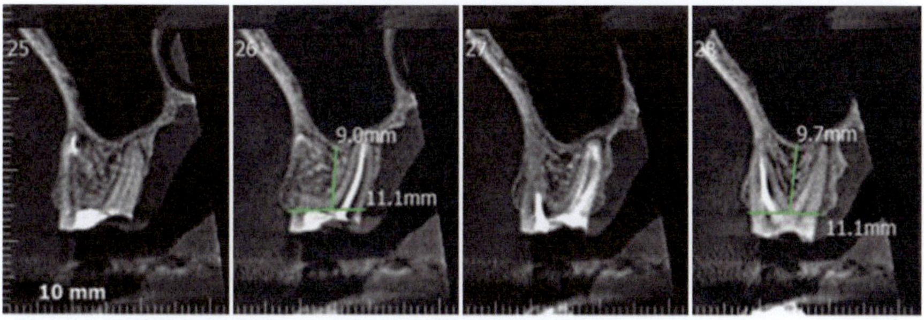

Fig. 3.23 CBCT showing cross-sectional view of a maxillary molar with adequate inter radicular bone

3.4 Contraindications

Choosing a wrong case could lead to failure of the treatment. Hence adhering to the principles of case selection and avoiding certain types of cases will increase predictability of the procedure.

The following are absolute contraindications for partial extraction therapies:

1. *Mobile teeth*: Success of socket shield procedure is dependent on the intact attachment of the labial root fragment (shield) to the labial bone. A mobile tooth is a contraindication for the procedure. A mobile shield would invariably lead to postoperative shield migration leading to a complication or a failure (Figs. 3.24 and 3.25).
2. *Absence of labial bone*: Firm teeth with dehiscence defects should also be avoided for performing a socket shield procedure. In the absence of any labial bone to hold the shield, postoperative mobility of the shield is inevitable and will lead to a failure (Fig. 3.26).

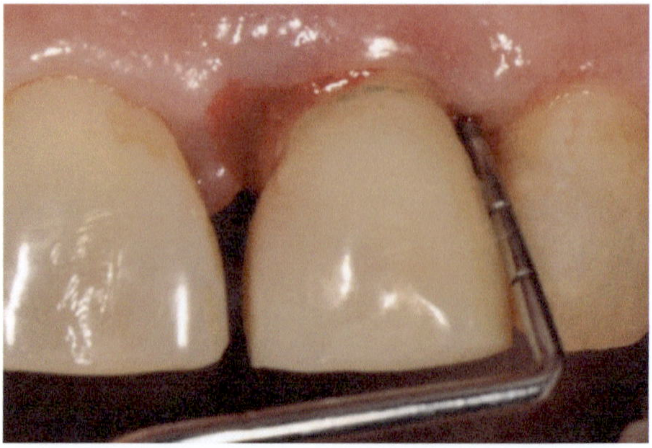

Fig. 3.24 Bleeding on probing due to periodontal disease

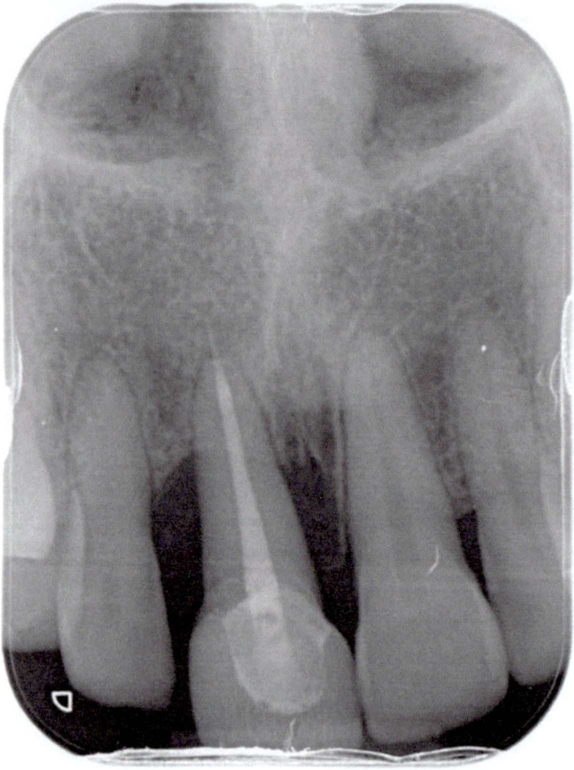

Fig. 3.25 Reduced interproximal height of bone

3. *Large periapical lesions*: Teeth with large cystic lesions and periapical pathology should also be ruled out for PET procedures. Eradication of pathology should be the primary objective of treatment. Inadequate access for removal of pathology may lead to a recurrence of the lesion. Such conditions should be treated using a conventional approach of extractions of teeth and surgical removal

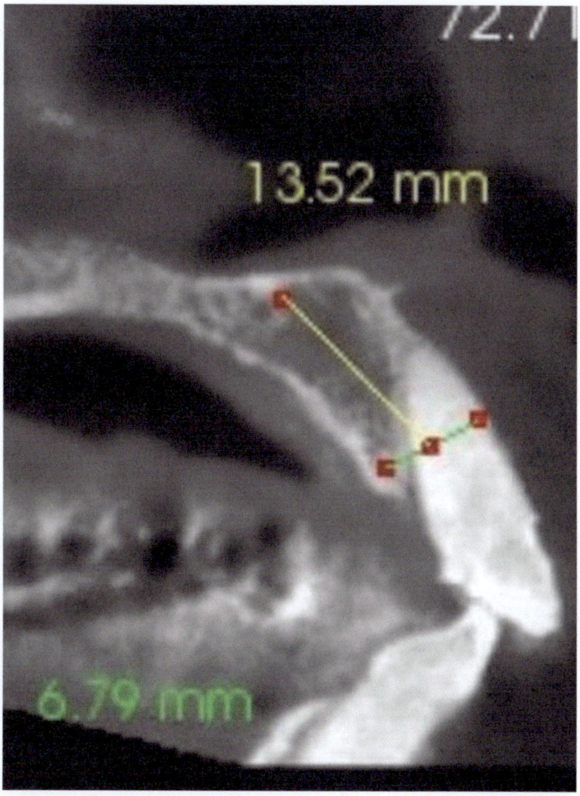

Fig. 3.26 Absence of labial bone seen on the CBCT

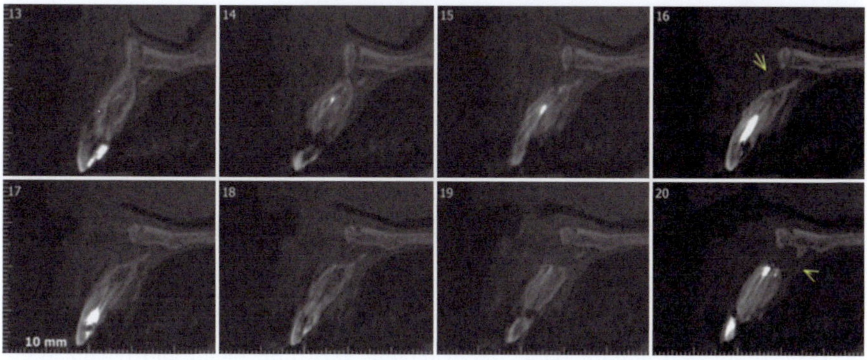

Fig. 3.27 Presence of a large cystic lesion seen on a CBCT

of the pathology (Fig. 3.27). Smaller lesions can be dealt with either through the socket or through a remote incision in the vestibule as described in Chap. 6.

4. *Internal resorption*: Teeth with internal resorption affecting the labial part of the root should be avoided for PET procedures (Fig. 3.28).

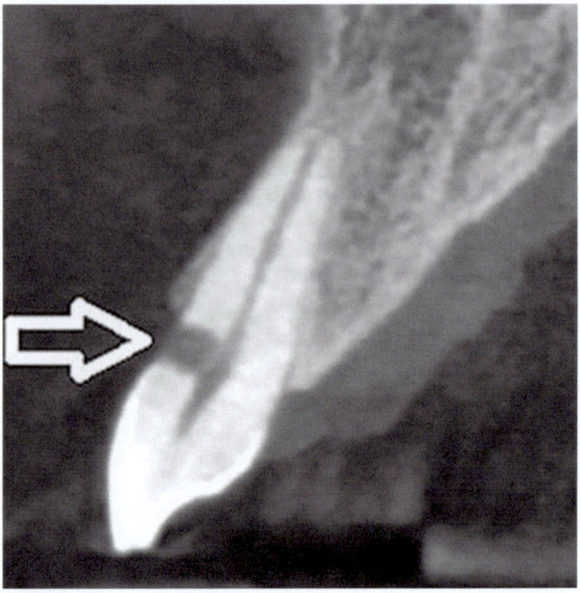

Fig. 3.28 Internal resorption on the labial part of the tooth seen in a CBCT

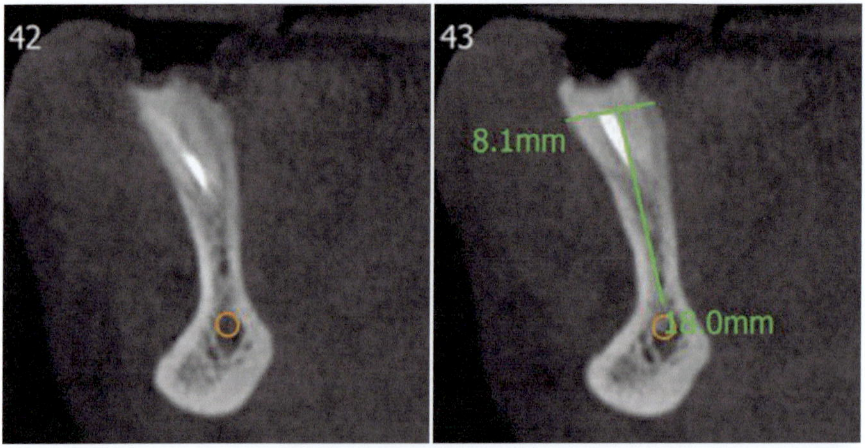

Fig. 3.29 Very thin labial and lingual bone in a mandibular premolar

5. *Thin labial and palatal bone*: Teeth having very thin facial and palatal bone should be considered as contraindications for any immediate implant placements [14]. Such a bone anatomy will not allow stability of the implant and will bring the implant too close to the shield. An intimate contact of the shield with the implant will lead to an inadvertent mobilization of the shield leading to a failure. Mandibular incisors and premolars have a high incidence of such anatomical findings. Hence socket shields in mandibular teeth should be undertaken with extreme caution after proper evaluation on CBCTs (Fig. 3.29).

3.5 Relative Contraindications

1. Discolored tooth root: Roots of nonvital teeth which have been heavily discolored overtime may pose an esthetic problem if retained. This will be more evident if the patient has a thin gingival biotype and a high lip line. The discolored root may show through the soft tissue leading to an esthetic failure. In such cases, a complete extraction of the root and conventional therapy should be considered (Fig. 3.30).
2. Teeth out of the arch: Malposed teeth needing extractions should ideally not be chosen for a postextraction immediate placement protocol. One of the conditions for a successful outcome of an implant-supported restoration is prosthetically driven placement. Placing an implant in the exact position of a malposed tooth will adversely affect the final esthetic and functional outcome of the treatment (Fig. 3.31).

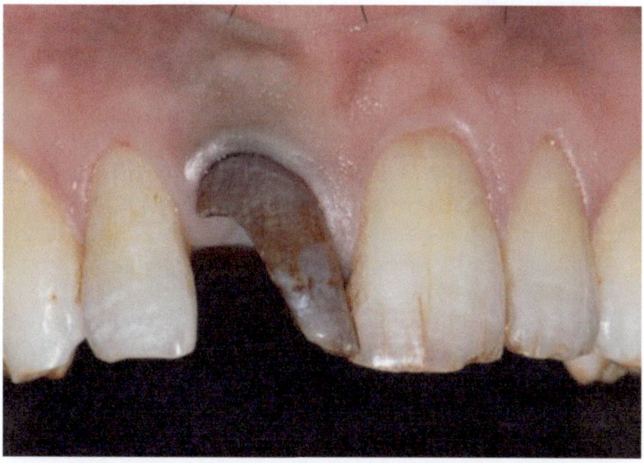

Fig. 3.30 Highly discolored tooth 11

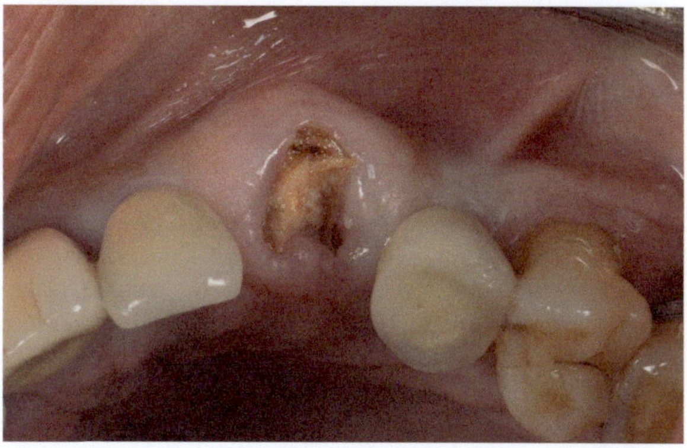

Fig. 3.31 Tooth 23 is out of the arch

3.6 Conclusion

The goal of partial extraction therapies is to help maintain the tissue contours and provide long-term health and stability with good esthetics. A thorough risk assessment will help identify the potential problems and thus avoid inadvertent complications with such procedures. Thorough understanding of the indications and contraindications are mandatory and their importance toward the success of partial extraction therapies cannot be overemphasized.

Acknowledgement Illustrations by: Udatta Kher.

References

1. Zitzmann N, Margolin M, Filippi A, Weiger R, Krastl G. Patient assessment and diagnosis in implant treatment. Aust Dent J. 2008;53:S3–Ss10.
2. Tjan AH, Miller GD. Some esthetic factors in a smile. J Prosthet Dent. 1984;51(1):24–8.
3. Frizzera F, Tonetto M, Cabral G, Shibli JA, Marcantonio E Jr. Periodontics, implantology, and prosthodontics integrated: the zenith-driven rehabilitation. Case Rep Dent. 2017;2017:1070292.
4. Kois JC. Predictable single tooth peri-implant aesthetics: five diagnostic keys. Compendium. 2004;25:895–905.
5. Salama H, Salama M, Kelly J. The orthodontic-periodontal connection in implant site development. Pract Periodontics Aesthet Dent. 1996;8:923–32.
6. Hinze M, Janousch R, Goldhahn S, Schlee M. Volumetric alterations around single-tooth implants using the socket-shield technique: preliminary results of a prospective case series. Int J Esthet Dent. 2018;13(2):146–70.
7. Becker W, Ochsenbein C, Tibbetts L, et al. Alveolar bone anatomic profiles as measured from dry skulls. Clinical ramifications. J Clin Periodontol. 1997;24:727–31.
8. Phillips K, Kois JC. Aesthetic peri-implant site development. The restorative connection. Dent Clin North Am. 1998;42:57–70.
9. Tarnow DP, Cho SC, Wallace SS. The effect of inter-implant distance on the height of inter-implant bone crest. J Periodontol. 2000;71:546–9.
10. Tarnow DP, Magner AW, Fletcher P. The effect of distance from the contact point to the crest of bone on the presence or absence of the interproximal dental papilla. J Periodontol. 1992;63:886–995.
11. Schwartz-Arad D, Chaushu G. The ways and wherefores of immediate placement of implants into fresh extraction sites: a literature review. J Periodontol. 1997;68:915–23.
12. Kan JY, Rungcharassaeng K. Immediate placement and provisionalization of maxillary anterior single implants: a surgical and prosthodontic rationale. Pract Periodontics Aesthet Dent. 2000;12:817–24.
13. Kan JY, Roe P, Rungcharassaeng K, Patel RD, Waki T, et al. Classification of sagittal root position in relation to the anterior maxillary osseous housing for immediate implant placement: a cone beam computed tomography study. Int J Oral Maxillofac Implants. 2011;26:873–6.
14. Gluckman H, Pontes CC, Du Toit J. Radial plane tooth position and bone wall dimensions in the anterior maxilla: a CBCT classification for immediate implant placement. J Prosthet Dent. 2018;120(1):50–6.
15. Elian N, Cho S-C, Froum S, Smith RB, Tarnow DP. A simplified socket classification and repair technique. Esthet Dent. 2007, 19:99–104.
16. Araújo MG, da Silva JC, de Mendonça AF, Lindhe J. Ridge alterations following grafting of fresh extraction sockets in man. A randomized clinical trial. Clin Oral Implants Res. 2015;26:407–12.

17. Khasnis SA, Kidiyoor KH, Patil AB, Kenganal SB. Vertical root fractures and their management. J Conserv Dent. 2014;17(2):103–10.
18. Cooney JP, Caputo AA, Trabert KC. Retention and stress distribution of tapered - end endodontic posts. J Prosthet Dent. 1986;55:540–6.
19. Fürhauser R, Florescu D, Benesch T, Haas R, Mailath G, Georg WC. Evaluation of soft tissue around single-tooth implant crowns: the pink esthetic score. Clin Oral Implants Res. 2005;16(6):639–44.
20. Zhao D, Wu Y, Xu C, Zhang F. Immediate dental implant placement into infected vs. noninfected sockets: a meta-analysis. Clin Oral Implants Res. 2016;27:1290–6.
21. Novaes AB Jr, Novaes AB. Immediate implants placed into infected sites: a clinical report. Int J Oral Maxillofac Implants. 1995;10:609–13.
22. Lee CT, Chuang SK, Stoupel J. Survival analysis and other clinical outcomes of immediate implant placement in sites with periapical lesions: systematic review. Int J Oral Maxillofac Implants. 2015;30:268–78.
23. Lang NP, Pun L, Lau KY, Li KY, Wong MC. A systematic review on survival and success rates of implants placed immediately into fresh extraction sockets after at least 1 year. Clin Oral Implants Res. 2012;23 Suppl 5:39–66.
24. Lioubavina-Hack N, Lang NP, Karring T. Significance of primary stability for osseointegration of dental implants. Clin Oral Implants Res. 2006;17:244–50.
25. Javed F, Ahmed HB, Crespi R, Romanos GE. Role of primary stability for successful osseointegration of dental implants: factors of influence and evaluation. Interv Med Appl Sci. 2013;5(4):162–7.
26. Kan JY, Rungcharassaeng K, Roe P, Mesquida J, Chatriyanuyoke P, Caruso JM. Maxillary central incisor – incisive canal relationship: a cone beam computed tomography study. Am J Esthet Dent. 2012;2013:180–7.
27. Dawson AB. The SAC classification in implant dentistry. Basel: ITI International Team for Implantology; 2009;1:172.
28. Baumer D, Zuhr O, Rebele S, Hürzeler M. Socket shield technique for immediate implant placement—clinical, radiographic and volumetric data after 5 years. Clin Oral Implants Res. 2017;28:1450–8.
29. Schwimer CW, et al. The socket-shield technique at molar sites: A proof-of-principle technique report. J Prosthet Dent. 2018;121(2):229–33.

4 Provisional Restorations in Partial Extraction Therapy

Ali Tunkiwala

Abstract

This chapter explains the various design principles associated with making provisional restorations for partial extraction therapy (PET) with implant placements. Detailed, step-by-step techniques are described and further simplified with well-designed graphics. This crucial step must be undertaken with a keen understanding.

4.1 Introduction

Implant therapy replaces missing teeth and should maintain the health of the surrounding alveolar bone and periodontium while doing so. When the bone and soft tissues surrounding the implant are healthy, the longevity of the implant therapy is enhanced. Provisional restorations connect the surgical site to the restorative arena and are a test drive for the proposed "pink and white" aesthetics. They also help to adapt and mold the gingival architecture to achieve the best emergence profile for the final restoration.

4.1.1 Designing Provisional Restorations

A well-designed provisional restoration is the key to achieving a successful outcome for any implant restoration in the aesthetic zone [1]. In cases where socket shield surgery is performed, it is necessary to plan for an immediate provisional restoration on the implant itself unless the (staged socket shield approach) Glocker approach [2] has been deployed. The main goal of the provisional restoration is to

A. Tunkiwala (✉)
Smiles by Design, Mumbai, India

U. Kher, A. Tunkiwala (eds.), *Partial Extraction Therapy in Implant Dentistry*,
https://doi.org/10.1007/978-3-030-33610-3_4

support the peri-implant soft tissue and provide a scaffold for the tissues to heal while establishing the emergence form for the final restoration [3].

The prerequisite for making a provisional restoration directly on the implant is high implant stability quotient or insertion torque of the implant [4]. In anterior implants, restorative procedures should ideally to be initiated immediately after implant placement. In cases where an intact soft tissue architecture is present around the implant site, an immediate provisional restoration helps immensely in maintaining it. This is more beneficial than having to perform techniques later on to recreate the soft tissue [5].

It is important to understand the management of soft tissue during the provisional restorative phase by modifying subgingival contours. Su et al. [6] classified these subgingival areas on implant restorations as having two distinct zones; namely, the critical and subcritical contour and showed that the modification of each of these zones can elicit soft tissue movement and provide the necessary support to the peri-implant soft tissue apparatus.

4.2 Principles of Design

4.2.1 Socket Shield Cases

In socket shield cases where the implant has been placed immediately after shield preparation, as discussed in the previous chapters, the provisional restoration must meet the following requirements:

(a) Its cervical cross-sectional shape must match that of the socket as seen at 1 mm below the free gingival margin. Positive support of the free gingival margin from the cervical contour of the provisional restoration is a prerequisite for successful soft tissue integration [6]. The cross section of the soft tissue architecture after atraumatic extraction may be oval, triangular, square, or trapezoidal [7]. The best way to accurately direct soft tissue around an extraction site is to mimic the shape of the cervical third of the tooth in question [6].

(b) The provisional restoration must not be in contact with the prepared shield. In fact, a space of at least 1.5 mm must be present between the provisional and the shield for the soft tissue to encapsulate the shield completely thereby protecting it from any contact with oral fluids. The contour of the provisional restoration as it emerges from the implant must take a gradual "S" shape as shown (Fig. 4.1). This allows the extra space needed to avoid contact with the shield.

    The buccolingual trajectory of the implant will govern this "S" shape and intensity (Fig. 4.2). The more labial the trajectory of the implant, the more concave (flatter) the emergence from the provisional must be (Fig. 4.3). The more palatal the implant is placed, the more acute (convex) the emergence will be, as the provisional will have to travel from the implant platform to the free gingival margin to support it (Fig. 4.4).

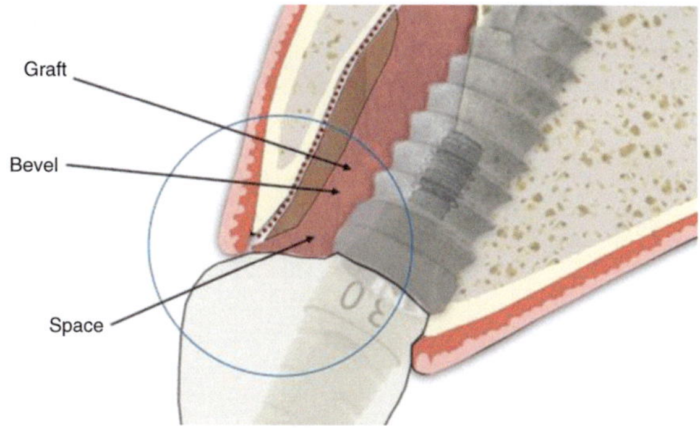

Fig. 4.1 Depicts the shaping of the provisional to maintain the space of 1.5 mm between itself and the shield

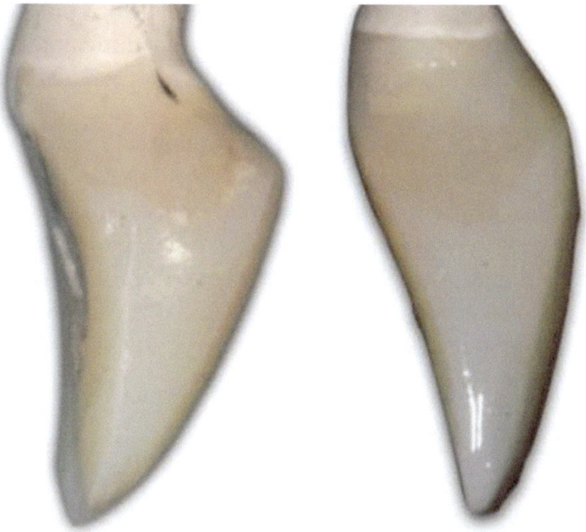

Fig. 4.2 The shape and intensity of the cervical contour of the provisional is governed by the implant trajectory

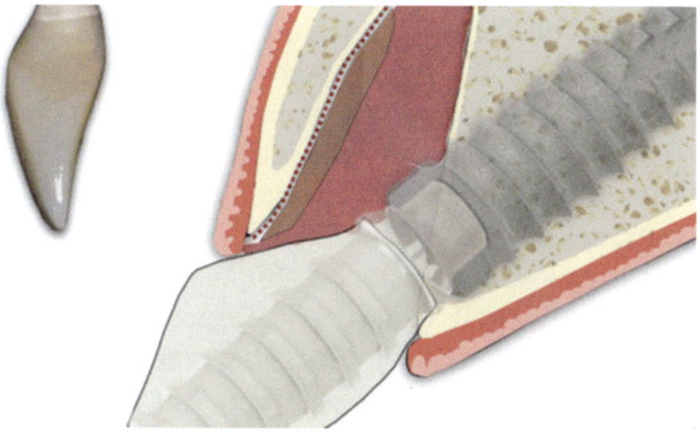

Fig. 4.3 Depicts the design of provisional with labial trajectory of implant placement

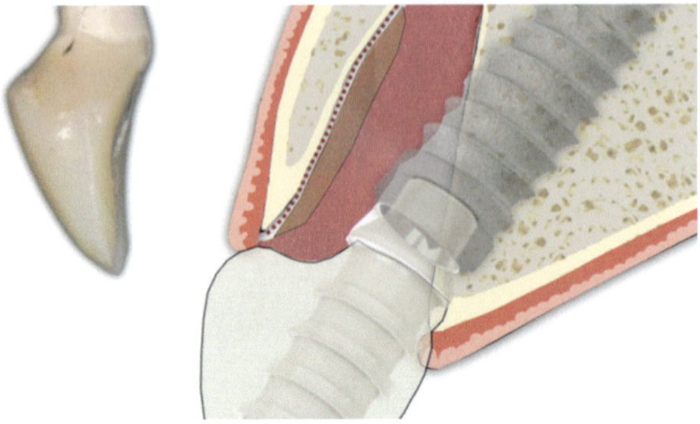

Fig. 4.4 Depicts the design of the provisional with extremely palatally placed implant

It is recommended to place the implant 3 mm below the facial crest of the free gingival margin to allow for adequate running room to enable the emergence from palatal placement to become more gradual and aesthetically acceptable [8].

In the case of "C"-shaped shield preparation, even the proximal subgingival aspect of the provisional restoration will need to be concave to maintain adequate distance (1.5 mm) from the shield.

(c) The provisional restoration on single teeth must not be in any occlusal contact with the opposing teeth in maximum intercuspation as well as in the chewing cycle. For meeting this requirement, it may be necessary to shorten the provisional at the incisal edge to allow it to escape from any eccentric contacts and the patient must not use it for any form of mastication [9].

4.2.2 Pontic Shield/Root Submergence Cases

The pontic shield is done when there is a periapical lesion and the apex of the extracted tooth needs to be removed but an implant is not placed in that socket.

In case of a pontic shield (Fig. 4.5), the provisional restoration must follow all the above rules. However, the cervical aspect of the design needs to be elaborated as there are several considerations. Historically, the term ovate pontic [10–12] was used where the pontic was inserted about 3 mm in the socket to allow for the creation of concave tissue in the socket as it healed. In contemporary times this depth of insertion into the socket is no longer warranted [13, 14]. The goal of the ovate pontic design was to create an illusion of the tooth emerging from within the socket as it happens in natural teeth. In pontic shield cases, the pontic is designed as an ovate pontic, but its labial cervical aspect is shaped in a similar 'S' shape emergence to allow for soft tissue thickness between the material and the shield.

In root submergence cases (Fig. 4.6) the root will be prepared to the level of bone. There must be at least 2 mm space between the submerged root and the tissue side of the well-polished convex provisional restoration. Figure 4.7 shows a radiographic appearance of a submerged root in relation to a definitive restoration with 2 mm space in between the two for the soft tissues.

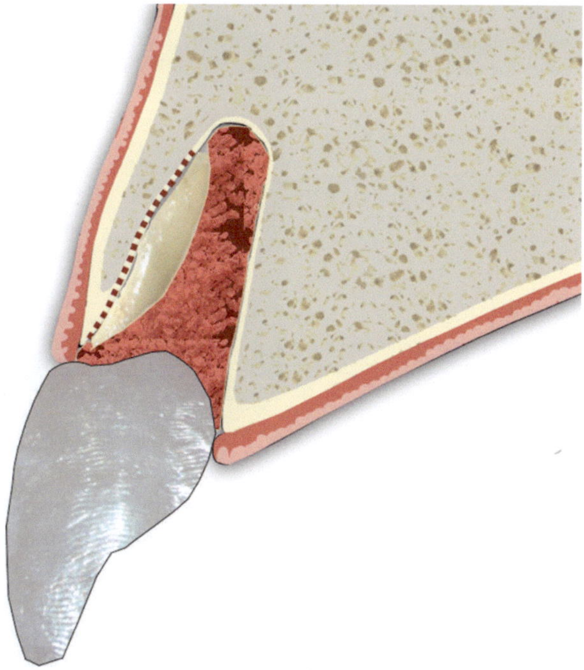

Fig. 4.5 Pontic shield design is similar to an ovate pontic in all respects except that its labial-cervical aspect is shaped to accommodate adequate soft tissue thickness between the provisional restoration and the prepared shield

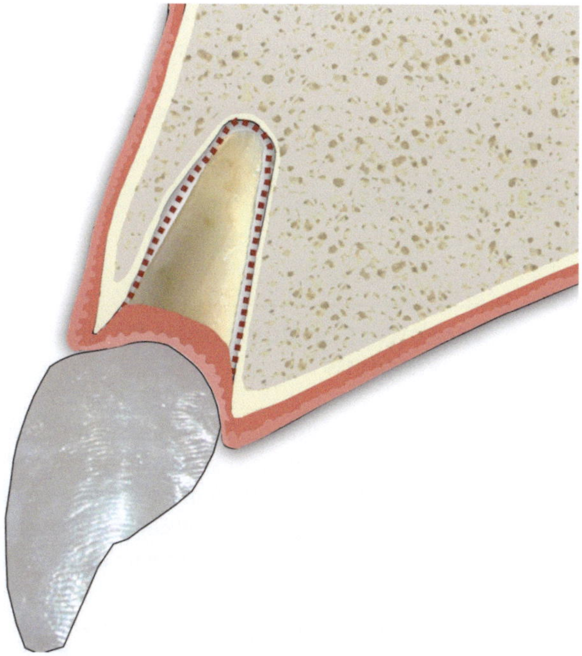

Fig. 4.6 Diagram: root submergence

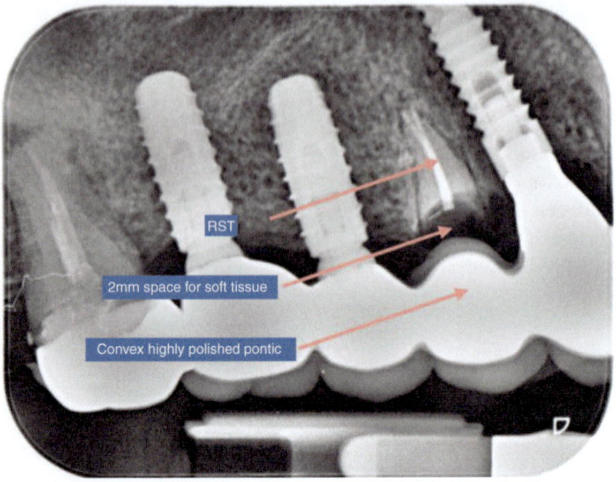

Fig. 4.7 Submerged root and its relation to pontic design for adequate soft tissue space in between the two

Adjunct procedures like a CT graft in pontic shield and root submergence cases [15] may be needed especially in thin gingival biotypes to allow for the creation of a robust soft tissue covering.

4.2.3 Techniques for Making a Provisional Restoration

There are several ways in which a provisional restoration can be fabricated on the implant after the socket shield procedure has been performed [16–18]. In such cases, it is now clear from the previous chapters that the shield must be prepared to the level of the buccal crest of the socket and not left supracrestal.

The provisional restorations can be:

(a) Cement-retained.
(b) Screw-retained.

4.3 Technical Considerations for Cement-Retained Provisionals

Cemented temporary resotrations though easier to fabricate pose certain risks when chosen for provisionalization, post surgically. Prefabricated abutments chosen for the cement-retained provisional restoration may place the restorative margin deep subgingivally. During cementation of the provisional restoration deep margins are difficult to clean thoroughly. Bleeding from the site may compromise visibility and any residual cement left behind is detrimental to the health of the tissues and even the survival of the implant [19]. Residual cement also has been attributed as a cause of peri-implantitis [20]. Another issue with cement-retained provisional restorations is that repeated removal and insertion of the provisional restorations can be cumbersome. Breakages are frequent, making remakes necessary.

It is for these reasons that the cement-retained provisional restoration is *not recommended* clinically, except in cases where the "one abutment one time" concept [21, 22] is followed. In this, the definitive abutment is selected and placed and torqued to its final position on the day of implant placement. On this abutment a cement-retained provisional is fabricated. At the end of 3–4 months, when osseointegration is confirmed, the cement-retained provisional is removed and an impression of the abutment is taken as it would be done for fixed prosthodontic work. The definitive restoration is then fabricated and cemented on this abutment that was placed on the day of surgery. In this concept, since the final abutment is fixed on the day of implant placement and not removed thereafter; it has been shown to have hemidesmosomal attachment [23, 24] to the surrounding tissues. This aids in better soft tissue integration as compared to the conventional protocols where repeated removal and reseating of the components on the implants can lead to mucosal recession. Apart from its use in such a onetime abutment concept, cement-retained provisional must be avoided or its use must be with extreme vigilance and caution.

4.3.1 Technique

For making cement-retained provisional restorations, the key principle is to make a putty index of the intact existing tooth or make a full contour wax up on the broken tooth. A putty matrix is fabricated on this, and can be used to carry the material for provisional restoration on the site. The materials used may be BisGMA-based chemically cured composite resins (Protemp 4, 3M ESPE) or auto-polymerizing acrylic resin. Due to the exothermic nature of the latter material and potential irritation of soft tissues from the residual monomers; the BisGMA-based resin materials are preferred for all provisional restorations that are made chairside.

The following case (Figs. 4.8, 4.9, 4.10, 4.11, 4.12, 4.13, 4.14, and 4.15) demonstrates the making of the cement-retained provisional restoration with direct chairside method for a single implant after partial extraction therapy. Here, a definitive abutment has been used as a onetime abutment on which the cement-retained provisional was fabricated and luted with a temporary cement [25, 26].

To prevent any migration of the material into the implant site a rubber dam sheet or a Teflon tape is recommended as shown (Fig. 4.16). This will prevent the material ingress and thus avoid the risk of particulate matter contaminating the implant site. Additionally, when using prefabricated abutments for cement-retained restorations, it is better to leave the restorative margins equigingival or if the lip lines permit, even supragingival to allow easy cleaning of the residual cement. If the restoration fit is very snug on the abutments, the cement can be avoided altogether.

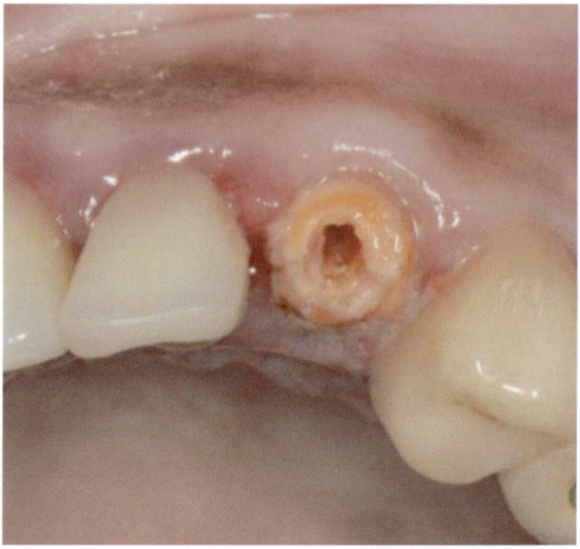

Fig. 4.8 Structurally poor tooth #23 slated for an extraction

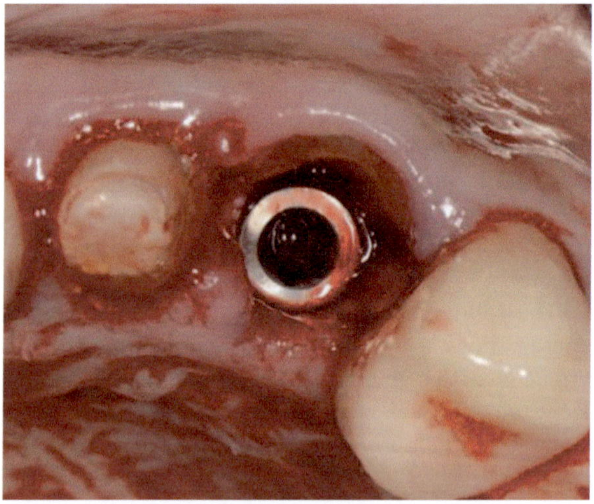

Fig. 4.9 Socket shield prepared and implant inserted in correct 3D position

4.4 Provisional Restorations for Adjacent Implant Sites

The following case (Figs. 4.17, 4.18, 4.19, and 4.20) demonstrates the making of the cement-retained provisional with direct chairside method for adjacent implants after partial extraction therapy.

In fabricating provisional restorations for adjacent teeth special attention should be given to the gingival embrasure and the interdental papilla it houses. Since most multiple adjacent implant provisional restorations are splinted (for strength) leaving

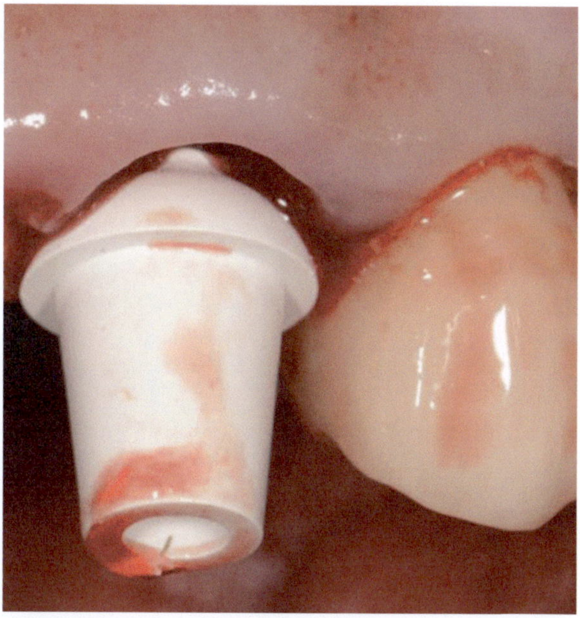

Fig. 4.10 Prefabricated reinforced PEEK abutment placed for try-in

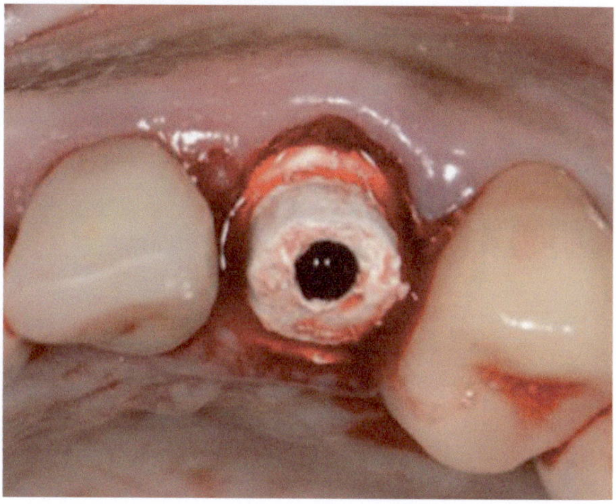

Fig. 4.11 Provisional abutment trimmed to size to provide sufficient room for final restoration

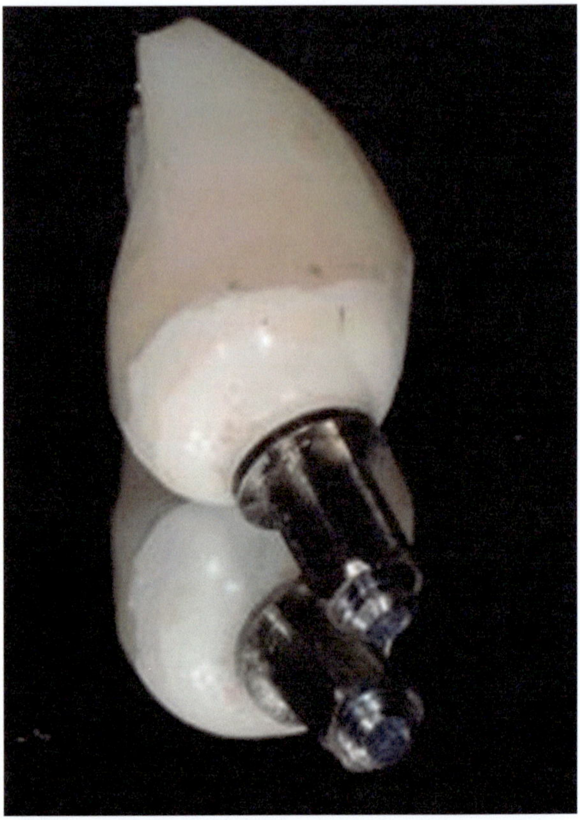

Fig. 4.12 Final shaping of the provisional restoration. Intaglio view

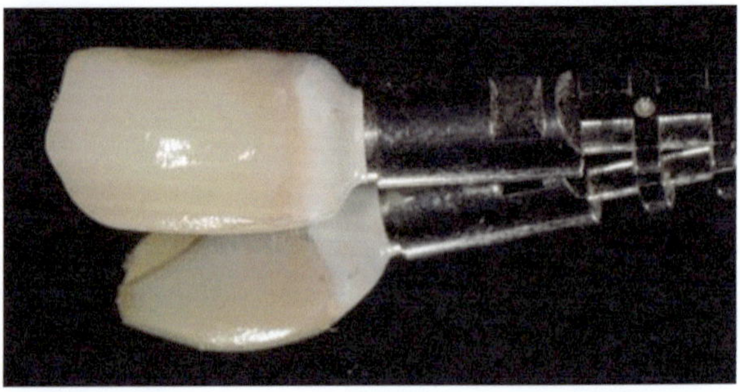

Fig. 4.13 Final shaping of the provisional restoration. Frontal view

adequate space for the interdental papillae is paramount. This allows better healing and reorganization of the papillae with a potential for interdental fill. However, if the ISQ values are high and the occlusion is favorable, individual adjacent implants may receive single, unsplinted provisional crowns.

When a provisional bridge has to be fabricated for a case that has had partial extraction therapy such as a pontic shield, the pontic design must be like a mini ovate with no contact on the shield area [9]. Figure 4.21 depicts the design of the provisional vis-a-vis the shield.

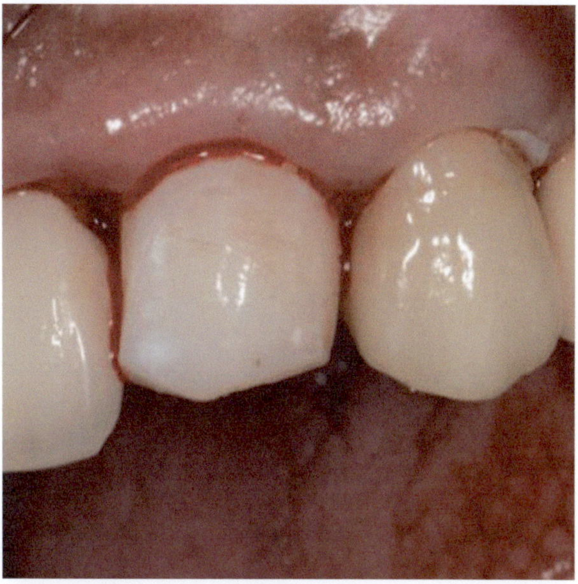

Fig. 4.14 Immediate Postoperative view after cementation of the provisional restoration

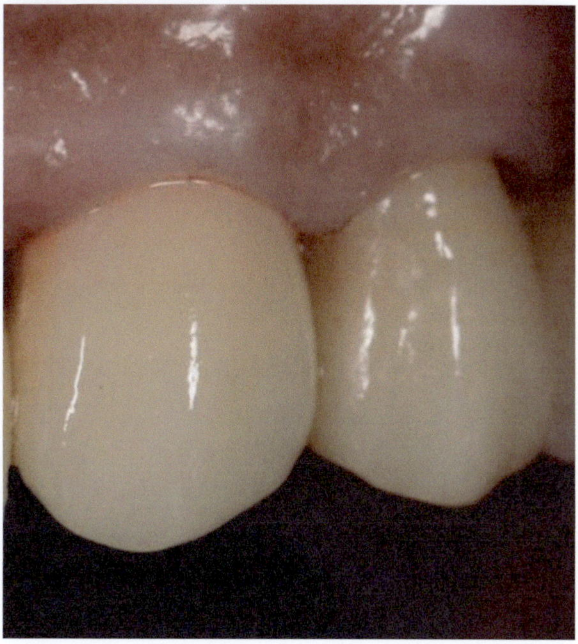

Fig. 4.15 Final restoration on #23

The following case illustrates making of a provisional restoration for socket shields on #13, #12, #21 and #22 and pontic shield on #11 (Figs. 4.22, 4.23, 4.24, 4.25, and 4.26).

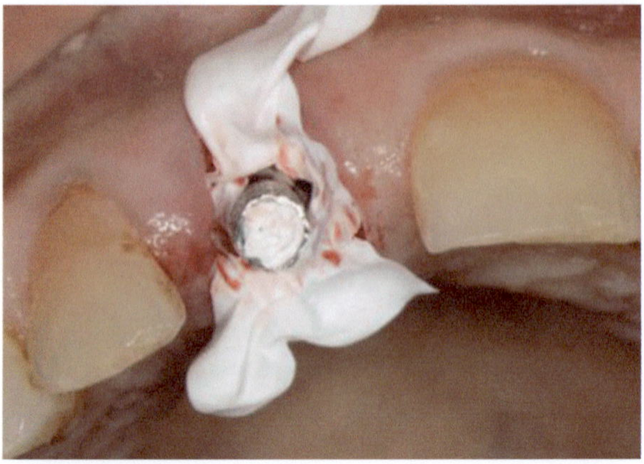

Fig. 4.16 Use a Teflon tape (or rubber dam sheet) to prevent ingress of material into the partial extraction site

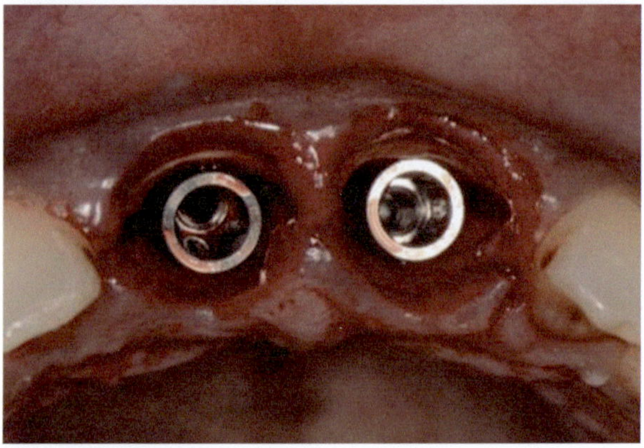

Fig. 4.17 Adjacent implants placed in central incisor sites with socket shields done

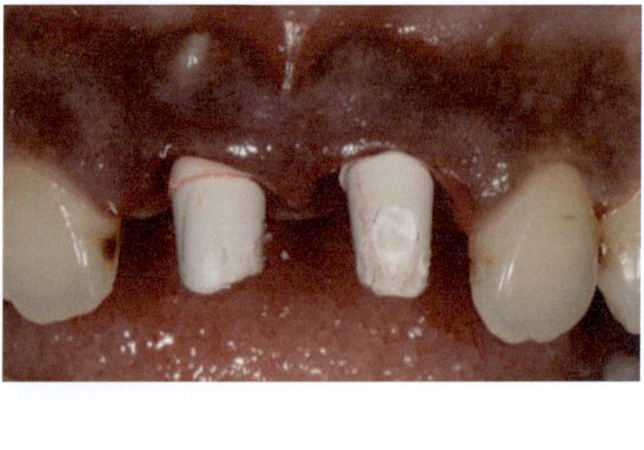

Fig. 4.18 Reinforced PEEK abutments placed and modified to receive a cement-retained provisional

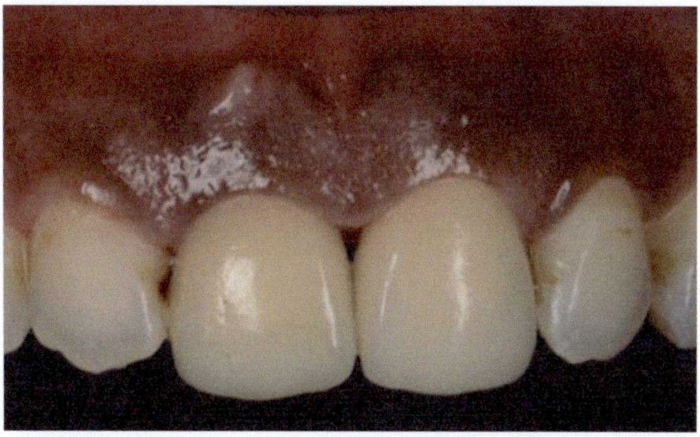

Fig. 4.19 Healed sites with provisional restorations depicting good tissue health

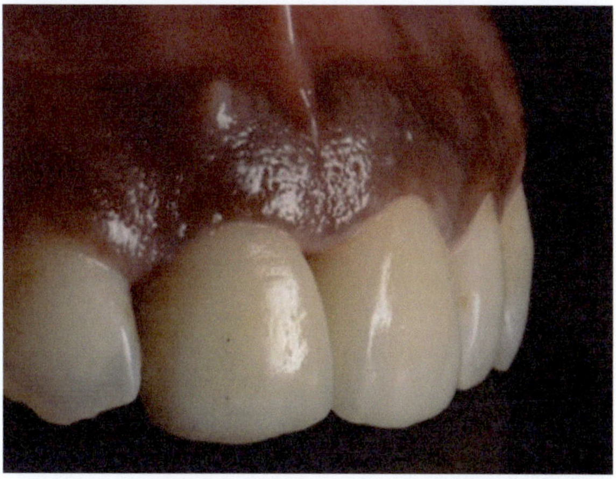

Fig. 4.20 The provisional restoration must exhibit ideal emergence profile

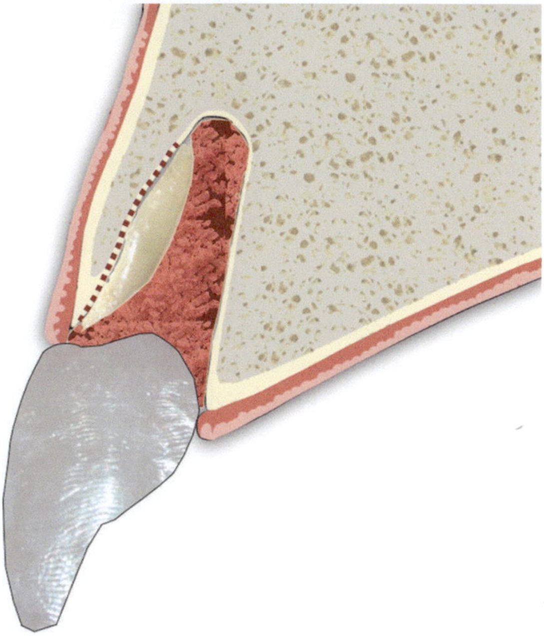

Fig. 4.21 Depicts the design of the ovate pontic in a case where pontic shield is prepared

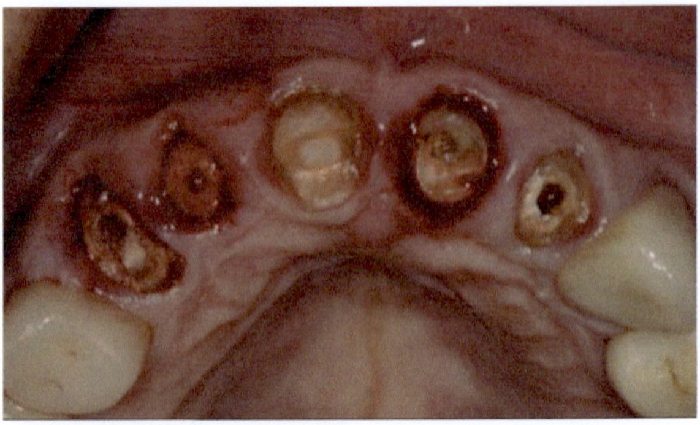

Fig. 4.22 Multiple PET sites after removal of weakened coronal structure

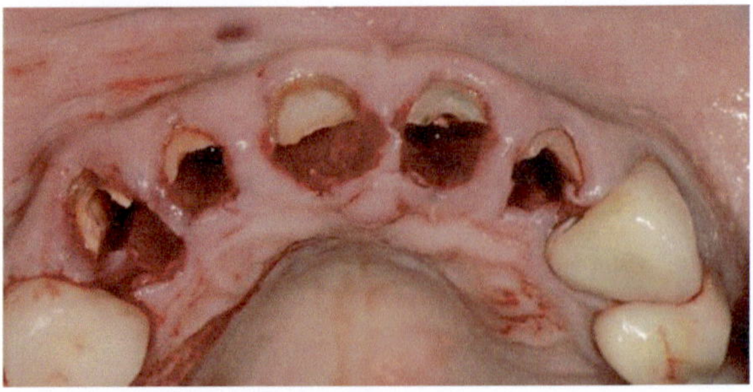

Fig. 4.23 Shields prepared to remove affected apex on all five teeth

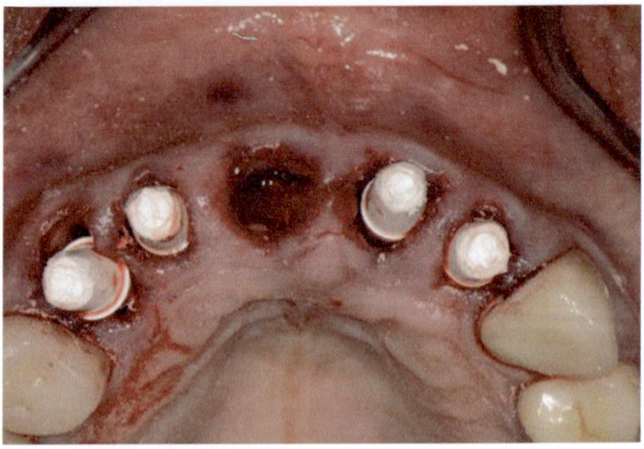

Fig. 4.24 Reinforced PEEK abutments for making immediate provisional restorations

A cement-retained restoration can also be fabricated by an indirect method where an impression can be taken of the implant and an abutment chosen to make the provisional restoration in the laboratory.

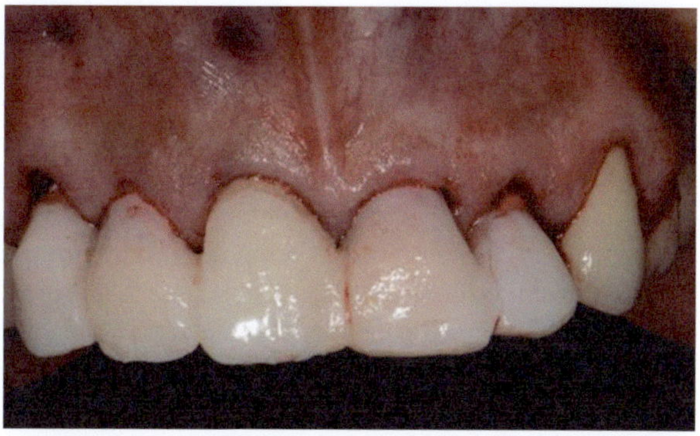

Fig. 4.25 Provisional restorations: immediate post-operative view

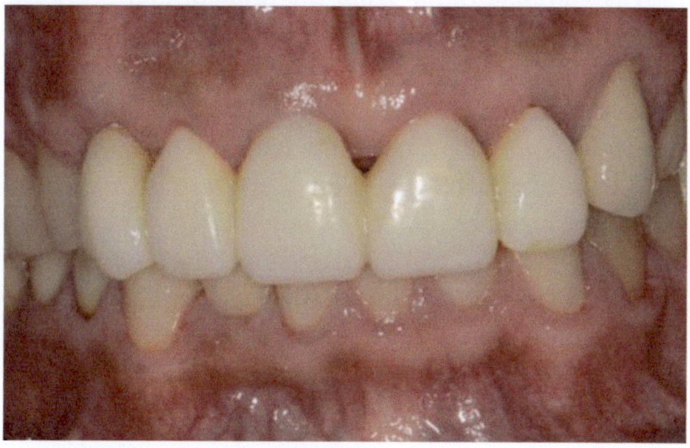

Fig. 4.26 Provisional restorations at 4 months with: one can appreciate the healthy tissues around the implants and the resotrations

4.5 Technical Considerations for Screw-Retained Provisional Restorations

Screw-retained provisional restorations offer the advantage of retrievability and negate the critical disadvantages of residual cement. Special attention during fabrication has to be paid to generate acceptable contours, fit and tissue support during fabrication of the provisional restoration.

There are various ways in which screw-retained restorations can be fabricated:

1. Direct method.
   (a) Temporary cylinder with resin build-up using a matrix.
   (b) Temporary cylinder with an available shell (polycarbonate crown/patient's own tooth/existing restoration).
2. Indirect method.

4.5.1 Direct Method

Temporary Cylinder with Resin Build Up

The following case (Figs. 4.27, 4.28, 4.29, 4.30, 4.31, 4.32, 4.33, 4.34, 4.35, 4.36, and 4.37) demonstrates the making of the screw-retained provisional restoration for a single implant after partial extraction therapy. A putty matrix is fabricated on the wax-up of the broken tooth. A temporary titanium or peek hollow cylinder can be used to make the screw-retained provisional restoration. Once the provisional material has set, the removal of the putty matrix will leave the Bis-GMA on the cylinder [27, 28]. A small access hole needs to be made in the provisional restoration based on the implant trajectory to unscrew the assembly from the implant. Flowable composite resin is then added to shape the gingival aspect, mainly the emergence of the provisional restoration from the implant platform. The subgingival contour of the provisional restoration is kept concave (S-shaped) as discussed earlier to allow greater soft tissue thickness in the area to cover the shield [9].

In several clinical cases of PET, based on the implant position vis-a-vis the socket morphology and the cross-sectional form of the gingival architecture, the provisional must be made concave as it emerges from the implant platform to accommodate the shield and have space to allow soft tissue to grow in. Figures 4.38 and 4.39 illustrate this aspect where the original design of the cervical part of the provisional restoration is too bulky or convex. An 'S'-shaped curve is created to achieve adequate concavity that will enable a gap between the shield and the tooth to allow space for soft tissue.

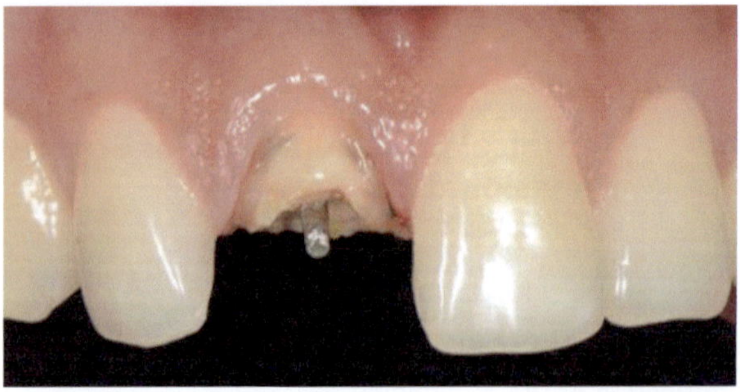

Fig. 4.27 Preoperative status of unrestorable tooth. Frontal view

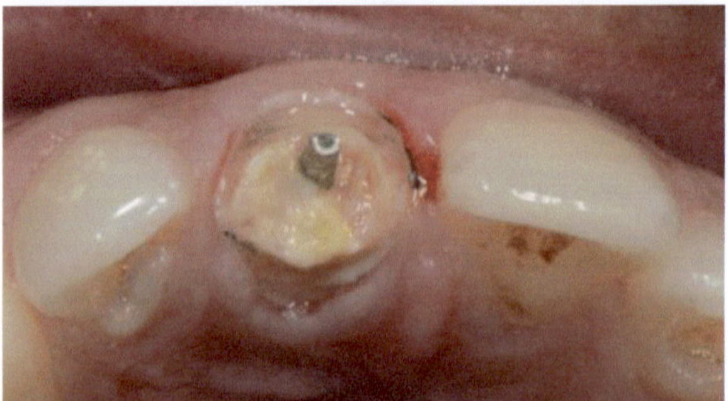

Fig. 4.28 Preoperative status of unrestorable tooth. Occlusal view

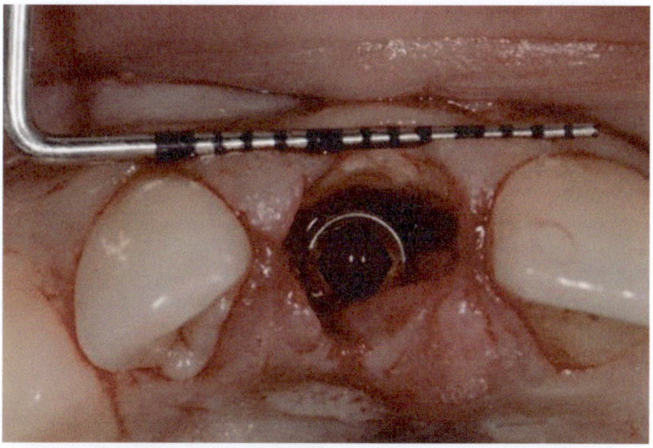

Fig. 4.29 Implant placed with no contact with the shield

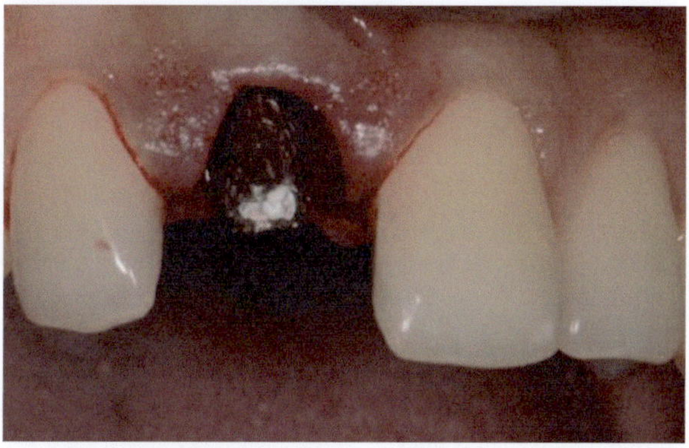

Fig. 4.30 Engaging temporary titanium cylinder attached to the implant

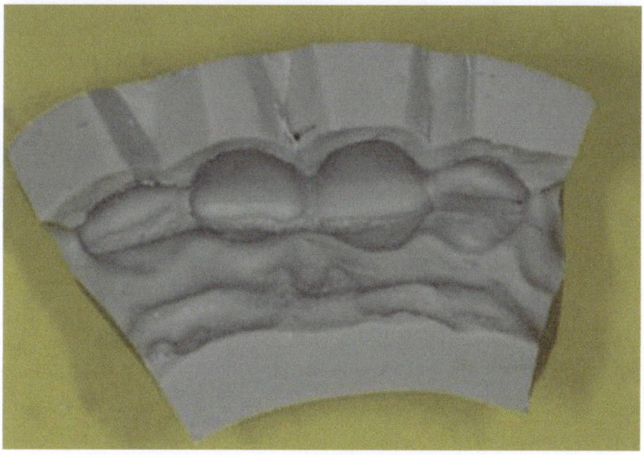

Fig. 4.31 Putty matrix from the preoperative wax-up

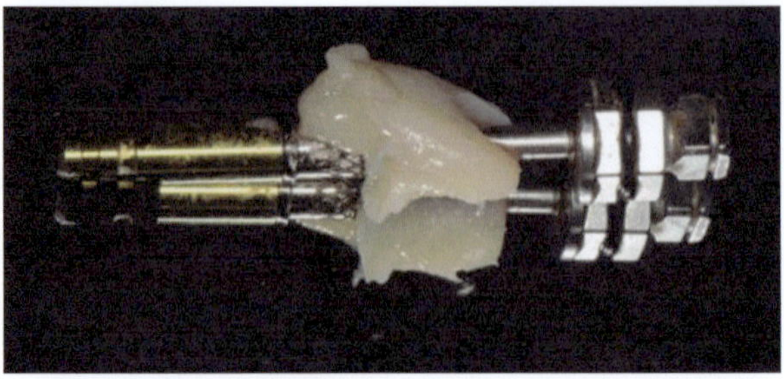

Fig. 4.32 The shell of provisional restoration attached intraorally to the cylinder using auto-polymerizing Bis-GMA resin loaded in the putty matrix

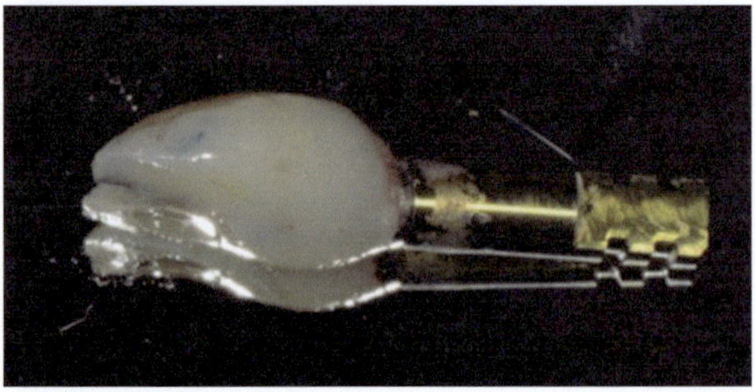

Fig. 4.33 Final shaping of the provisional restoration

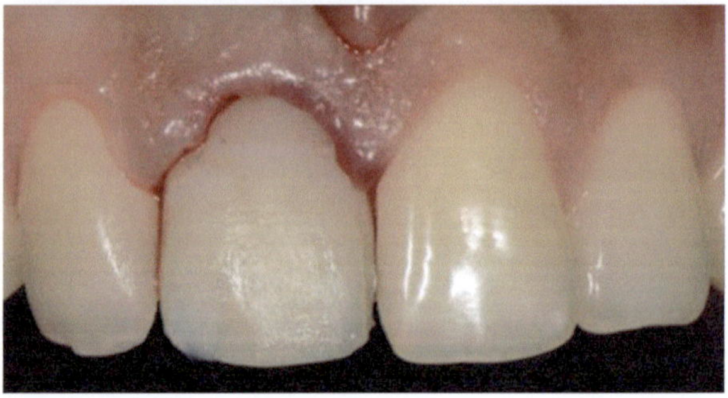

Fig. 4.34 Screw-retained provisional restoration delivered immediately after implant placement

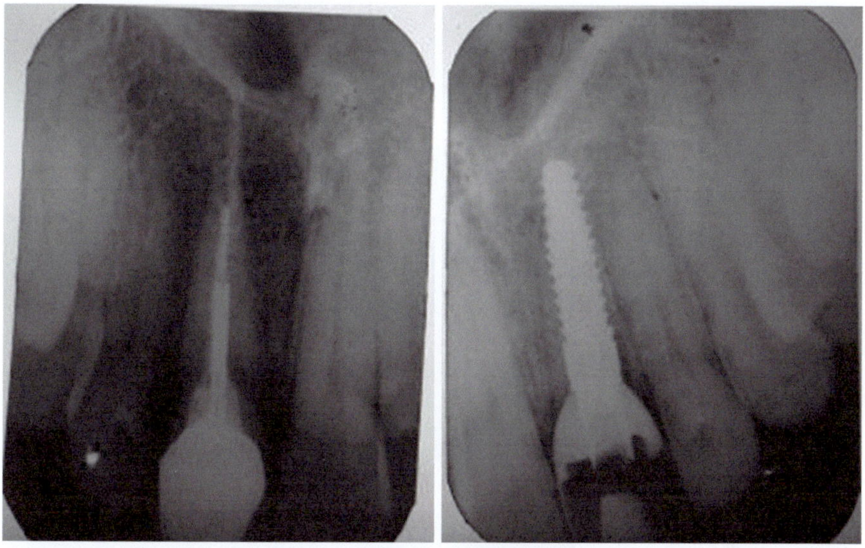

Fig. 4.35 Preoperative and post implant radiograph with provisional restoration

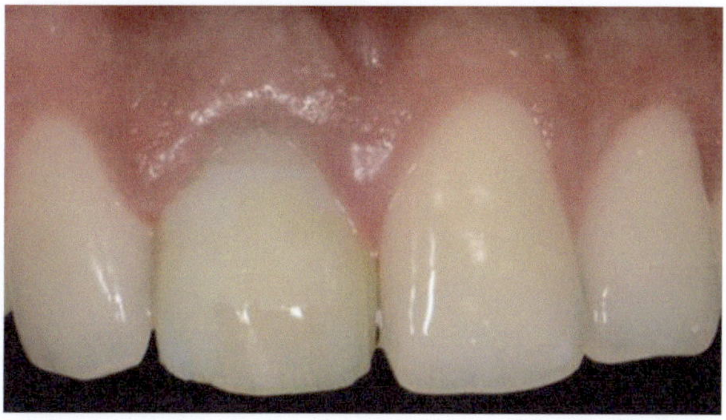

Fig. 4.36 Healed site with provisional restoration at 4 months

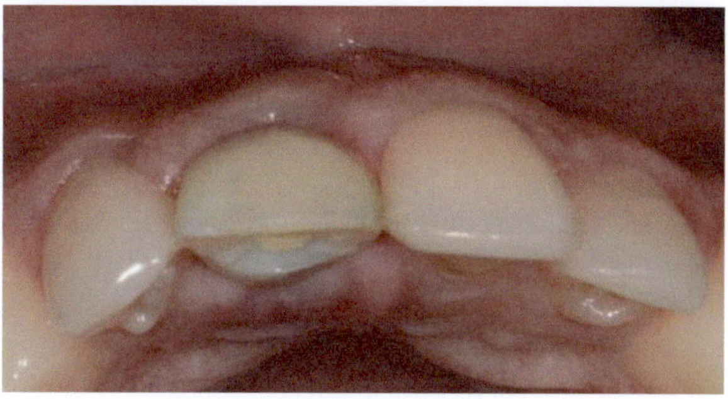

Fig. 4.37 Healed site with provisional restoration at 4 months with excellent tissue contours

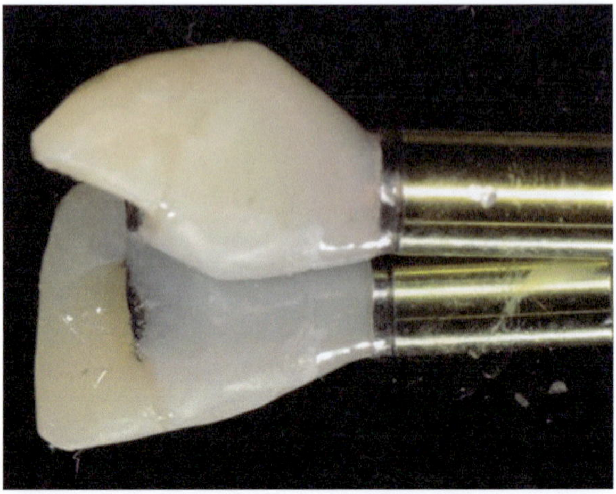

Fig. 4.38 Provisional with over-contoured subgingival contour

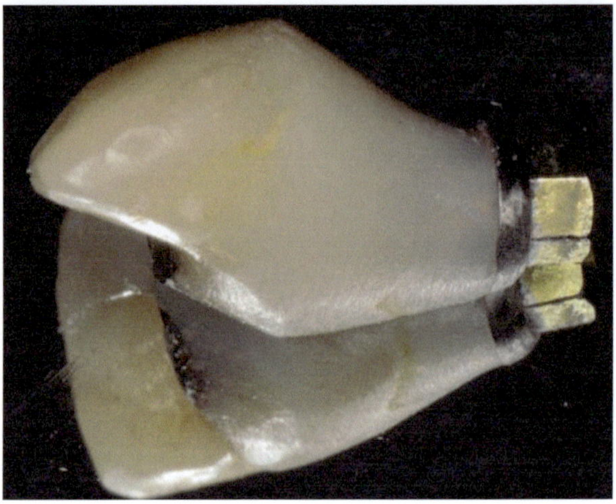

Fig. 4.39 Provisional with contour corrected and made more concave to have space for the soft tissue

Su et al. [6] explained in their article the need for demarcating the subgingival contour into two distinct zones called the critical contour and the subcritical contour. The critical contour is the area of implant abutment and crown located immediately apical to the gingival margin with an approximate range of 1 mm. The subcritical contour is located apical to the critical contour up to the implant platform. The subcritical contour may be convex, flat, or concave. Within physiologic limits, making the facial subcritical contour more convex can lead to coronal migration of gingival margin. However, all these discussions are pertaining to the anterior implant placement when the entire tooth has been extracted. In cases of socket shield, the presence of the labial sliver of tooth that has been shaped as discussed in the chapter on surgical considerations will allow the bone and soft tissue levels to be maintained very well around the implant site. Hence, the role of critical contour is reduced to providing support to the free gingival margin. The subcritical contour must *always be concave or flat* in these socket/pontic shield cases to maintain adequate space from the shield. Modification of subcritical contour and making it more convex to influence the gingival architecture may have detrimental effects due to lack of restorative space between the shield and the provisional. Thus, all principles of gingival architecture molding that we learn in immediate (total) extraction and implant cases may not be valid and should not be blindly applied without due consideration to the effect it will have on the shield stability and success of the partial extraction therapy. In most cases the maintenance of gingival architecture is easily achieved with the partial extraction cases as the labial bone resorption and its detrimental effects are avoided if case selection is appropriate.

The following case (Figs. 4.40, 4.41, 4.42, 4.43, 4.44, 4.45, 4.46, 4.47, 4.48, and 4.49) illustrates the making of screw-retained provisionals for adjacent implants after PET. In cases where some teeth are not salvageable and an implant is not needed in that area, a root submergence/pontic shield can be done to preserve tissue contour.

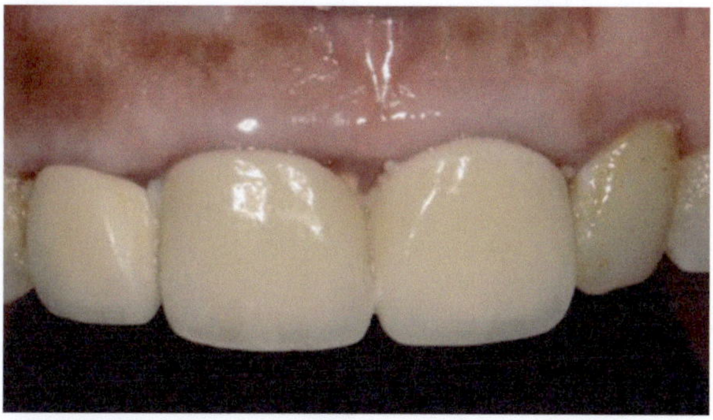

Fig. 4.40 Preoperative condition with structurally questionable incisors

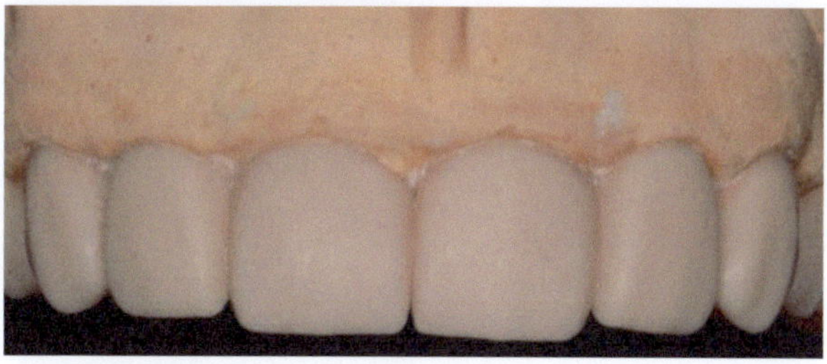

Fig. 4.41 Wax-up for the final smile

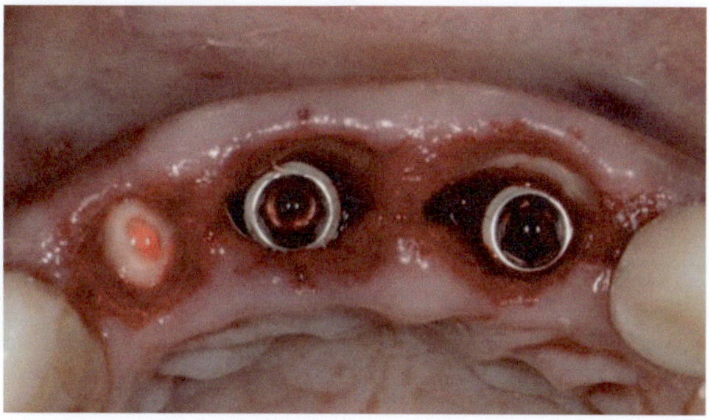

Fig. 4.42 Implants placed with shield preparation in #11 and #21. Root submergence in #12

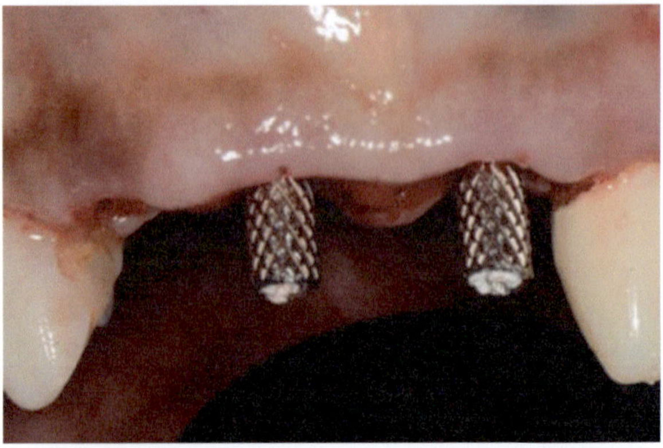

Fig. 4.43 Non-engaging temp cylinders ready to receive auto-polymerizing Bis-GMA on the putty matrix made from the wax-up

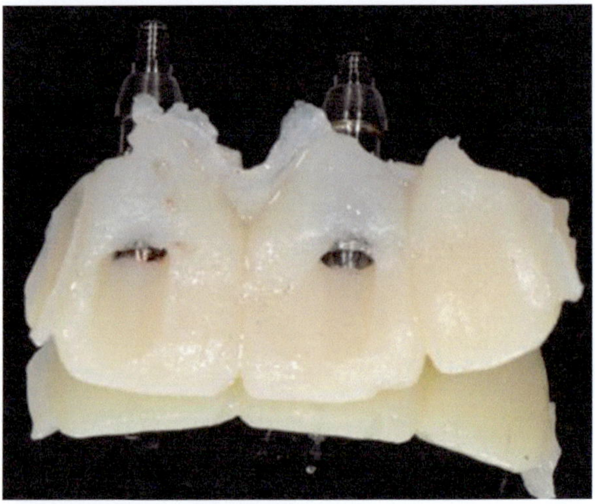

Fig. 4.44 Provisional restoration shell fixated on the temporary titanium cylinders. The cervical aspect will need to be worked upon by addition and shaping of flowable composite resin. The contour will be corrected and made more concave to have space for the soft tissue

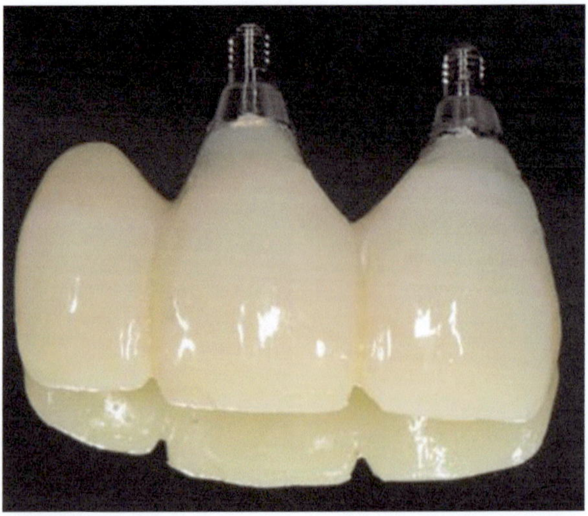

Fig. 4.45 Provisional restoration shaped and ready to be screwed onto the two implants. Note the ovate pontic design on #12

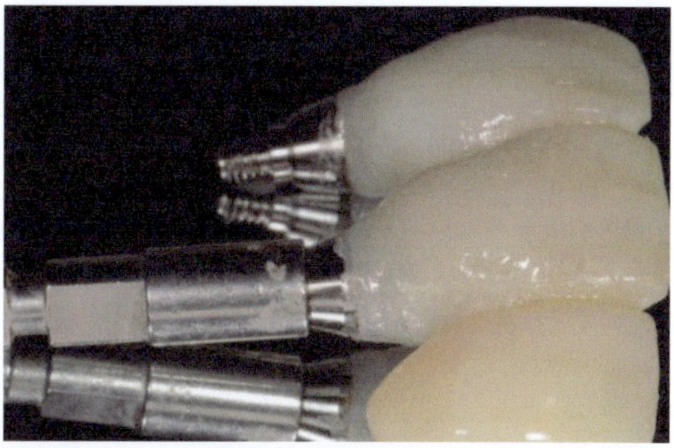

Fig. 4.46 Profile view of finished provisional restoration with ideal labial emergence profile

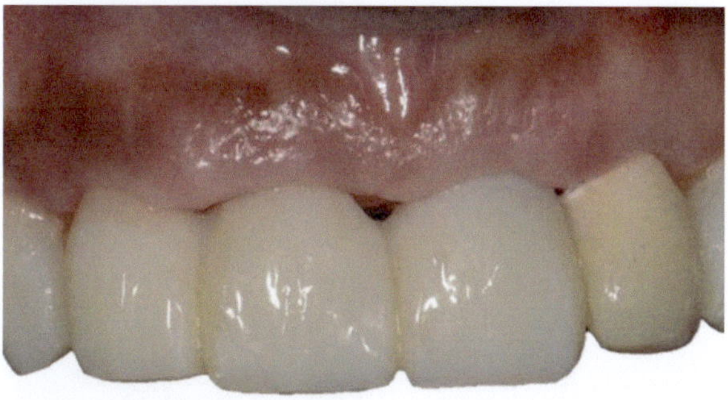

Fig. 4.47 Provisional restoration screwed onto the implants and torqued to 30 N cm

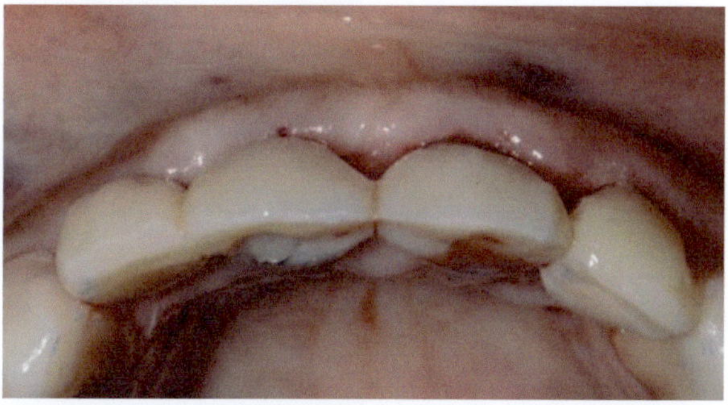

Fig. 4.48 Excellent tissue contours maintained at the end of the surgical phase

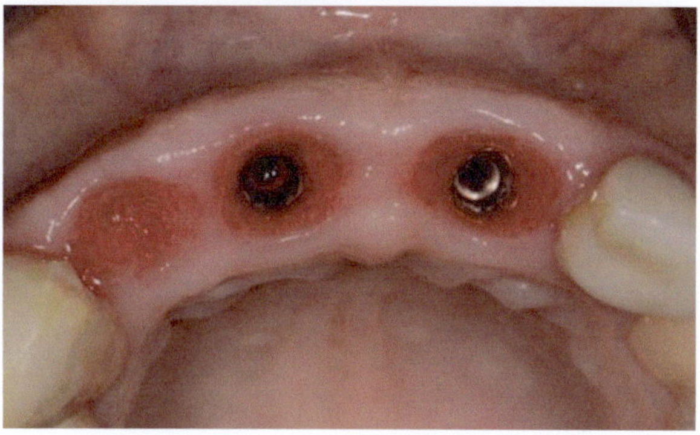

Fig. 4.49 Tissue contours as seen 4 months after surgery when the provisional was unscrewed. Note the complete soft tissue closure at the #12 site where root submergence was carried out

Temporary Cylinder with Patients Own Tooth/Existing Restoration

Case 1: In certain cases, the coronal part of the existing tooth that requires extraction can be salvaged and used as a shell to make a screw-retained provisional. After extraction, the tooth is sectioned at the CEJ to remove any root remnants and then the internal part of the coronal portion is cleaned out to make a hollow shell that can be relined with composite resin after etching and bonding. The following case demonstrates this method (Figs. 4.50, 4.51, 4.52, 4.53, 4.54, 4.55, 4.56, 4.57, 4.58, and 4.59).

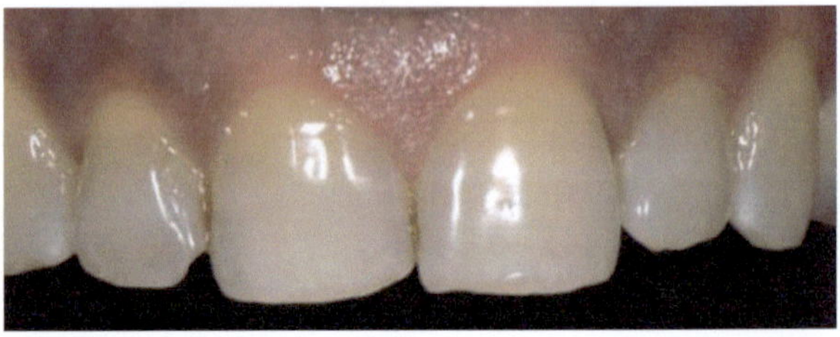

Fig. 4.50 Preoperative status of #21 having internal resorption and needing extraction

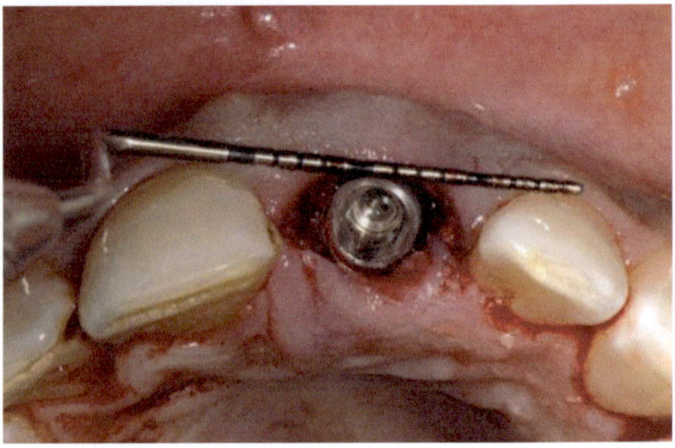

Fig. 4.51 Implant placed in correct 3D position

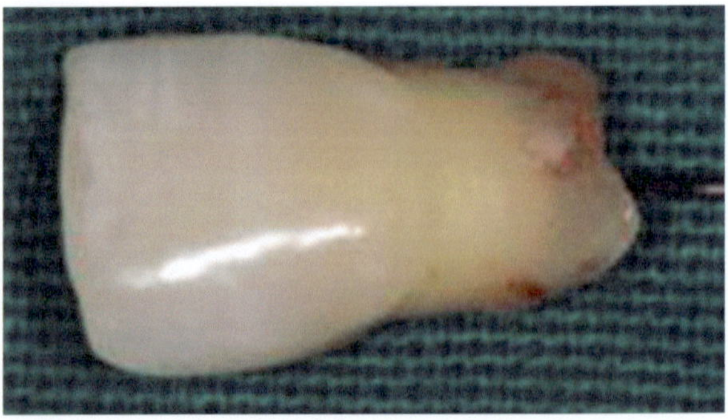

Fig. 4.52 The offending tooth with intact coronal structure that can be used to make a provisional restoration

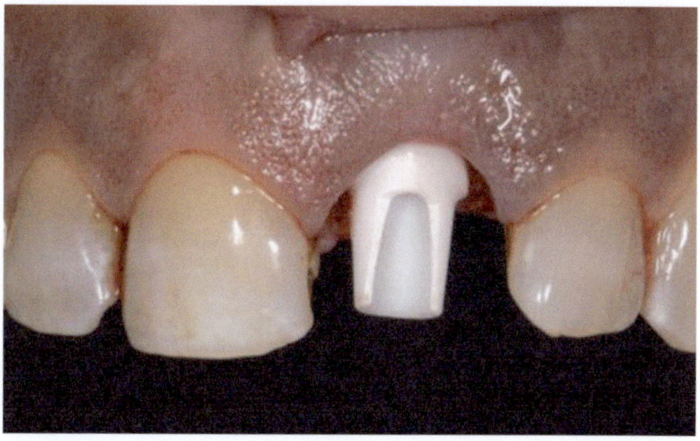

Fig. 4.53 Abutment on which the existing tooth will be relined and retrofitted

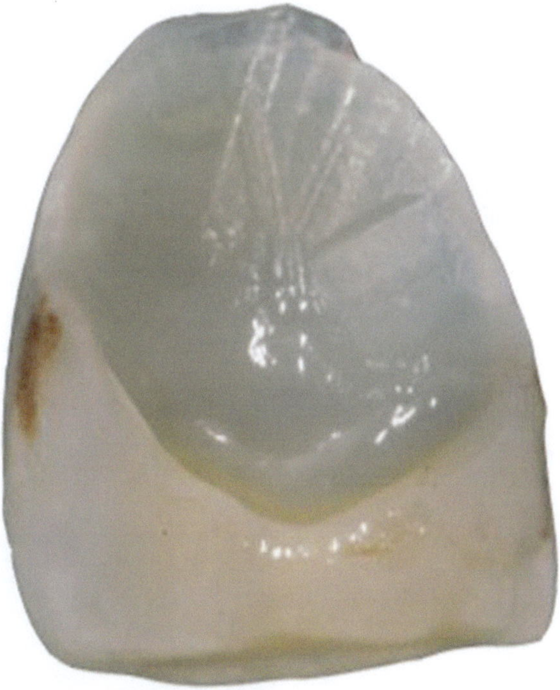

Fig. 4.54 The coronal part of extracted tooth cleaned up and made into a shell

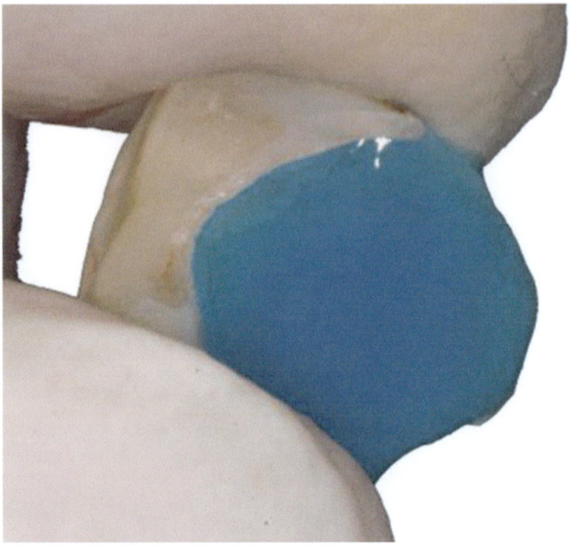

Fig. 4.55 The prepared shell is etched on internal surface

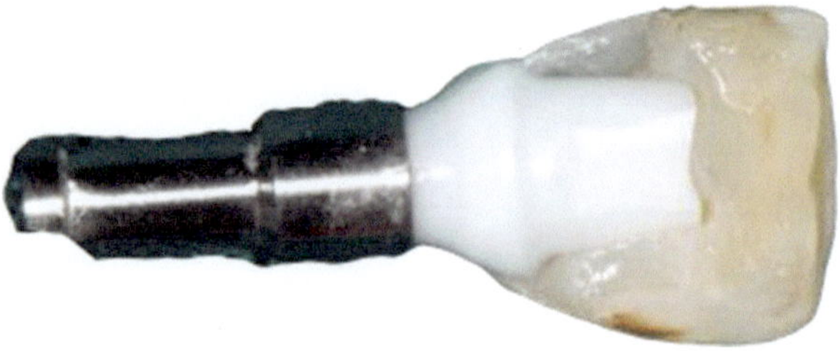

Fig. 4.56 The shell ready to be relined with composite resin

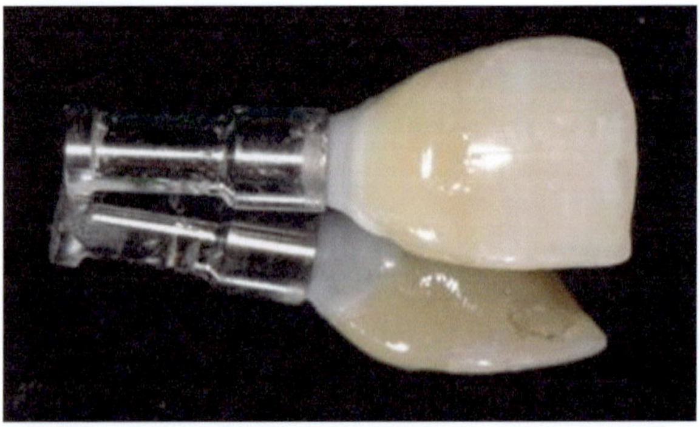

Fig. 4.57 Provisional restoration using the patient's own tooth, with its final contour

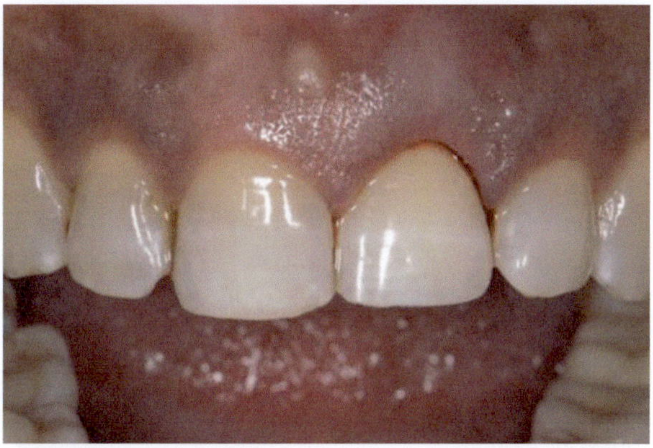

Fig. 4.58 Provisional restoration delivered immediately after implant placement

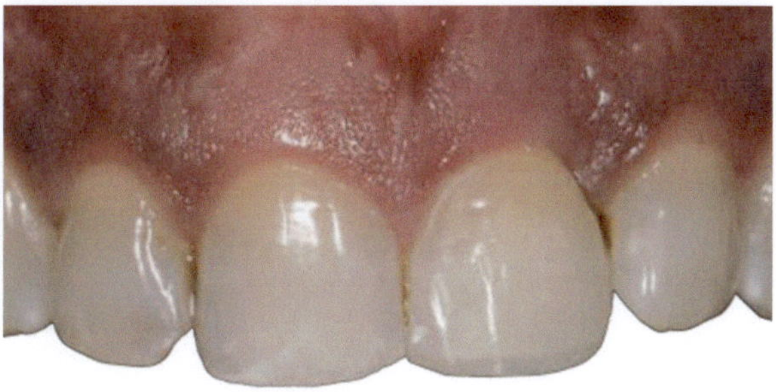

Fig. 4.59 Provisional restoration with healed site at 4 months

Case2: Temporary cylinder with polycarbonate crown shell.*

Just as a tooth shell can be relined, a polycarbonate crown too can be relined and used as a provisional restoration. The following case demonstrates the clinical technique (Figs. 4.60, 4.61, 4.62, 4.63, 4.64, 4.65, 4.66, and 4.67).

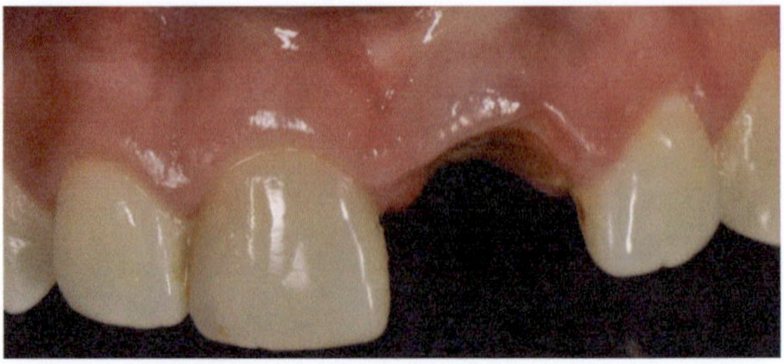

Fig. 4.60 Preoperative condition of structurally poor #21

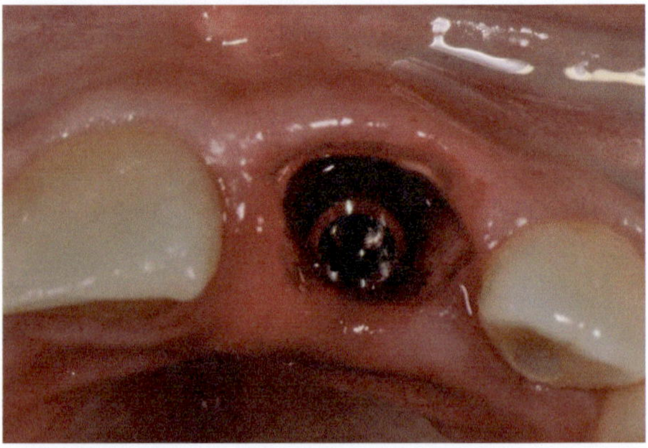

Fig. 4.61 Shield prepared and implant placed in correct 3D position

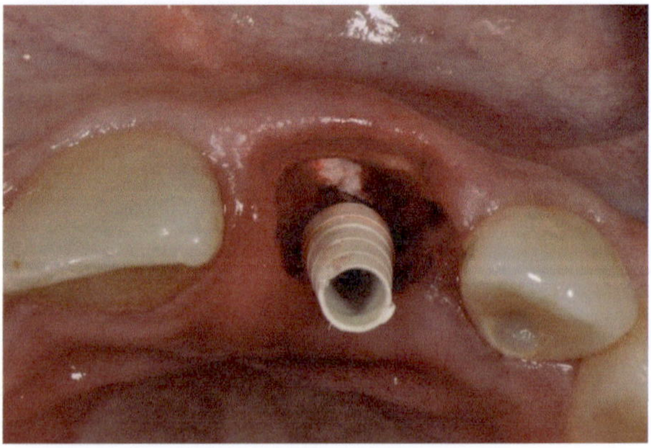

Fig. 4.62 Engaging PEEK temp cylinder will enable making of a screw-retained provisional

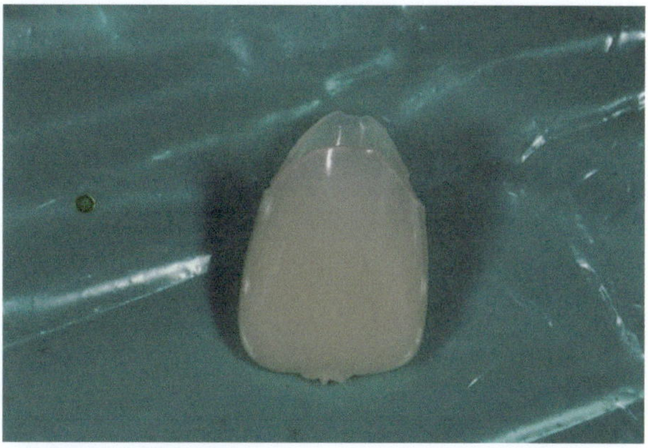

Fig. 4.63 Polycarbonate crown selected for the site

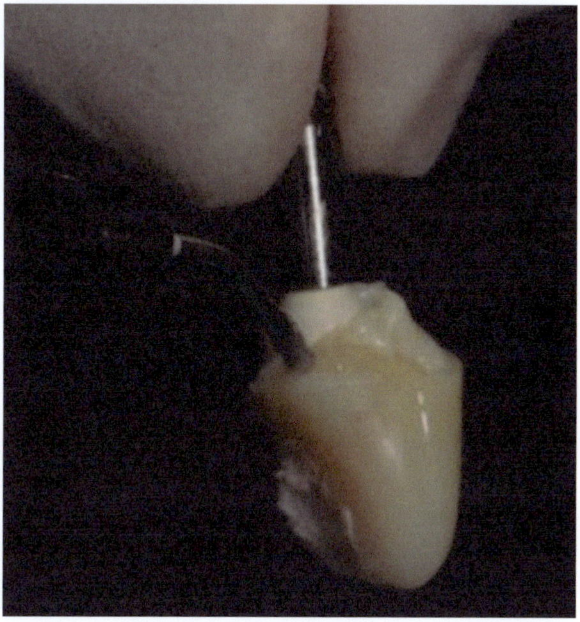

Fig. 4.64 Flowable composite used to reline and fix the shell to the temporary cylinder

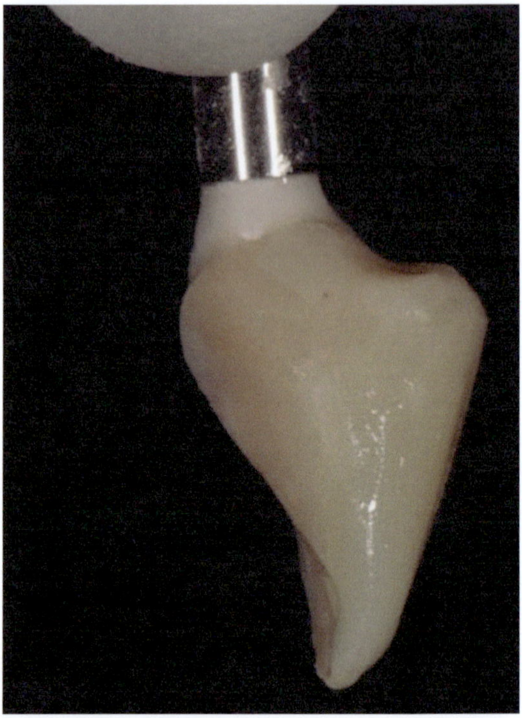

Fig. 4.65 Provisional with concave subcritical contour

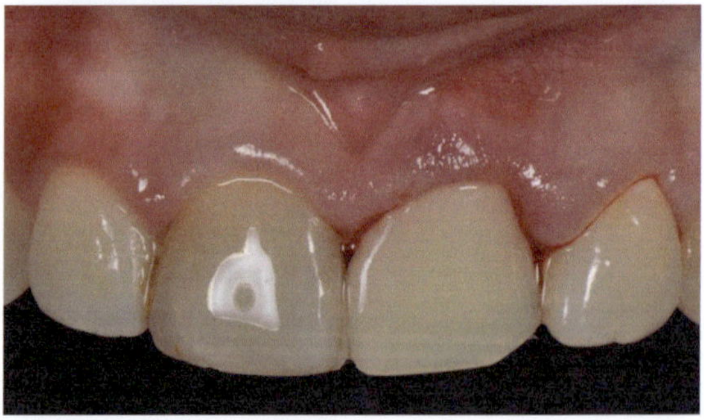

Fig. 4.66 Provisional screw-retained restoration on the implant on day of placement

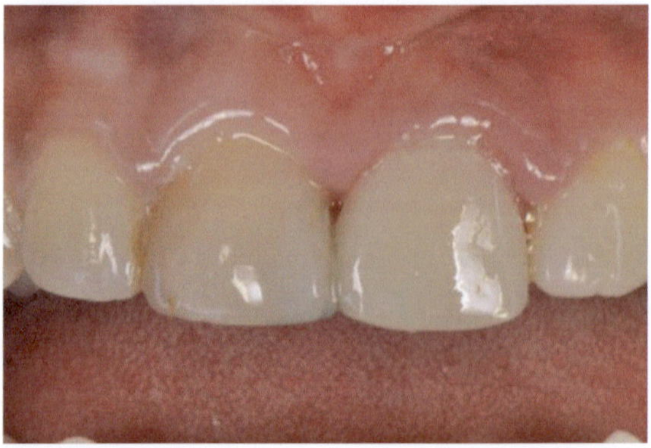

Fig. 4.67 Provisional restoration at 4 months with healed site showing excellent tissue contours

*Case 3: Converting existing restoration to a screw-retained provisional crown**. In cases where an intact existing restoration is present and the weak coronal aspect of the tooth is fractured, the existing restoration can be converted and used as a provisional shell. Figures 4.68, 4.69, 4.70, 4.71, 4.72, 4.73, 4.74, 4.75, 4.76, 4.77, 4.78, 4.79, and 4.80 depict a case in which this procedure was carried out.

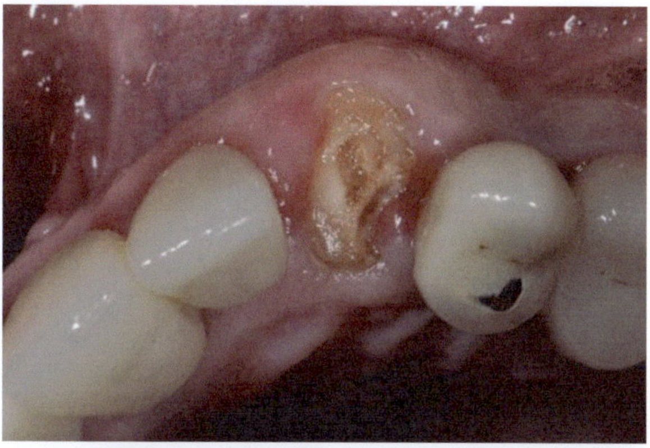

Fig. 4.68 Fractured nonrestorable tooth #23. The patient reported with coronal fracture with the restoration in form of a lithium disilicate crown intact

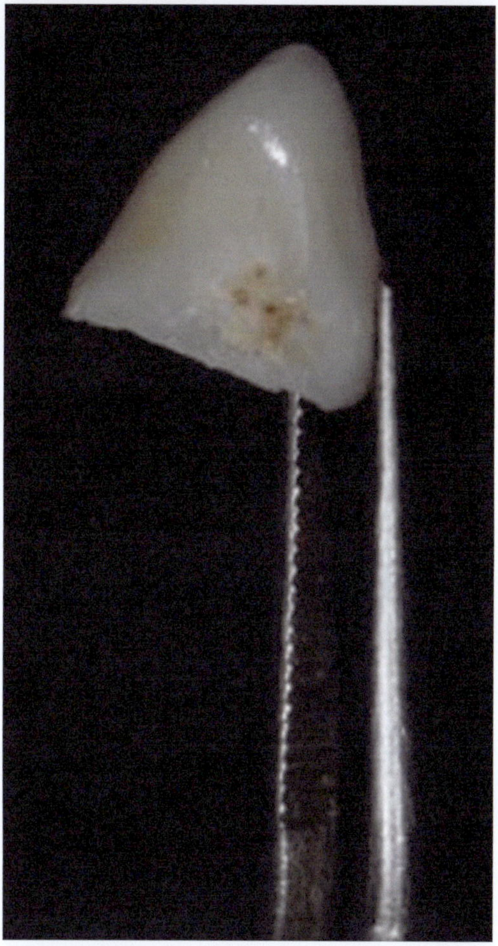

Fig. 4.69 Existing lithium disilicate crown cleaned up to act as a provisional restoration shell

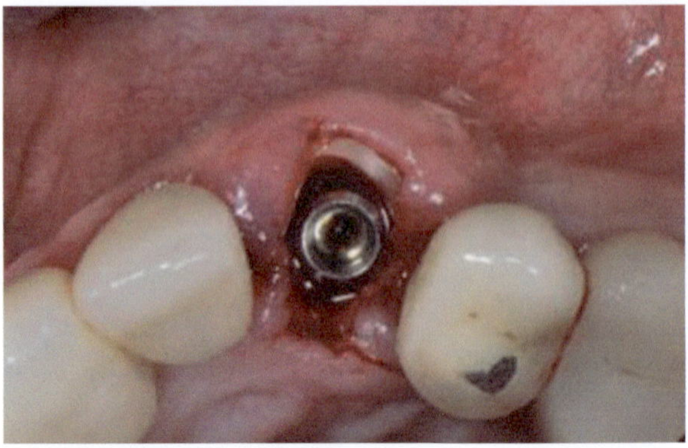

Fig. 4.70 Socket shield prepared and implant placement carried out with high ISQ value

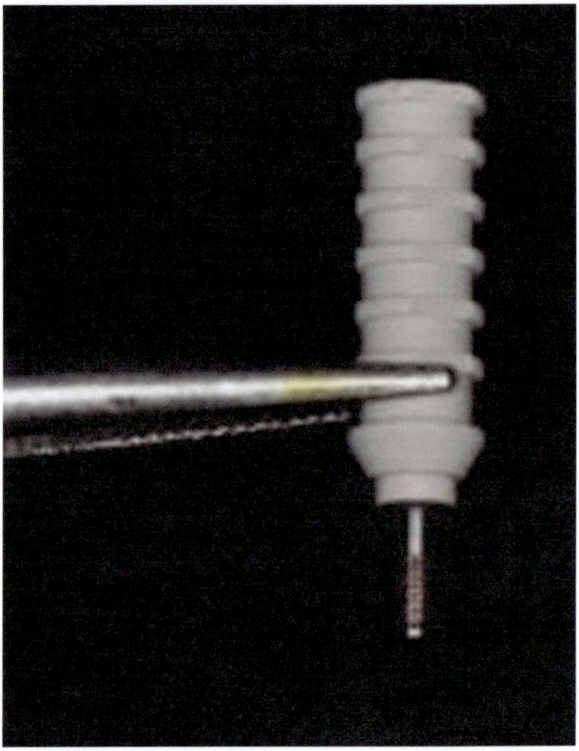

Fig. 4.71 PEEK temporary cylinder

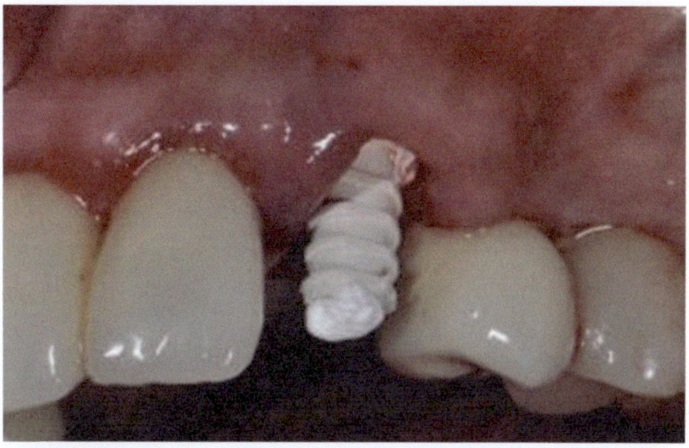

Fig. 4.72 PEEK temporary cylinder fixed over implant. Teflon tape used to protect socket and plug screw channel

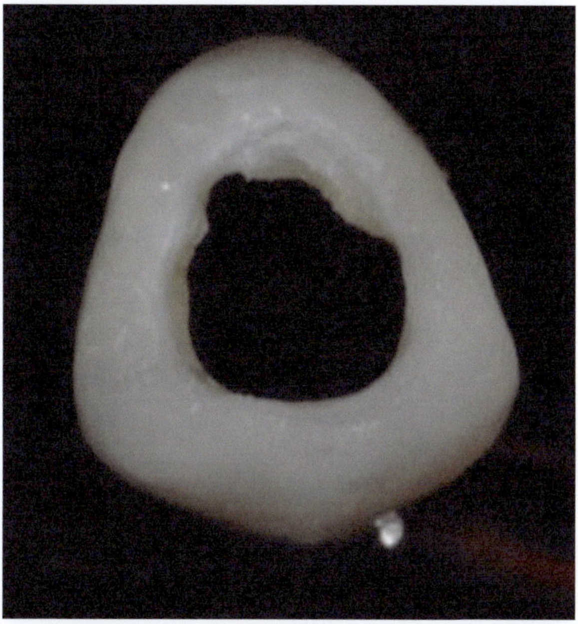

Fig. 4.73 Existing restoration hollowed out on palatal side

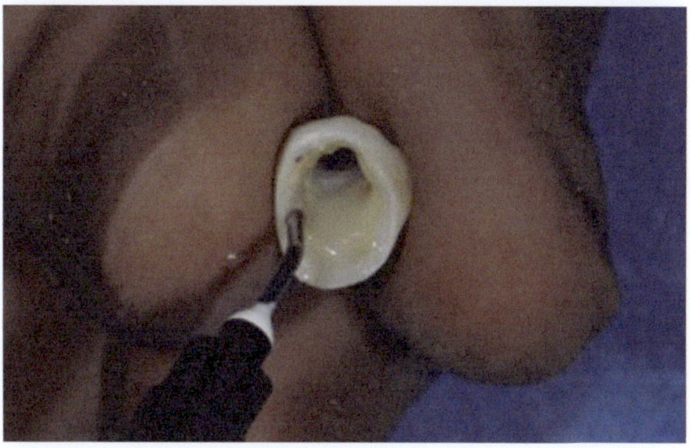

Fig. 4.74 Flowable resin used after etching and bonding internal surface of the crown

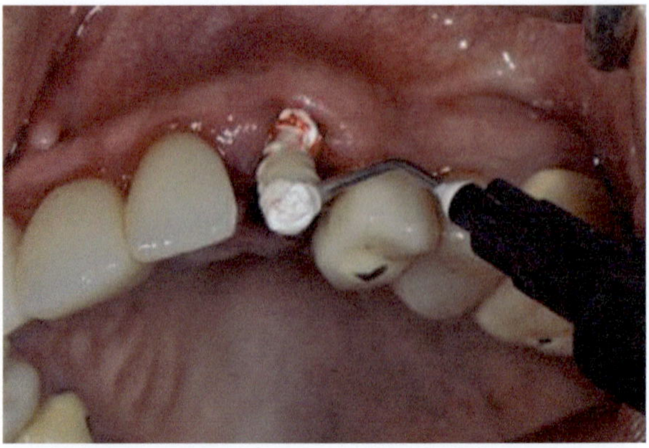

Fig. 4.75 Applying flowable resin on temporary abutment

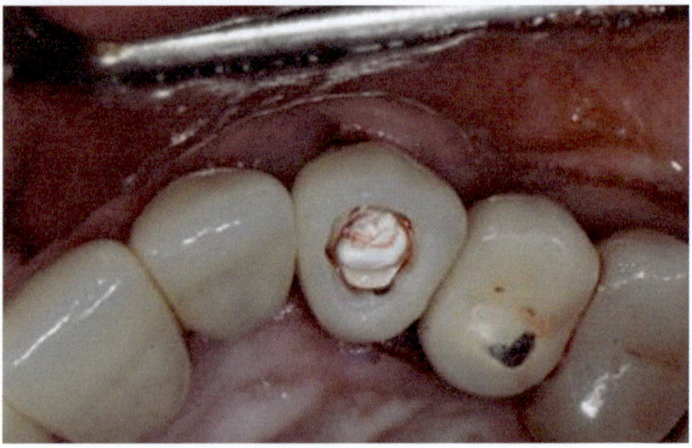

Fig. 4.76 Inserting old restoration over the abutment followed by light cure

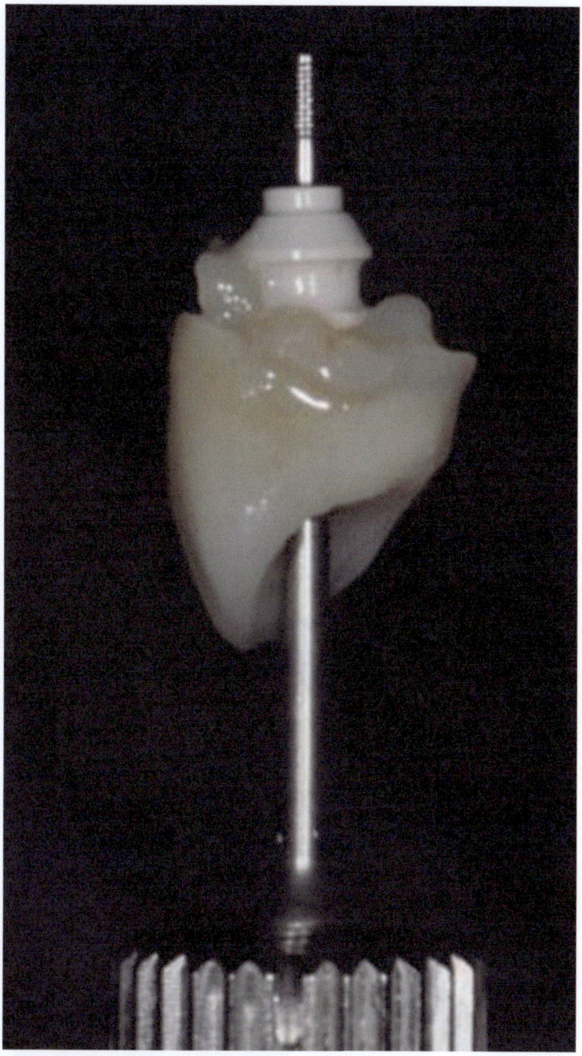

Fig. 4.77 Abutment and restoration shell picked up

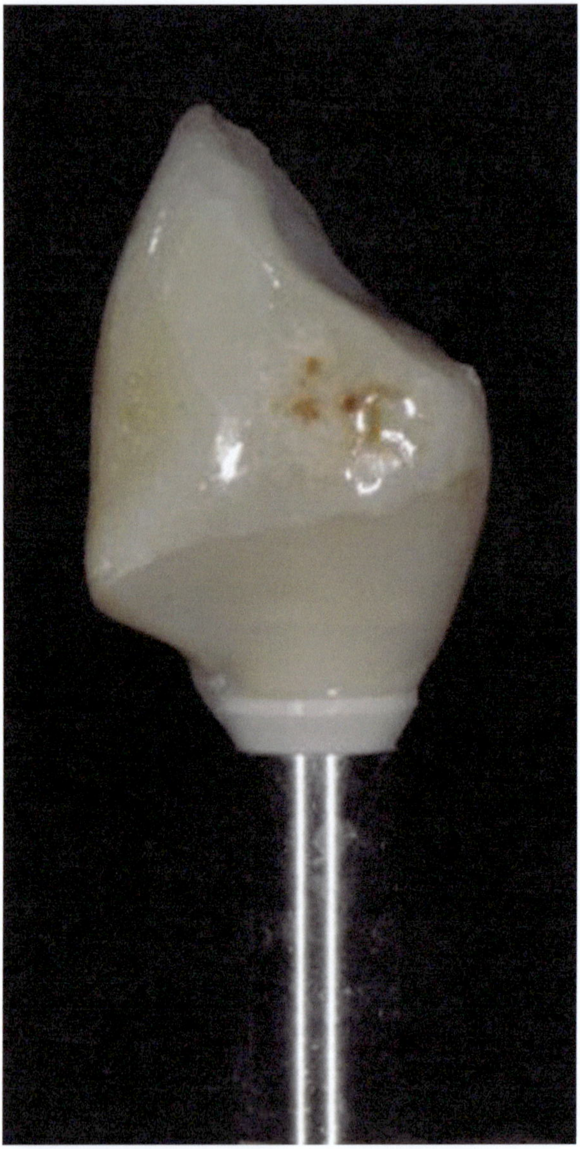

Fig. 4.78 Addition of flowable composite for contouring the cervical aspect. Note the concave subcritical contour to allow space for the shield

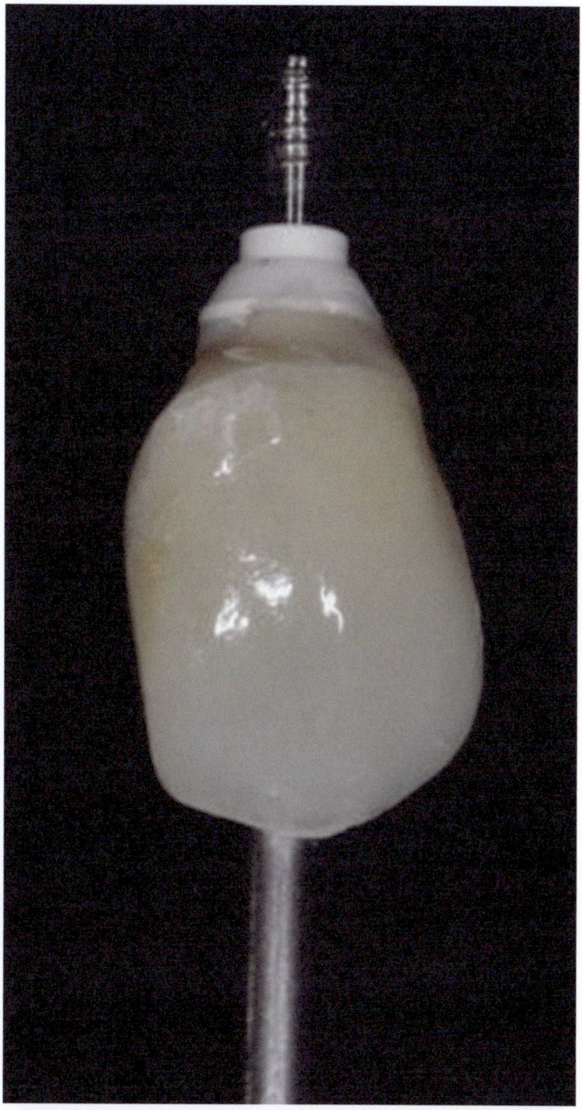

Fig. 4.79 Screw-retained provisional crown made from existing restoration

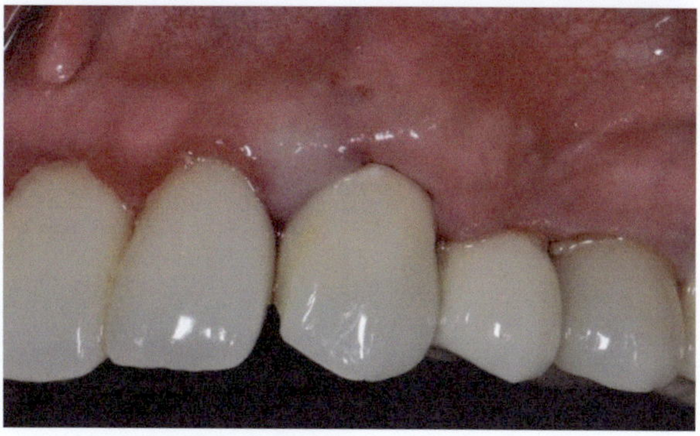

Fig. 4.80 Immediate postinsertion view of the screw-retained provisional crown

4.5.2 Indirect Method for Making Screw-Retained Provisional Restorations

A screw-retained provisional can also be made with indirect technique where an impression is made after the implant placement and sent to the laboratory for fabrication. The following case illustrates the detailed steps for the same (Figs. 4.81, 4.82, 4.83, 4.84, and 4.85)*.

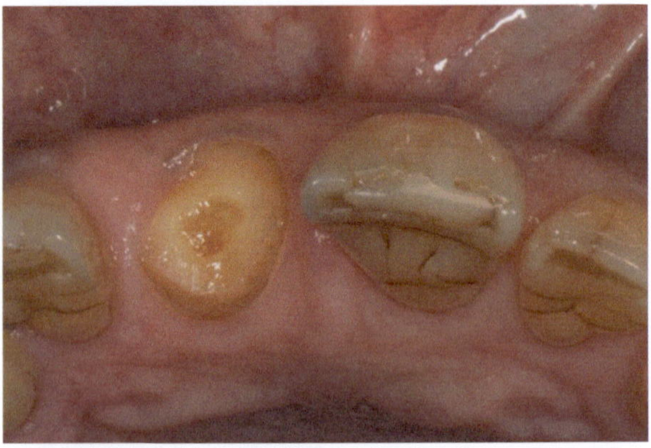

Fig. 4.81 Unrestorable #11

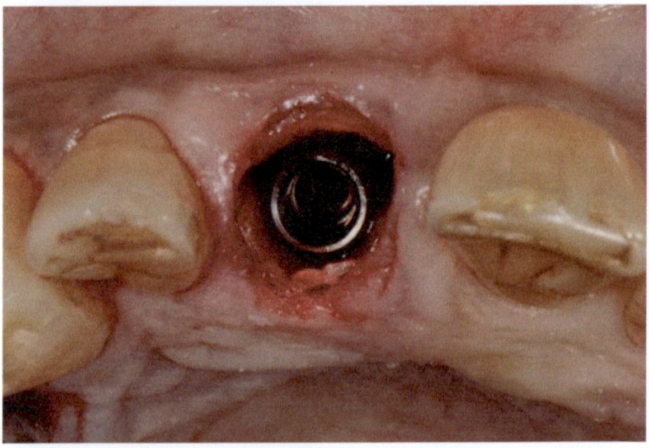

Fig. 4.82 Shield prepared and implant placed in correct 3D position

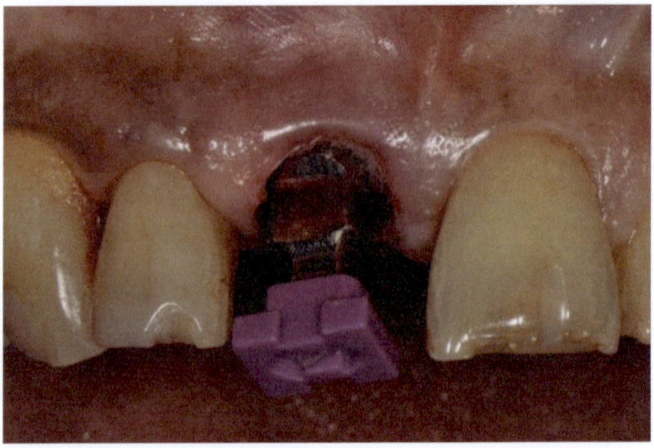

Fig. 4.83 Impression taken with snap coping

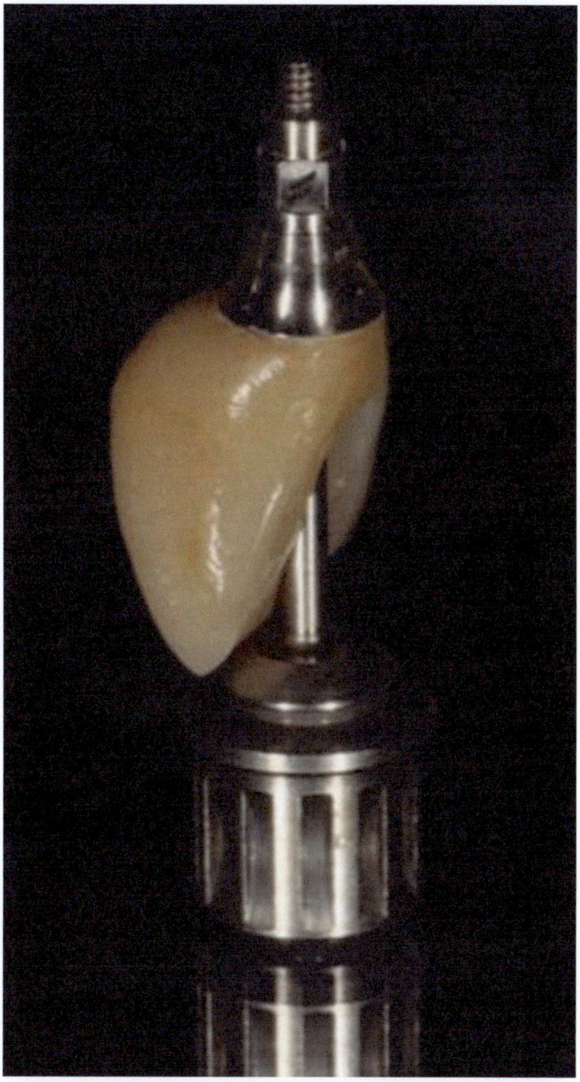

Fig. 4.84 Lab-fabricated provisional restoration with correctly shaped cervical contours

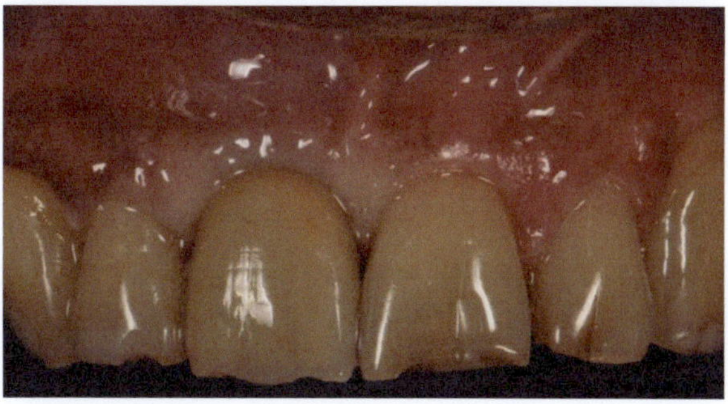

Fig. 4.85 Provisional restoration made in lab and delivered within 24 h

4.6 Conclusion

The provisional restorations play a key role in harnessing the health and shape of the soft tissues around the implant placed with partial extraction therapy protocols [20]. Customization of the emergence of the final restoration can be done with a well-made provisional restoration. This will also provide an adequate preview of the final result [21]. The added advantage of these provisional restorations on the implants is the immediate aesthetic replacement it provides to the patient.

Acknowledgement Illustrations by: Udatta Kher.
*Case Courtesy: Dr Udatta Kher (Fig. 4.60 Onwards)

References

1. Cardaropoli D, Tamagnone L, Roffredo A, Gaveglio L. Soft tissue contour changes at immediate postextraction single-tooth implants with immediate restoration: a 12-month prospective cohort study. Int J Periodontics Restorative Dent. 2015;35(2):191–8.
2. Glocker M, Attin T, Schmidlin P. Ridge preservation with modified "socket-shield" technique: methodological case series. Dent J. 2014;2:11–21.
3. Kan J, Runcharassaeng K. Immediate placement and provisionalization of maxillary anterior single implants: a surgical and prosthodontic rationale. Pract Periodontics Aesthet Dent. 2000;12(9):817–24.
4. Kan J, Rungcharassaeng K, Deflorian M, Winstein T, Wang H, Testori T. Immediate implant placement and provisionalization of maxillary anterior single implants. Periodontol 2000. 2018;77(1):197–212.
5. Kois JC, Kan JY. Predictable peri implant gingival aesthetics: surgical and prosthodontic rationales. Pract Proced Aesthet Dent. 2001;13:691–8.
6. Su H, González-Martín O, Weisgold A, Lee E. Considerations of implant abutment and crown contour: critical contour and subcritical contour. Int J Periodontics Restorative Dent. 2010;30(4):335–43.
7. Clavijo V, Blasi A. Decision making process for restoring single implants. Quintessence Dent Technol. 2017;2017:66–88.
8. Gluckman H, Salama M, Jonathan DT. Partial extraction therapies (PET). Part 2: procedures and technical aspects. Int J Periodontics Restorative Dent. 2017;37(3):377–85.
9. Gluckman H, Nagy K, Toit D. Prosthetic management of implants placed with the socket-shield technique. J Prosthet Dent. 2018;121–4:581–5.
10. Dewey KW, Zugsmith R. An experimental study of tissue reactions about porcelain roots. J Dent Res. 1933;13:459–72.
11. Abrams L. Augmentation of the deformed residual edentulous ridge for fixed prosthesis. Compend Contin Educ Gen Dent. 1980;1:205–13.
12. Edelhoff D, Spiekermann H, Yildirim M. A review of esthetic pontic design options. Quintessence Int 1985. 2002;33:736–46.
13. Spear FM. The use of implants and ovate pontics in the esthetic zone. Compend Contin Educ Dent. 2008;29:72–4.
14. Magne P, Magne M, Belser U. The esthetic width in fixed prosthodontics. J Prosthodont. 1999;8:106–18.
15. Salama M, Ishikawa T, Salama H, Funato A, Garber D. Advantages of the root submergence technique for pontic site development in esthetic implant therapy. Int J Periodontics Restorative Dent. 2007;27-6:521–7.

16. Priest G. Esthetic potential of single-implant provisional restorations: selection criteria of available alternatives. J Esthet Restor Dent. 2006;18(6):326–38.
17. Santosa R. Provisional restoration options in implant dentistry. Aust Dent J. 2007;52:234–42.
18. Wittneben J, Buser D, Belser U, Brägger U. Peri-implant soft tissue conditioning with provisional restorations in the esthetic zone: the dynamic compression technique. Int J Periodontics Restorative Dent. 2013;33:447–55.
19. Hirayama H, Kang K, Oishi Y. The modification of interim cylinders for the fabrication of cement-retained implant-supported provisional restorations. J Prosthet Dent. 2003;90(4):406–9.
20. Thomas GW. The positive relationship between excess cement and peri-implant disease: a prospective clinical endoscopic study. J Periodontol. 2009;80(9):1388–92.
21. Degidi M, Nardi D, Piattelli A. One abutment at one time: non-removal of an immediate abutment and its effect on bone healing around subcrestal tapered implants. Clin Oral Implants Res. 2011;22:1303–7.
22. Kupeyan K, Herman B, May K. Implant and provisional crown placement: a one stage protocol. Implant Dent. 1998;7:213–9.
23. Momen A, Smith AT, Nabeel A, Ma S, Warwick D. The "one abutment – one time" protocol: a systematic review and meta-analysis. J Periodontol. 2017;88:1–19.
24. Atsuta I, Ayukawa Y, Kondo R, Wakana O, Matsuura Y, Furuhashi A, Tsukiyama Y, Koyano K. Soft tissue sealing around dental implants based on histological interpretation. J Prosthodont Res. 2016, 60:3–11.
25. Seong WJ, Birdi HS, Hinrichs J. Fabricating a versatile cement-retained implant provisional restoration with a customized temporary abutment. J Dent Health Oral Disord Ther. 2017;6(6):00220.
26. Lemongello GJ. Customized provisional abutment and provisional restoration for an immediately-placed implant. Pract Proced Aesthet Dent. 2007;19-7:419–24.
27. Touati B, Guez G. Immediate implantation with provisionalization: from literature to clinical implications. Pract Proced Aesthet Dent. 2002;14:699–707.
28. Frizzera F, Tonetto M, Cabral G, Shibli JA, Marcantonio E Jr. Periodontics, implantology, and prosthodontics integrated: the zenith-driven rehabilitation. Case Rep Dent. 2017;2017:Article ID 1070292.

PET for Multirooted Teeth

5

Udatta Kher

Abstract

The immense success in achieving excellent soft tissue contours around implants placed in the esthetic zone with the PET procedures has opened up the possibility of performing it on multirooted teeth. However, the presence of two or more roots adds to the complexity of the case and special attention is needed to achieve consistent results. In this chapter, the authors share their clinical experiences and describe the step-by-step procedure of performing socket shield procedures in premolars and molars. Case selection and risk factors are explained to prevent complications and failures.

5.1 Introduction

Post-extraction alteration of the alveolar ridge is not a phenomenon restricted to the anterior maxilla. Loss of labial bone following extraction continues even after placement of an implant, both in the anterior and posterior regions of the alveolar ridge [1–3]. Often contour augmentation by performing a guided bone regeneration procedure is suggested to compensate for this buccal bone collapse [4, 5]. Performing the socket shield procedure for posterior teeth has similar benefits as the anterior teeth [6]. It helps in maintaining the integrity of the buccal bone and helps in preserving the attached mucosa around the osseointegrated implant [7]. This has a positive impact on the long-term maintenance of the peri-implant tissues. Buccal collapse, if not augmented by a bone graft and/or a soft tissue graft, results in poor emergence profile of the prosthesis. Buccal collapse results in food entrapment and

U. Kher (✉)
Only Smiles Dental Centre, Mumbai, India

U. Kher, A. Tunkiwala (eds.), *Partial Extraction Therapy in Implant Dentistry*,
https://doi.org/10.1007/978-3-030-33610-3_5

creates a non-self-cleansing area. It may also result in loss of vestibule, loss of attached keratinized gingiva, and difficulty in plaque control.

A socket shield procedure for a posterior tooth will prevent all the above troubles and help in long-term maintenance of the peri-implant tissues [6].

A proof of principle for a molar socket shield was published in a case report by Schwimer et al. [8].

5.2 PET for the Maxillary First Molar

The maxillary molar poses a few challenges for the execution of a PET procedure. The site usually has limited access for effective sectioning of the roots. Anatomical factors such as root configuration and the proximity to the sinus floor play an important role in case selection for a molar PET [9, 10]. Achieving primary closure after a molar PET is usually not possible and the fabrication of a customized healing abutment becomes a necessity, adding to the complexity of the treatment procedure [11, 12].

Multirooted teeth sockets have been classified by Smith et al. into three types [13] (Fig. 5.1).

Type A: The implant is completely housed in the inter-radicular bone (Fig. 5.2).

Type B: The implant is partly surrounded by the inter-radicular bone and partly has no bone contact within the socket (Fig. 5.3).

Type C: there is no available inter-radicular bone for implant placement (Fig. 5.4).

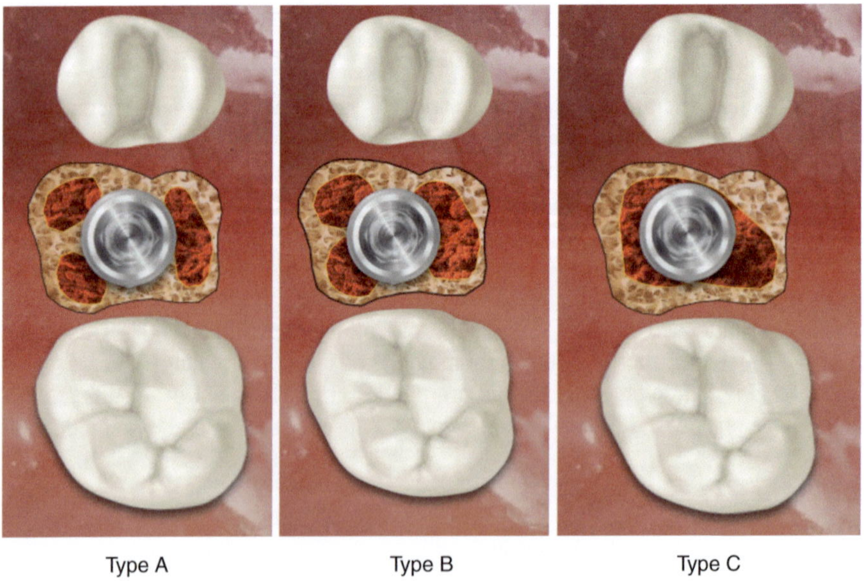

Fig. 5.1 Classification of multirooted teeth sockets

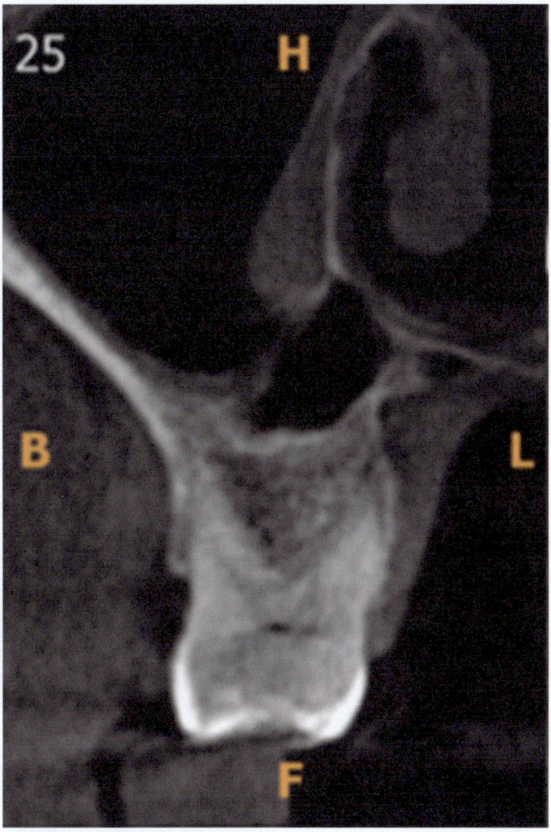

Fig. 5.2 Adequate inter radicular bone for housing the implant (Type A socket)

5.2.1 Case Selection

The following factors must be considered while choosing a case for a maxillary molar PET procedure.

Indications

1. Firm unrestorable maxillary molar: Broken down teeth which were previously endodontically treated and are unrestorable with a long-term definitive crown due to a lack of ferrule should be selected.
2. Absence of a periapical lesion: The selected teeth should not have a periapical lesion. A small periapical lesion in relation to the palatal root maybe acceptable since the palatal root will be completely extracted during the process [14].
3. Divergent roots with adequate inter-radicular bone. A correct prosthetically driven position for a maxillary molar is such that the implant trajectory emerges from the central fossa of the tooth to be replaced [4, 15]. To successfully achieve that, a robust inter-radicular bone is necessary to place the implant in that position and achieve good primary stability for the implant [16–18]. Type A or type B socket would be ideally suited for a PET procedure [13] (Figs. 5.5 and 5.6).

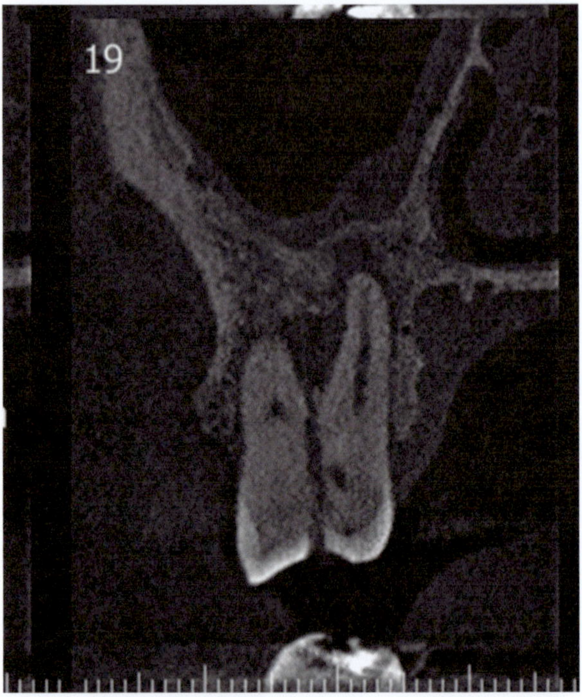

Fig. 5.3 Less inter radicular bone for housing the implant (Type B socket)

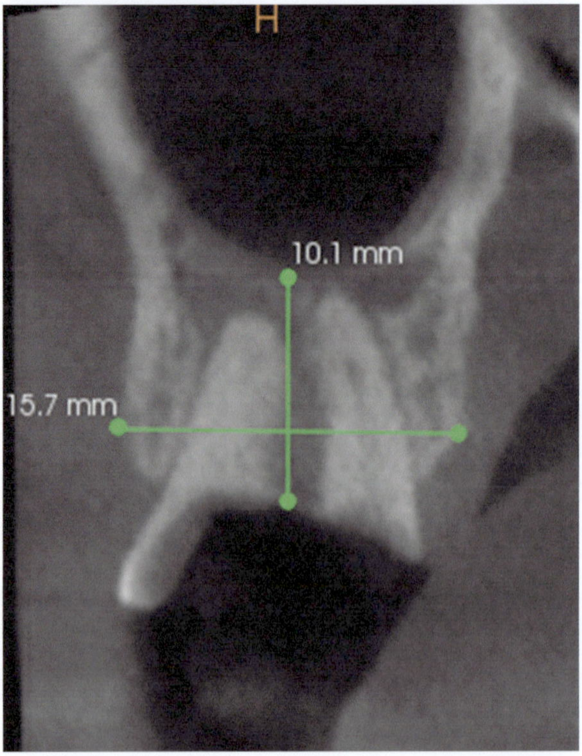

Fig. 5.4 Absence of any inter radicular bone (Type C socket)

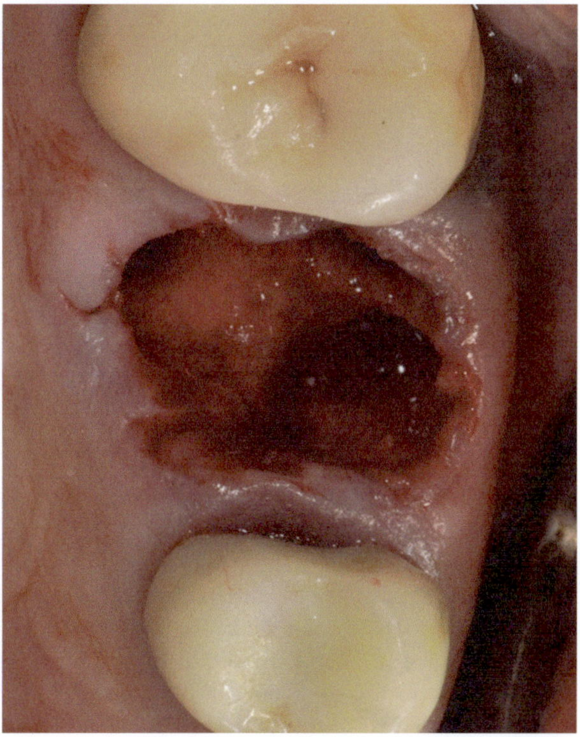

Fig. 5.5 Example of adequate inter-radicular bone in a maxillary molar

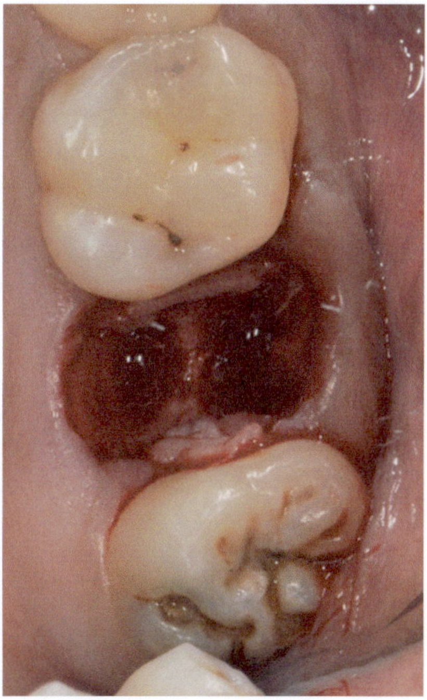

Fig. 5.6 Example of insufficient inter-radicular bone

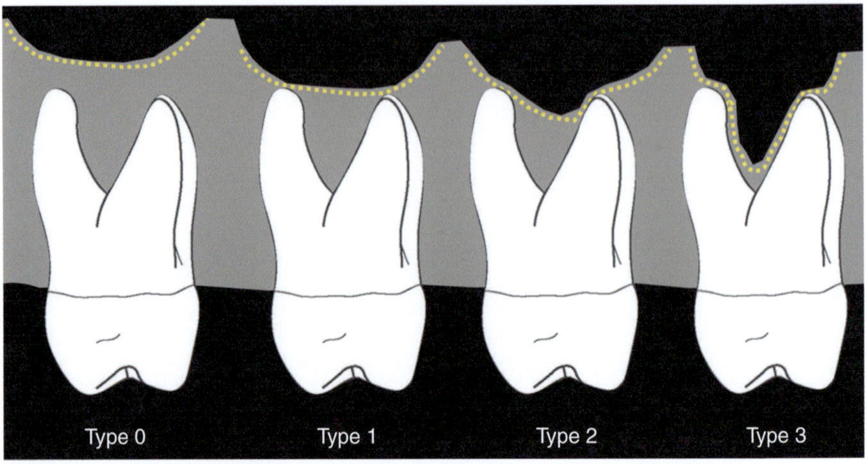

Fig. 5.7 Relationship between maxillary molar roots and maxillary sinus floor [10]

4. Adequate bone apical to the roots below the floor of the sinus: Since a large part of the implant may not be surrounded by native bone at the time of placement, it is necessary to have adequate bone apical to the roots to achieve primary stability of the implant [19, 20]. Jung and Cho have classified the relationship between the floor of the maxillary sinus and its proximity to the roots of maxillary molars. Type 0 and Type 1 as illustrated in Fig. 5.7 are suitable for an immediate implant placement in the molar [10]. Whereas Type 2 and Type 3 would require a simultaneous sinus lift and grafting procedure along with the post-extraction immediate implant placement.

Contraindications

1. Mobile teeth: As for single-rooted teeth, periodontally compromised teeth with mobility are absolute contraindications for a PET procedure [21].
2. Absence of buccal bone: The success of the socket shield procedure is dependent on the intactness of the buccal bone to support the buccal roots after sectioning [22]. In the absence of buccal bone, the shield has a high risk of becoming mobile after the sectioning, leading to an inevitable failure.
3. Heavily pneumatized maxillary sinuses: Pneumatization of the sinus floor brings the sinus floor closer to the roots of the maxillary teeth [23, 24]. This limits the amount of bone available for immediate post-extraction implant placement (Fig. 5.8). An indirect sinus lift and augmentation is necessary in such situations, which adds to the overall complexity of the case. The authors are not in favor of this modality to minimize the risks of complications and failures. However, a staged socket shield procedure as suggested by Glocker et al. can be attempted along with socket grafting. Implant placement can be delayed in such scenarios until bone regeneration is achieved in the socket.

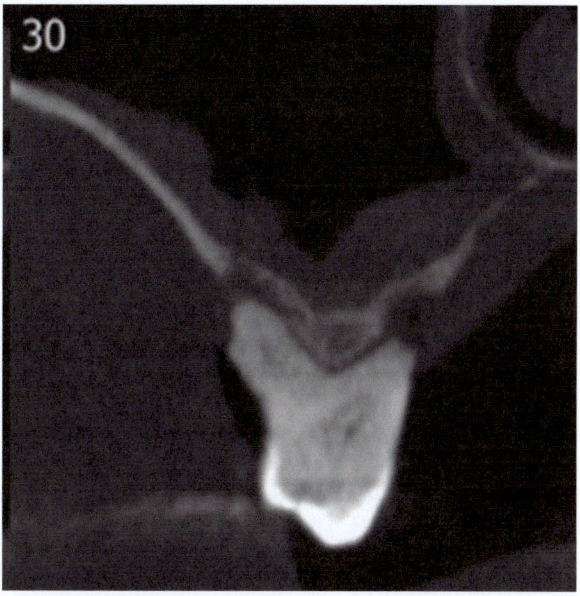

Fig. 5.8 Example of a molar with periapical lesion, absence of labial bone, and a pneumatized maxillary sinus

4. Fused teeth roots with little palatal bone: Closely approximated roots or completely fused roots (Type C socket) also limit the amount of available bone for placing the implant and for achieving adequate primary stability.

5.2.2 Step by Step Procedure

The step-by-step procedure for a maxillary molar socket shield is as follows:

1. Decoronation of the tooth is carried out up to the level of marginal gingiva using a carbide bur on a high-speed water-cooled drill.
2. A long shank carbide bur is used to section the palatal root from the buccal roots. The cut is made in the mesiodistal direction to completely separate the tooth into two halves.
3. A second cut is made in the bucco-palatal direction to separate the mesio-buccal root from the disto-buccal root.
4. The palatal root is carefully extracted using fine-tipped elevators and root forceps.
5. The following steps can be performed after raising a small flap for better visualization. However, the authors prefer a flapless approach [25].
6. The buccal roots are trimmed down to the level of the bone using large diamond burs on a high-speed drill.
7. The buccal roots are further sectioned in the mesio-distal direction to create a buccal and a palatal section using long shank carbide drills. The section should pass through the root canal space so as to reach the apex of the roots.
8. The palatal sections of both roots are carefully mobilized using periotomes or very fine-tipped elevators.

9. The palatal fragments of the two buccal roots are extracted.
10. The buccal shields are now thinned out using round diamond burs all the way to the apex.
11. A radiograph is taken to verify that the gutta percha is completely removed and that the apices of the roots are eliminated during the shield preparation [26].
12. A bevel is made on the internal aspect of the shields to provide space for the prosthesis [8].
13. The buccal shields are carefully checked for their intactness. In case any shield is mobile, it should be extracted and the case should be treated like a conventional post-extraction implant placement [27].
14. The socket is curetted and rinsed thoroughly with normal saline.
15. The inter-radicular bone is probed to verify its integrity.
16. The osteotomy preparation is initiated in the furcation to get the implant in the most suitable prosthetically driven position. A surgical stent maybe used at this stage to aid in achieving the right position and angulation.
17. The authors prefer using the osseodensification drills for preparation of the implant sites [28]. The use of these drills optimizes the osteotomy sites by densifying the bone surrounding the osteotomy. Alternatively, the dedicated drills recommended by the implant manufactures could be used for implant site preparation.
18. After the osteotomy is complete, the implant is placed in its final position under controlled torque.
19. The implant stability is measured using an ISQ device.
20. The depth of the implant should be at the level of the furcation or approximately 1 mm below the level of the buccal bone and shields.
21. A bone substitute material may be placed in the remaining socket space. The authors choose not to graft the gap and have not found any significant compromise in the final outcome [29]. A collagen sponge can be placed instead of a bone graft, which will help in retaining the blood clot.
22. A wide healing abutment or a customized healing abutment is fixed over the implant to seal the periphery of the socket.
23. If a flap is raised, it is sutured using monofilament suture material.
24. A postoperative radiograph is taken to verify the implant position.

Postoperatively, the patient is put on a 0.12% chlorhexidine mouth rinse for 2 weeks. Sutures are removed after 8–10 days.

After 3 months the implant stability is checked using the ISQ device. If found to be satisfactory, a definitive restoration is fabricated.

5.3 PET Case for the Maxillary First Molar

The following case presents a socket shield procedure for a maxillary first molar and a maxillary first premolar that were indicated for extractions (Fig. 5.9, 5.10, 5.11, 5.12, 5.13, 5.14, 5.15, 5.16, 5.17, 5.18, 5.19, 5.20, 5.21, 5.22, and 5.23).

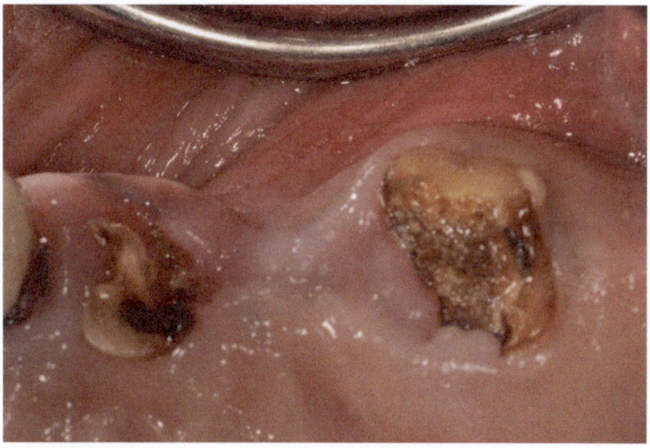

Fig. 5.9 Preoperative situation. Fractured unrestorable teeth 25 and 27

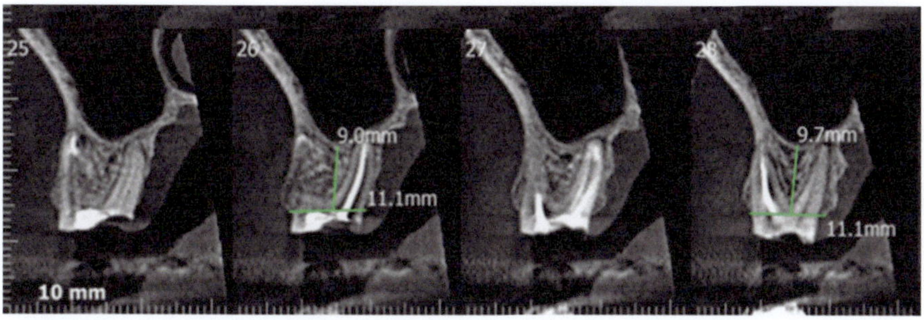

Fig. 5.10 Cross-sectional view of tooth 26

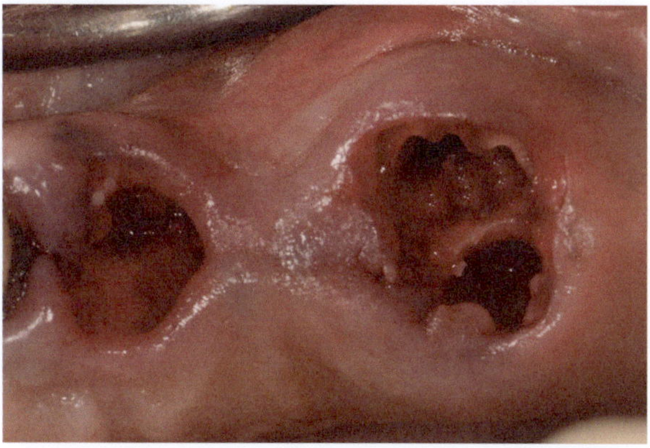

Fig. 5.11 After extraction of palatal root and shield preparation of buccal roots

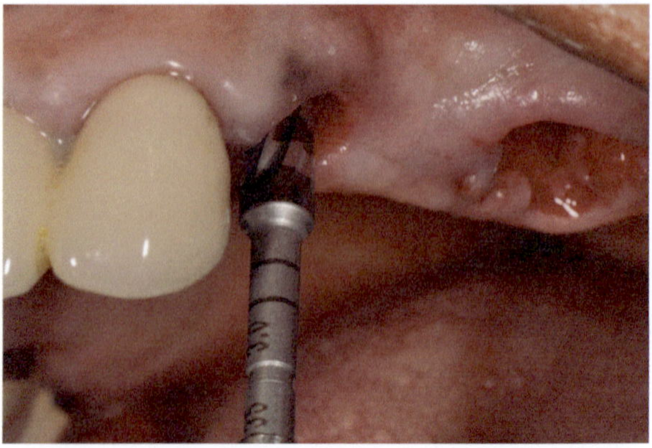

Fig. 5.12 Implant site preparation using Densah drills (Vesah Inc., U.S.A.)

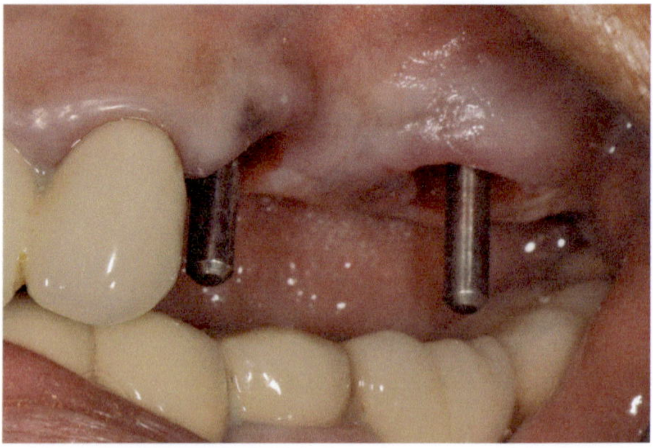

Fig. 5.13 Prosthetically driven position

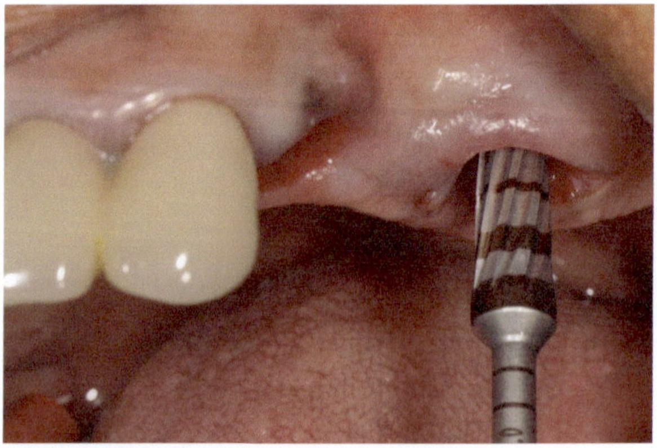

Fig. 5.14 Site optimization using Densah drills (Versah Inc., U.S.A.)

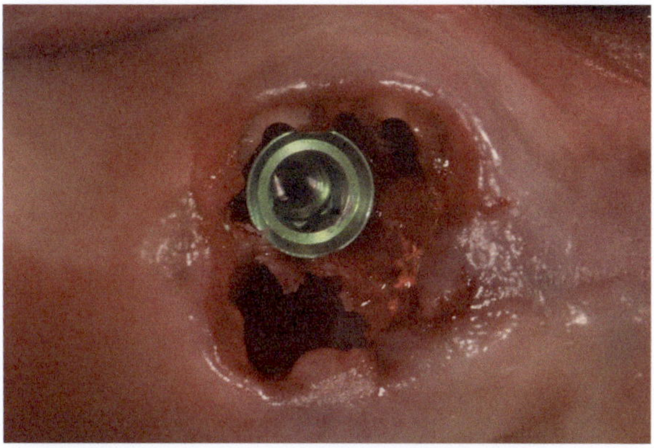

Fig. 5.15 Implant placed in furcation bone (Biohorizons Inc., U.S.A.)

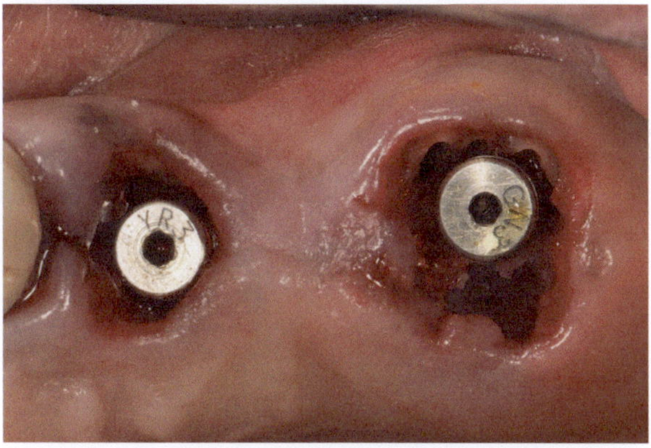

Fig. 5.16 Healing abutments

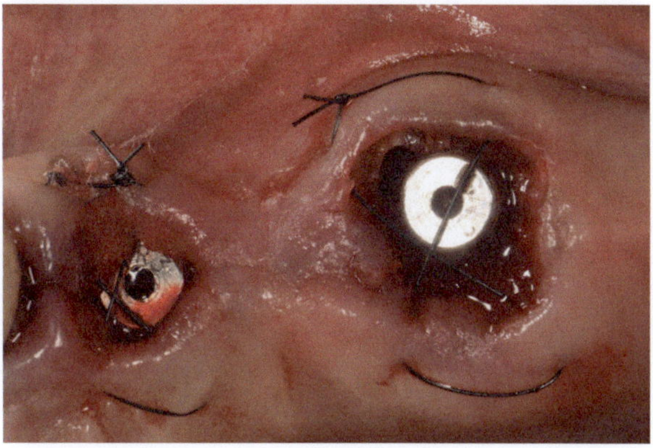

Fig. 5.17 Collagen sponge and sutures

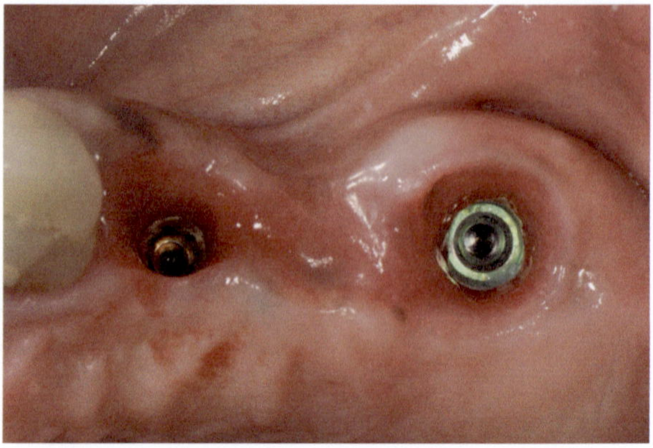

Fig. 5.18 Healing after 3 months

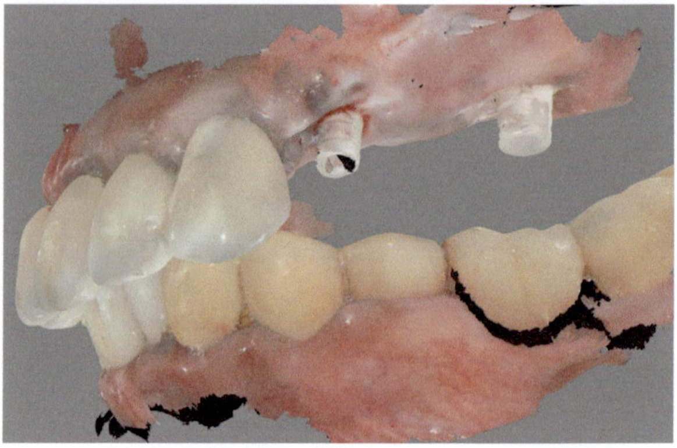

Fig. 5.19 Digital impression for the fabrication of the final restoration

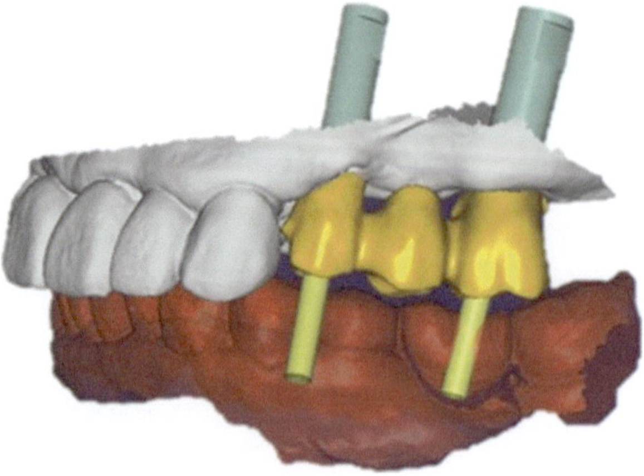

Fig. 5.20 Planning for final restoration

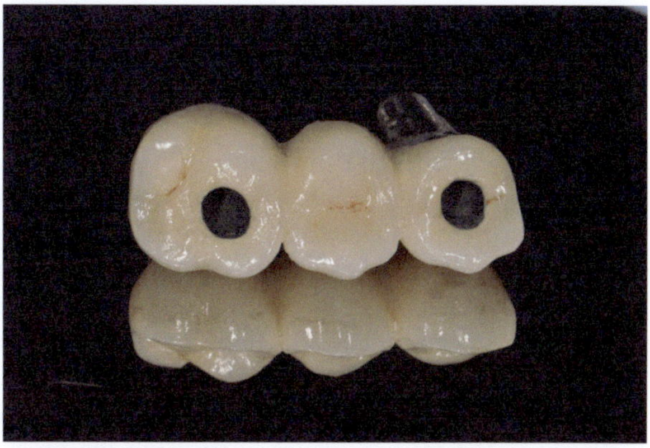

Fig. 5.21 Screw-retained metal-ceramic restoration

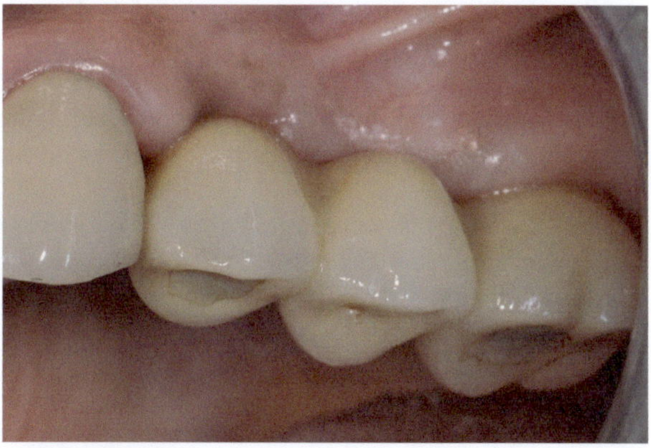

Fig. 5.22 Definitive restoration. Note good tissue contours around implant sites

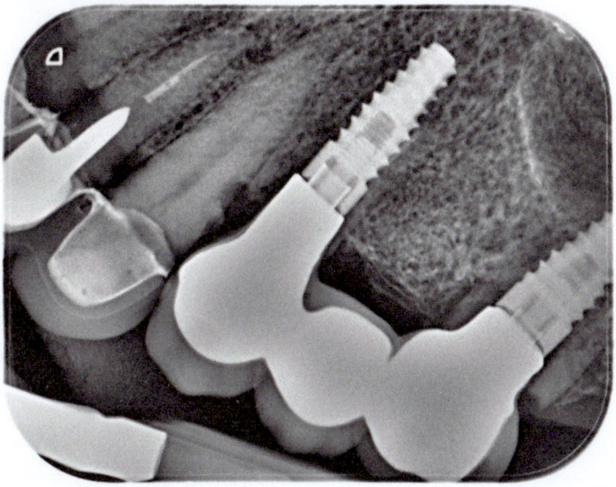

Fig. 5.23 Postoperative radiograph

5.4 PET for the Mandibular Molar

The PET procedure for the mandibular molar also follows a similar sequence like the maxillary first molar. The only difference is the number of roots present. The procedure is carried out using a flapless approach or with the help of a mini flap design. Adequate bone volume beyond the apex of the root should be present to avoid inadvertent damage to the inferior alvolar nerve. In cases where the inferior alveolar nerve is close to the apices of the teeth, an immediate placement should be avoided. Instead a staged socket shield procedure (Glocker's technique) should be considered (Chap. 6). In the mandibular molar, both roots are sectioned mesiodistally and the lingual fragments are carefully extracted. A good amount of inter-radicular bone is necessary for implant placement. The implant is placed in the inter-radicular bone using the osseodensification procedure in order to preserve the available bone. This helps in achieving adequate primary stability. Following this step, a customized healing abutment or a wide design of a stock healing abutment is chosen. The gap between the implant and shield can be filled with a piece of collagen sponge, which will help in retaining the blood clot for future bone formation within the socket. Alternatively, a bone substitute material, which will completely resorb, is placed and covered with a collagen membrane.

The following case demonstrates the socket shield procedure for a mandibular first molar, indicated for extraction. Adequate amount of inter-radicular bone allowed immediate implant placement (Figs. 5.24, 5.25, 5.26, 5.27, 5.28, 5.29, 5.30, 5.31, 5.32, and 5.33).

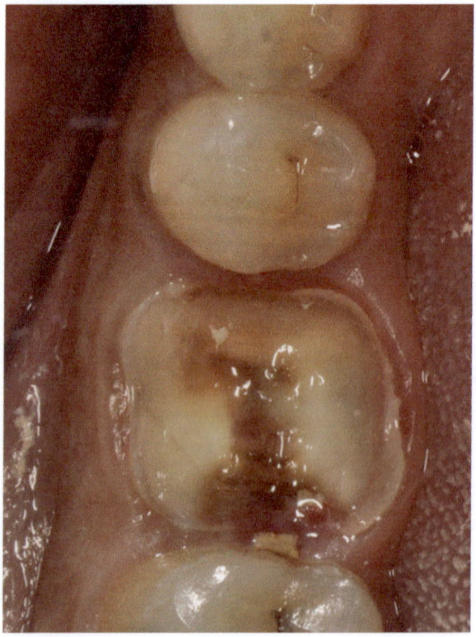

Fig. 5.24 Badly broken down non-restorable mandibular first molar

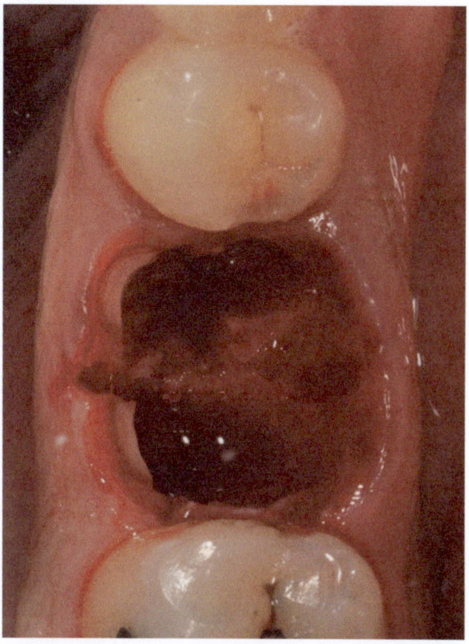

Fig. 5.25 Extraction of lingual part of the roots and shield preparation

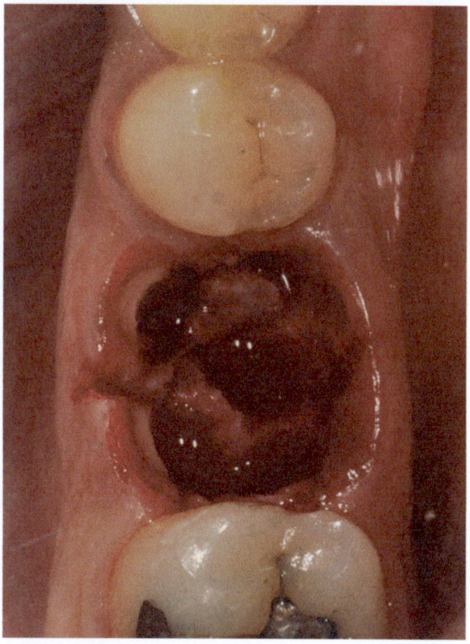

Fig. 5.26 Ossteotomy preparation in inter-radicular bone

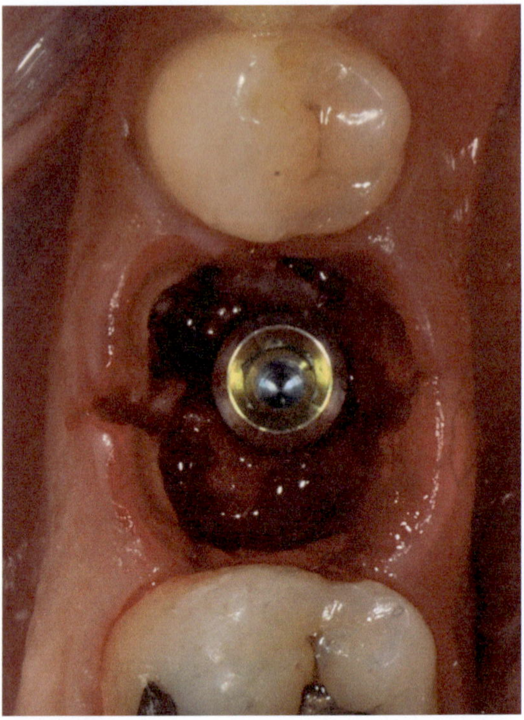

Fig. 5.27 Prosthetically driven implant placement in the inter-radicular bone (Biohorizons Inc., U.S.A.)

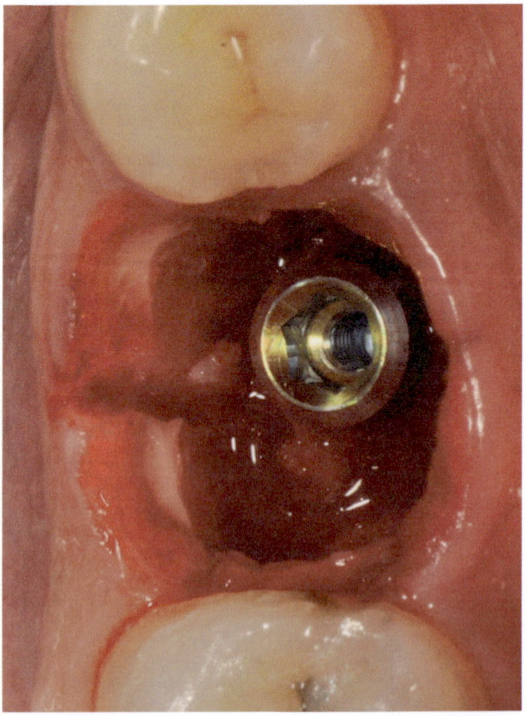

Fig. 5.28 Adequate space between shield and implant surface to allow bone fill

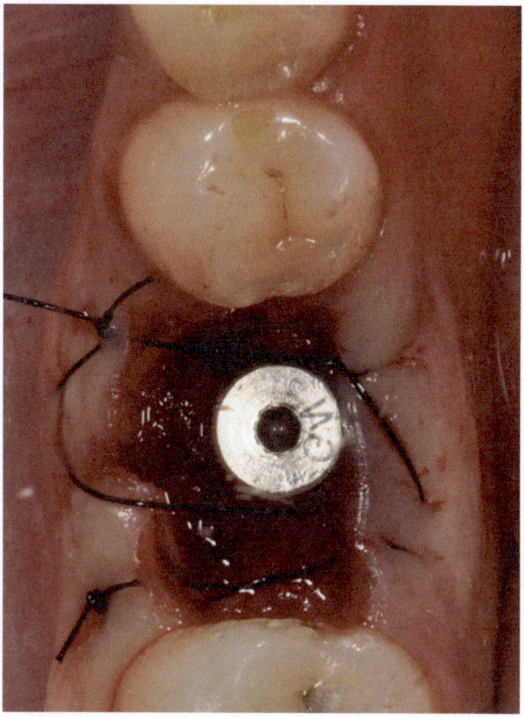

Fig. 5.29 Collagen plug in socket, healing abutment on the implant and horizontal mattress sutures

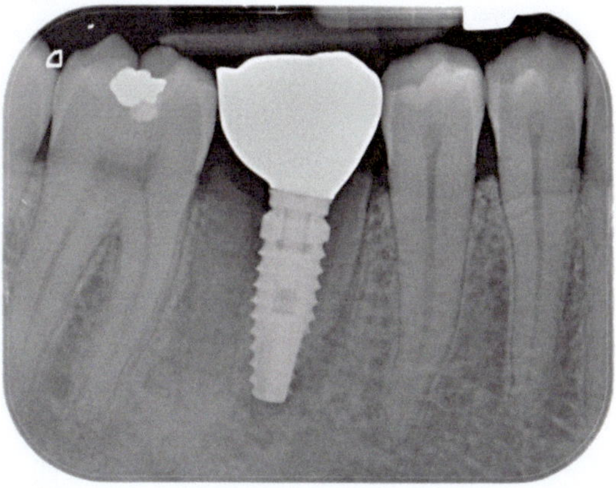

Fig. 5.30 Postoperative radiograph depicting implant placement and the shields

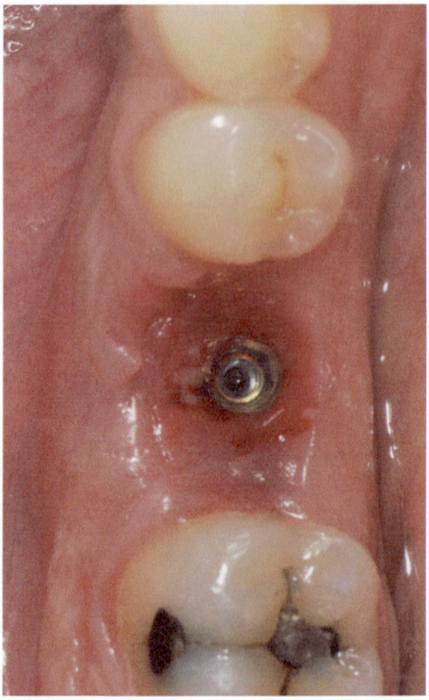

Fig. 5.31 Healed site 3 months after implant placement displaying absence of any buccal collapse of tissue

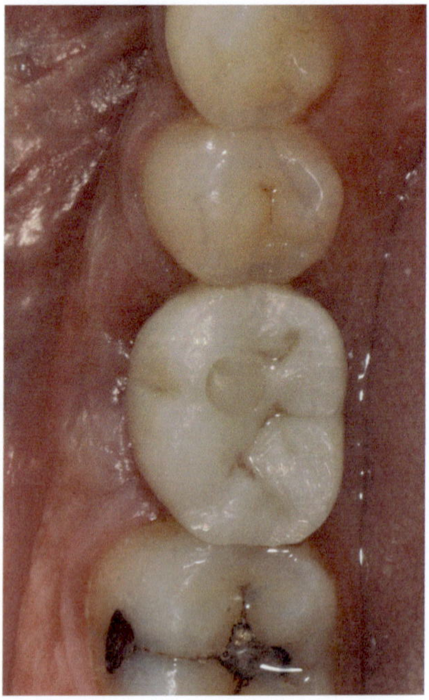

Fig. 5.32 Screw retained zirconia crown

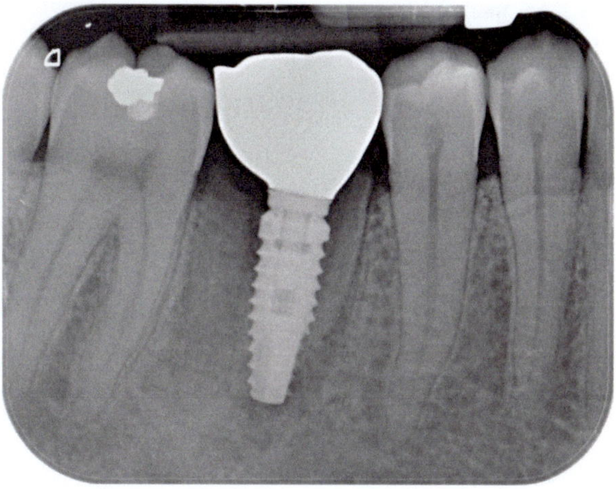

Fig. 5.33 Post operative radiograph

5.5 PET for the Maxillary First Premolar

Maxillary first premolars can have a single root or two roots. The procedure for the maxillary first premolar with two roots is similar to the molar. The palatal root is extracted. This is followed by the shield preparation of the buccal root and placement of the implant in the furcal bone. Since the first premolar is within the esthetic zone, an accurate three-dimensional placement is critical for achieving a good emergence profile and a satisfactory esthetic outcome of the final restoration. A chairside provisional restoration can be fabricated if the patient desires. However, the crown should be kept well short of the opposing dentition to avoid detrimental forces, which could result in a failure.

The definitive restoration can replace the provisional restoration after 3 months (Figs. 5.34, 5.35, 5.36, 5.37, 5.38, and 5.39).

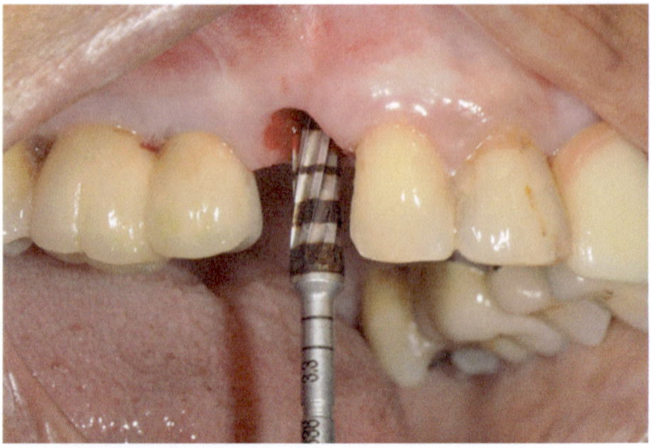

Fig. 5.34 Implant site preparation with the Densah drills (Versah Inc., U.S.A.)

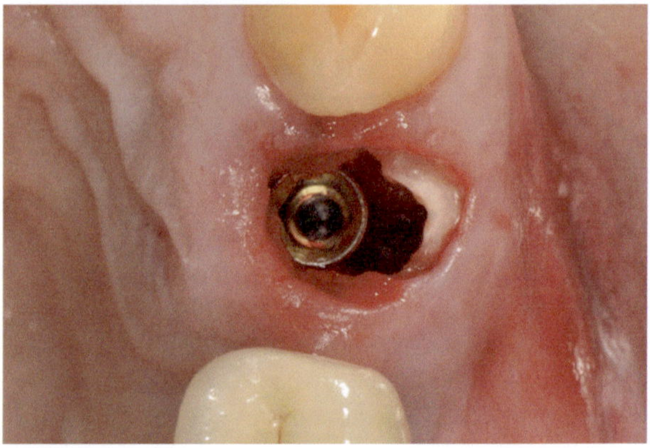

Fig. 5.35 Implant in its final position (Biohorizons Inc., U.S.A.)

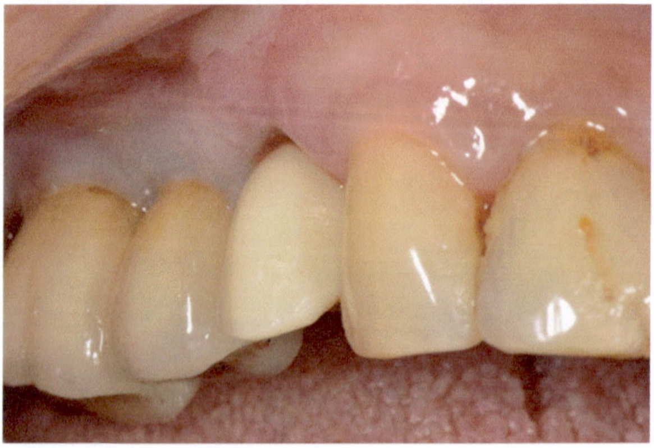

Fig. 5.36 Screw-retained acrylic provisional restoration

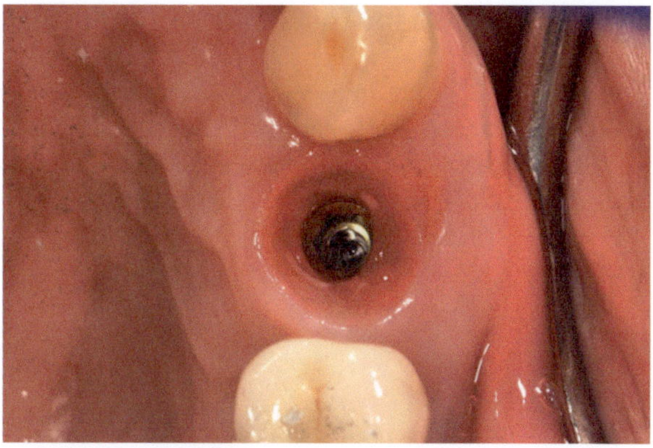

Fig. 5.37 After 3 months

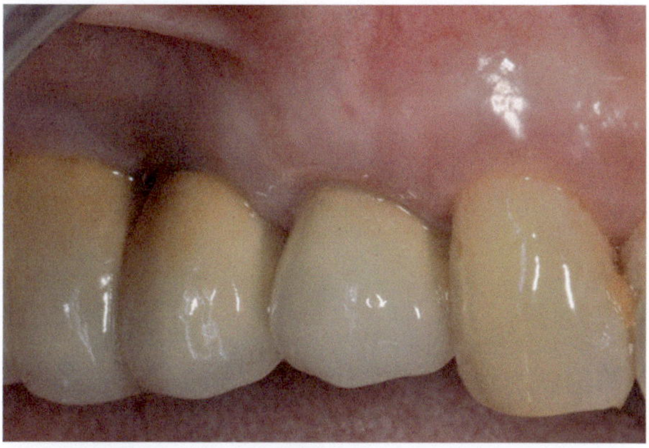

Fig. 5.38 Definitive screw-retained metal-ceramic restoration

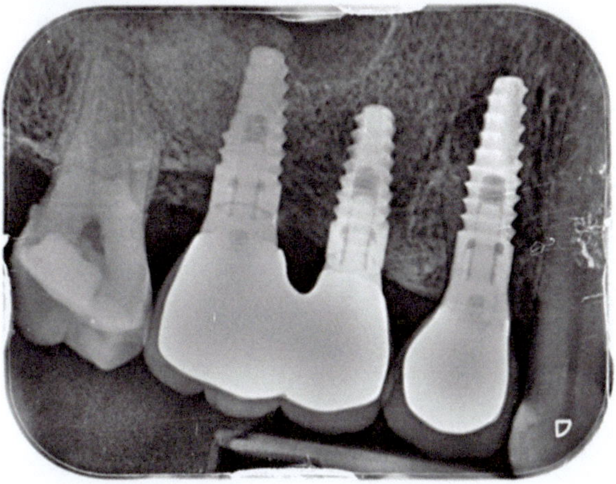

Fig. 5.39 Postoperative radiograph

5.6 PET Case for Two Maxillary Premolars

Teeth 24 and 25 were indicated for extractions. A mini flap was raised to enable good visualization of the interdental peak of bone and to allow accurate shield preparation. After shield preparations on both teeth, implants were placed in the socket in a prosthetically driven position. Healing abutments were placed and the mini flap was sutured (Figs. 5.40 and 5.41).

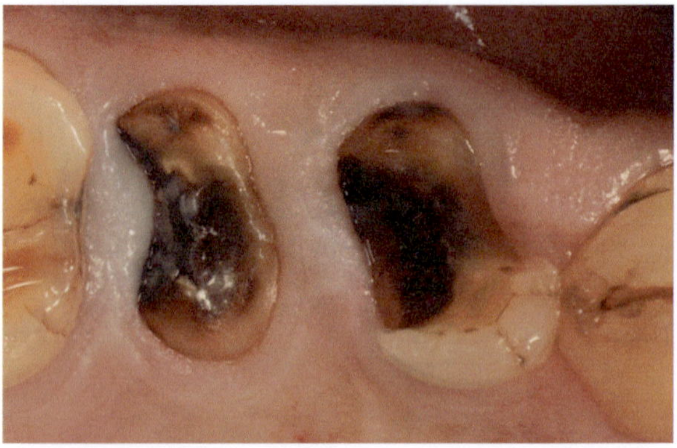

Fig. 5.40 Unrestorable maxillary premolars

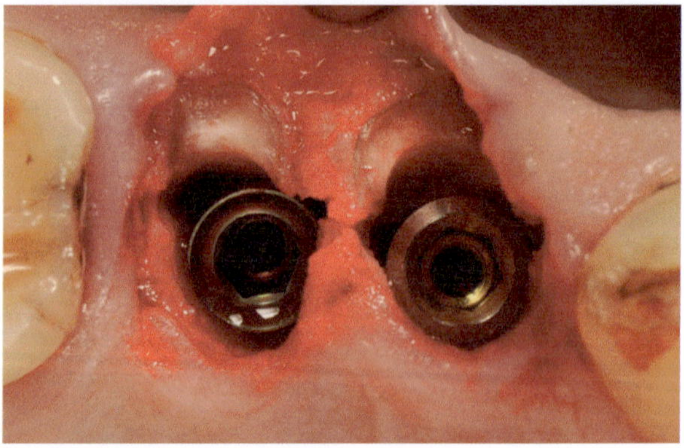

Fig. 5.41 Mini flap design for shield preparation and implant placement allows good visualization of the operative field

5.7 Conclusion

Prevention of crestal and horizontal bone loss has been on the top of the wish list for clinicians. Even in the posterior segments of the mouth, preservation of the bone around implants plays a crucial role in long-term maintenance of healthy tissues. Utilizing PET concepts for multirooted teeth is an effective and economical way of attaining this goal.

Achieving prosthetically driven positions for post-extraction implant placements in maxillary molar and premolar sites requires high degree of expertise. Such a procedure should be attempted only by clinicians who have previous experience with immediate post-extraction implant placements in multirooted teeth and with PET procedures in single-rooted teeth.

Acknowledgement Illustrations by: Udatta Kher.

References

1. Araujo MG, Lindhe J. Dimensional ridge alterations following tooth extraction. An experimental study in the dog. J Clin Periodontol. 2005;32:212–8.
2. Araujo M, Sukekava F, Wennstrom J, Lindhe J. Ridge alterations following implant placement in fresh extraction sockets: an experimental study in the dog. J Clin Periodontol. 2006;32:645–52.
3. Cardaropoli G, Araujo M, Lindhe J. Dynamics of bone tissue formation in tooth extraction sites: an experimental study in dogs. J Clin Periodontol. 2003;30:809.
4. Fugazzotto PA. Implant placement at the time of maxillary molar extraction: technique and report of preliminary results of 83 sites. J Periodontol. 2006;77:302.
5. Cardaropoli D, Tamagnone L, Roffredo A, et al. Relationship between the buccal bone plate thickness and the healing of postextraction sockets with/without ridge preservation. Int J Periodont Restor Dent. 2014;34:211.
6. Bäumer D, Zuhr O, Rebele S, Hürzeler M. Socket shield technique for immediate implant placement – clinical, radiographic and volumetric data after 5 years. Clin Oral Implants Res. 2017;28(11):1450–8.
7. Zhang Z, Dong Y, Yang J, Xu R, Deng F. Effect of socket-shield technique on alveolar ridge soft and hard tissue in dogs. J Clin Periodontol. 2019;46:256–63.
8. Schwimer CW, et al. The socket-shield technique at molar sites: a proof-of-principle technique report. J Prosthet Dent. 2019;121(2):229–33.
9. Kilic C, Kamburoglu K, Yuksel SP, Ozen T. An assessment of the relationship between the maxillary sinus floor and the maxillary posterior teeth root tips using dental cone-beam computerized tomography. Eur J Dent. 2010;4:462–7.
10. Jung YH, Cho BH. Assessment of the relationship between the maxillary molars and adjacent structures using cone beam computed tomography. Imaging Sci Dent. 2012;42(4):219–24.
11. Akin R. A new concept in maintaining the emergence profile in immediate posterior implant placement: the anatomic harmony abutment. J Oral Maxillofac Surg. 2016;74(12):2385–92.
12. Finelle G, Sanz-Martín I, Knafo B, Figué M, Popelut A. Digitalized CAD/CAM protocol for the fabrication of customized sealing socket healing abutments in mmediate implants in molar sites. Int J Comput Dent. 2019;22(2):187–204.
13. Smith RB, Tarnow DP. Classification of molar extraction sites for immediate dental implant placement: technical note. Int J Oral Maxillofac Implants. 2013;28:911.

14. Quirynen M. An infected jawbone site compromising successful osseointegration. Periodontol. 2003;33:129–44.
15. Clarizio LF. Techniques for ideal implant placement in the mandibular first molar position. Compend Contin Educ Dent. 1995;16(8):806–13.
16. Rebele SF, Zuhr O, Hürzeler MB. Pre-extractive interradicular implant bed preparation: case presentations of a novel approach to immediate implant placement at multirooted molar sites. Int J Periodontics Restorative Dent. 2013;33(1):88–95.
17. Fugazzotto PA. Implant placement at the time of maxillary molar extraction: treatment protocols and report of results. J Periodontol. 2008;79(2):216–23.
18. Tizcareño MH, Bravo-Flores C. Anatomically guided implant site preparation technique at molar sites. Implant Dent. 2009;18(5):393–401.
19. Romanos GE. Surgical and prosthetic concepts for predictable immediate loading of oral implants. J Calif Dent Assoc. 2004;32:991–1001.
20. Amato F, Polara G. Immediate implant placement in single-tooth molar extraction sockets: a 1- to 6-year retrospective clinical study. Int J Periodontics Restorative Dent. 2018;38(4):495–501.
21. Mitsias ME, Siormpas KD, Kotsakis GA, Ganz SD, Mangano C, Iezzi G. The root membrane technique: human histologic evidence after five years of function. Biomed Res Int. 2017;2017:7269467.
22. Elian N, Cho S-C, Froum S, Smith RB, Tarnow DP. Simplified socket classification and repair technique esthetic dentistry. PPAD. 2007;19:99–104.
23. Del Fabro M, Testori T. Maxillary sinus surgery and alternatives in treatment: anatomy of the maxillary sinus. Berlin: Quintessence; 2009.
24. Sharan A, Madjar D. Maxillary sinus pneumatization following extractions: a radiographic study. Int J Oral Maxillofac Implants. 2008;23:48–56.
25. Bersani E, Coppede AR, de Paula Pinto Prata HH. Immediate loading of implants placed in fresh extraction sockets in the molar area with flapless and graftless procedures: a case series. Int J Periodontics Restorative Dent. 2010;30:291–9.
26. Gluckman H, Salama M, Du Toit J. Partial extraction therapies (PET). Part 1: maintaining alveolar ridge contour at pontic and immediate implant sites. Int J Periodontics Restorative Dent. 2016;36:681–7.
27. Gluckman H, Du Toit J, Salama M. The socket-shield technique to support buccofacial tissues at immediate implant placement: a case report and review of the literature. Int Dent Africa Ed. 2015;5:1–7.
28. Huwais S, Meyer EG. A novel osseous densification approach in implant osteotomy preparation to increase biomechanical primary stability, bone mineral density, and bone-to-implant contact. Int J Oral Maxillofac Implants. 2017;32:27–36.
29. Kumar PR, Kher U. Shield the socket: procedure, case report and classification. J Indian Soc Periodontol. 2018;22(3):266–72.

Variations of the Socket Shield Procedure

6

Udatta Kher and Payal Rajender Kumar

Abstract

The socket shield procedure has seen numerous modifications in the technique to suit different clinical situations. Cuspids, which have extra-long roots, require special attention during sectioning and implant placement. A variation in the socket shield technique is necessary while treating adjacent teeth needing PET procedures. Small peri-apical lesions in teeth needing PET procedures can be managed successfully with a modified approach. A C-shaped socket shield is a departure from the conventional shield design, but has significant benefits while replacing 2 adjacent teeth with implants. A staged socket shield procedure is indicated in a few cases where simultaneous implant placement is not feasible. This chapter deals with all the deviations from the original technique and will help the reader understand the finer nuances of the procedure.

6.1 Introduction

The socket shield technique is constantly evolving, and its applications are now increasing beyond the maxillary incisors. With the success of the procedure being clinically validated with numerous cases for maxillary incisors, it is crucial to expand the scope of the technique and apply it to other teeth as well. Also, as time has passed by, minor variations in shield preparation have been proposed that can help achieve better interdental fill of gingival tissues and even allow infected sites to be incorporated within the gamut of the procedure.

U. Kher (✉)
Only Smiles Dental Centre, Mumbai, India

P. Rajender Kumar
Private Practice, New Delhi, India

U. Kher, A. Tunkiwala (eds.), *Partial Extraction Therapy in Implant Dentistry*,
https://doi.org/10.1007/978-3-030-33610-3_6

The following clinical situations require a slightly different approach from the one mentioned in the previous chapter.

1. Socket shield technique for maxillary canines.
2. SS for management of a fenestration defect.
3. C shaped shields for adjacent implant sites.
4. Adjacent teeth socket shields.
5. Staged socket shield procedure(Glocker's technique).

6.2 Socket Shield Procedure for Maxillary Canines

The canine roots pose a unique challenge while performing a socket shield procedure. The length of the roots is often too long [1] for sectioning with conventional long shank burs on a contra-angled handpiece (Table 6.1).

Generally, the head of the contra-angled handpiece tends to come in contact with adjacent teeth, which then acts as an obstruction to the further advancement of the long shank bur. There are various ways in which this can be tackled. Firstly, a straight carbide bur on a straight handpiece can be used to section the extra-long root. Alternatively, the apical tip of the canine can be drilled away by accessing it through an esthetic buccal flap [3, 4]. The length of the root that can be accessed with the long shank bur, is first cut away. Then the apex of the canine is removed by accessing it through a remote incision, as is done for an apicoectomy surgery.

Another challenge in shield preparation for maxillary cuspids is that the length of the root often exceeds the length of the implants (Table 6.1). Hence achieving primary stability in such cases can be quite challenging. Having good palatal bone for anchoring the implant is mandatory in such situations [5]. An extra-long root and absence of adequate palatal bone will complicate the procedure since the implant may come very close to the shield while being torqued in place.

6.2.1 Case 1

The following cases demonstrate the methods used to overcome the challenges posed by maxillary cuspids.

A 40-year-old female patient reported with a fractured maxillary canine. The tooth had been previously restored with a post, core, and a crown. It was nonrestorable and needed to be extracted. A socket shield procedure with a simultaneous

Table 6.1 Average length of human teeth (mms) [2]

	Maxilla	Mandible
Central incisors	22.5	20.7
Lateral incisors	22.0	21.1
Canines	26.5	25.6
First premolars	20.6	21.6
Second premolars	21.5	22.3
First molars	20.8	21.0
Second molars	20.0	19.8

implant placement and provisional crown was performed. The provisional restoration was replaced with a porcelain fused to metal restoration after osseointegration (Figs. 6.1, 6.2, 6.3, 6.4, 6.5, 6.6 and 6.7).

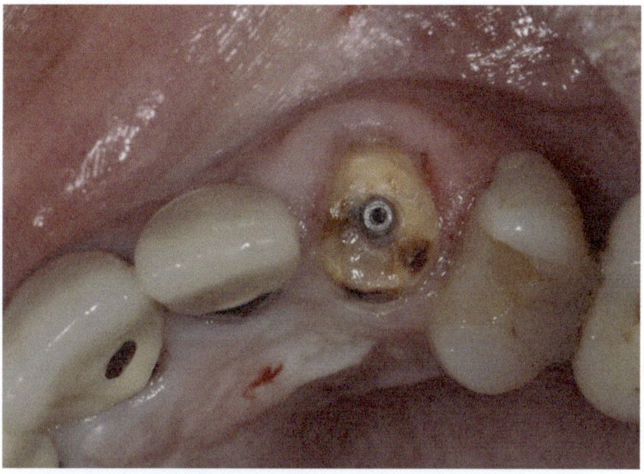

Fig. 6.1 Fractured maxillary canine

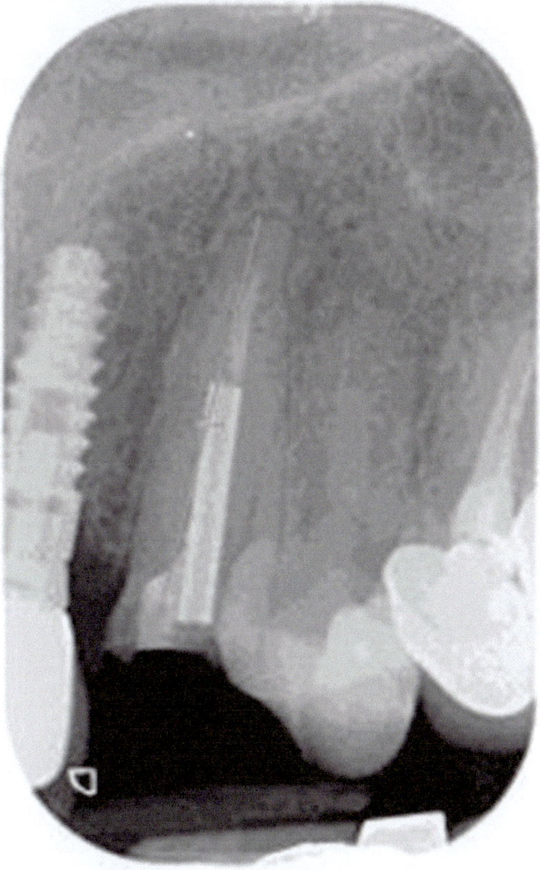

Fig. 6.2 Extra-long canine root

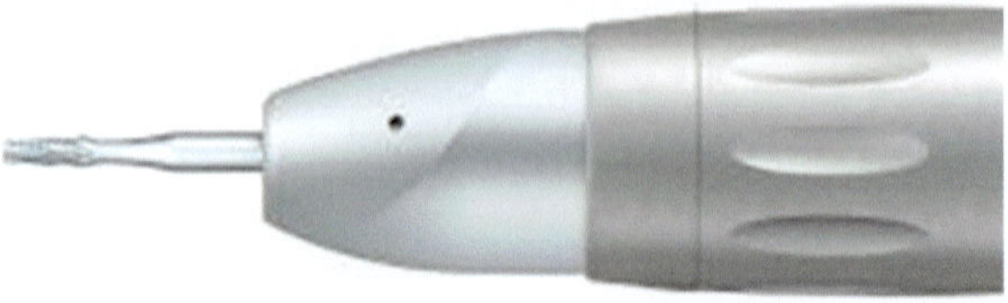

Fig. 6.3 Straight handpiece and straight carbide bur

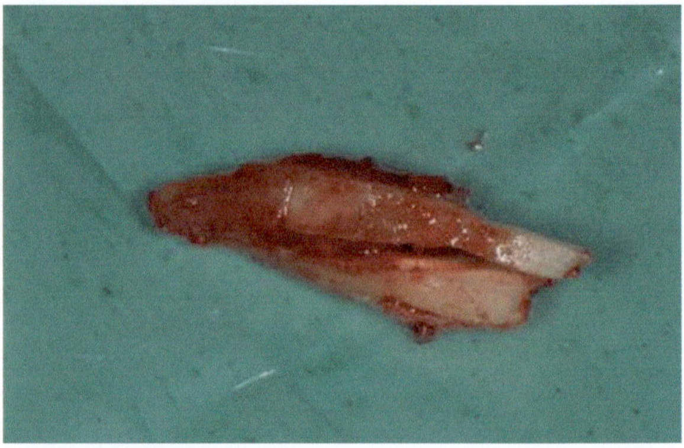

Fig. 6.4 After sectioning and extraction. Note apex of root in the palatal root section

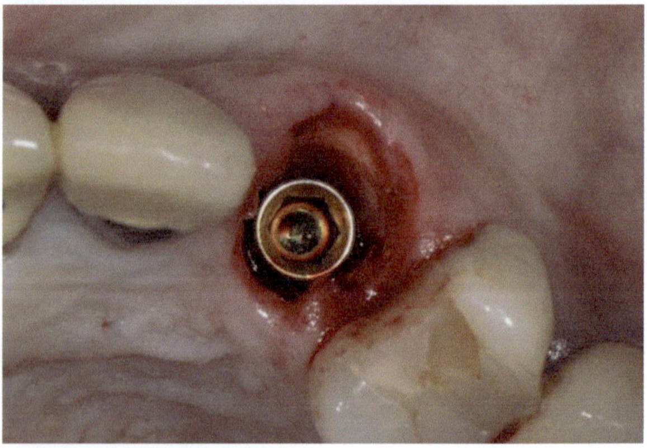

Fig. 6.5 Implant placed in palatal bone

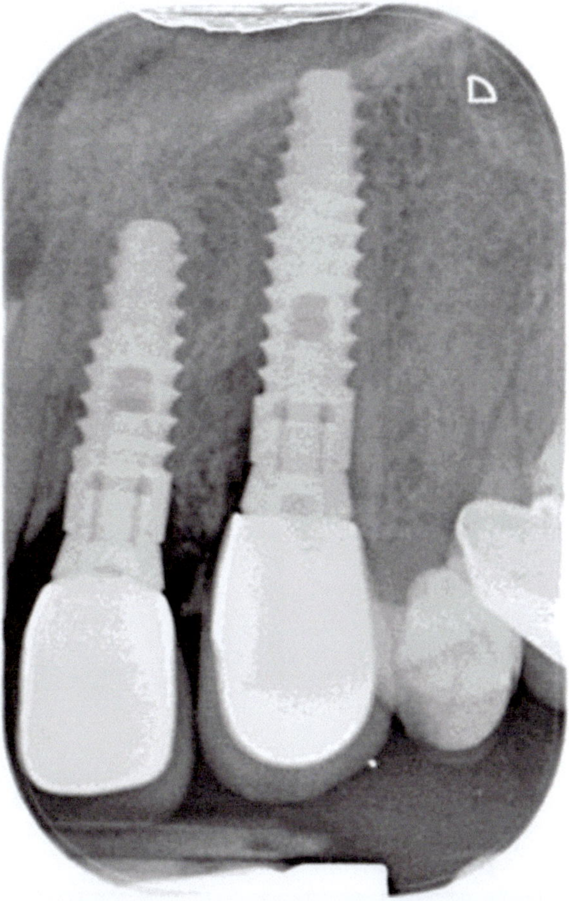

Fig. 6.6 Postoperative radiograph after placement of definitive restoration

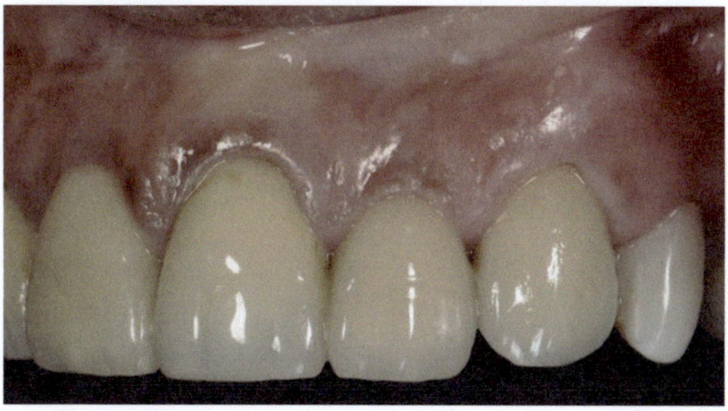

Fig. 6.7 Screw-retained metal ceramic restoration

6.2.2 Case 2

In the following case the apex of the canine could not be accessed even with the longest drill. Hence a vestibular flap was used to extract the apex of the root. Implant placement was done in the palatal wall of the socket. The apical defect created was grafted using a bone substitute material and a collagen membrane. A semilunar incision is made in the vestibule similar to the apicectomy incision. An apicectomy in conjunction with debridement of the peri-apical lesion can be accomplished using this approach [3, 4]. The defect can be grafted using a bone substitute material and a collagen membrane (Figs. 6.8, 6.9, 6.10, 6.11 and 6.12).

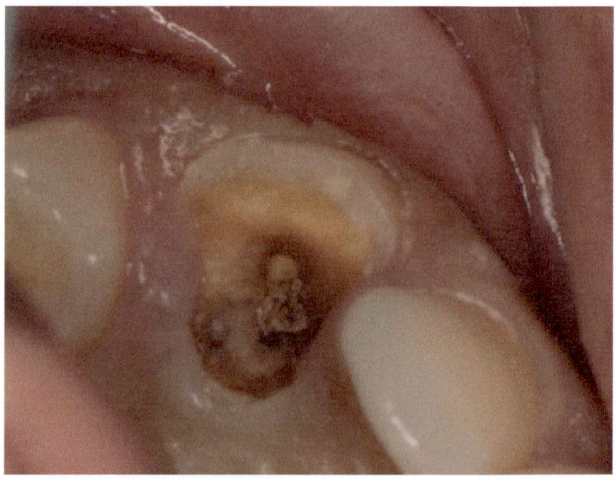

Fig. 6.8 Fractured canine

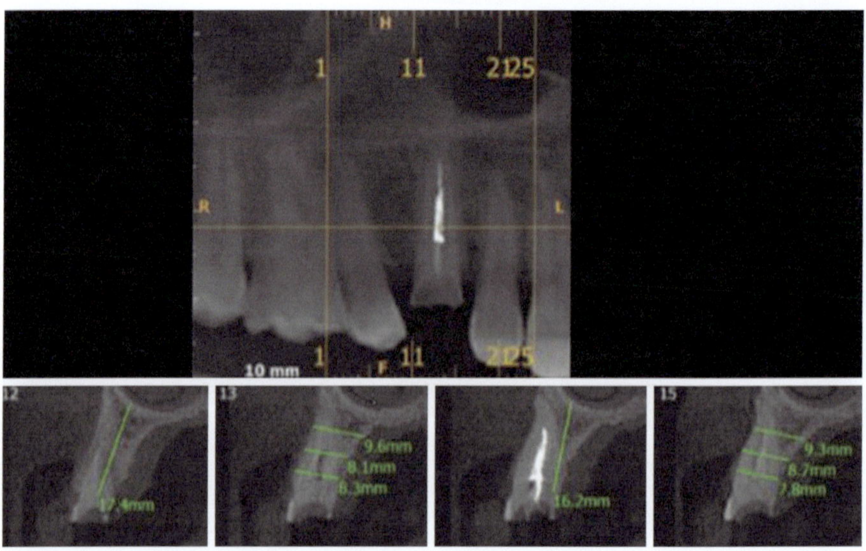

Fig. 6.9 Long canine root

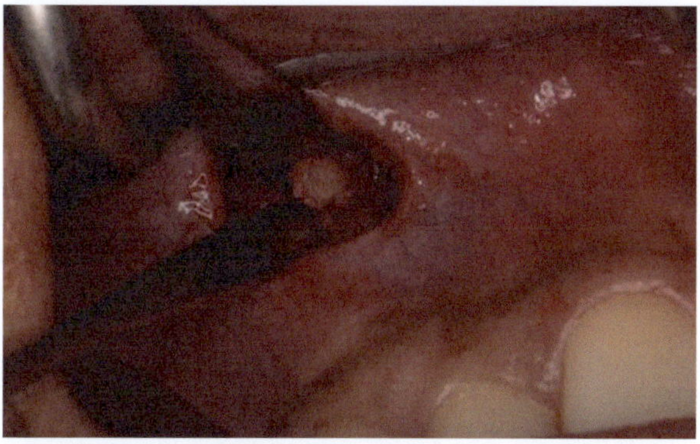

Fig. 6.10 Apicoectomy of canine root tip through a vestibular incision

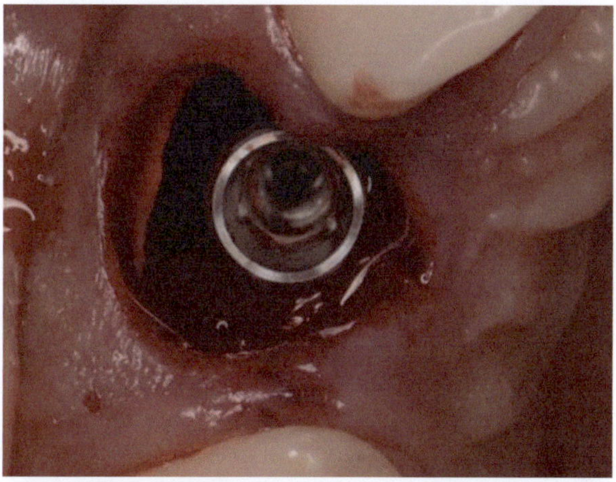

Fig. 6.11 Socket shield and implant placement

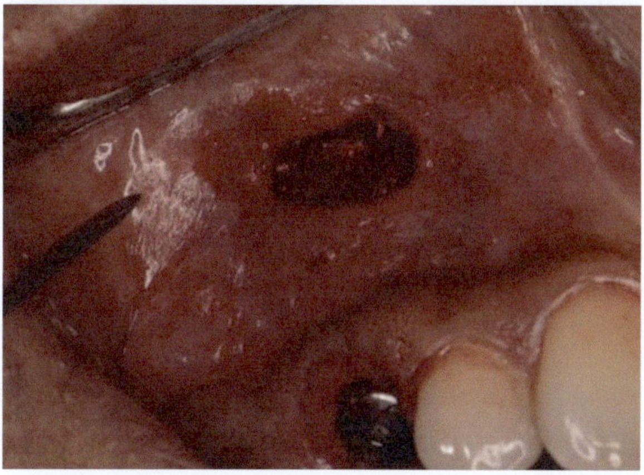

Fig. 6.12 Grafting apical defect with an allograft

6.3 Socket Shield for a Fenestration Defect

Removal of the apex of the root and thorough curettage of the peri-apical lesion is mandatory for the success of the procedure. Leaving behind pathology will severely affect the outcome of the treatment [6]. In case of a peri-apical lesion, it may be challenging to completely remove it through the socket after preparation of the shield. In such cases, an esthetic buccal flap maybe utilized to gain access to the apical region [7–9].

6.3.1 Case 3

The following case report demonstrates the application of the esthetic buccal flap for the management of a fenestration defect in conjunction with a socket shield procedure.

A 62-year-old lady reported with pain in maxillary left central incisor. The affected tooth was previously endodontically treated and had a crown with open margins. The peri-apical X-ray and CBCT revealed a well-circumscribed peri-apical lesion approximately 4 mm in diameter. The marginal labial bone was intact. The apical area had a fenestration.

The tooth was firm and had healthy periodontium. The treatment plan was to perform a socket shield procedure with implant placement and an immediate provisional restoration.

The challenge in the case was to completely remove the apical portion of the root and carry out the peri-apical debridement.

The partial extraction and preparation of the shield was performed as described in Chap. 2. After that a semilunar incision was made 2 mm below the mucogingival junction curving superiorly into the vestibular area. A full thickness mucoperiosteal flap was raised to expose the fenestration defect. Using a round diamond bur on a high-speed handpiece, the apical tip of the root was sectioned. Following that, a thorough curettage of the peri-apical are area was done.

The implant site was prepared on the palatal wall of the socket following the conventional technique of immediate implant placement and a tapered internal hex implant (Biohorizons Inc., U.S.A.) was placed. The apical defect was grafted with a Xenograft (Biooss, Geistlisch, Switzerland) and a collagen membrane (Bioguide, Geistlisch, Switzerland) was trimmed and adapted over it. The closure of the semilunar incision was carried out using 4.0 PTFE sutures (Cytoplast, Osteogenics, U.S.A.).

A temporary PEEK abutment (Biohorizons Inc., U.S.A.) was attached to the implant. The screw access hole was blocked with a piece of PTFE and a provisional crown was fabricated out of a silicone index and Protemp 4 (3M Inc., U.S.A.). The temporary crown was trimmed and polished. The gap between the implant and the shield did not receive any graft material. The crown was torqued over the implant at 20 Ncm. The access hole was blocked with PTFE tape and flowable composite resin (3M Inc., U.S.A.).

After 6 months of healing time the definitive restoration was fabricated. The healing of the marginal tissues was excellent and there was complete resolution of the peri-apical infection as seen on the postoperative radiograph (Figs. 6.13, 6.14, 6.15, 6.16, 6.17, 6.18, 6.19, 6.20, 6.21, 6.22, 6.23, 6.24, 6.25, 6.26 and 6.27).

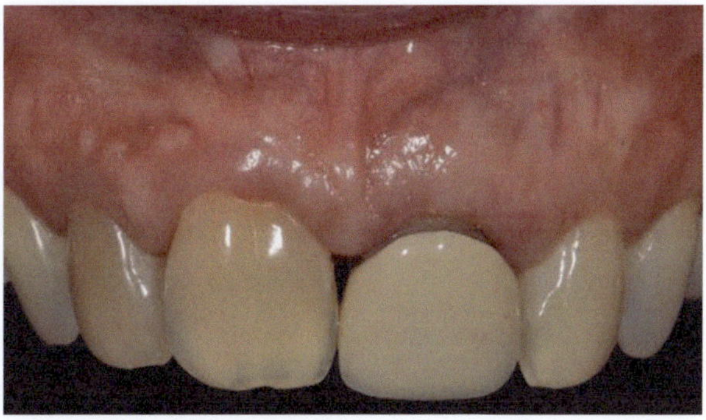

Fig. 6.13 Preoperative situation. Failing tooth #21

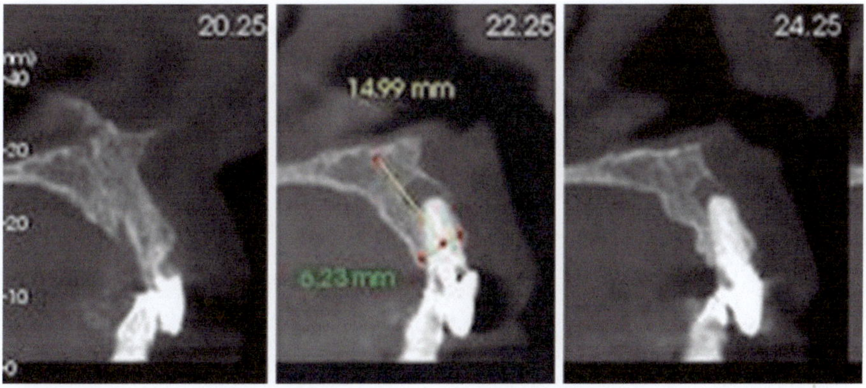

Fig. 6.14 Peri-apical infection in relation with tooth #21

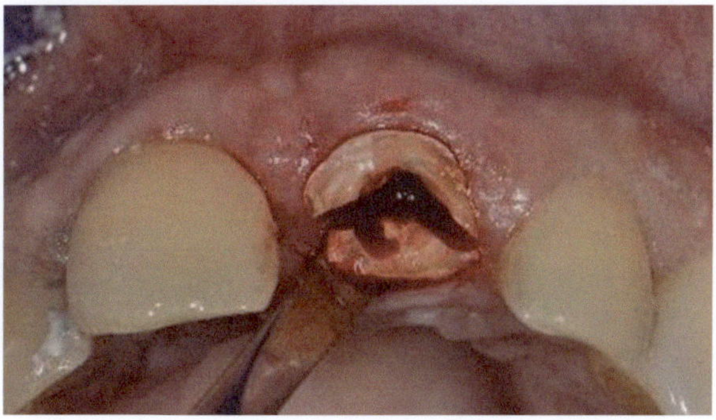

Fig. 6.15 Tooth sectioned and palatal fragment extracted

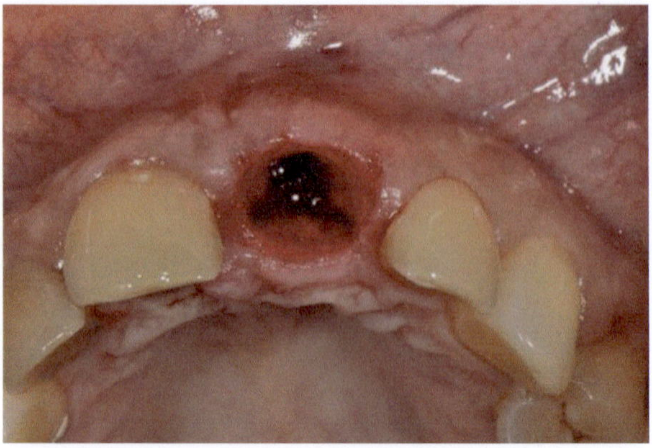

Fig. 6.16 Shield preparation completed

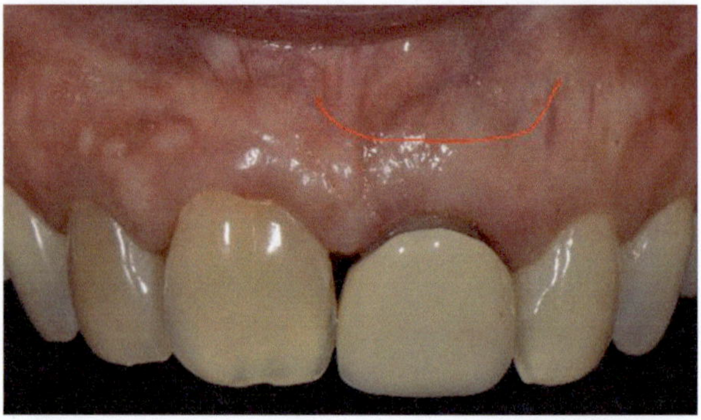

Fig. 6.17 Esthetic buccal flap incision outline

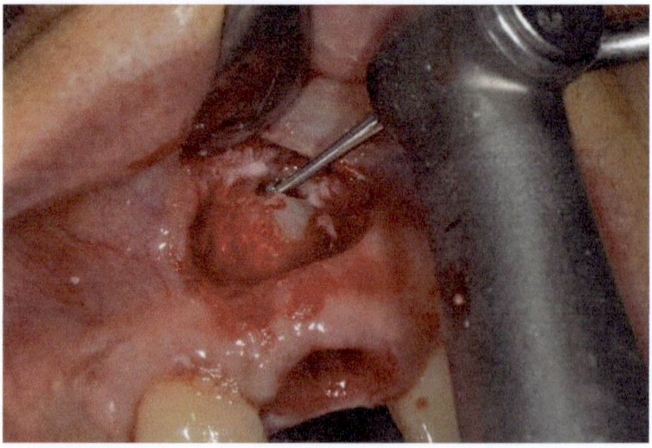

Fig. 6.18 Removal of root tip

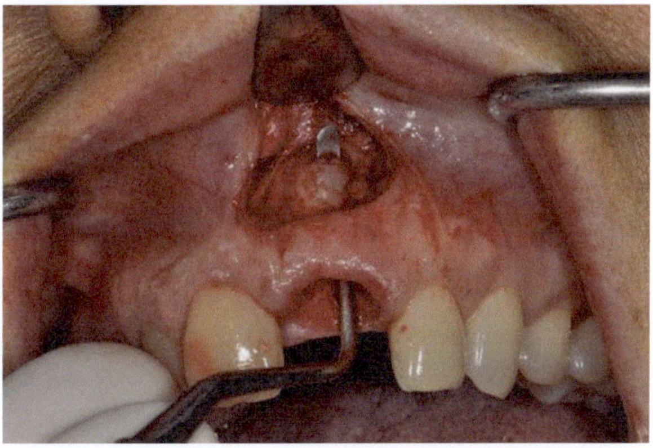

Fig. 6.19 Curettage of peri-apical granulomatous tissue

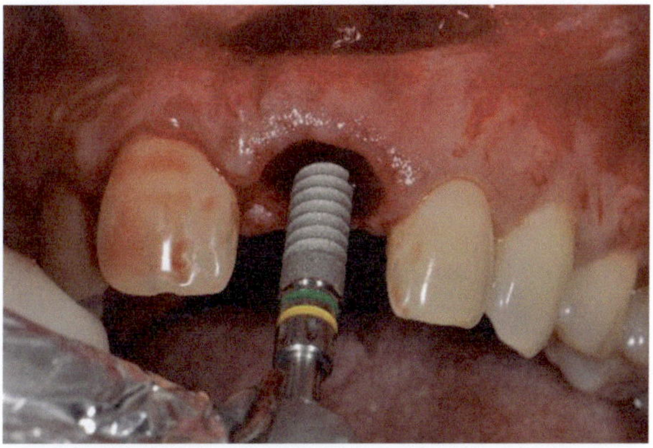

Fig. 6.20 Implant placement (Biohorizons Inc., U.S.A.)

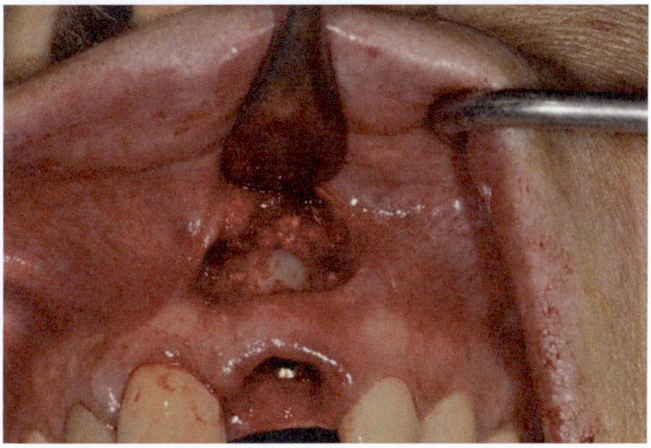

Fig. 6.21 Grafting of apical defect

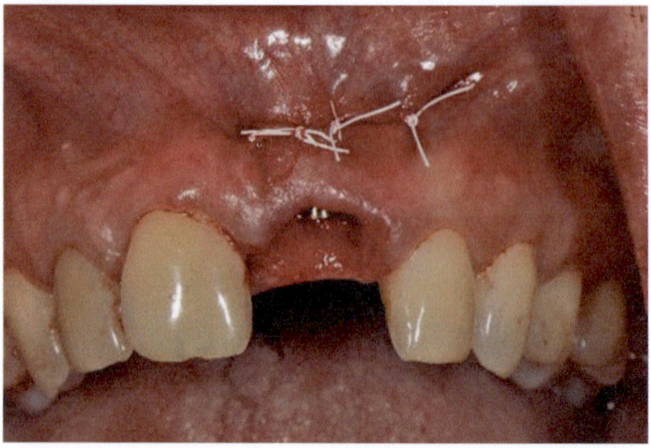

Fig. 6.22 Closure with interrupted sutures

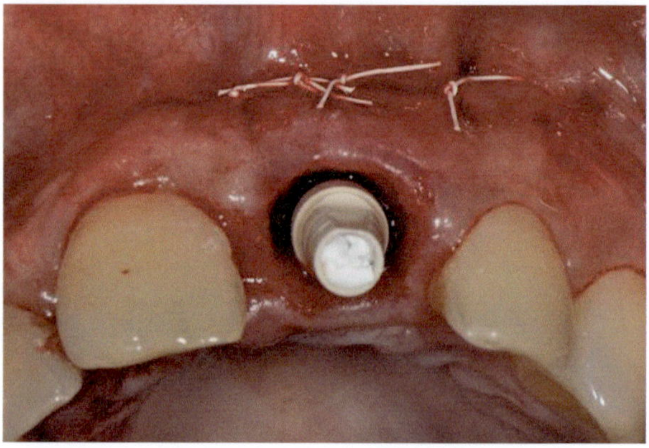

Fig. 6.23 Temporary PEEK abutment

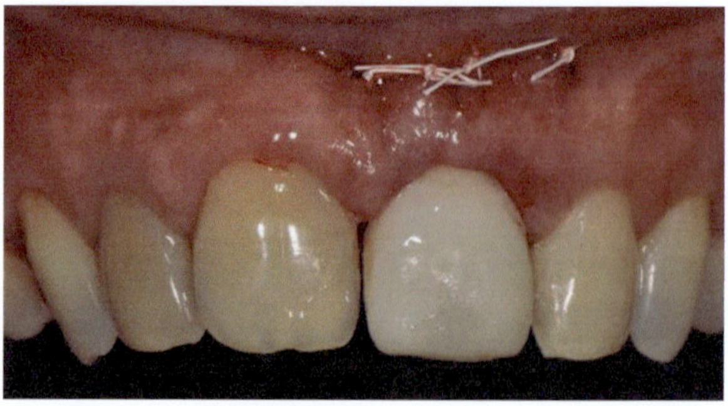

Fig. 6.24 Screw-retained provisional restoration

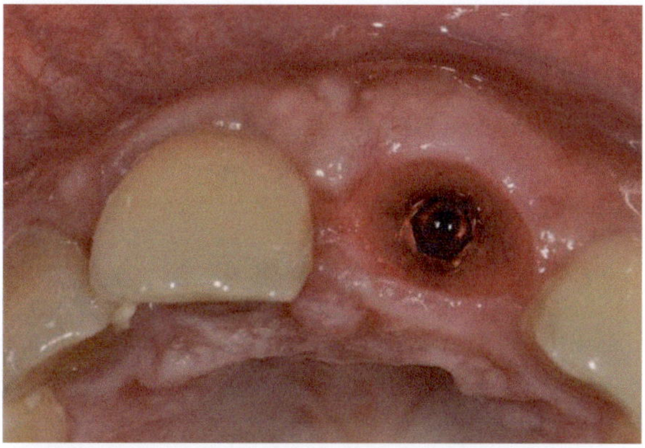

Fig. 6.25 Healing after 6 months

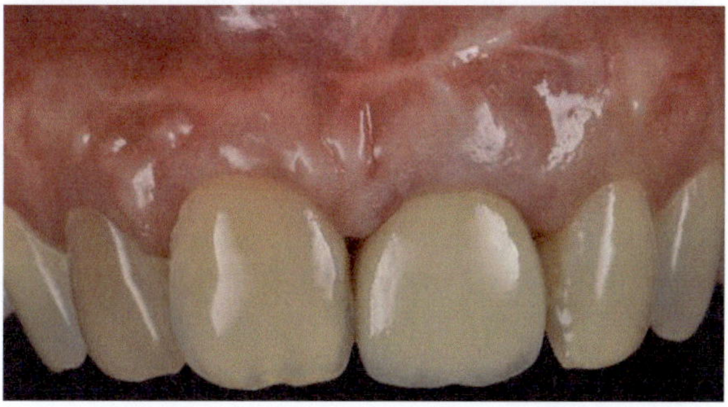

Fig. 6.26 Definitive restoration

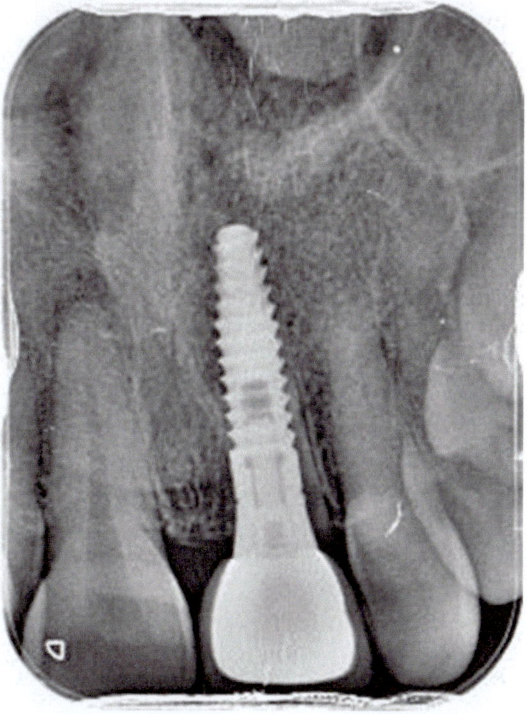

Fig. 6.27 Postoperative radiograph

6.4 Adjacent Teeth Socket Shields

One of the most useful indications for PET is when multiple adjacent teeth in the arch are involved [10]. The biggest challenges faced by clinicians is maintenance of the interdental papilla between adjacent implants [11]. The loss of bone peak between 2 adjacent implants leads to tissue loss resulting in the absence of the interdental papilla [12, 13]. Another issue with adjacent teeth missing is the loss of labial tissue contour. Very often such cases result in an esthetic failure due to the inevitable appearance of a dark triangle between adjacent crowns. To overcome the problem of dark triangles, clinicians need to resort to making the prostheses on adjacent implants with long connectors between them. This makes the teeth look unnatural and unaesthetic [14–16].

Various strategies such as use of scalloped implant designs [17–19] and staged implant placements done along with soft tissue grafting procedures have been suggested in literature to overcome the difficulties in maintaining interdental papilla between two adjacent implants [20–24]. The strategic placement of one implant and an adjacent pontic site with soft tissue grafting and an ovate pontic design has also been suggested [25, 26]. However, all these techniques have had limited success in clinical practice.

Adjacent teeth needing extractions managed with PET allows the preservation of the interdental bone, thus improving the prospects of having an intact papilla.

6.4.1 Case 4

The following case demonstrates the successful maintenance of the interdental tissue and good soft tissue contours between a lateral incisor and a canine needing extractions and implant supported restorations (Figs. 6.28, 6.29, 6.30, 6.31 and 6.32).

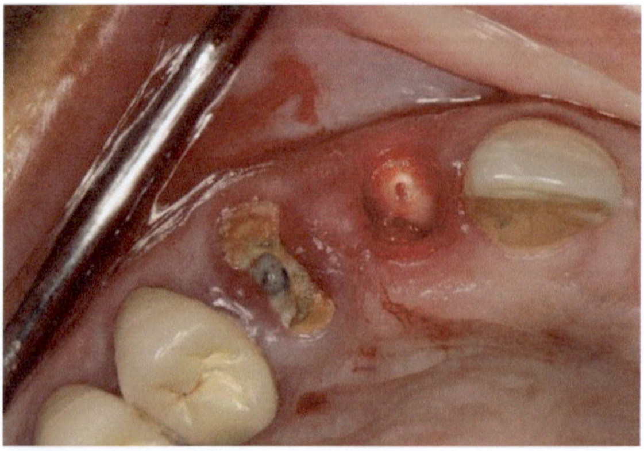

Fig. 6.28 Unrestorable teeth 12 and 13

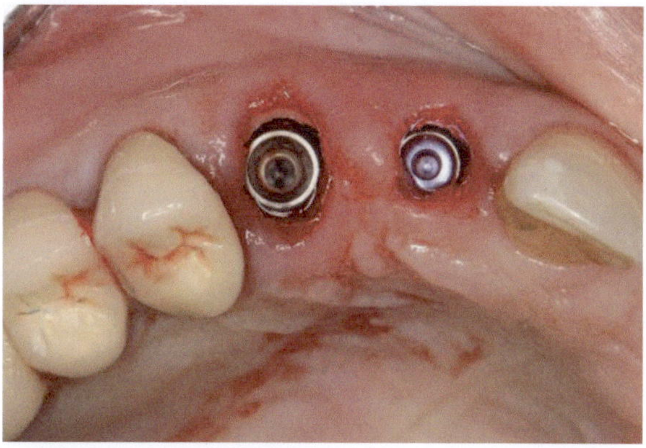

Fig. 6.29 Conventional shield preparation and implant placement (Osstem Implant Co., South Korea)

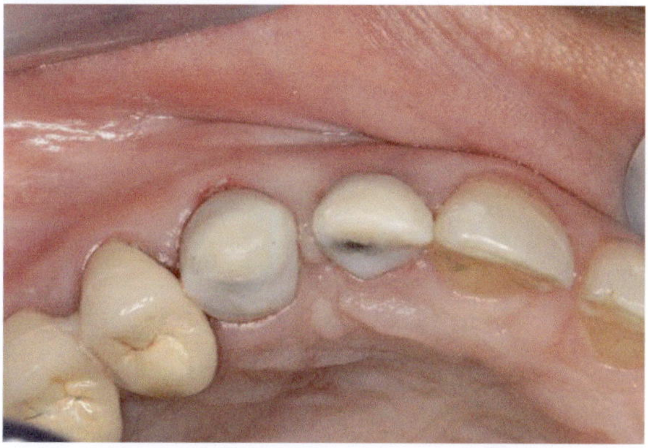

Fig. 6.30 Individual screw-retained provisional restorations made to support peri-implant soft tissue and interdental papilla

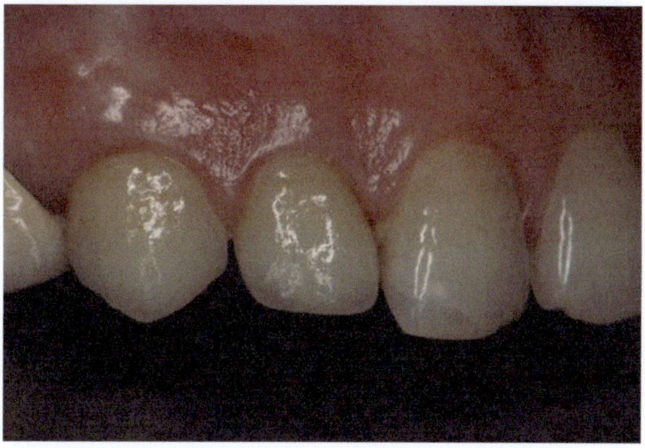

Fig. 6.31 Definitive crowns displaying excellent tissue health and contours

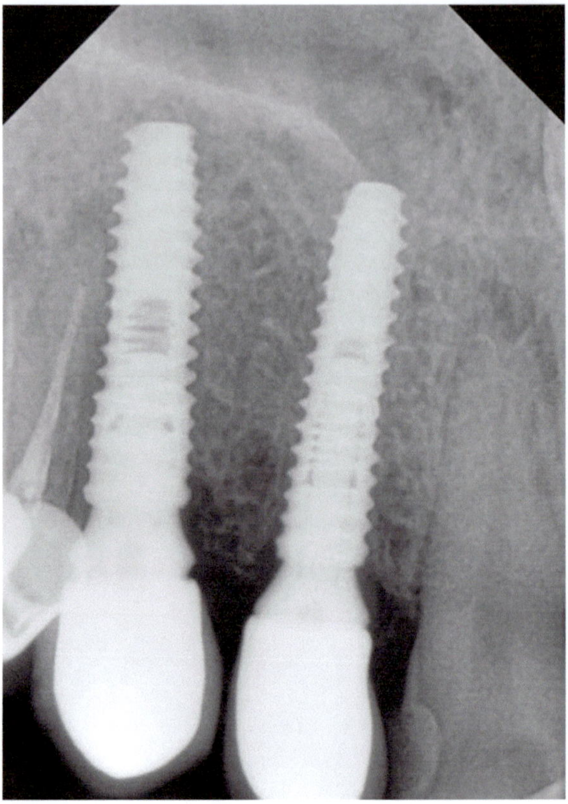

Fig. 6.32 Postoperative radiograph showing good bone level between 2 adjacent implant sites

6.4.2 Case 5

Restorations of 2 central incisors with implant-supported restoration is one of the most challenging clinical situations. The following case was executed by performing socket shields with implant placement and chairside provisional crowns. The healing after 4 months was remarkable. Natural tissue contours were maintained along with the interdental papilla around the definitive restorations (Figs. 6.33, 6.34, 6.35, 6.36 and 6.37).

The two cases displayed above demonstrate how the interdental tissue has been maintained while restoring adjacent implants in the esthetic zone with the socket shield technique. The remarkable feature of the technique is that these results could be achieved without the use of any biomaterial or any invasive surgical technique.

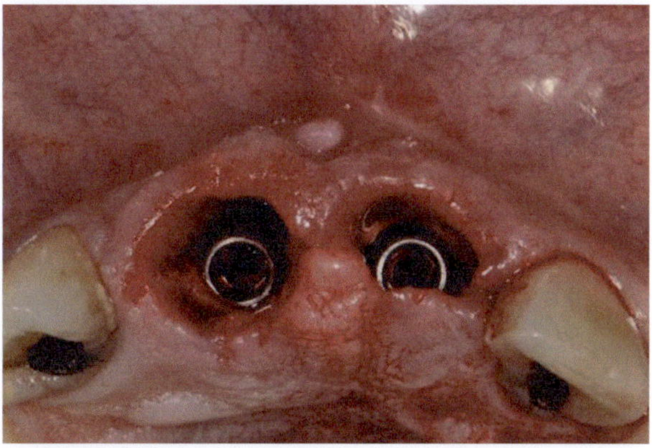

Fig. 6.33 Socket shield procedure with implant placements for 2 maxillary central incisors

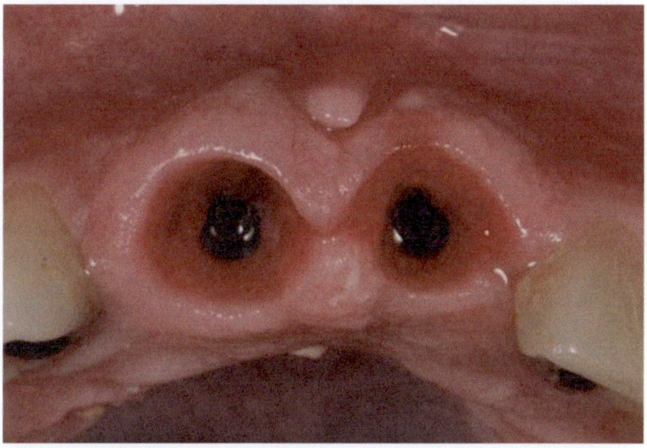

Fig. 6.34 Soft tissue contours on removal of the provisional restoration after 4 months

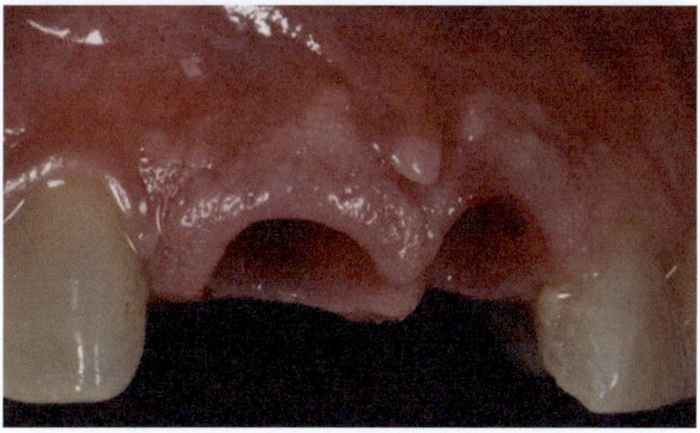

Fig. 6.35 Note good tissue contours

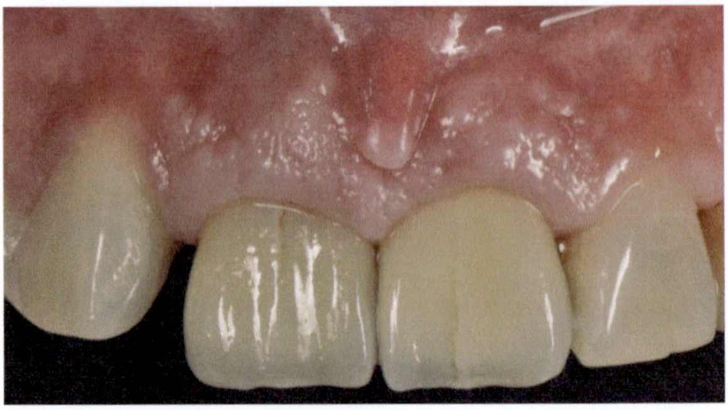

Fig. 6.36 Definitive metal ceramic restoration

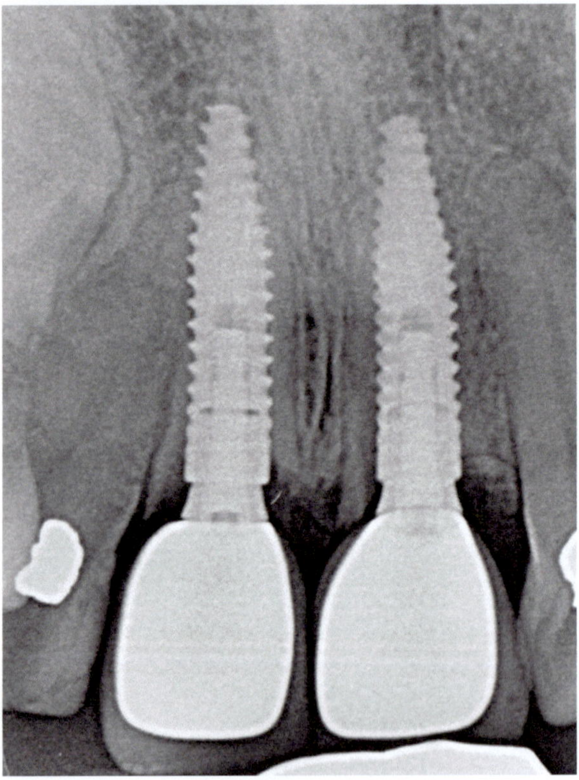

Fig. 6.37 One year postoperative radiograph

6.5 C-Shaped Shield

The significant benefit of the socket shield procedure is the long-term maintenance of the labial bone due to the presence of the periodontal ligament [26, 27]. It is hypothesized that extending the shield interproximally may help in maintaining the interdental bone crest [7, 10]. This concept is more applicable in clinical situations where there are adjacent socket shields as the absence of the periodontal ligament may lead to crestal bone loss which in turn may cause absence or shortening of the interdental papilla.

A C-shaped shield will prevent the interdental bony peak from resorption, thus maintaining the height of the interdental papilla [11].

6.5.1 Case 6

A 32-year-old female patient reported with fractured anterior crowns due to a traumatic injury. The teeth 11, 21, 22 had been endodontically treated 8 years ago. C-shaped socket shields were made followed by immediate chairside provisional restorations. The soft tissue architecture was well maintained at the end of the healing phase. The C-shaped shields supported the interdental papillae and prevented a post-restoration dark triangles (Figs. 6.38, 6.39, 6.40, 6.41, 6.42 and 6.43).

One of the issues with the C-shaped shield is that the overall area of native bone surrounding the implant is limited. This can be a concern in smaller sockets such as the lateral incisors. In such situations, an intimate contact of the implant with the shields is inevitable. In the experience of the authors, the C-shaped shield is best

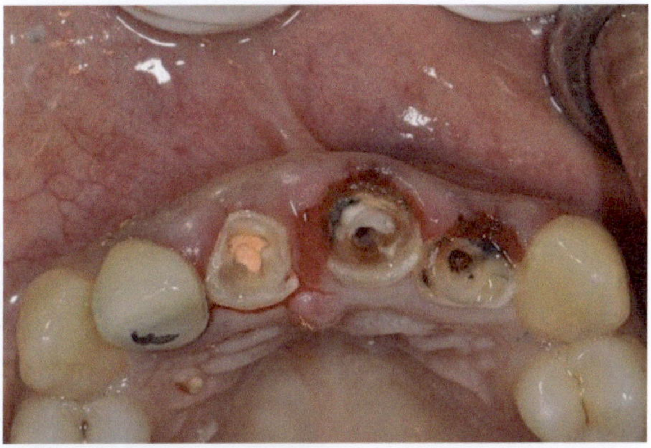

Fig. 6.38 Preoperative situation. Fractured teeth 11, 21, 22

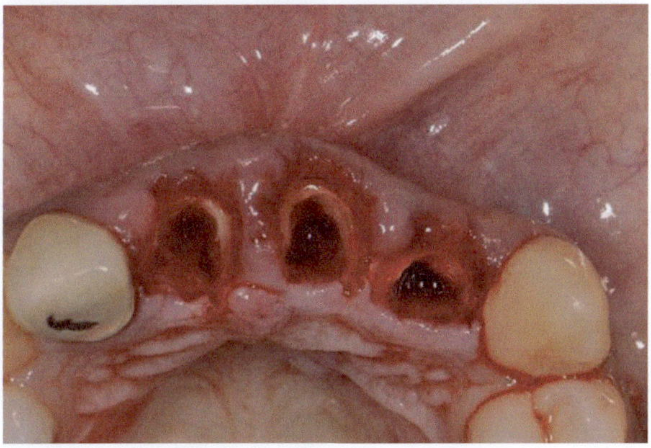

Fig. 6.39 C-shaped shield designed to maintain interproximal tissue height and contour

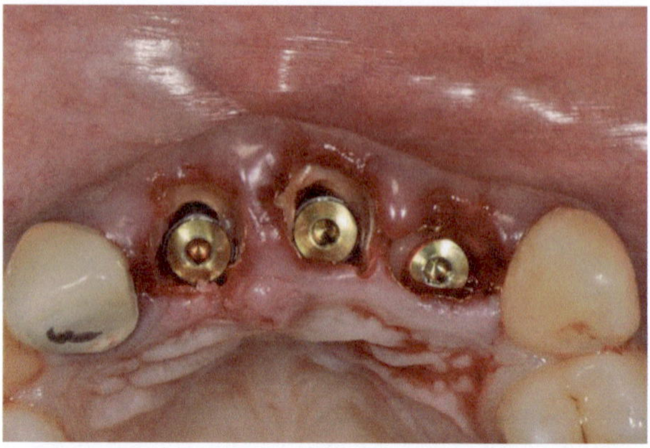

Fig. 6.40 Immediate implant placements (Biohorizons Inc., U.S.A.) in the palatal wall of the socket

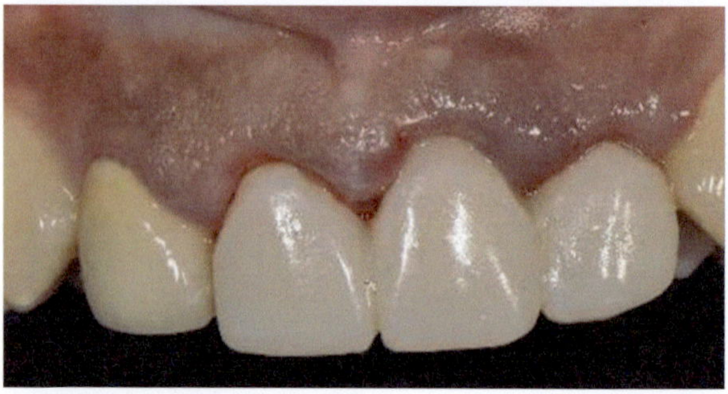

Fig. 6.41 Screw-retained provisional restorations

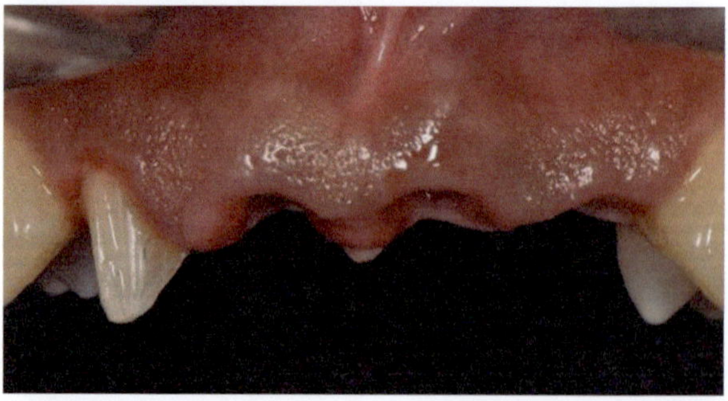

Fig. 6.42 Four months postoperative view after removal of the provisional restoration. Note the maintenance of tissue contours

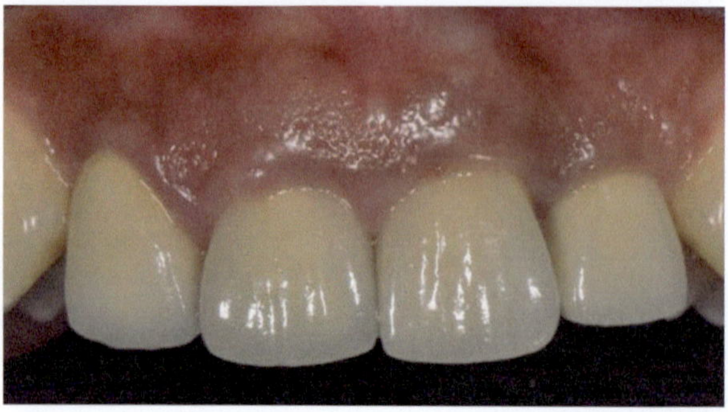

Fig. 6.43 Definitive metal ceramic restorations displaying good tissue contours, interdental papilla, and absence of dark triangles

suited for central incisors and canines, since the mesiodistal width of these teeth is wide enough to accommodate a suitable implant diameter without contacting the prepared shield. Since the available data on the success of a C-shaped shields is very limited, it cannot be considered as a routine method for shield preparation.

6.6 Staged Socket Shield Procedure (GLOCKER'S Technique)

A variation of the protocol is to stage the implant placement, following shield preparation. A simultaneous approach of shield preparation and implant placement would save the overall treatment time. However, in certain clinical situations, it may be more prudent to place the implant at a later date to allow healing and bone fill in the socket [28].

The indications for a staged approach over immediate placement are as follows:

1. Anatomical factors: The bone anatomy after the partial extraction may not be suitable for an immediate implant placement. In such a situation, trying to place the implant on the day of the partial extraction may result in the implant being placed in an inappropriate position or angulation, which does not comply with the prosthetic plan. This is especially relevant in multirooted teeth like the maxillary premolars or molars. At times it is prudent to stage the implant placement even for extra-long maxillary canines. The length of the longest available implant is often shorter than the length of a maxillary canine root.

   Sometimes the root apices of maxillary canines and premolars and molars communicate with sinus. In such cases extraction of the apex along with the palatal part leads to formation of oro-antral opening that should be allowed to heal before implant placement.

   Attempting a simultaneous placement in such cases may not be possible due to lack of apical bone, which is necessary to achieve primary stability of the implant [29, 30]. By allowing complete healing, a more straightforward procedure of implant placement can be executed.
2. Apical infection: Though post-extraction immediate implant placements in teeth with peri-apical lesions have been successfully documented in literature, they do have the inherent risk factor associated with the protocol [31, 32]. Allowing complete resolution of the peri-apical infection may be prudent in some cases. Hence in cases where there is a small- to moderate-sized lesion, extraction followed by a thorough curettage and a delayed implant placement will reduce the likelihood of a postoperative complication. Waiting for 12 weeks or more following the partial extraction and shield preparation will provide the clinician a sterile and healthy environment to place the implant. It will also provide the clinician with additional soft tissue for manipulation and primary closure. The presence of the labial shield prevents the loss of the labial bone [33]. Hence implant placement can be delayed in specific clinical situations without the fear of an alveolar ridge collapse. This is a great advantage since in early placement after complete extraction, a contour augmentation with a biomaterial is mandatory to replace the lost labial bone. In the Glocker technique, the use of a biomaterial could be avoided.

3. Adolescent patients: Implant placements should be delayed in young patients whose skeletal growth is incomplete [34, 35]. Extractions of teeth in such patients leads to a complete collapse of the alveolar ridge by the time they are ready for implant placement. Performing a partial extraction of the root will prevent any alveolar ridge alteration and maintain the bucco-palatal width and vertical height of bone for future implant placement.
4. Operator preference: For the inexperienced operator, an immediate placement protocol, shield preparation followed by implant placement and fabrication of the provisional crown can be quite intimidating. Breaking down the procedure into 2 stages reduces the complexity of the procedure.

6.6.1 Surgical Technique

1. After administration of local anesthesia, the palatal section of the root is extracted utilizing the same technique and armamentarium described in Chap. 2.
2. The procedure can be carried out using a flapless or a flapped approach depending on several factors discussed in that chapter. The shield preparation is done following the usual protocols.
3. The remaining socket is filled with a piece of collagen sponge and suture is placed to retain it. No attempt is made to achieve any primary closure of the wound. However, the authors have experienced soft tissue ingress in the socket during the socket healing phase.
4. Alternatively, a bone substitute material is packed into the socket and covered with a small piece of free gingival graft to seal the socket. The authors have encountered better bone condition post healing when a bone substitute material has been used to graft the socket.
5. An early implant placement (after 6 weeks of healing) or a delayed implant placement (after 12 weeks of healing) strategy can be employed depending on the clinical situation. If there is adequate bone for placing the implant in the prosthetically driven position, an early implant placement can be performed. In case of a bony defect in the peri-apical region due to a previous pathology, it is prudent to wait for complete bone fill in the sockets before attempting an implant placement.
6. The implant placement is carried out using the usual protocols for correct prosthetically driven 3D placement as discussed in Chap. 2.
7. The use of Densah drills (Versah Inc., U.S.A.) to compact the bone between the implant and the shield is crucial in Glocker technique [36]. The drills, when used in a reverse direction, following the manufacturer's instructions can result in preserving existing bone within the osteotomy site and simultaneously creating a zone of dense bone surrounding the osteotomy. This helps in achieving better stability for the implant. The authors experience a significant benefit in utilizing this approach.
8. A provisional restoration or a healing abutment can be fixed over the implant.
9. Definitive restoration is fabricated after osteointegration of the implant.

6.6.2 Case 7

A 44–year-old male reported with a fractured tooth 14. The tooth was badly decayed and needed to be extracted. Since the inter-radicular bone was very thin and delicate, achieving good primary stability during immediate implant placement would have been challenging. Hence a staged socket shield procedure was planned, wherein only a partial extraction was performed along with preparation of the socket shield. The implant placement was done after 6 weeks of healing. On the day of implant placement, a healing abutment was placed. The healing was uneventful and good tissue contours were noticed on removal of the healing abutment after 3 months (Figs. 6.44, 6.45, 6.46, 6.47, 6.48, 6.49, 6.50, 6.51, 6.52, 6.53, 6.54, 6.55, 6.56, 6.57, 6.58 and 6.59).

The Glocker technique of performing the socket shield followed by staged implant placement is a practical and effective way of treating difficult clinical situations without any compromise in the end result. The authors recommend this approach for clinicians new to partial extraction therapies treatment modality, to ease out the surgical procedure and shorten the learning curve.

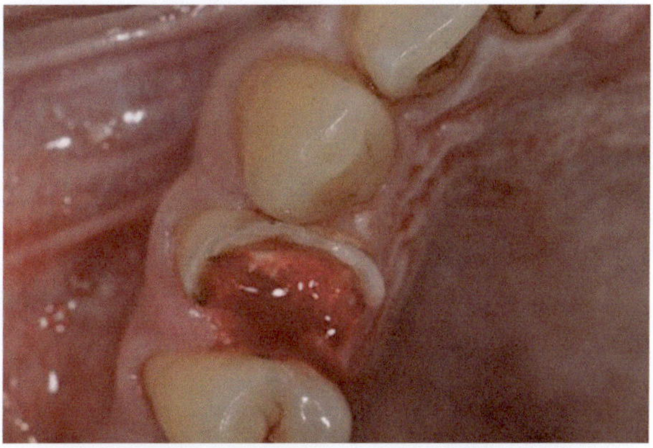

Fig. 6.44 Preoperative situation. Fractured and unrestorable tooth 14

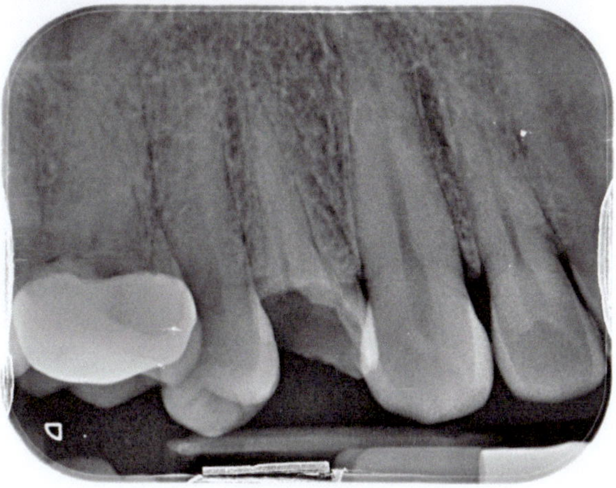

Fig. 6.45 Radiograph of the fractured tooth 14

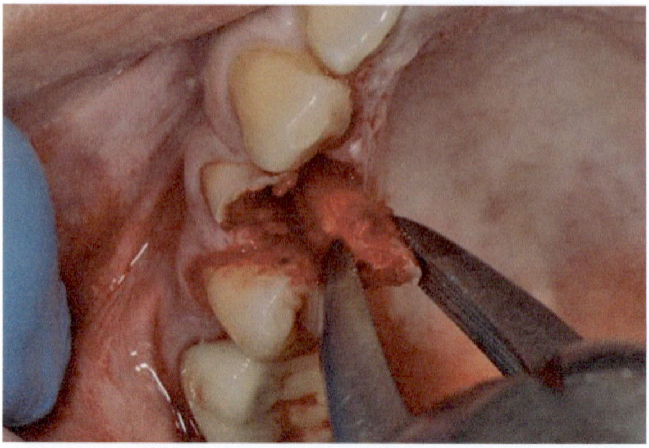

Fig. 6.46 Extraction of the palatal root

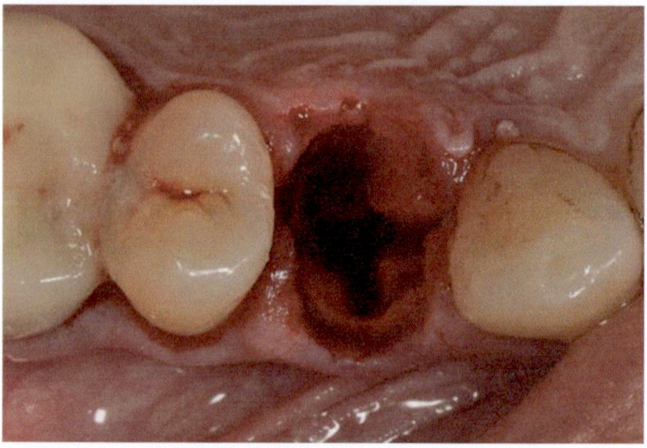

Fig. 6.47 Shield preparation

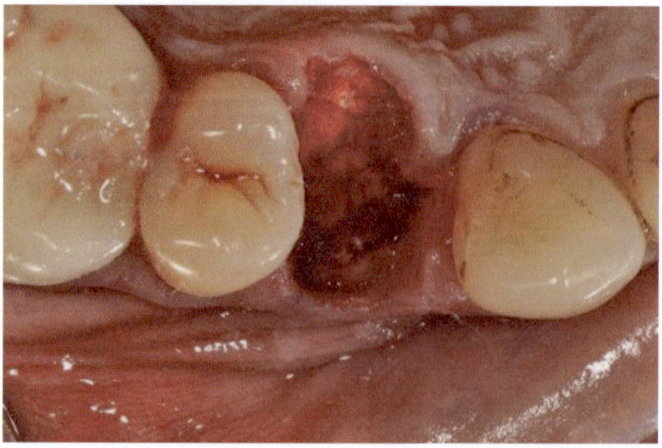

Fig. 6.48 Collagen sponge placed in the socket

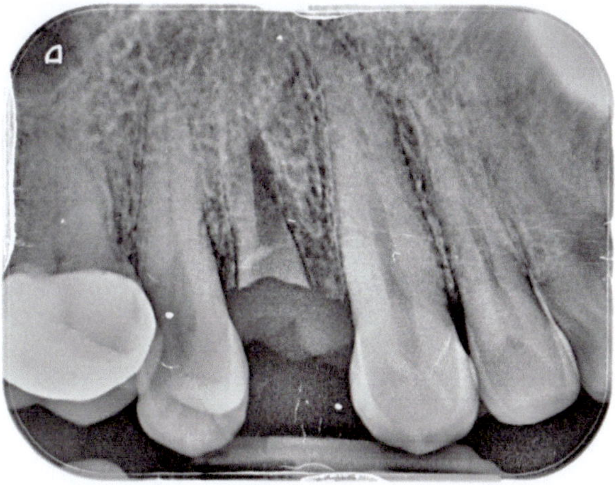

Fig. 6.49 Radiograph showing prepared shield

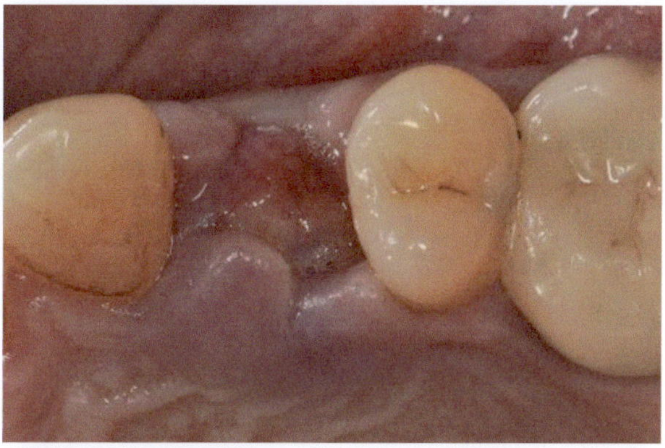

Fig. 6.50 Healing after 6 weeks

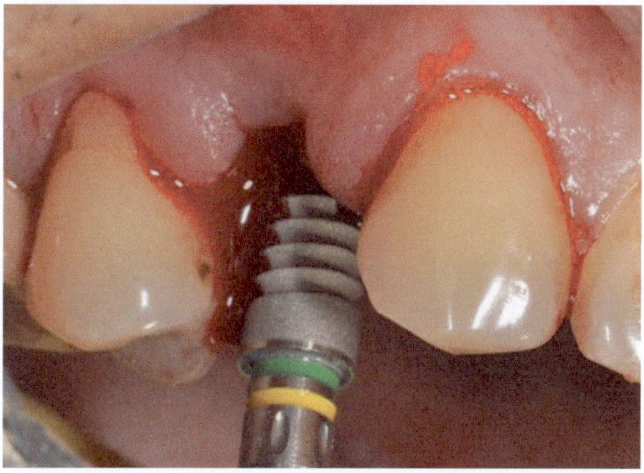

Fig. 6.51 Implant placement (Biohorizons Inc., U.S.A.)

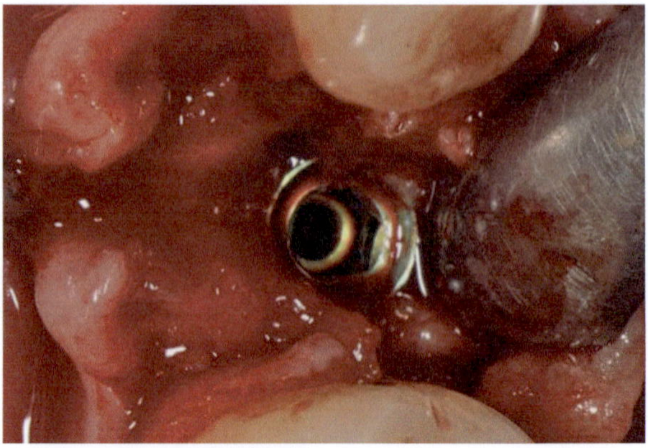

Fig. 6.52 Implant placed in the correct prosthetically driven position

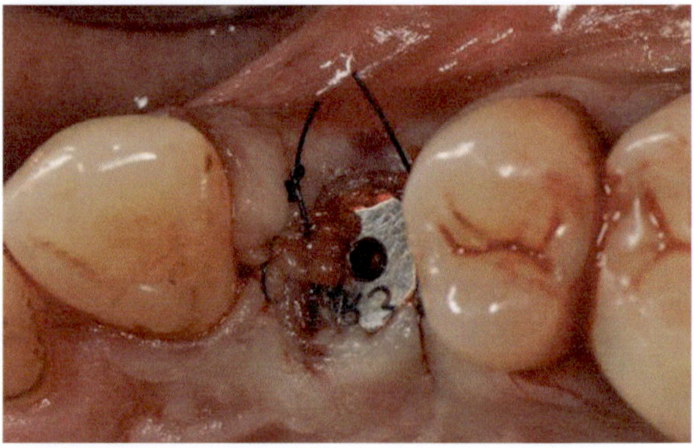

Fig. 6.53 Placement of healing abutment and closure of the mini-flap

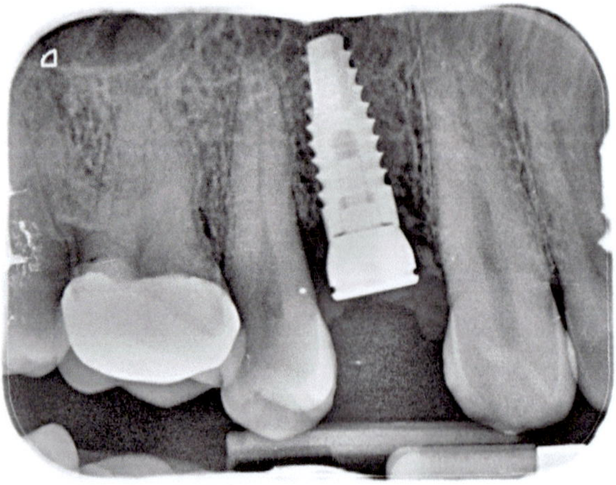

Fig. 6.54 Immediate postoperative radiograph after implant placement

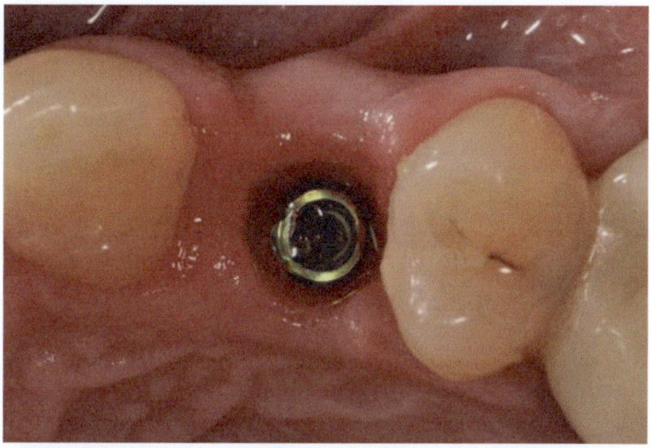

Fig. 6.55 Healing after 4 months

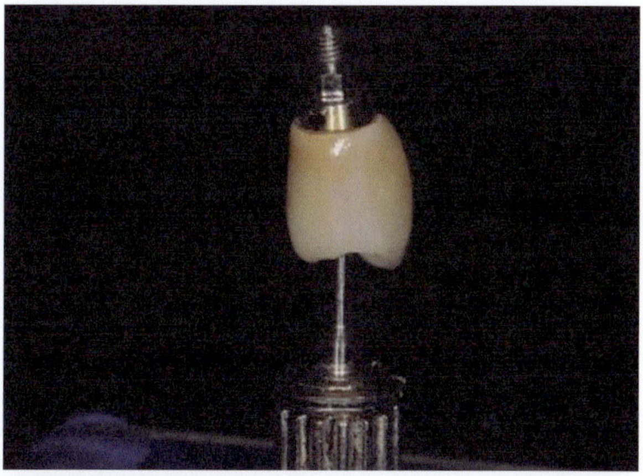

Fig. 6.56 Screw-retained Zirconia crown on a titanium-based abutment

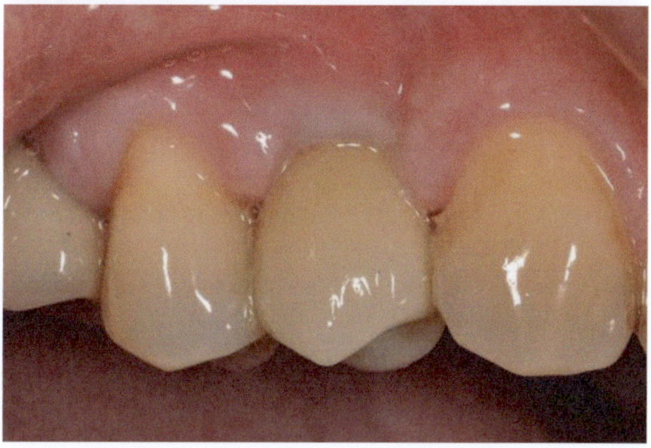

Fig. 6.57 Postoperative view of the definitive restoration

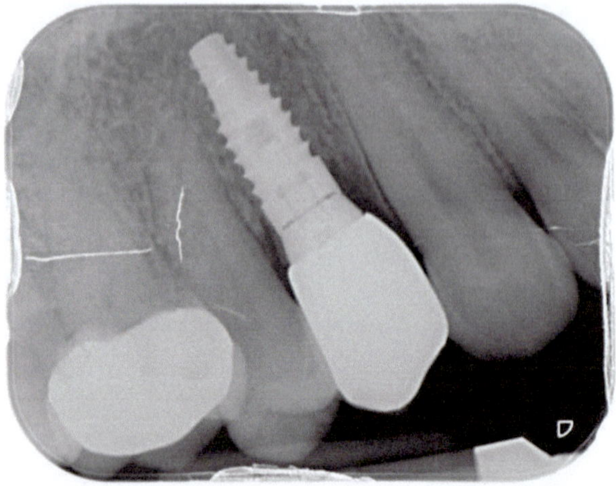

Fig. 6.58 Postoperative radiograph

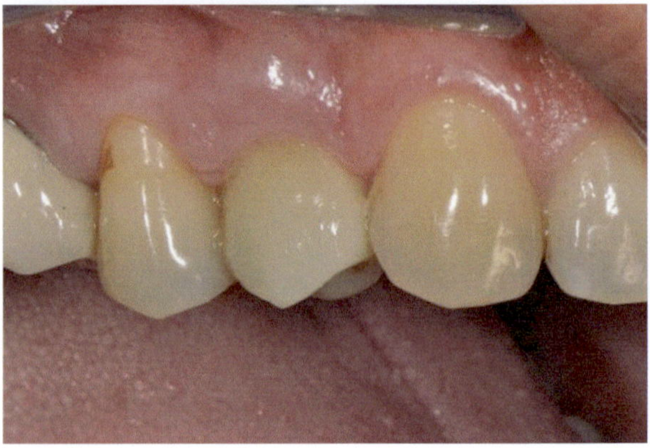

Fig. 6.59 One year follow-up view displaying healthy peri-implant soft tissue contours

6.7 Conclusion

The partial extraction therapies are an evolving science. As the collective experience of the fraternity increases in this field, there will be variations of the classic approach. The clinicians practicing this science need to update their knowledge in this field and look out for ways to make the procedure safer, faster, and more predictable.

Acknowledgement Case 2 (Sect. 6.2) Courtesy: Dr T. V. Narayan. Case 4 (Sect. 6.4) Courtesy: Dr Sameer Karavkar, Navi Mumbai

References

1. Ash MM, Nelson SJ. The permanent canines: maxillary and mandibular. In: Wheeler's dental anatomy, physiology, and occlusion. 8th ed. St. Louis, Mo: Elsevier; 2007. p. 191–214.
2. Black GV. Descriptive anatomy of the human teeth. 4th ed. Philadelphia: Hansebooks; 1902.

3. Gutmann JL. Surgical endodontics: past, present, and future. Endod Top. 2014;30(1):29–43.
4. Grandi C, Pacifici L. The ratio in choosing access flap for surgical endodontics: a review. Oral Implantol (Rome). 2009;2(1):37–52.
5. Buser D, Chappuis V, Belser UC, Chen S. Implant placement post extraction in esthetic single tooth sites: when immediate, when early, when late? Periodontol. 2017;73:84–102.
6. Gluckman H, Salama M, Du Toit J. Partial extraction therapies (PET) part 1: maintaining alveolar ridge contour at Pontic and immediate implant sites. Int J Periodontics Restorative Dent. 2016;36:681–7. https://doi.org/10.11607/prd.2783.
7. Cherel F, Etienne D. Papilla preservation between two implants: a modifiedsocket-shield technique to maintain the scalloped anatomy? A case report. Quintessence Int. 2014;45(1):23–30.
8. Marius Steigmann, Hom-Lay Wang, (2006) Esthetic Buccal Flap for Correction of Buccal Fenestration Defects During Flapless Immediate Implant Surgery. Journal of Periodontology 77:(3):517–522
9. Udatta Kher, Aliasger Tunkiwala, Zerxis Umrigar, (2015) Management of Fenestration Defects During Flapless Immediate Implant Placement in the Esthetic Zone. The International Journal of Periodontics & Restorative Dentistry 35 (6):e90-e96
10. Kan JY, Rungcharassaeng K. Proximal socket shield for interimplant papilla preservation in the esthetic zone. Int J Periodontics Restorative Dent. 2013;33:e24–31.
11. Kumar PR, Kher U. Shield the socket: procedure, case report and classification. J Indian Soc Periodontol. 2018;22(3):266–72.
12. Tarnow DP, Cho SC, Wallace SS. The effect of inter-implant distance on the height of inter-implant bone crest. J Periodontol. 2000;71:546–9.
13. Salama H, Salama MA, Garber D, Adar P. The interproximal height of bone: a guidepost to predictable aesthetic strategies and soft tissue contours in anterior tooth replacement. Pract Periodontics Aesthet Dent. 1998;10:1131–41.
14. Buser D, Martin W, Belser UC. Optimizing esthetics for implant restorations in the anterior maxilla: anatomic and surgical considerations. Int J Oral Maxillofac Implants. 2004;19:43–61.
15. Palmer RM, Palmer PJ, Newton JT. Dealing with esthetic demands in the anterior maxilla. Periodontology. 2003;2000(33):105–18.
16. Zetu L, Wang H-L. Management of inter-dental/interimplant papilla. J Clin Periodontol. 2005;32:831–9.
17. Holt RL, Rosenberg MM, Zinser PJ, Ganeles J. Concept for a biologically derived, parabolic implant design. Int J Periodontics Restorative Dent. 2002;22:473–81.
18. Gadhia MH, Holt RL. A new implant design for optimal esthetics and retention of interproximal papillae. Implant Dent. 2003;12:164–9.
19. Wohrle PS. NobelPerfect™ esthetic scalloped implant: rationale for a new design. Clin Implant Dent Relat Res. 2003;5(Suppl 1):64–73.
20. Grunder U. The inlay-graft technique to create papillae between implants. J Esthet Dent. 1997;9:165–8.
21. Palacci P. Papilla regeneration technique. In: Palacci P, Ericsson I, Engstrand P, Rangert B, editors. Optimal implant positioning & soft tissue management for the Branemark system. Chicago: Quintessence Pub. Co; 1995. p. 59–70.
22. Misch CE, Al-Shammari KF, Wang HL. Creation of interimplant papillae through a split-finger technique. Implant Dent. 2004;13:20–7.
23. Tinti C, Benfenati SP. The ramp mattress suture: a new suturing technique combined with a surgical procedure to obtain papillae between implants in the buccal area. Int J Periodontics Restorative Dent. 2002;22:63–9.
24. Shahidi P, Jacobson Z, Dibart S, Pourati J, Nunn ME, Barouch K, et al. Efficacy of a new papilla generation technique in implant dentistry: a preliminary study. Int J Oral Maxillofac Implants. 2008;23:926–34.
25. Spear FM. The use of implants and ovate pontics in the esthetic zone. Compend Contin Educ Dent. 2008;29:72–4, 76–80; quiz 81, 94

26. Hurzeler MB, Zuhr O, Schupbach P, et al. The socket-shield technique: a proof-of-principle report. J Clin Periodontol. 2010;37:855–62.
27. Baumer D, Zuhr O, Rebele S, et al. The socket-shield technique: first histological, clinical, and volumetrical observations after separation of the buccal tooth segment—a pilot study. Clin Implant Dent Relat Res. 2015;17:71–82.
28. Glocker M, Attin T, Schmidlin P. Ridge preservation with modified "socket-shield" technique: a methodological case series. Dent J. 2014;2:11–21.
29. Lazzara RJ. Immediate implant placement into extraction sites: surgical and restorative advantages. Int J Periodontics Restorative Dent. 1989;9:332–43.
30. Nemcovsky CE, Artzi Z, Moses O, et al. Healing of marginal defects at implants placed in fresh extraction sockets or after 4–6 weeks of healing. A comparative study. Clin Oral Implants Res. 2002;13:410–9.
31. Tolman DE, Keller EE. Endosseous implant placement immediately following dental extraction and alveoloplasty: preliminary report with 6-year follow-up. Int J Oral Maxillofac Implants. 1991;6:24–8.
32. Koh RU, Rudek I, Wang HL. Immediate implant placement:positives and negatives. Implant Dent. 2010;19(2):98–108.
33. Gluckman H, Du Toit J, Salama M. The Pontic-shield: partial extraction therapy for ridge preservation and Pontic site development. Int J Periodontics Restorative Dent. 2016;36(3):417–23.
34. Oesterle LJ, Cronin RJ Jr, Ranly DM. Maxillary implants and the growing patient. Int J Oral Maxillofac Implants. 1993;8:377–87.
35. Westwood RM, Duncan JM. Implants in adolescents: a literature review and case reports. Int J Oral Maxillofac Implants. 1996;11:750–5.
36. Huwais S, Meyer EG. A novel osseous densification approach in implant osteotomy preparation to increase biomechanical primary stability, bone mineral density, and bone-to-implant contact. Int J Oral Maxillofac Implants. 2017;32:27–36.

Pontic Site Management

7

Tarun Kumar, Sudhindra Kulkarni, and Udatta Kher

Abstract

Alveolar bone loss begins as soon as teeth are extracted. Root submergence technique (RST) and pontic shield (PS) embody the partial extraction therapy philosophy. The retention of a root or its part has benefited in the maintenance of hard and soft tissues. RST is a procedure wherein an entire root is left behind. The PS is a procedure wherein the shield is prepared similar to a socket shield, and only the buccal aspect of the root is left behind. RST was the first technique under the umbrella of PET. The current chapter discusses the indications, preparation aspects, complications, and management of these two concepts.

7.1 Introduction

The root submergence technique (RST) and the pontic shield technique (PS) are an intergral part of the partial extraction therapy (PET). Both procedures are performed only when a tooth or root is indicated for an extraction. Both procedures aid in the maintenance of alveolar ridge architecture under pontic sites. Whilst the RST is chosen when the root indicated for extraction is healthy, the PS is indicated when there is a small periapical lesion around the root (Fig. 7.1).

T. Kumar
Department of Implantology, Bapuji Dental College, Davanagere, Karnataka, India

S. Kulkarni
Department of Implantology, SDM Dental College, Sri Dharmasthala Manjunatheshwara University, Dharwad, Karnataka, India

Private Practice, Hubli, Karnataka, India

U. Kher (✉)
Only Smiles Dental Centre, Mumbai, India

U. Kher, A. Tunkiwala (eds.), *Partial Extraction Therapy in Implant Dentistry*,
https://doi.org/10.1007/978-3-030-33610-3_7

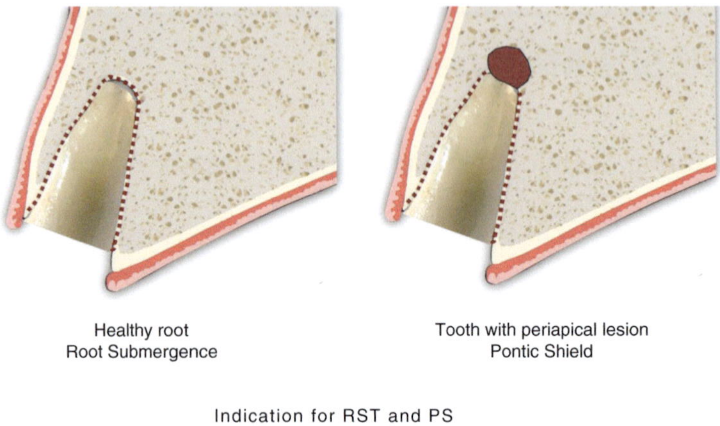

Fig. 7.1 Indications for Root Submergence Technique and Pontic Shield technique

7.2 Root Submergence Technique

Extraction of a tooth triggers a cascade of events that results in alveolar bone loss up to 56% in the first 3 months and usually continues throughout life [1]. Bone loss following tooth extraction is inevitable and progressive (Chap. 1). The buccal bone loss that occurs post extraction leads to changes in the horizontal and vertical dimension overtime [2, 3]. This has been a matter of concern in esthetic and restorative dentistry because of the challenges in achieving good emergence profiles for pontic sites (Fig. 7.2).

Complex hard and soft tissue reconstruction procedures are needed to achieve esthetically pleasing results. Remodeling of bone is expected in spite of ridge preservation or socket grafting procedures [4].

At times the progressive bone loss beneath the pontic sites creates an esthetic compromise in restorations after a few years. It also leads to issues pertaining to maintenance of hygiene. Salama et al. [5, 6] and Gluckman et al. [7] proposed retention of the root or its part for maintenance of hard and soft tissue during extraction. Retaining the tooth root or part of it, aided in the retention of the periodontal ligament attachment to the alveolar bone, thus maintaining the vascular supply to the bundle bone. Retaining roots beneath full removable dentures to maintain the alveolar ridge, termed as root submergence technique (RST), was proposed by Howell in 1970 [8].

Root submergence is a technique of retaining the radicular portion of the root within the confines of the alveolar housing to prevent alveolar bone loss, thereby preserving the ridge contours.

This technique was reported by Malmgren et al. [9, 10] as far back as 1970, with successful bone regeneration around submerged tooth roots. Howell observed that the endodontically treated roots decreased alveolar bone loss under complete dentures [8]. The concept evolved over the years for the development of pontic sites beneath fixed partial dentures. Submerging the whole root or a part of it is decided largely based on the status of the root and requirement for maintaining the ridge architecture at the pontic sites under fixed restorations.

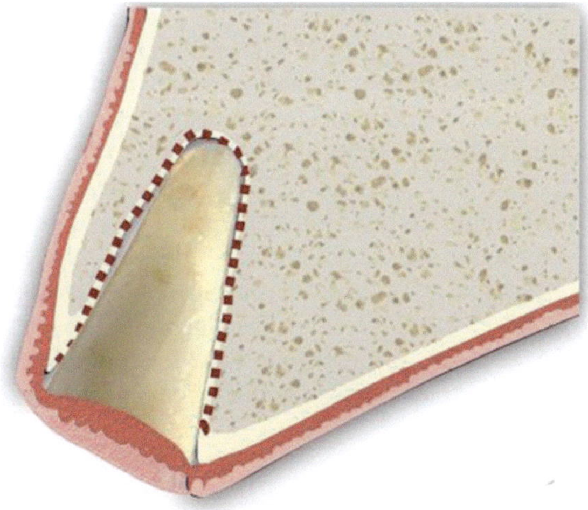

Fig. 7.2 Submerged root covered with soft tissue

7.3 RST Timeline

Howell F 1970: Retention of alveolar bone by endodontic root treatment [8]

Whitaker 1974: A Study of the Histological Reaction of Submerged Root Segments [11]

Levin 1974: Intentional Submergence of Nonvital Roots [12]

Guyer SE 1975: Selectively retained vital roots for partial support of overdentures [13]

Plata RL 1976: Intentional retention of vital submerged roots in dogs. [14]

O'Neal RB 1978: Submergence of endodontically treated roots for alveolar bone preservation. [15]

Welker WA 1978: Preventive Prosthodontics-mucosal coverage of roots [16]

Garver DG, 1980: Vital root retention in humans: a final report [17]

Von Wowern 1981: 4 year followup study of RST for alveolar ridge preservation [18]

Garver DG 1983: The retention of vital submucosal roots under immediate dentures [19]

Lambert 1984: Autogenous dermal graft coverage of submerged roots in dog [20]

Harper K 2002: Submerged an endodontically treated root to preserve the alveolar ridge under a bridge. [21]

Salama MA 2007: RST for pontic site development in esthetic implant therapy. [6]

Howard Gluckman 2016: Introduced a new term Partial Extraction Therapy (PET) into the literature , review of these ridge preservation therapies, provided a classification of PET and a guide to their application. [7]

7.3.1 Indications

Only teeth without periapical infections which are indicated for extractions should be chosen for root submergence technique. The RST can be performed in the following clinical situations:

1. As pontic sites under teeth-supported fixed partial dentures.
2. As pontic sites under implant-supported fixed partial dentures.
3. Under removable prosthesis to maintain alveolar ridge dimension.
4. Under a cantilevered implant-supported prosthesis.
5. As a means of preserving bone for future implant sites in adolescent patients whose skeletal growth is still incomplete.

7.3.2 Contraindications

RST should be strictly avoided in some clinical situations. Conventional treatment procedure of complete extraction along with bone and soft tissue graft should be performed in these scenarios. These include:

1. Teeth with periapical infections.
2. Vertically fractured teeth.
3. Mobile teeth.
4. Teeth with internal or external resorption.

7.3.3 Clinical Considerations

Armamentarium

High-speed handpiece with irrigation, straight and round carbide burs, round diamond finishing bur, gingival protection instrument.

Teeth with minor periapical infections have to be endodontically treated prior to RST. Vital RST procedure can be considered if the root is covered with soft tissue after sectioning, in order to maintain the blood supply. Endodontic treatment should be carried out for vital teeth with unhealthy pulp tissue if the root is to be submerged [6].

7.4 Surgical Technique

1. The tooth is decoronated using the high-speed drill at the buccal gingival level.
2. The soft tissues at the crest should be protected using a gingiva protecting instrument.
3. Using a flame-shaped or round diamond bur the root is trimmed to the level of the alveolar bone crest (Figs. 7.3 and 7.4).

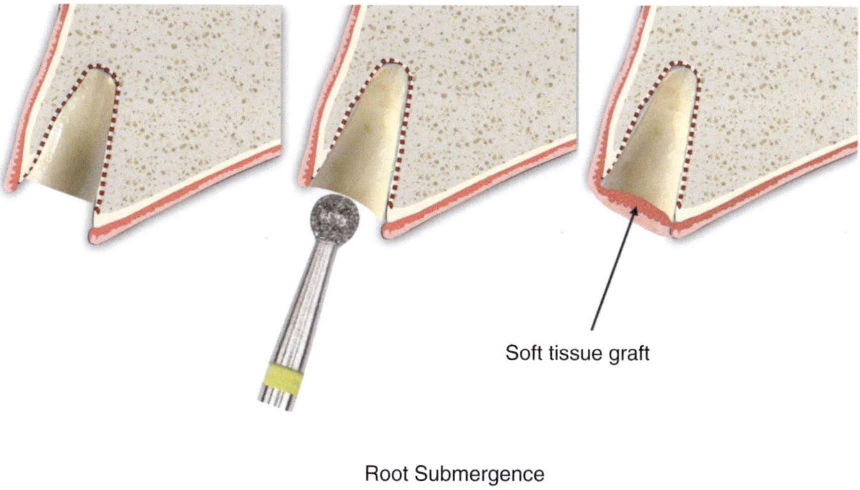

Fig. 7.3 Preparation of the root for Root Submergence technique

Fig. 7.4 Post-restoration radiograph depicting the correctly contoured RST and convex pontic and the optimum space for soft tissue between the two

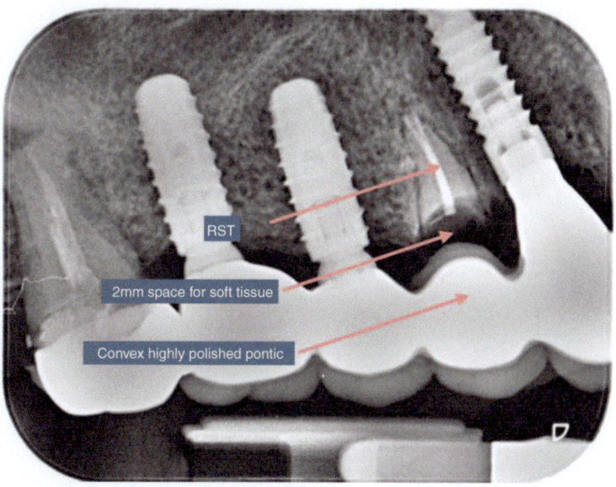

4. The center of the root is further hollowed out using a round diamond bur under irrigation to create additional space for soft tissue below the future pontic site. The hollowing prevents exposure of the roots during the healing phase. A minimum of 2 mm of soft tissue should be present above the submerged root to prevent it from future migration and exposure [2].
5. To ensure healing by primary intention soft tissue closure is achieved by one of the following methods.
   (a) A: Buccal advancement of the flap to achieve primary closure.
   (b) B: Free gingival graft (FGG) harvested with a tissue punch from the palate or tuberosity.
   (c) C: Free connective tissue graft (CTG) harvested from the palate or tuberosity.
   (d) D: Palatal pedicled flap.

7.5 Cases

The cases below exhibit root submergence technique with soft tissue augmentation techniques.

7.5.1 Case 1

A 26-year-old male suffered a traumatic injury that led to the fractures of 3 anterior teeth. Extractions followed by immediate implant placements were done for teeth 11 and 22. The root of tooth 21 was endodontically treated and submerged. A subepithelial palatal pedicled flap was used to cover the root. The submerged root helped in attaining excellent soft tissue profile for the pontic site under the definitive metal ceramic restoration which was supported on the 2 implants (Figs. 7.5, 7.6, 7.7, 7.8, 7.9, 7.10, 7.11, 7.12 and 7.13).

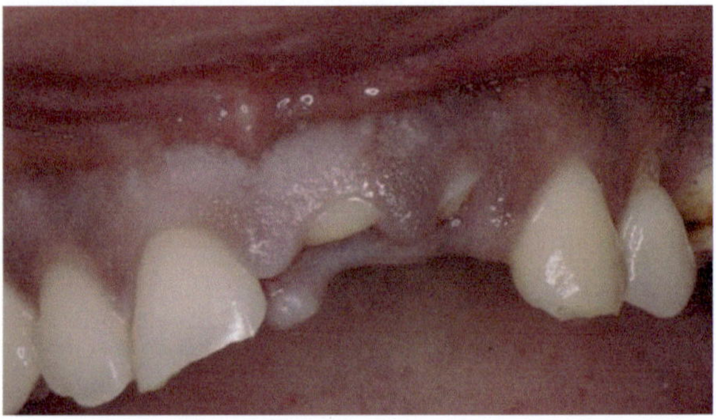

Fig. 7.5 Fractured teeth 11, 21, and 22. Teeth 11 and 22 are implant sites whereas 21 is a pontic site

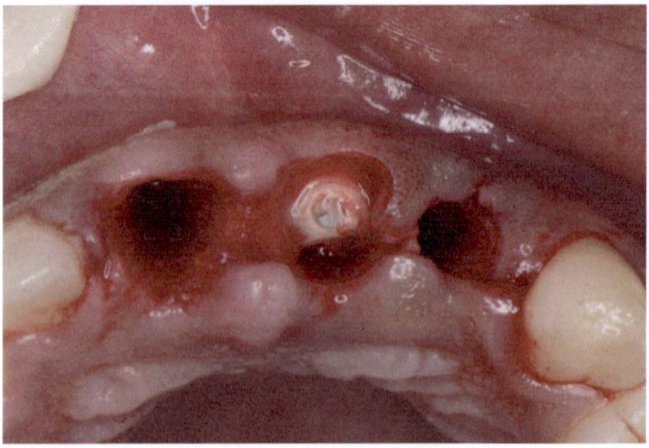

Fig. 7.6 Teeth 11 and 22 extracted and prepared for implant, 21 endodontically treated and decoronated to receive the pontic

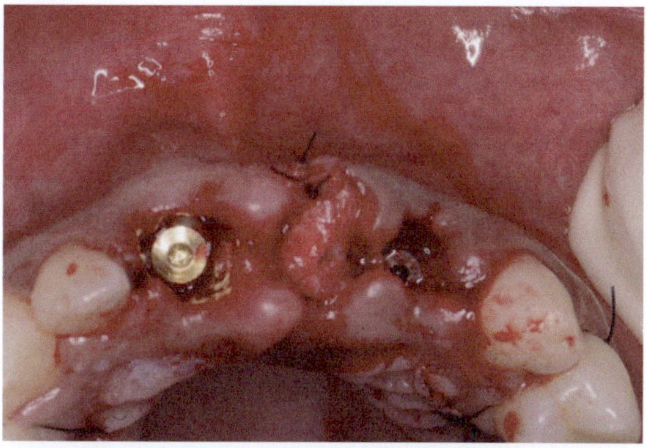

Fig. 7.7 The site 21 covered with connective tissue graft (CTG) harvested from palate

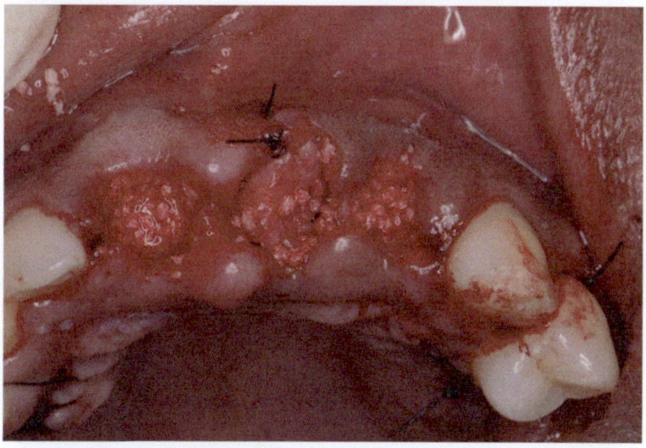

Fig. 7.8 Bone graft and CTG covering above the implant platform for sites 11 and 22

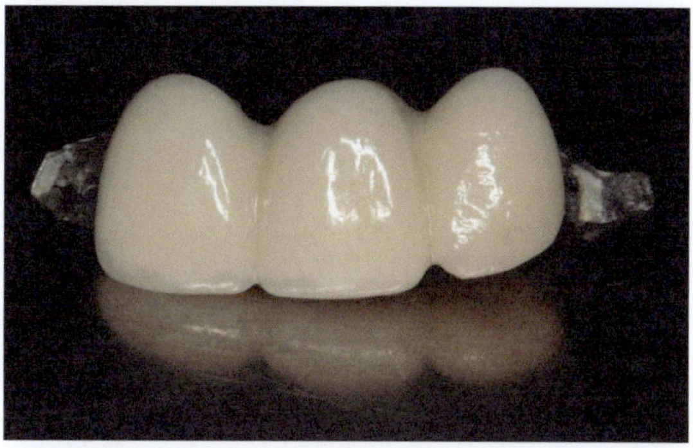

Fig. 7.9 Maryland prosthesis used as temporary restoration

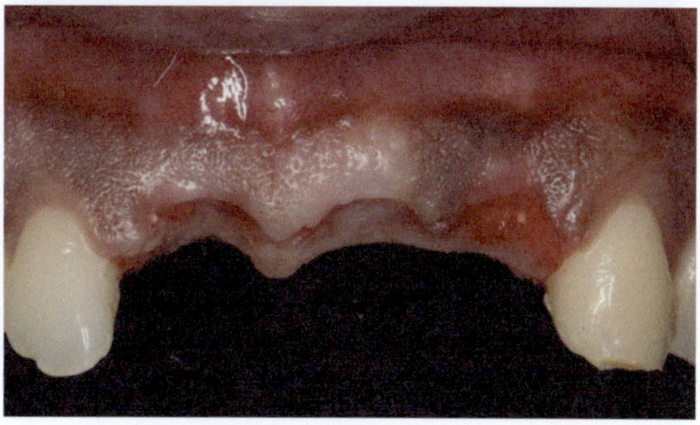

Fig. 7.10 The temporary prosthesis aided in developing the tissue contours. The submerged root is covered by the soft tissue

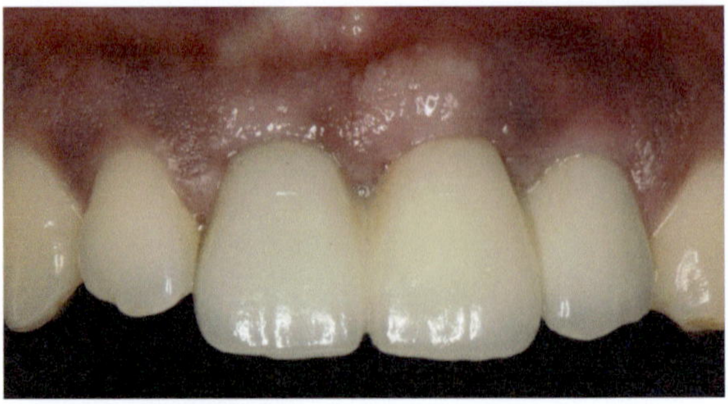

Fig. 7.11 Final prosthesis. The natural emergence of the restorations at the implant as well as the pontic sites is appreciable

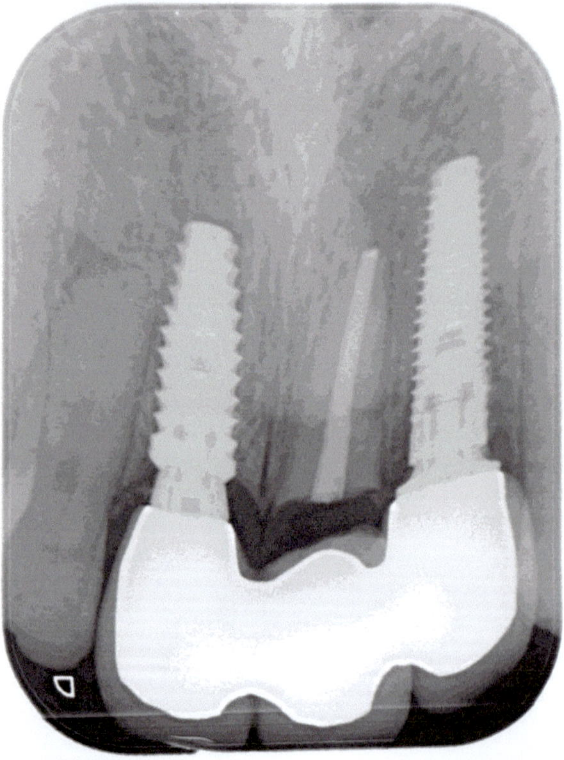

Fig. 7.12 The radiograph shows the osseointergrated implants and the submerged root

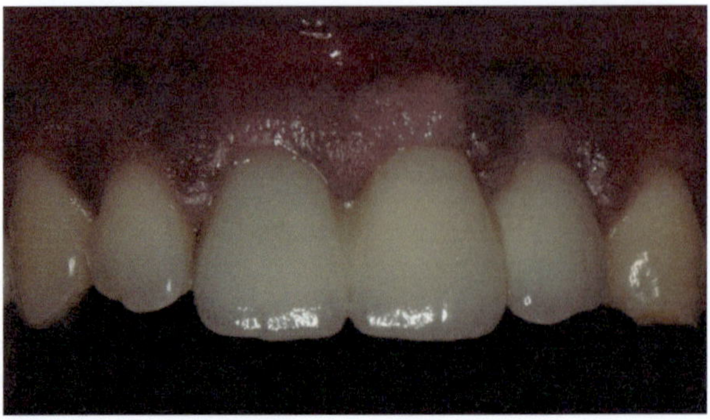

Fig. 7.13 At one-year recall: satisfactory contours around the implants and the pontic sites. One can appreciate the stippling on the implant as well as the pontic sites indicating optimal health

7.5.2 Case 2

In the following case, a root submergence was done for tooth 13 to maintain the soft tissue contours which helped in achieving excellent emergence profile for the pontic site (Figs. 7.14, 7.15 and 7.16).

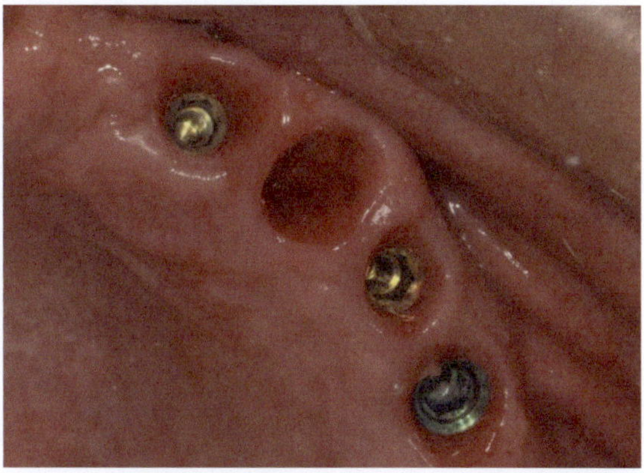

Fig. 7.14 A healthy pontic site having a submerged root

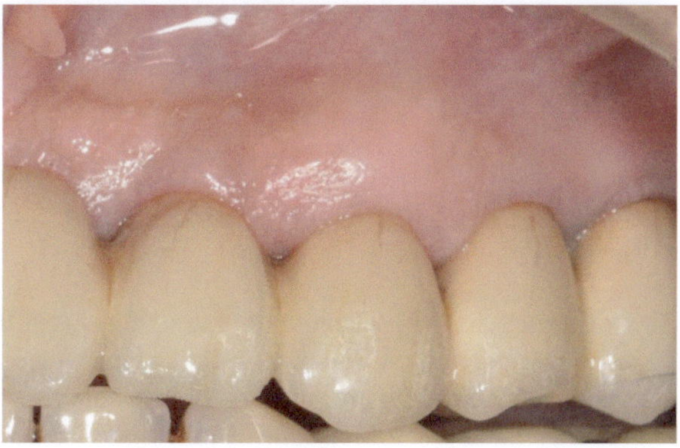

Fig. 7.15 Excellent emergence profile for the canine pontic

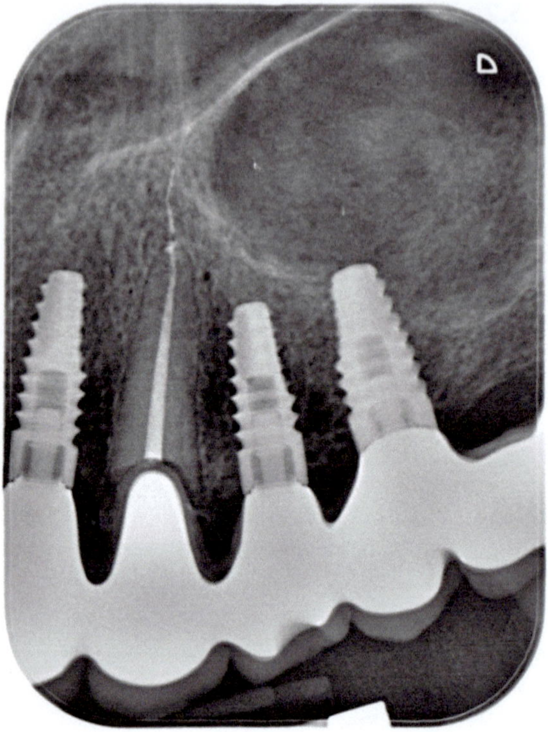

Fig. 7.16 Radiograph showing a healthy submerged root under a screw-retained implant supported restoration

7.5.3 Case 3

The following case was planned for extractions of all the teeth followed by a fixed restoration supported on 6 implants. The canines were endodontically treated, decoronated, and the roots were submerged. Implants were placed at strategic locations to provide a fixed restoration. The canine roots retained the surrounding soft tissue architecture and prevented the inevitable buccal collapse that occurs after extraction. The final screw-retained prosthesis exhibited satisfactory contours at the canine pontic sites because of the submerged roots (Figs. 7.17, 7.18, 7.19 and 7.20).

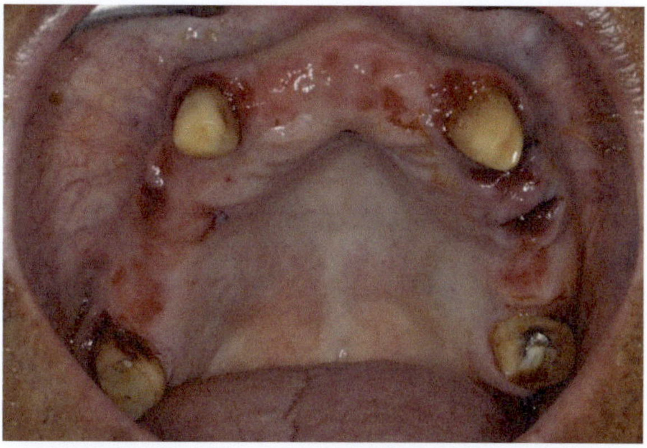

Fig. 7.17 Preoperative status showing a failing maxillary dentition

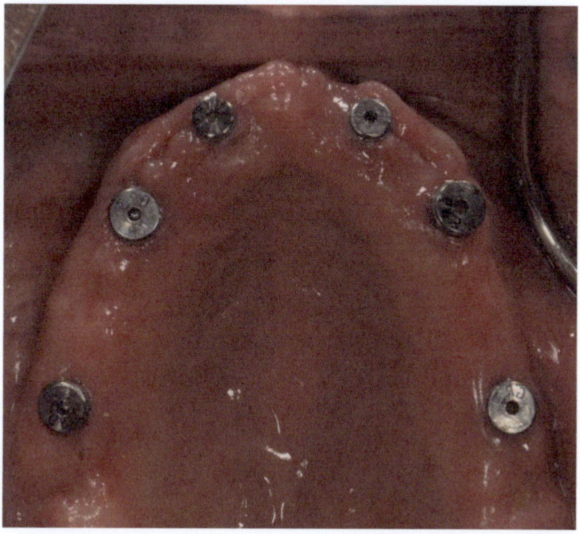

Fig. 7.18 Occlusal view of the completely healed sites. Note the healthy contours in sites 13 and 23 due to the submerged roots

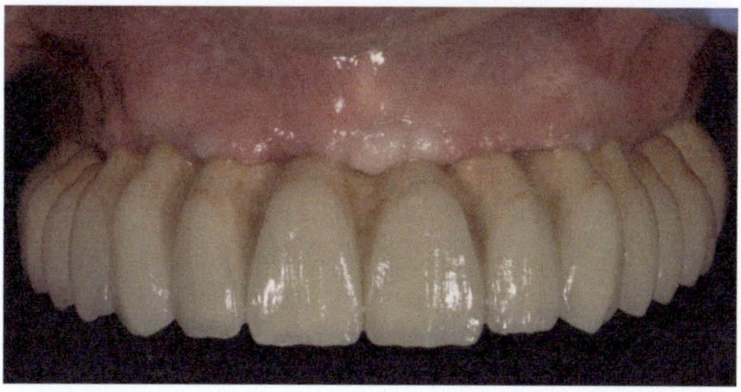

Fig. 7.19 Definitive screw-retained prosthesis. Note the excellent emergence profile at the 2 pontic sites in relation to tooth #13 and #23

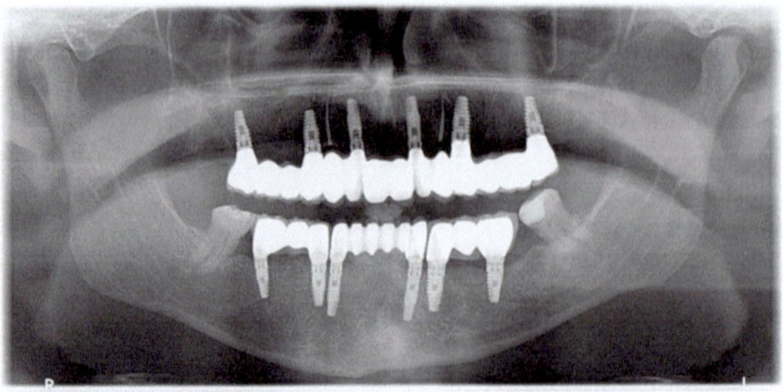

Fig. 7.20 Radiograph showing submerged roots of the both the maxillary canines

7.6 RST Complications and Management

7.6.1 Root Exposure

One of the frequent complications of the root submergence is the exposure of the coronal part of the root through the soft tissue. The exposed part of the root is prone to caries, periodontal disease or periapical infections if left untreated [6].

Cause

It is caused due to inadequate soft tissue coverage over the root surface.

Prevention

This can be prevented by adequately submerging the root below the level of the crestal bone and creating a concavity for soft tissue to creep. A soft tissue graft over the submerged root will reduce the probability of such root exposures. Care should be taken not to exert pressure from the pontic of the provisional restoration during the healing phase. The presence of a removable denture over the submerged roots can also contribute to thinning of the overlying soft tissue and inadvertent exposure.

Management

The management of such exposures entails reduction of the height of the root by trimming it down below the bone crest followed by a connective tissue graft coverage.

7.6.2 Infection

Periodontal or a periapical infection of the root piece is a potential threat to the long-term prognosis of the RST.

Cause

This is usually caused due to improper assessment of the preoperative situation. A pre-existing infection may be overlooked during the initial diagnosis and radiographic evaluation, and may manifest at a later date following the final restoration.

Prevention

Such complications can be prevented by a thorough preoperative clinical and radiographical evaluation of the health of the root prior to commencement of the procedure. The presence of a periapical infection leading to a future complication can be prevented by endodontically treating the root to be submerged [22, 23].

Management

A mild periapical infection can be treated by removal of the restoration, raising a flap to expose the root, and performing endodontic treatment. At times even an apical surgery may be considered. The restoration can be refixed over the implants after completion of the therapy and elimination of pathology. A moderate infection can be managed by converting the root submergence into a pontic shield preparation. By doing so, the apical contents of the root are completely eliminated, thus allowing a resolution of the infection. A severe infection leading to mobility of the root should be managed by a complete extraction of the root piece followed by a thorough debridement of the socket and a socket grafting procedure [21].

7.6.3 Migration of the Root

In rare cases a coronal migration of the root may occur.

Cause

This is usually caused due to mobilization of the root during the surgical procedure or improper selection of the case for submergence. Migration of the root is unlikely if the root was firm at the commencement of the treatment and was not inadvertently mobilized during the preparation.

Prevention

Adequate submergence of the root to ensure complete soft tissue coverage will reduce the chances of such complications.

Management

If the root piece which has migrated coronally but is found to be firm, trimming it down and covering with a soft tissue graft will help in managing the problem. In cases where the root is mobile, it will be prudent to extract it and cover the defect with a soft or hard tissue graft to maintain the tissue contours.

The main advantage of RST over other techniques is the ability to convert the situation to either a pontic shield procedure or a socket grafting procedure in case of a failure.

7.7 Case

An exposure of the root was observed in the following case of an attempted RST. A small part of the root was visible in the tooth #11 site after removal of the provisional restoration. The root was trimmed below the level of the crestal bone and a palatal pedicled flap was mobilized and sutured to cover the root (Figs. 7.21, 7.22, 7.23 and 7.24).

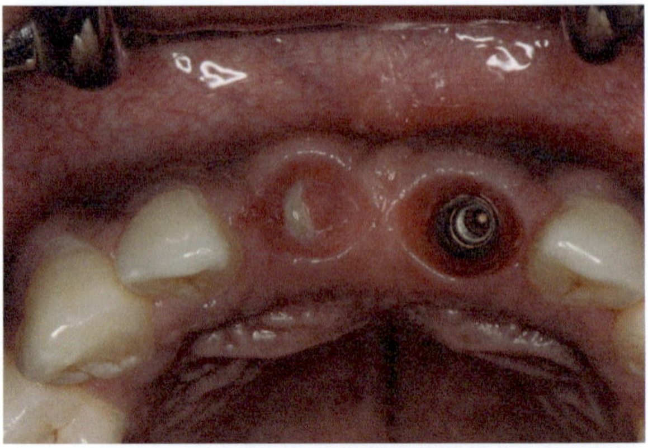

Fig. 7.21 Internal exposure of the submerged root

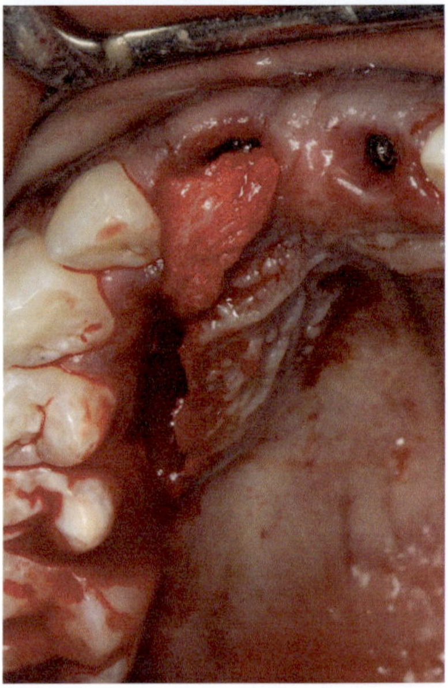

Fig. 7.22 Vascularized interpositional pedicled connective tissue graft (VIP-CT) palatal pedicle connective tissue to cover the exposed root

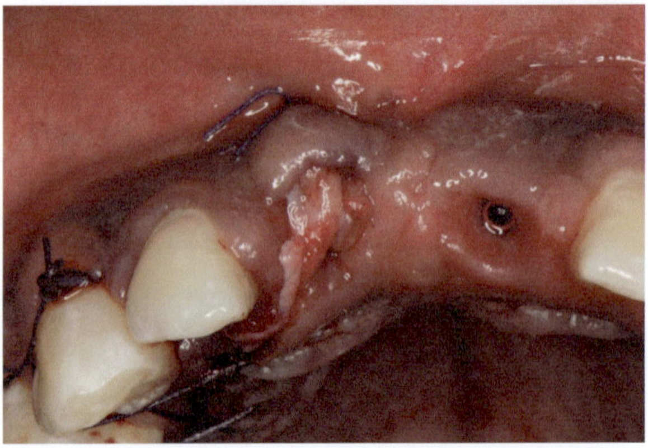

Fig. 7.23 The VIP-CT covering the exposed root

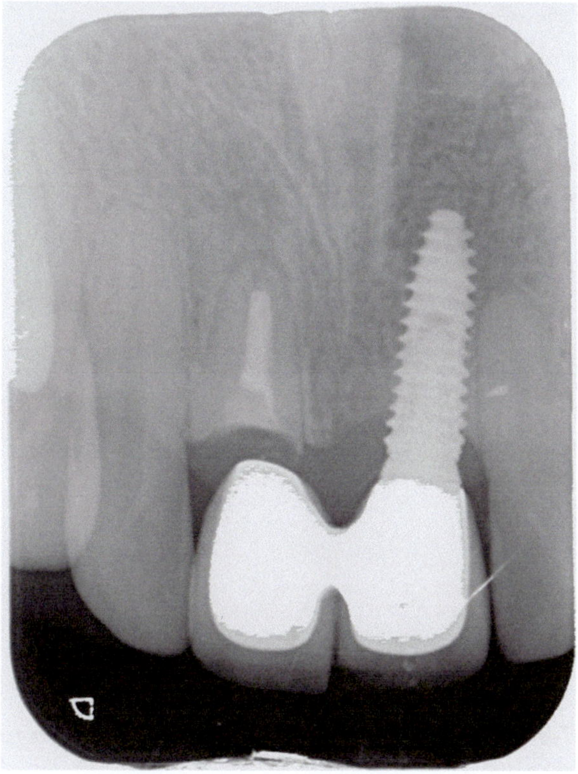

Fig. 7.24 Radiograph of the final restoration

7.8 Pontic Shield

7.8.1 Evolution of Pontic Shield Technique

One of the contraindications of the RST is the presence of an apical infection in the root to be submerged. To overcome this limitation, Gluckman et al. proposed a novel technique called the pontic shield (PS) which is a part of the partial extraction therapies [6, 7].

The procedure entails preparing the root exactly like the socket shield procedure and leaving it under a pontic. The advantage of this is to maintain the soft tissue contours which will allow excellent emergence profile for the pontic. It will also maintain the alveolar ridge dimension and prevents its potential collapse overtime (Fig. 7.25).

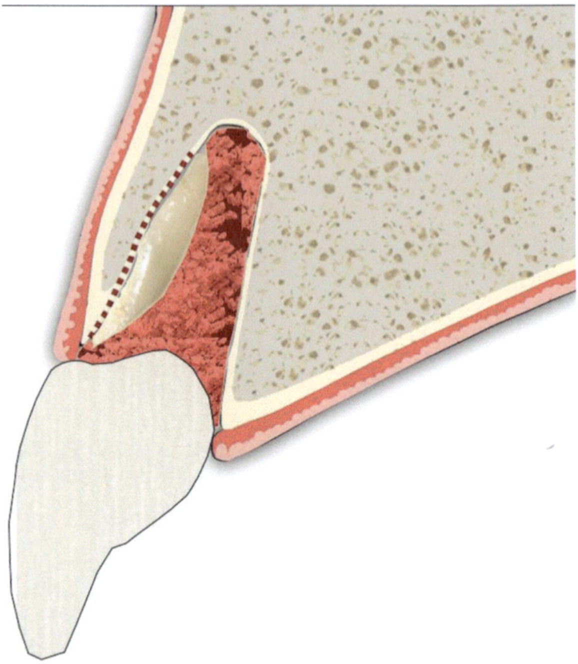

Fig. 7.25 Pontic shield

7.8.2 Indications for Pontic Shield Technique

A tooth that is indicated for an extraction could potentially be converted into a pontic shield. The prepared pontic shield could be used under an implant supported bridge. Roots with a small periapical lesion are chosen for pontic shield technique. Healthy roots without a periapical lesion are better suited for the root submergence technique.

The following are absolute contraindications for the pontic shield technique:

1. Mobile root: A mobile root is likely to migrate or erupt overtime and should not be chosen for a PS technique.
2. A root that is vertically fractured buccolingually: A fracture in the mesiodistal direction will be suitable for PS since the palatal fragment can be extracted and the labial fragment (if firm) can be retained for the shield preparation. A buccolingually fractured root should be extracted.
3. Very narrow or severely curved roots: Technical difficulties will be encountered during the shield preparation if the roots are curved or too narrow like the lower incisors.

4. Roots close to adjacent teeth: The inadvertent damage to the apex of the adjacent root is likely to occur if it is in close proximity to the root to be prepared. Hence such roots should not be selected for shield preparation.
5. External resorption on buccal aspect: The external resorption on the labial aspect of the root may continue even after shield preparation leading to a failure of the treatment.

7.9 Pontic Shield: Surgical Technique

The preparation of the root for the pontic shield follows the exact guidelines as the socket shield technique described in details in Chap. 2 [24–26].

Following shield preparation the socket may or may not be grafted. No consensus exists to date on the need to use a bone substitute material in the remaining part of socket. Some degree of soft tissue invagination may occur due to lack of a bone graft material. This may not negatively impact the final outcome, since no implant is being placed in that site. The labial shield helps in maintaining the labial contours. However, placement of a bone graft will ensure a complete bone fill which may be beneficial if that site is to be used for an implant placement in future.

After shield preparation and socket grafting, soft tissue closure is achieved with the help of an autogeneous soft tissue grafting procedure similar to that for an RST, explained earlier in this chapter (Fig. 7.26).

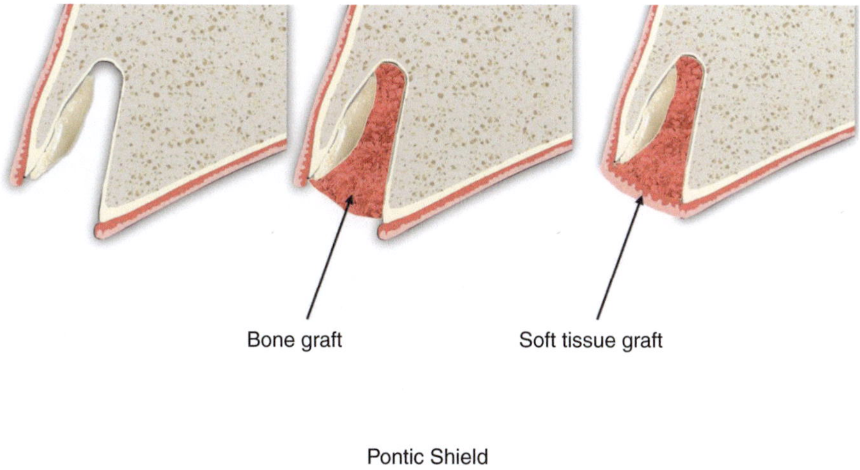

Fig. 7.26 Steps for the pontic shield procedure

7.10 Cases

The following are a few cases in which the sites have been preserved to achieve good emergence profiles for future pontics using the pontic shield technique [7].

Five different techniques of closure of the socket following shield preparation are illustrated in these cases. Whilst the shield preparation technique remains the same in all cases the method of achieving closure over the socket differs in each case.

7.10.1 Case 1

Case illustrating pontic shield in relation to a maxillary second premolar between two implants in maxillary first premolar and maxillary molar. Primary closure was achieved in this case by a buccal advancement flap and horizontal mattress sutures (Figs. 7.27, 7.28, 7.29, 7.30, 7.31, 7.32, 7.33 and 7.34).

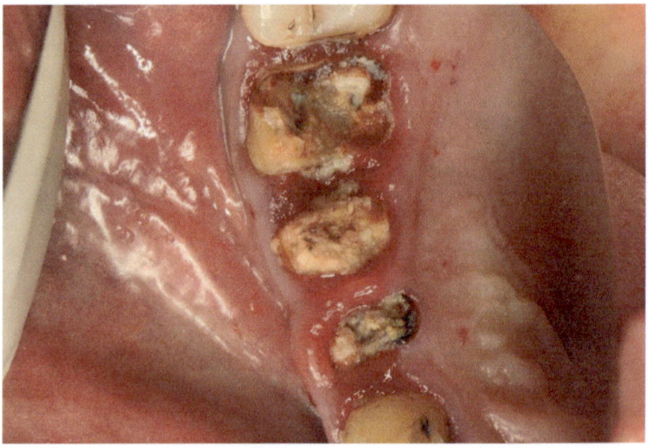

Fig. 7.27 Fractured non-restorable maxillary posterior teeth #14, #15, and #16

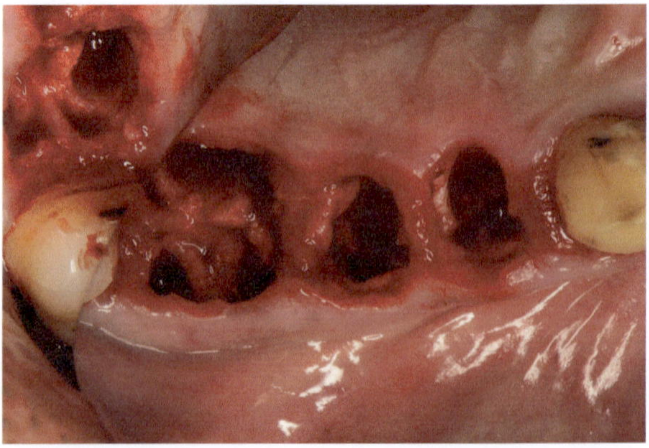

Fig. 7.28 Shields prepared similar to the socket shield in the premolar sockets

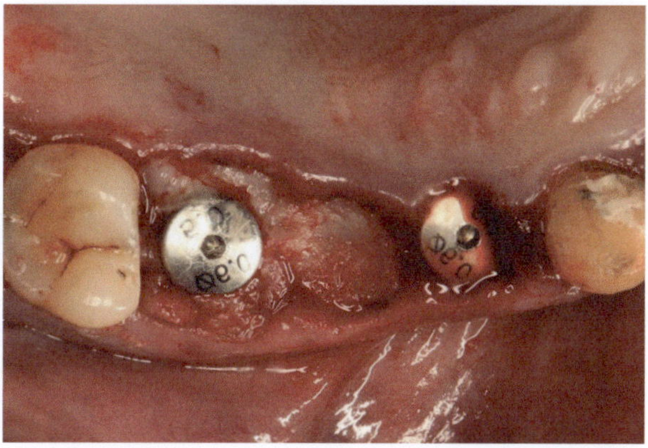

Fig. 7.29 Immediate post-extraction implant placed in the molar area and implant placed with SS in tooth #14 area. For tooth #15 site the shield is left in-situ and the socket is filled with calcium phosphosilicate putty bone graft (Novabone Inc., U.S.A.)

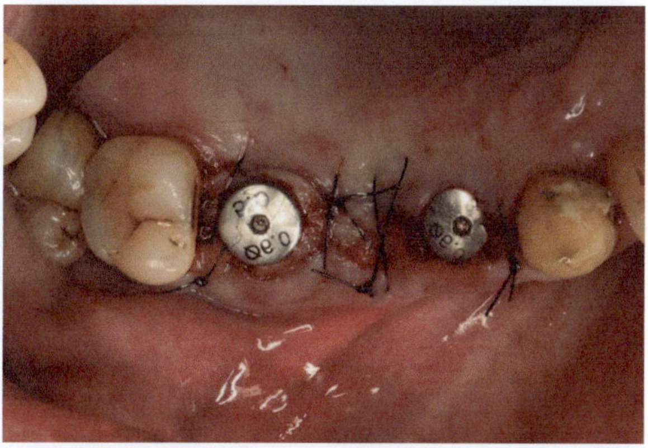

Fig. 7.30 Primary closure to prevent extrusion of graft material

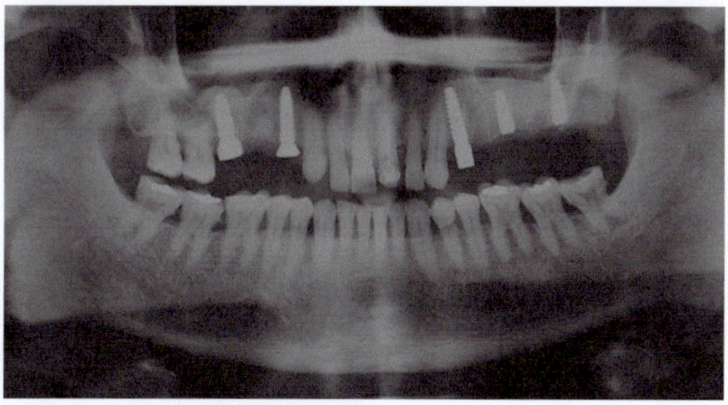

Fig. 7.31 Radiograph taken immediate post-implant placement

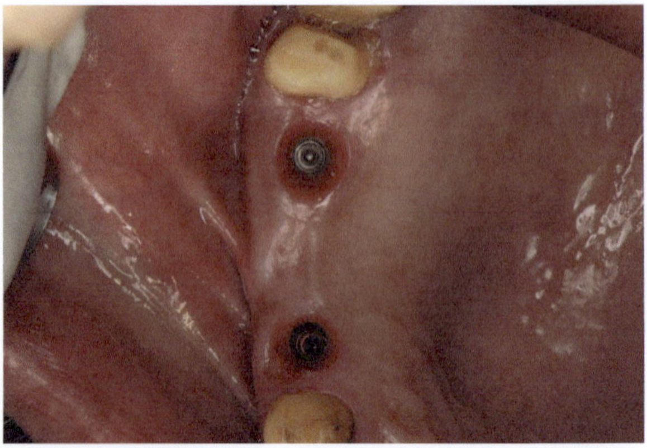

Fig. 7.32 Note the intact contour of teeth 14 and 15 sites. The soft tissue on the ridge as well as on the buccal aspect appear well contoured

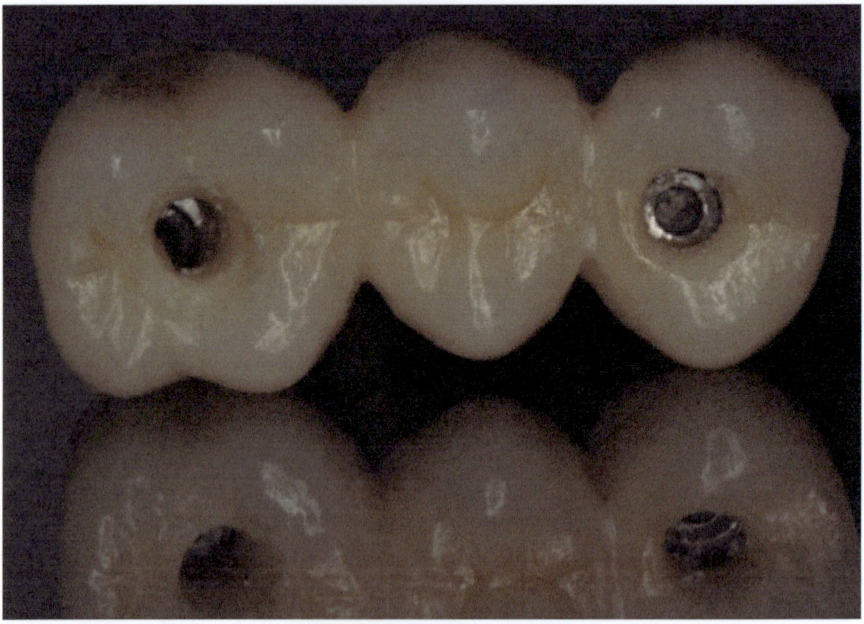

Fig. 7.33 The final prosthesis: screw-retained metal-ceramic bridge

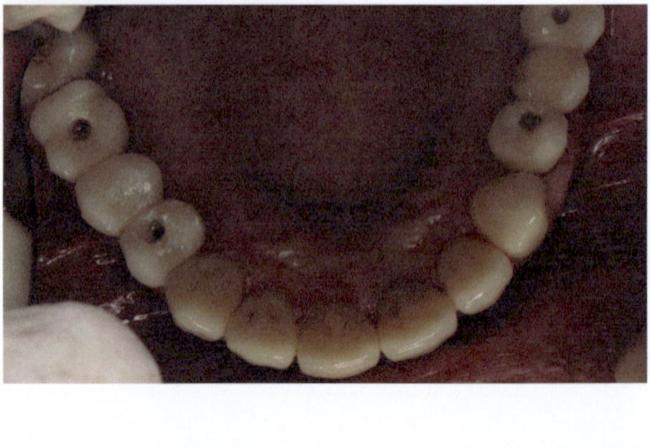

Fig. 7.34 Final screw-retained restoration

7.10.2 Case 2

The following case required multiple implant placements after socket shield procedure in the anterior maxilla. The pontic shields were prepared at the sites where no implants needed to be placed. Calcium phosphosilicate putty (Novabone Inc., USA) was used to graft the sockets and was covered with collagen sponge and figure of 8 sutures (Figs. 7.35, 7.36, 7.37, 7.38 and 7.39).

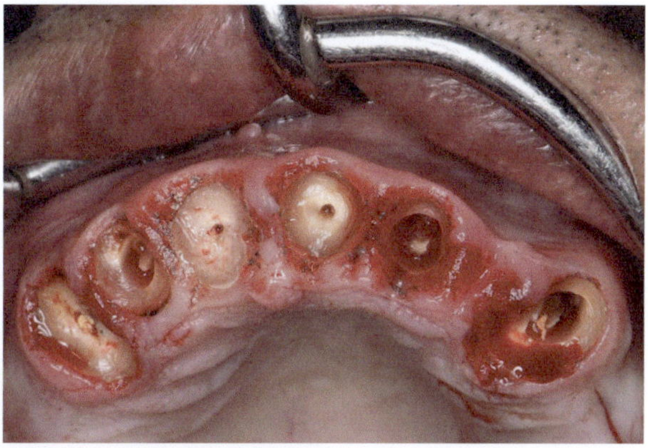

Fig. 7.35 Multiple pontic sites situation in the maxilla extending from tooth 13 to 23 after de-coronation

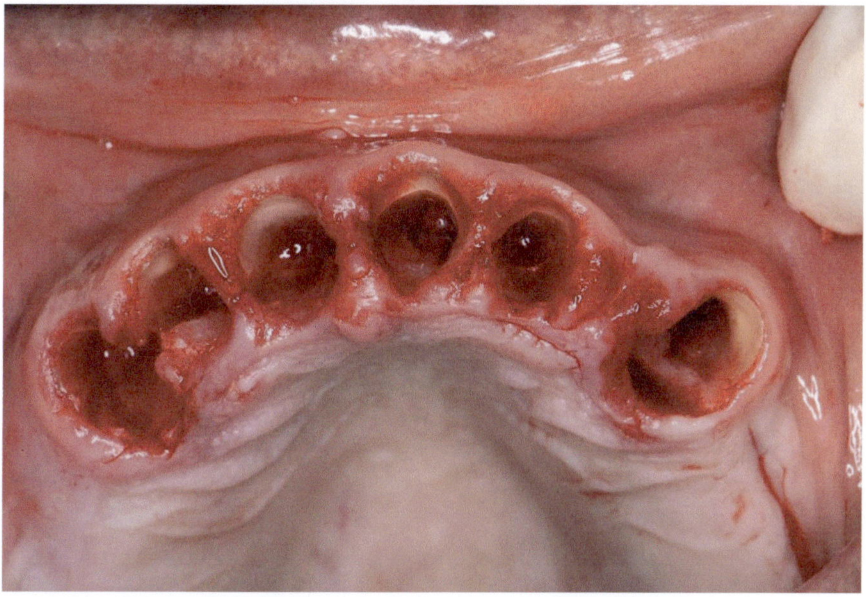

Fig. 7.36 Multiple shields prepared

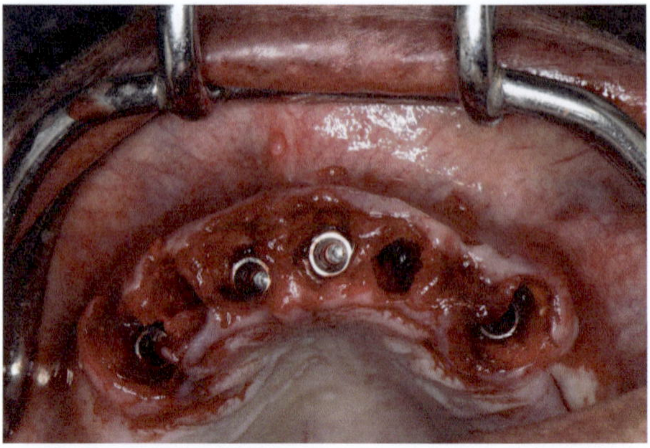

Fig. 7.37 Implant placement done in relation to sites 13, 11, 21, 23 and pontic shield in relation to sites 12, 22

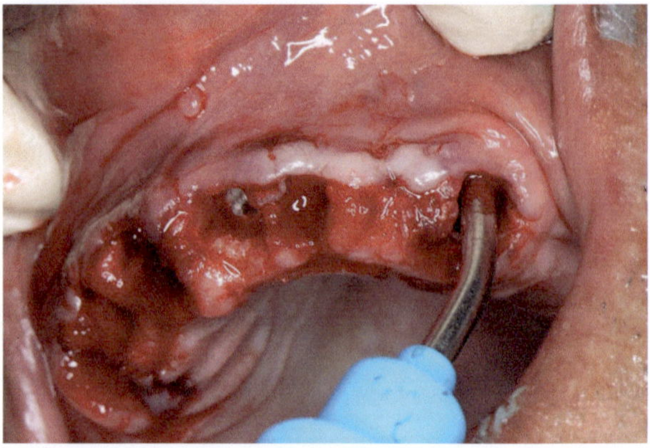

Fig. 7.38 Grafting of gaps and pontic shield area with a bone substitute material

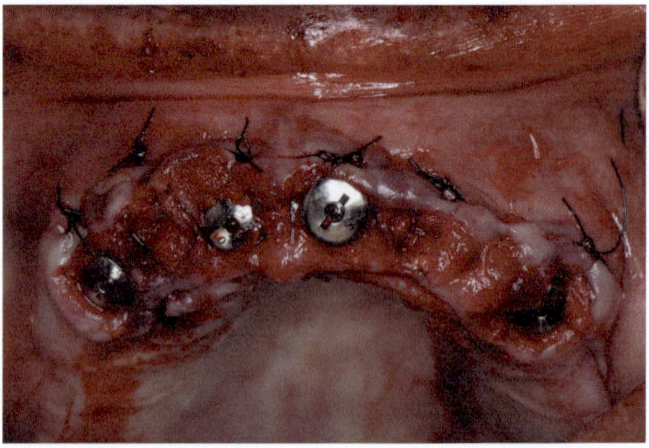

Fig. 7.39 Post-implant placement; collagen sponge placed and suturing done

7.10.3 Case 3

In the following case the pontic site for the maxillary central incisor was filled with platelet-rich fibrin (A-PRF) and allowed to heal by secondary intention (Figs. 7.40, 7.41, 7.42, 7.43, 7.44, 7.45 and 7.46).

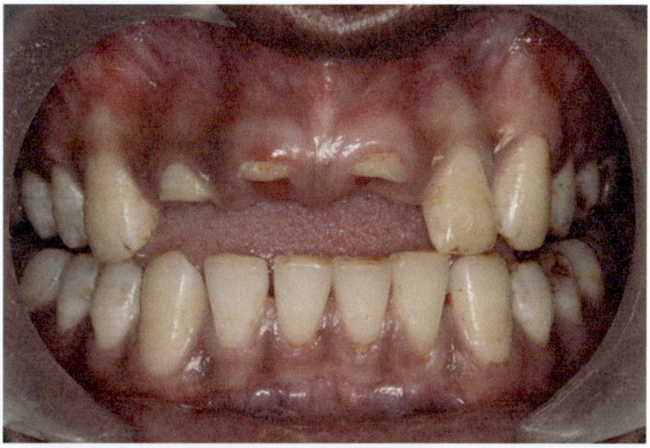

Fig. 7.40 Cantilever pontic site (between two implants)—indication for PS, fractured teeth 11, 12, and 21

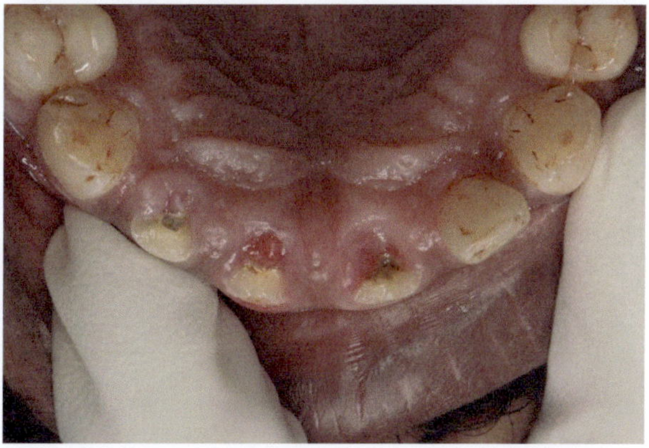

Fig. 7.41 Occlusal view showing non restorable fractured teeth

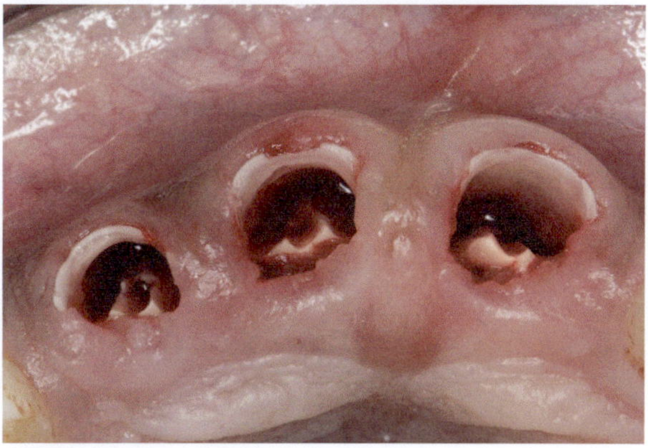

Fig. 7.42 Partial root removal and shield preparation

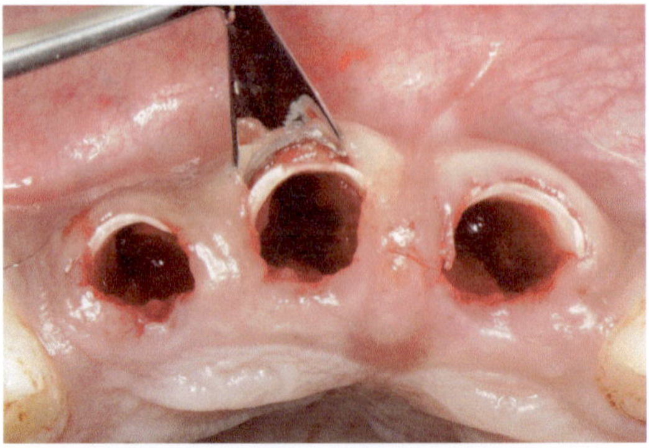

Fig. 7.43 Socket shields re-contoured to the level of the crestal bone

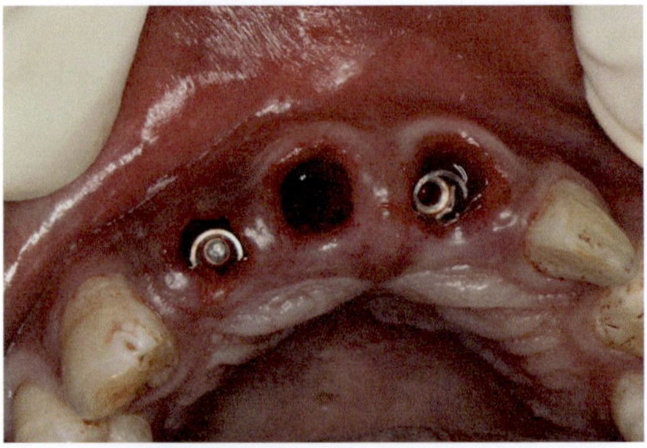

Fig. 7.44 Pontic shield in relation to tooth 11 and SS with teeth 12 and 21

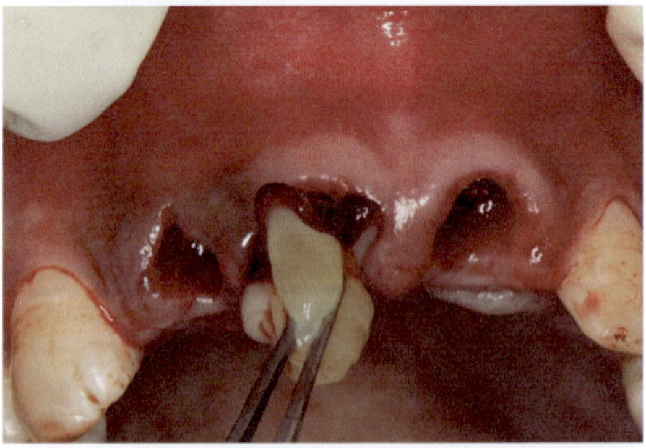

Fig. 7.45 A-PRF™ (platelet-rich fibrin) plugged in the sockets

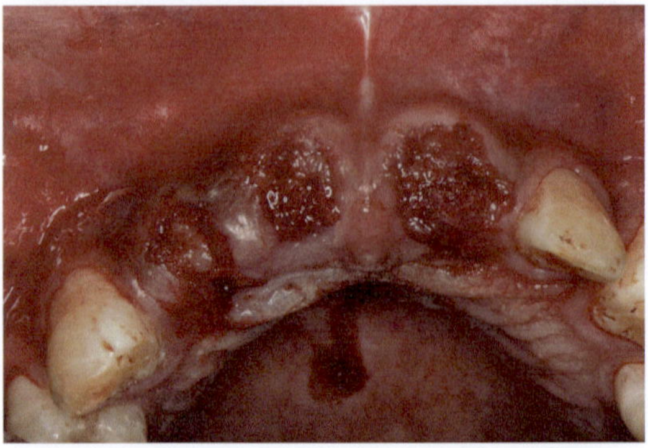

Fig. 7.46 Sockets sealed with PRF plugs

7.10.4 Case 4

The following case demonstrates the use of a pedicled palatal flap to achieve complete closure of the pontic site. A-PRF was used to graft the remainder of the socket after pontic shield preparation (Figs. 7.47, 7.48, 7.49, 7.50, 7.51, 7.52, 7.53 and 7.54).

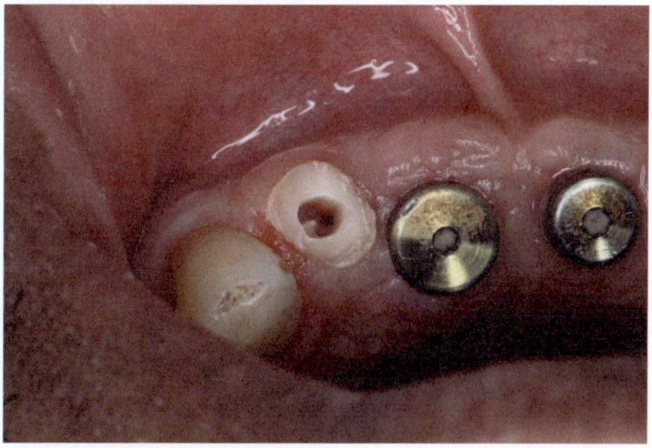

Fig. 7.47 De-coronation of tooth 12

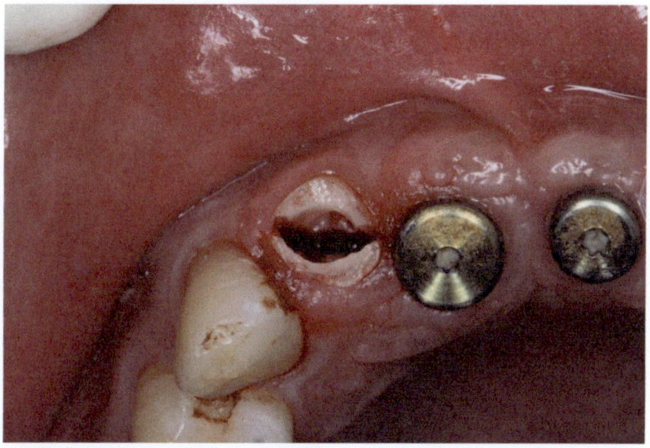

Fig. 7.48 Sectioning of the tooth

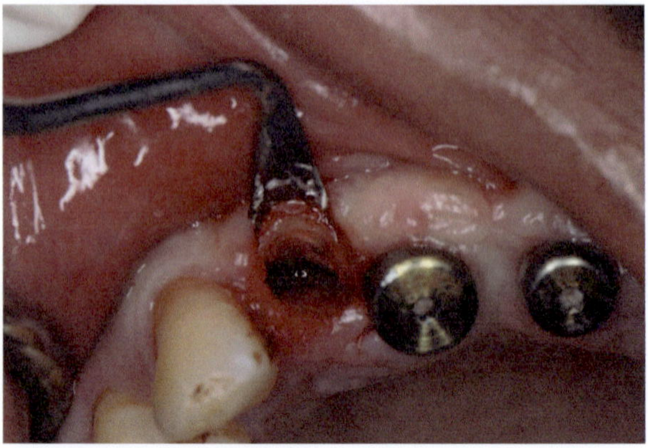

Fig. 7.49 Partial root removal and contouring of remaining root to the level of the crestal bone

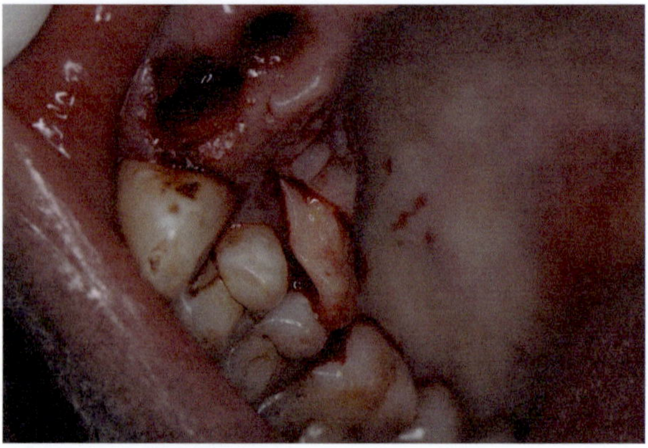

Fig. 7.50 Mobilizing a pedicled graft from the palate

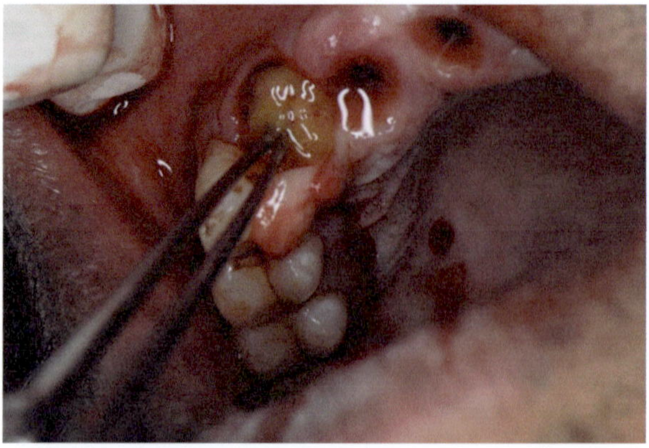

Fig. 7.51 A-PRF™ placed in the tooth 12 socket

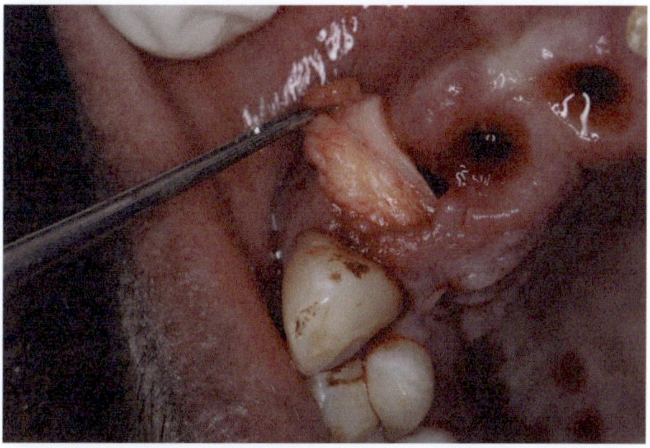

Fig. 7.52 VIP-CT flap for soft tissue coverage

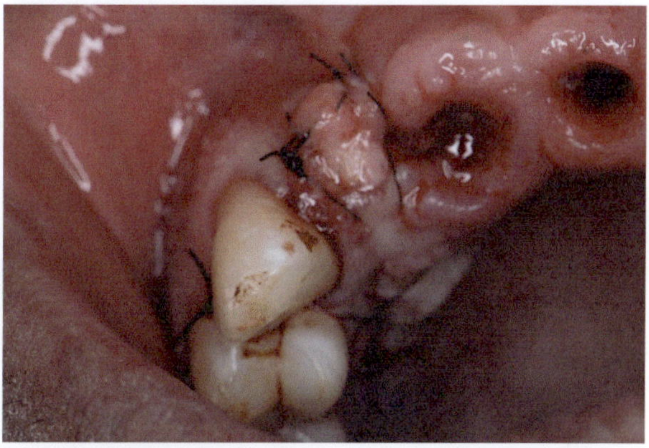

Fig. 7.53 Flap approximated and closed

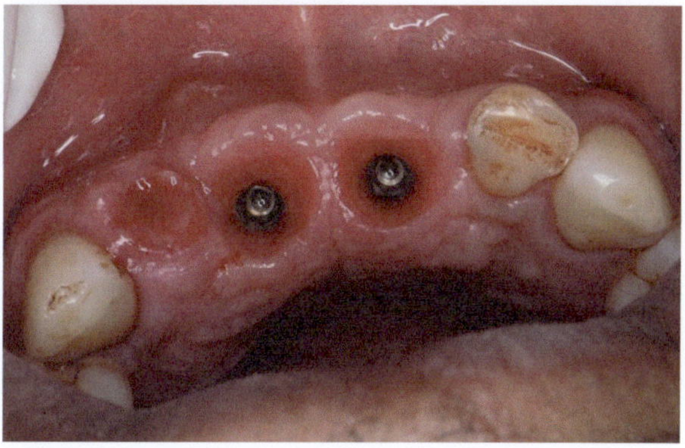

Fig. 7.54 Healed implant and pontic site at 3 months

7.10.5 Case 5

In the following case no attempt was made to graft the pontic shield site with any bone substitute material. Also, no soft tissue closure procedure was carried out. Socket healing by secondary intention, like a conventional extraction socket was achieved* (Figs. 7.55, 7.56, 7.57 and 7.58).

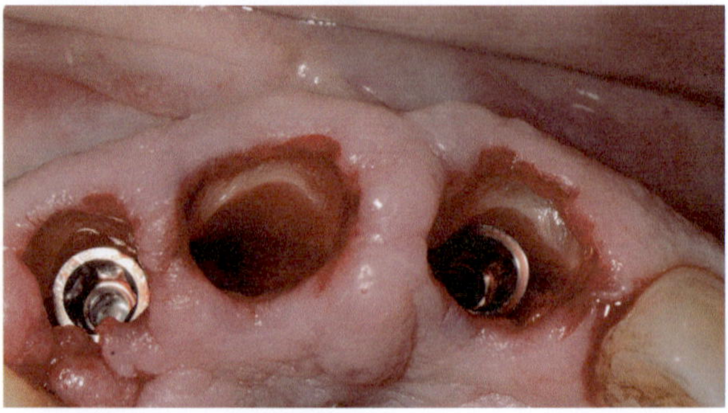

Fig. 7.55 Socket shield procedure for teeth 12 and 21. Pontic shield preparation for tooth 11

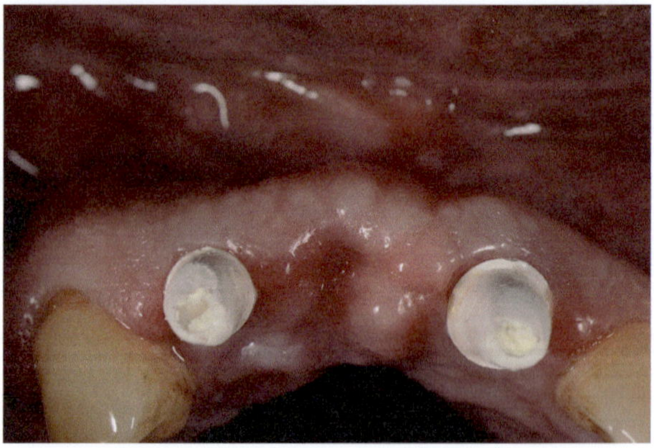

Fig. 7.56 After healing. Note complete closure of pontic shield site with soft tissue

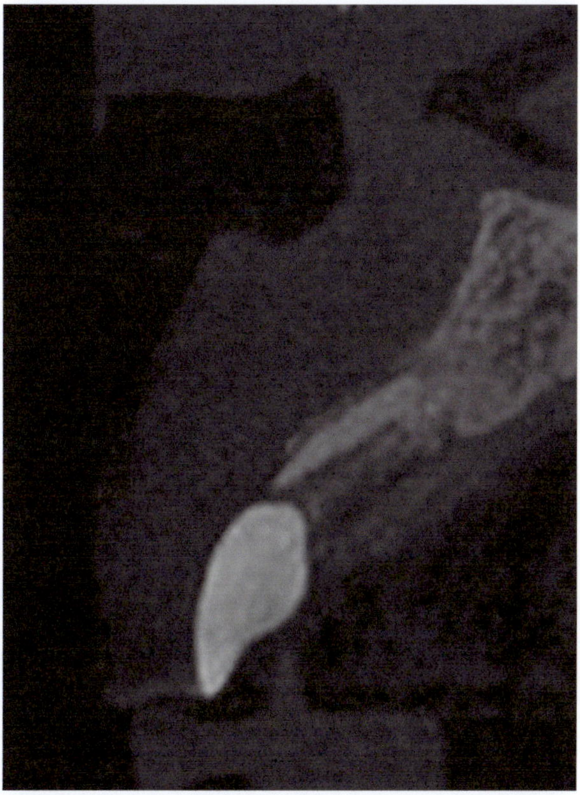

Fig. 7.57 Postoperative CBCT showing pontic shield and the completely healed socket

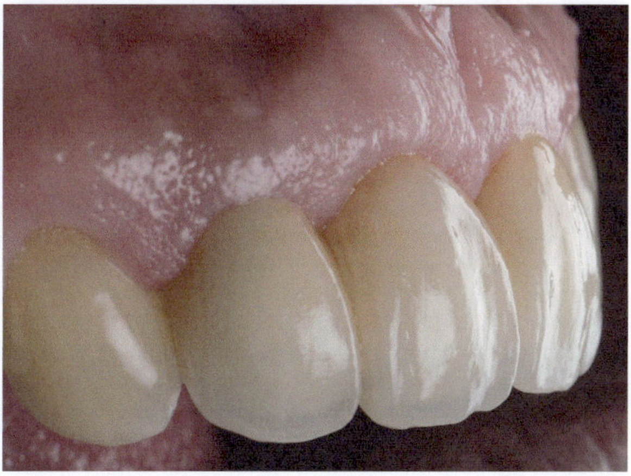

Fig. 7.58 Post-restoration view of the implant supported bridge with excellent tissue contours below the pontic

7.11 Conclusion

The procedures of root submergence and pontic shield preparation are convenient for preparing pontic sites for restorations, either with implant supported prosthesis or under conventional prosthesis. The retention of the root or only the buccal aspect of the root holds up the sensitive buccal cortical plate, and thus maintains the morphology of the alveolus. This procedure aids in optimizing esthetic outcomes in pontic sites, especially in the anterior maxilla by providing ideal emergence contours for the restorations.

Acknowledgement Illustrations by: Udatta Kher
*Case 5 Courtesy: Dr Ali Tunkiwala

References

1. Araujo MG, Lindhe J. Dimensional ridge alterations following tooth extraction. An experimental study in the dog. J Clin Periodontol. 2005;32:212–8.
2. Schropp L, Wenzel A, Kostopoulos KT. Bone healing and soft tissue contour changes following single tooth extraction: A clinical and radiographic 12-month prospective study. Int J Periodontics Restorative Dent. 2003;23:313–23.
3. Araujo M, Sukekava F, Wennstrom J, Lindhe J. Ridge alterations following implant placement in fresh extraction sockets: an experimental study in the dog. J Clin Periodontol. 2006;32:645–52.
4. Nevins M, Camelo M, De Paoli S, et al. A study of the fate of the buccal wall of extraction sockets of teeth with prominent roots. Int J Periodontics Restorative Dent. 2006;26:19–29.
5. Salama H, Salama MA, Garber D, Adar P. The inter-proximal height of bone: A guidepost to predictable aesthetic strategies and soft tissue contours in anterior tooth replacement. Pract Periodontics Aesthet Dent. 1998;10:1131–41.
6. Salama M, Ishikawa T, Salama H, Funato A, Garber D. Advantages of the root sub-mergence technique for pontic site development in esthetic implant therapy. Int J Periodontics Restorative Dent. 2007;27:521–7.
7. Gluckman H, Salama M, Du Toit J. Partial extraction therapies (PET) part 1: maintaining alveolar ridge contour at pontic and immediate implant sites. Int J Periodontics Restorative Dent. 2016;36(5):681–7.
8. Howell F. Retention of alveolar bone by endodontic root treatment. Seminario Annual del Grupo de Estudios Dentales U.S.C de Mexico 23, May 1970
9. Malmgren B, Cvek M, Lundberg M, Frykholm A. Surgical treatment of ankylosed andinfrapositioned reimplanted incisors in adolescents. Scand J Dent Res. 1984;92:391–9.
10. Malmgren B, Malmgren O, Andreasen JO. Alveolar bone development after decoro-nation of ankylosed teeth. Endod Topics. 2006;14:35–40.
11. Whitaker DD, Shankle RJ. A study of the histologic reaction of submerged root segments. Oral Surg Oral Med Oral Pathol. 1974;37:919e35.
12. Levin MP, Getter L, Cutright DE, Bhaskar SN. Intentional submucosal submergence of nonvital roots. J Oral Surg. 1974;32(11):834–9.
13. Guyer SE. Selectively retained vital roots for partial support of overdentures: A patient report. J Prosthet Dent. 1975;33:258–63.
14. Plata RL, Kelln EE, Linda L. Intentional retention of vital submerged roots in dogs. Oral Surg Oral Med Oral Pathol. 1976;42:100–8.
15. O'Neal R, Gound T, Levin MP, del Rio BCE. Submergence of roots for alveolar bone preservation. I. Endodontically treated roots. Oral Surg Oral Med Oral Pathol. 1978;45:803–10.

16. Welker WA, Jividen GJ, Kramer DC. Preventive prosthodonticsDOUBLEHYPHENmucosal coverage of roots. J Prosthet Dent. 1978;40:619–21.
17. Garver DG, Fenster RK. Vital root retention in humans: a final report. J Prosthet Dent. 1980;43:368–73.
18. Von Wowern N, Winther S. Submergence of roots for alveolar ridge preservation. A failure (4-year follow-up study). Int J Oral Surg. 1981;10:247–50.
19. Garver DG, Muir TE. The retention of vital submucosal roots under immediate dentures: a surgical procedure. J Prosthet Dent. 1983 Dec;50(6):753–6. PubMed PMID: 6581289
20. Lambert PM, et al. Autogenous dermal graft coverage of submerged roots in the dog. J Oral Maxillofac Surg. 42(9):595–9.
21. Harper KA. Submerging an endodontically treated root to preserve the alveolar ridge under a bridge—A case report. Dent Update. 2002;29:200–3.
22. Wong KM, Chneh CM, Ang CW. Modified root submergence technique for multiple implant-supported maxillary anterior restorations in a patient with thin gingival biotype: a clinical report. J Prosthet Dent. 2012;107:349–52.
23. Gongloff RK. Vital root retention. A 5-year experience. Int J Oral MaxillofacSurg. 1986;15:33–8.
24. Gluckman H, Salama M, Du Toit J. Partial extraction therapies (PET) part 2: procedures and technical aspects. Int J Periodontics Restorative Dent. 2017;37(3):377–85.
25. Glocker M, Attin T, Schmidlin P. Ridge preservation with modified "Socket- Shield" technique: methodological case series. Dent J. 2014;2:11–21.
26. Dohan DM, Choukroun J, Diss A, et al. Platelet-rich fibrin (PRF): a second-generation platelet concentrate. Part II : Plateletrelated biologic features. Oral Surg Oral Med Oral Pathol Oral Radiol Endod. 2006;101:E45–50.

PET for Multiple Teeth and Full-Arch Implant-Supported Reconstructions

8

Udatta Kher

Abstract

Over the past few years, clinicians from various parts of the world have experienced a high level of success with the PET procedures for single teeth in the esthetic zone. It is time to explore the possibilities of PET procedures for multiple implant sites and full-arch implant-supported restorations. Ridge alterations and loss of hard and soft tissue is far more pronounced in cases where multiple teeth are extracted. Using a combination of the socket shield, pontic shield and, root submergence procedures, clinicians can now predictably achieve satisfactory contours around implants. Preserving healthy parts of the roots and eliminating only the diseased portions can go a long way in avoiding advanced grafting procedures for long span implant cases and full-arch implant-supported rehabilitations. This chapter pushes the boundaries of PET procedures in complicated cases requiring multiple teeth extractions and simultaneous implant placements.

8.1 Introduction

Full-arch reconstruction with implant-supported restorations is a complex treatment procedure wherein the clinician is faced with numerous challenges. One of the biggest limitations with long-standing edentulous ridges is finding adequate bone for implant placements. Ridge alteration after extractions of all teeth is commonly observed [1–3]. Pneumatization of the sinus is one of the most common post-extraction complications in posterior maxilla that limits the available bone for the implant placement [4]. Another common occurrence is the limited amount of attached keratinized tissue around implants placed in fully edentulous jaws [5]. It is

U. Kher (✉)
Only Smiles Dental Centre, Mumbai, India

U. Kher, A. Tunkiwala (eds.), *Partial Extraction Therapy in Implant Dentistry*,
https://doi.org/10.1007/978-3-030-33610-3_8

well established that implants are at a higher risk of bone loss and peri-implantitis when there is deficient attached tissues around implants [6]. Extensive amount of hard and soft tissue augmentation procedures are required in cases where teeth have been completely extracted [7–10]. The other challenge during the restorative phase is to create good emergence profiles around implants abutments and pontic sites. Improper emergence profiles lead to a poor esthetic result and difficulty in long-term maintenance of the implant-supported restoration [11].

Socket shield procedures, performed by preserving the labial part of the roots, have been successfully done for single teeth implant-supported restorations [12, 13]. Extending the scope of partial extraction therapies to multiple sites needing post-extraction immediate implant placements will have a significant benefit in maintaining the alveolar ridge architecture around the implants [14, 15]. In the past clinicians have found it extremely challenging to reconstruct loss of alveolus and surrounding teeth structures after extractions of multiple teeth in the esthetic zone. Hard and soft tissue augmentation for multiple implant sites is a complex treatment procedure [9, 10, 16]. Vertical augmentation has limited long-term success rate as reported in literature. Hence an alternative protocol which is aimed at preserving bone and soft tissue instead of reconstructing tissues could be the solution to these problems.

Performing multiple PETs on adjacent sites needing post-extraction implant placements should be undertaken by clinicians after getting comfortable with PET procedures on single teeth. The rationale for doing socket shield procedures for adjacent implant sites was highlighted in Chap. 5. By extending this scope further to involve more number of teeth along with the applications of pontic shields and root submergence technique, the clinician can handle more challenging situations in treating multiple implant sites and full-arch implant-supported reconstructions [15, 17–19]. A high level of clinical expertise and experience in single teeth PET procedures is required for clinicians to undertake such complex cases [20].

8.2 Challenges in Multiple Sites Treated with PET

1. Time-consuming process for partial extractions of roots: Partial extractions of multiple roots can take much longer than extracting the whole tooth. This may increase the overall surgical time for the procedure.
2. Prosthetically driven implant placements: Placing multiple implants in ideal locations is simpler when one does post-extraction immediate placements, since the sockets provide the exact locations for insertion of implants. However, managing implant trajectories and depth of placements can be quite challenging. Guided implant placements using CT-guided stents will be helpful to overcome this difficulty.
3. Fabrication of a fixed temporary restoration: Fabricating a fixed provisional restoration on the day of the surgery is also a time-consuming process and needs the services of the restorative dentist and the laboratory.

4. Management of minor healing complications like internal and external shield exposures: With more shields to prepare in full-arch cases, the incidence of minor complications like internal and external exposures is likely to be more and management of these complications during the healing phase is an additional burden on the clinician [21].

8.3 Case 1

The following case utilizes all the PET procedures for a maxillary full-arch implant-supported reconstruction.

A 65-year-old healthy non-smoker male reported with repeated debonding of his crowns which were done 15 years ago. The underlying teeth were badly destroyed due to secondary caries under the crowns and were non-restorable. A decision was made to extract the teeth and provide him with an implant-supported fixed denture. The periodontal status was satisfactory. He desired a fixed provisional restoration during the healing phase of his treatment. His treatment was divided into 3 phases.

8.3.1 Phase 1: Socket Shields and Tooth-Supported Provisional Restorations

In the first phase of treatment, a well-adjusted fixed provisional restoration was fabricated on the existing teeth after removal of the old restorations. The provisional restoration was designed to adapt to desirable function, phonetics, and esthetics. Thereafter, socket shield procedures were performed on teeth 12, 13, 21, and 23 utilizing the technique described in Chap. 2. The implants placed after the socket shield procedures were kept submerged. Few strategic teeth were chosen to support the fixed provisional restoration (Figs. 8.1, 8.2, 8.3, 8.4, 8.5 and 8.6).

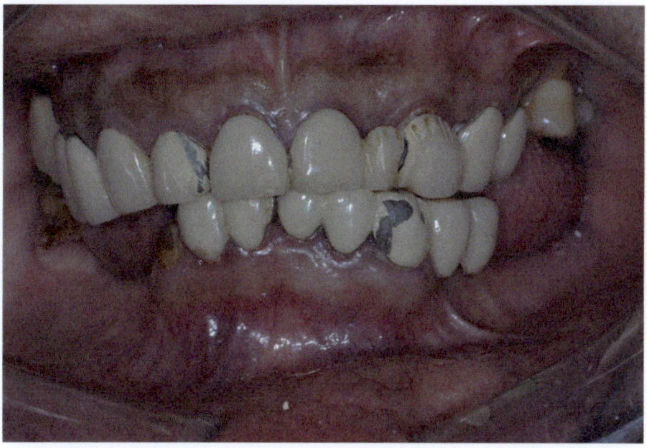

Fig. 8.1 Preoperative situation. Failing upper dentition

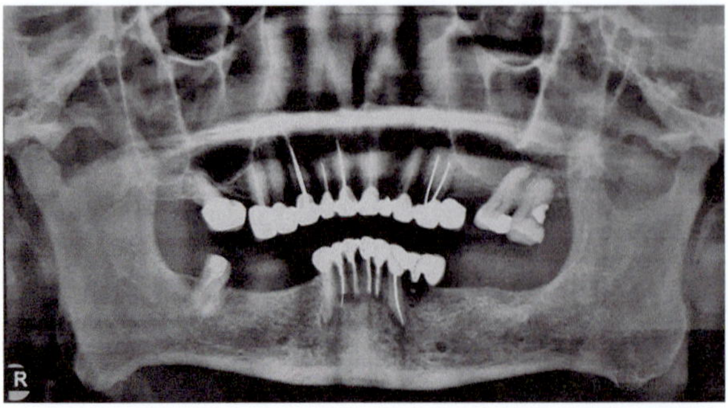

Fig. 8.2 Radiograph showing endodontically treated teeth with post and cores having periapical lesions

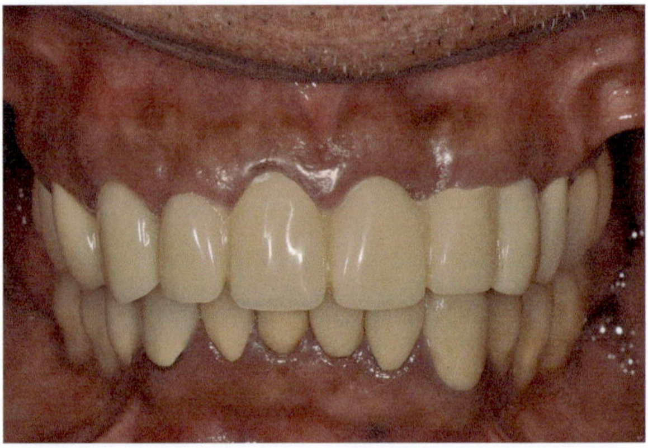

Fig. 8.3 Fixed provisional restorations fabricated on natural teeth

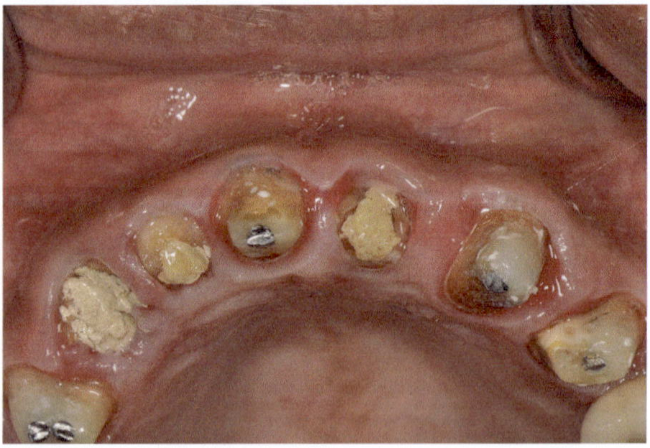

Fig. 8.4 Condition of underlying natural teeth

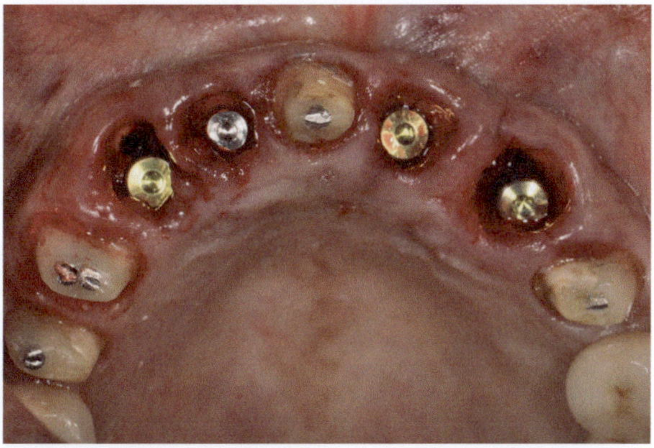

Fig. 8.5 Partial Extraction Therapies on 4 anterior teeth. Socket shields with implant placement in teeth 12, 13, 21, and 23

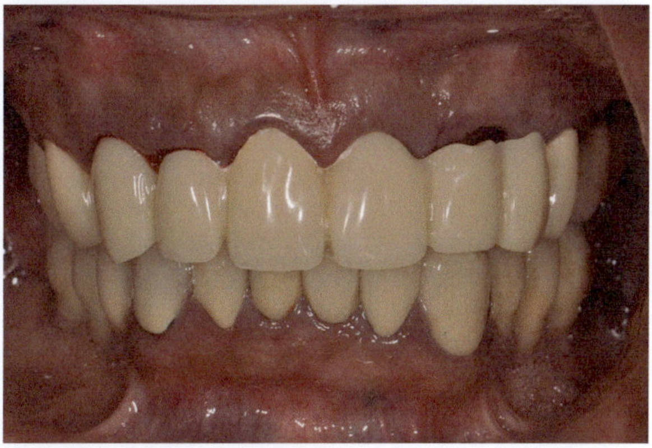

Fig. 8.6 Fixed provisional restoration on the remaining natural teeth

8.3.2 Phase 2: Pontic Shield, Root Submergence Technique, and Implant-Supported Provisional Restorations

After 3 months of healing time, the provisional restoration was removed. The submerged implants were surgically exposed and temporary titanium abutments were attached onto these implants. Tooth 11 was prepared for a pontic shield since it had a minor periapical lesion. Care was taken to completely remove the apex of the root and the periapical area was thoroughly debrided using small tipped bone curettes. A small piece of collagen plug was placed in the socket to help in retaining the blood clot.

Teeth 14, 15, and 24 were prepared for root submergence as described in Chap. 7. The roots were kept at the level of the crestal bone and the tissue around them was allowed to close by secondary healing.

A putty index was prepared before the removal of the existing tooth-supported provisional restoration, which provided the form for fabrication of the implant-supported fixed temporary restoration. The openings of the temporary titanium abutments were filled with cotton. An auto-polymerizing composite material was used to fabricate the implant-supported provisional restoration with the help of the putty index. After setting of the material, the cotton pieces were removed from the abutments and the internal screws were loosened. The provisional restoration attached to the titanium abutments were removed from the mouth and voids were filled using light-cured flowable resin material. Finishing and polishing was done and the provisional screw-retained restoration was fixed over the implants. Occlusal adjustments were done so as to achieve uniform contacts of equal intensity across all the teeth in the arch (Figs. 8.7, 8.8, 8.9, 8.10, 8.11 and 8.12).

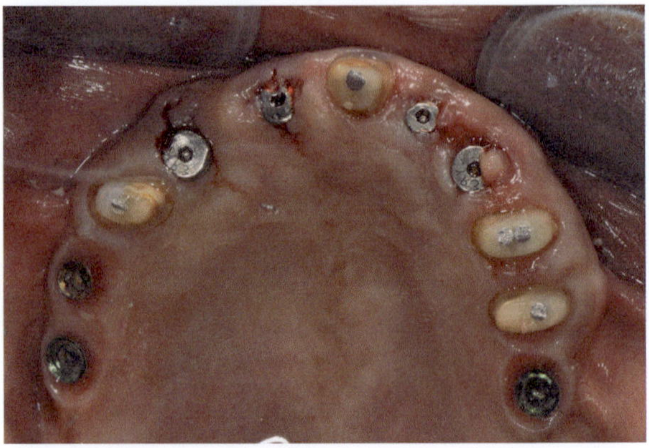

Fig. 8.7 Surgical exposure of osseointegrated implants

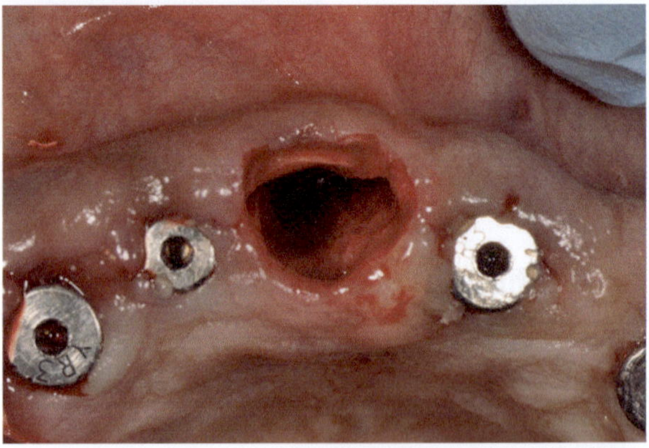

Fig. 8.8 Pontic shield preparation for tooth 11

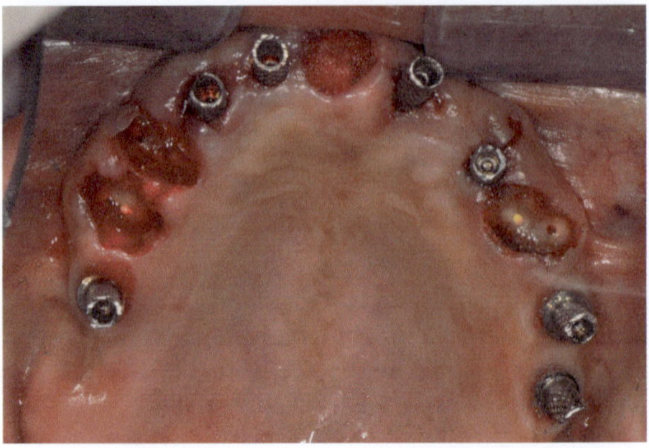

Fig. 8.9 Root submergence technique for teeth 14, 15, and 24. Temporary titanium abutments for supporting a screw-retained fixed provisional restoration

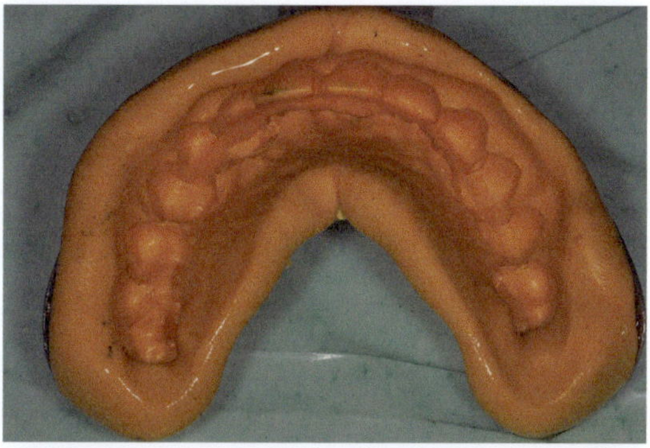

Fig. 8.10 Silicone index of the provisional restoration

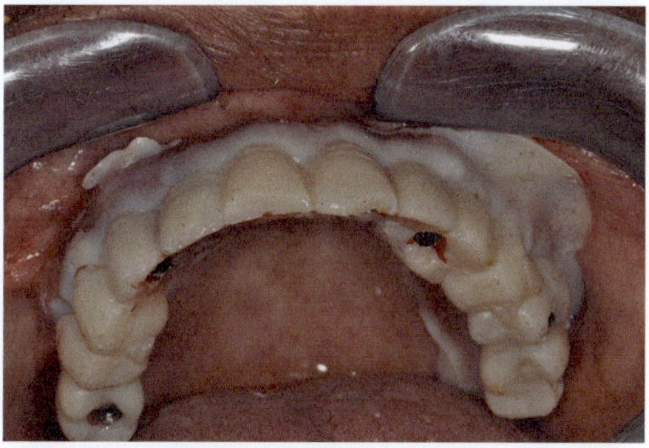

Fig. 8.11 Fabrication of a screw-retained fixed provisional restoration on osseointegrated implants

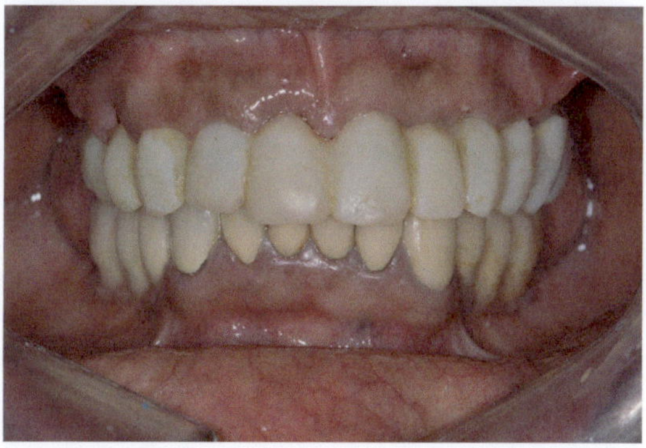

Fig. 8.12 Maxillary screw-retained restoration on all the osseointegrated implants

8.3.3 Phase 3: Definitive Restoration

After 4 weeks of healing time, the provisional restoration was removed and the fabrication of the definitive restoration was initiated. The soft tissue contours developed with the provisional restoration were found to be satisfactory. The final restoration was a screw-retained porcelain fused to metal prosthesis. The internal screws of the prosthesis were torqued at 30 Ncm as recommended by the manufacturer. Occlusal adjustments were done and the screw accesses were sealed using composite resin (Figs. 8.13, 8.14, 8.15, 8.16, 8.17 and 8.18). *

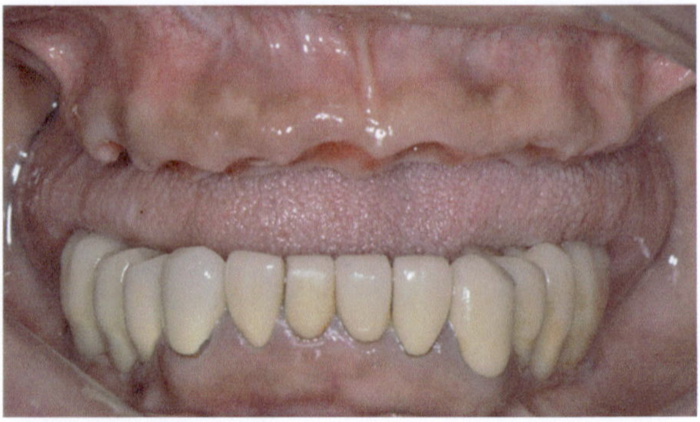

Fig. 8.13 Soft tissue architecture seen after removal of the provisional restoration

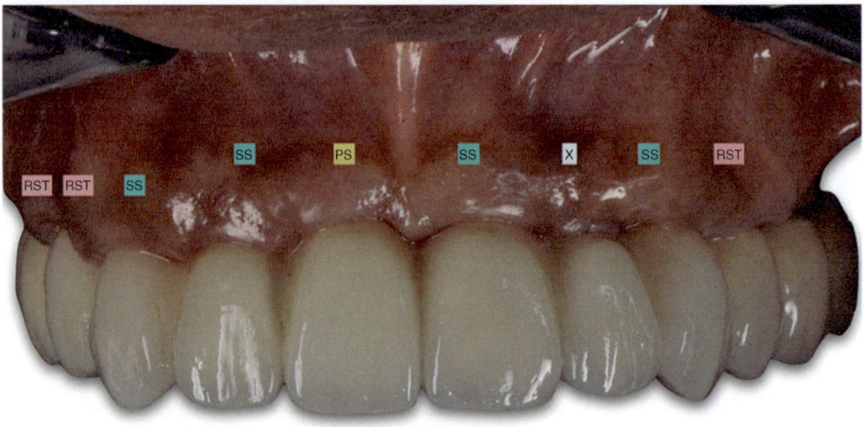

Fig. 8.14 Screw-retained porcelain fused to metal fixed restoration

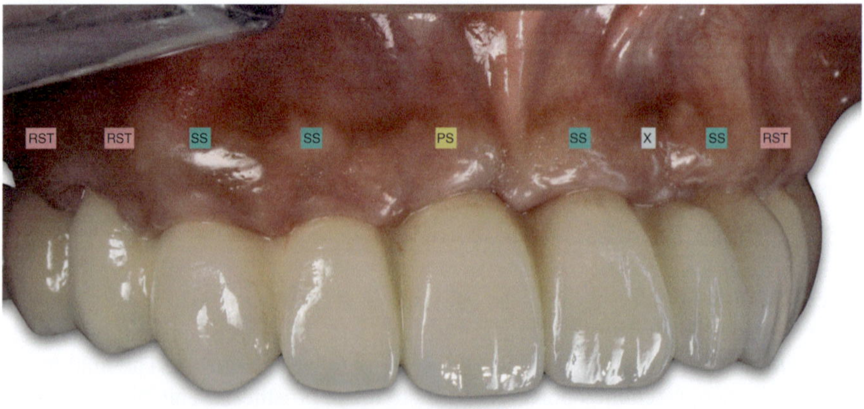

Fig. 8.15 Right lateral view of the definitive screw-retained fixed restoration

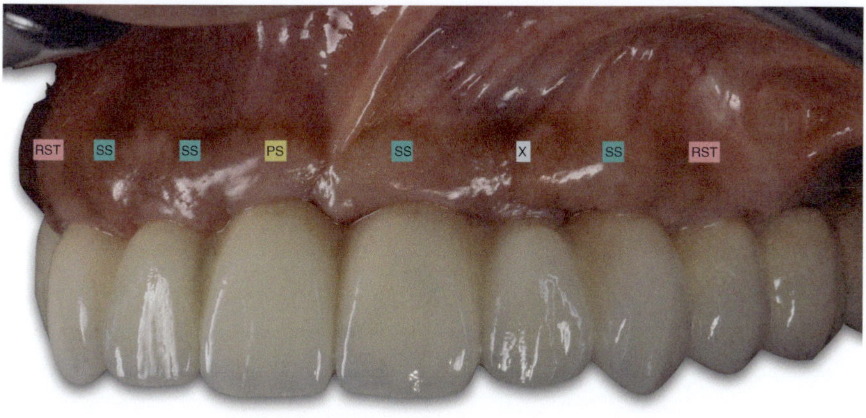

Fig. 8.16 Left lateral view of the definitive screw-retained fixed restoration

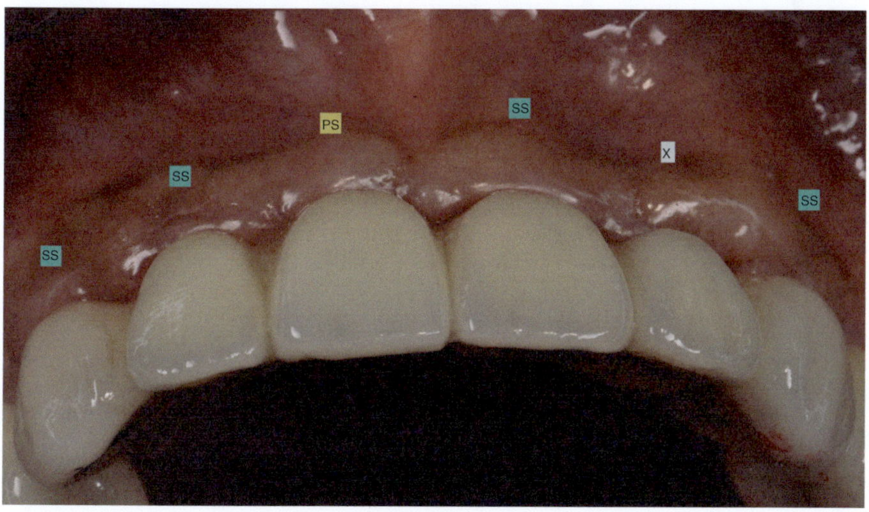

Fig. 8.17 Close-up view displaying healthy peri-implant soft tissue contours

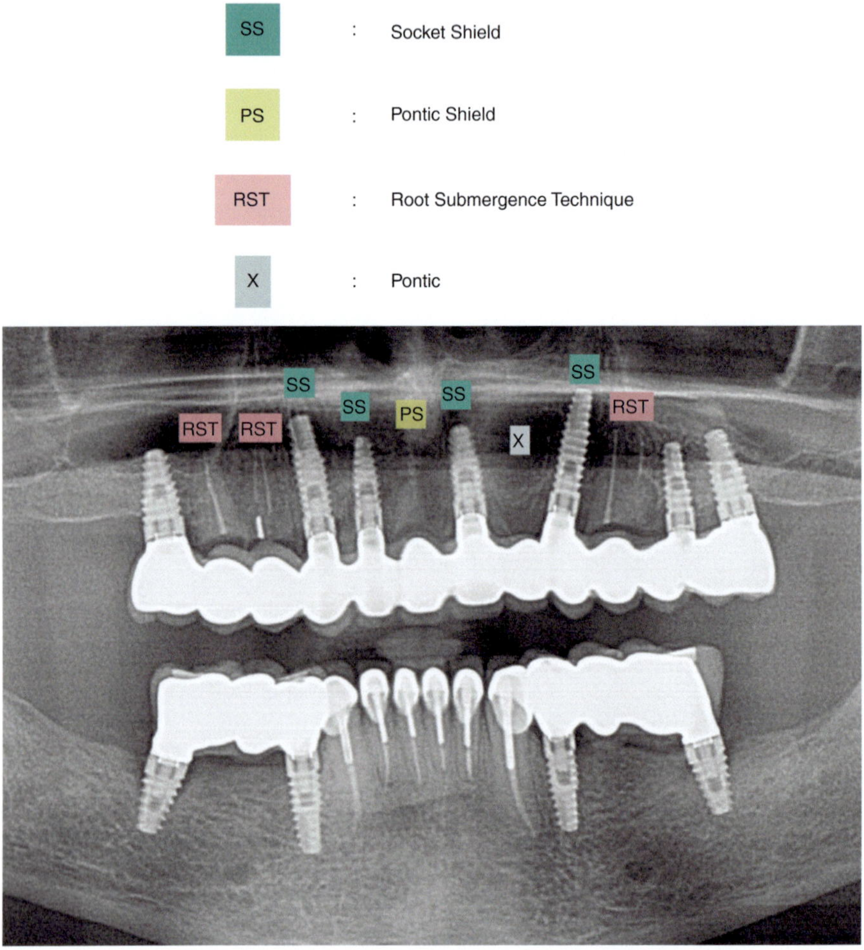

Fig. 8.18 Postoperative radiograph of the upper full-arch implant-supported restoration with multiple PET sites

8.4 Case 2

A 74-year-old man with history of controlled diabetes mellitus reported with missing teeth 14, 15, 16, 17 and badly carious teeth 11, 12, 13, 22, 23. The carious teeth were extensively decayed and were non-restorable. The treatment plan was to perform PET on all the five anterior teeth and place 3 implants in the extraction sockets. Two additional implants were planned for sites in 14 and 16 region. The final prosthesis planned was screw-retained porcelain fused to metal fixed bridge (Figs. 8.19, 8.20, 8.21, 8.22 and 8.23).

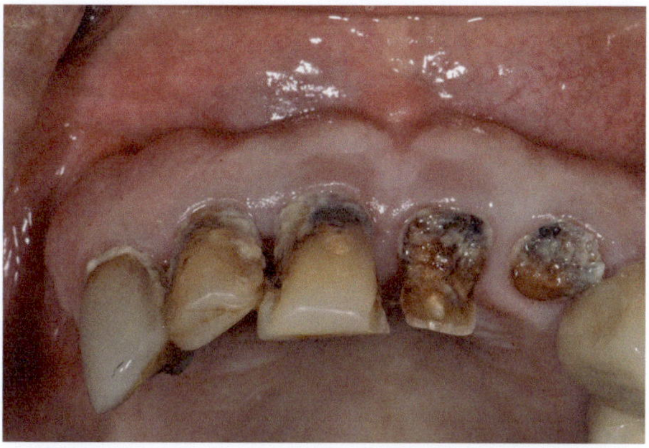

Fig. 8.19 Preoperative status showing badly decayed anterior teeth

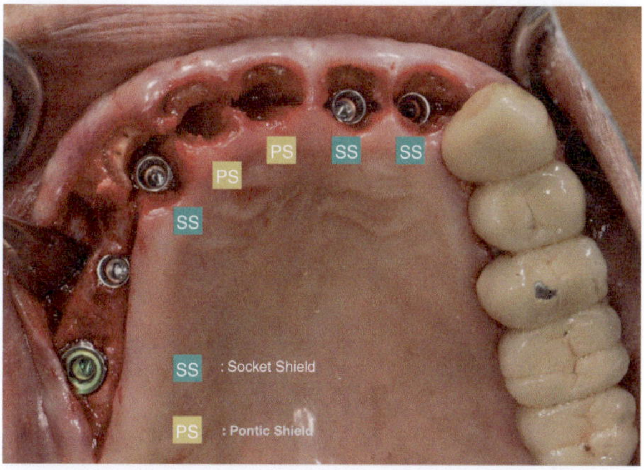

Fig. 8.20 Partial extractions with implant placements

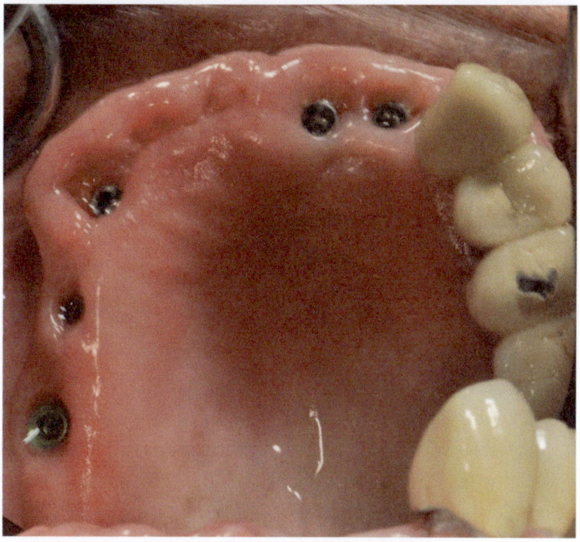

Fig. 8.21 Tissues after healing after 5 months

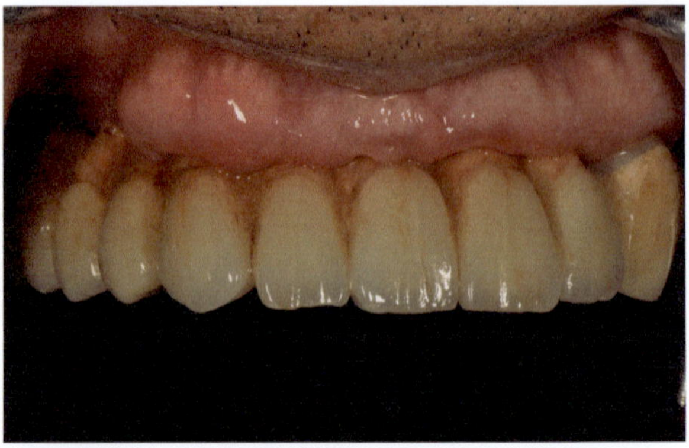

Fig. 8.22 Screw-retained metal ceramic restoration

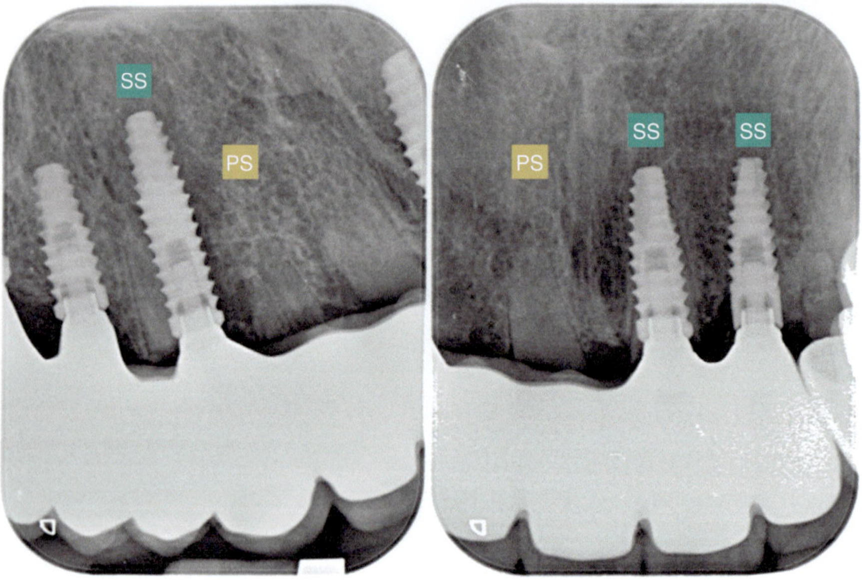

Fig. 8.23 Radiographic image of final restoration with PET procedures. Definitive screw-retained restoration on five implants.

8.5 Case 3

A 55-year-old female patient reported with frequent debonding of her crowns and bridges. Teeth in both the posterior quadrants were missing. Tooth 13 had a cystic lesion. The underlying teeth were extensively decayed and broken down. Since all the teeth lacked a proper ferrule, a decision was made to extract teeth and provide the patient with an implant-supported fixed restoration. Cystic ennucleation was done for tooth 13.

Multiple PET procedures were performed along with simultaneous implant placements and fixed provisional restorations.

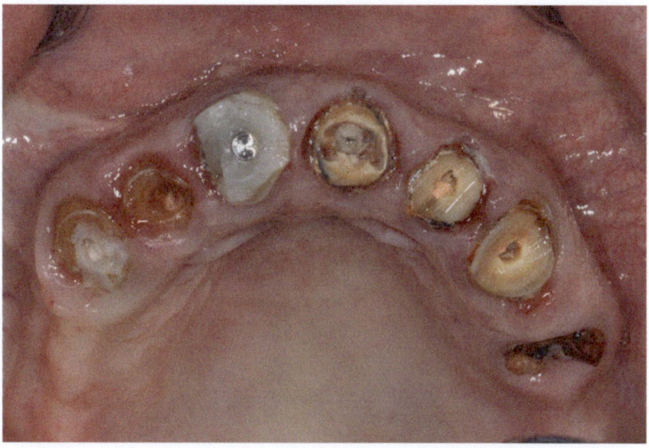

Fig. 8.24 Preoperative situation

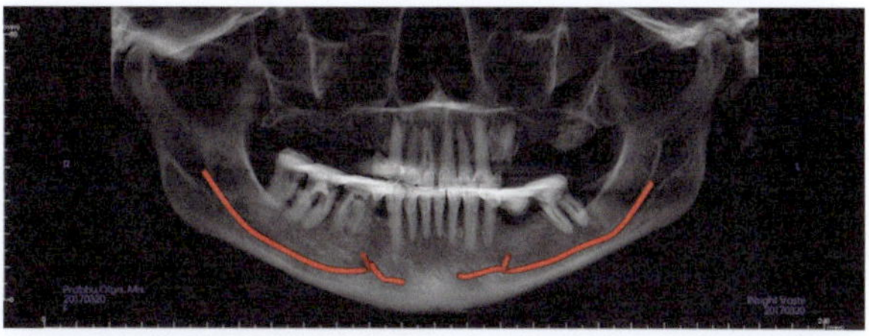

Fig. 8.25 Preoperative radiograph

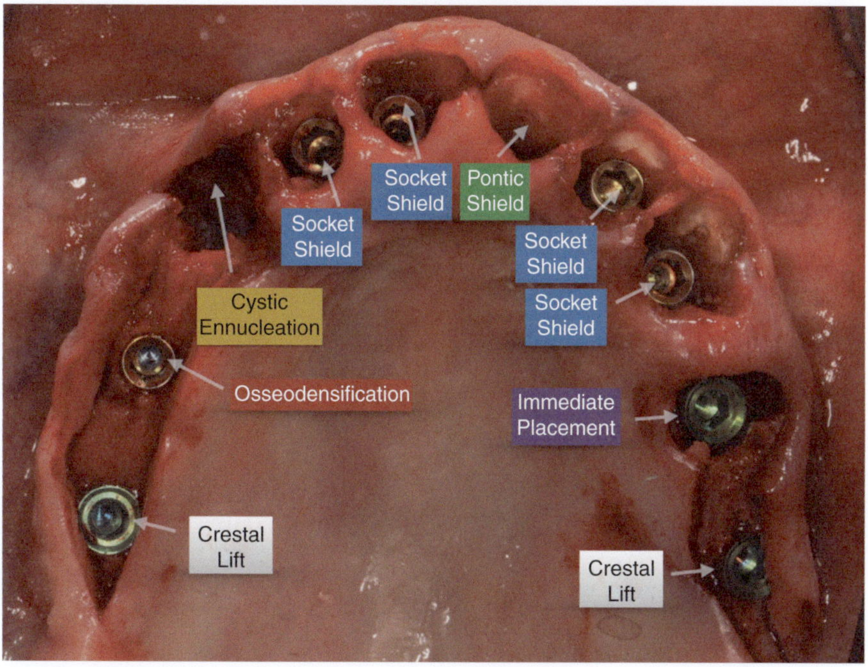

Fig. 8.26 Multiple PET sites with immediate implant placement

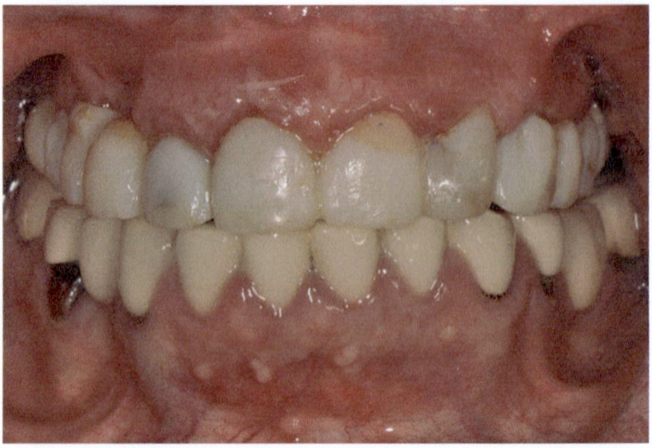

Fig. 8.27 View of peri implant soft tissue on removal of the provision restorations after 4 months of healing

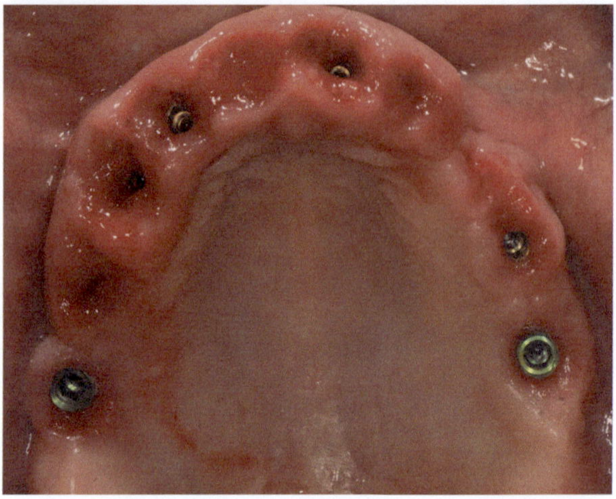

Fig. 8.28 Screw-retained provisional restoration

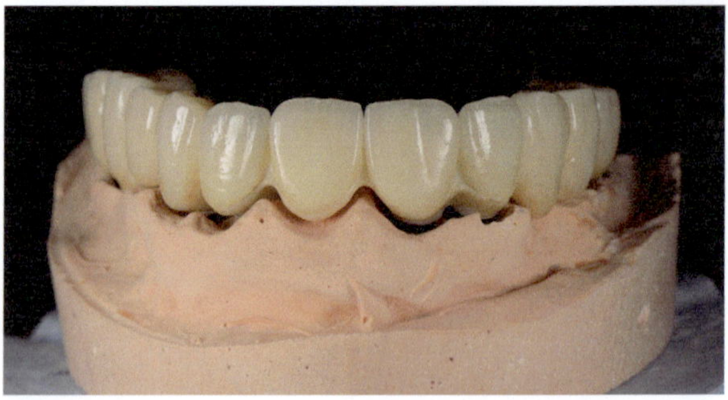

Fig. 8.29 Definitive Zirconia prosthesis with ceramic layering. Labwork credit: Katara Dental, Pune

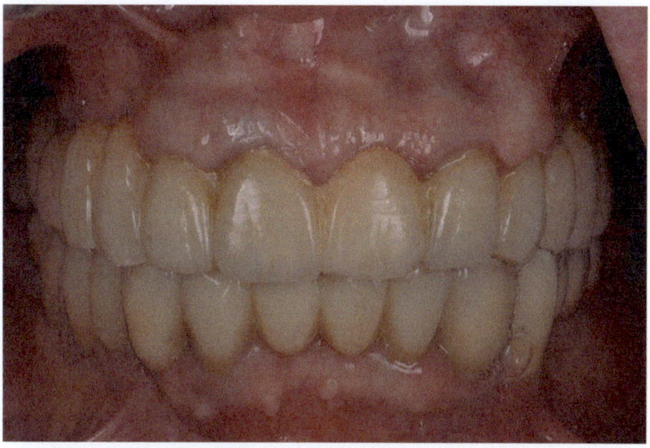

Fig. 8.30 Screw-retained upper and lower fixed restorations

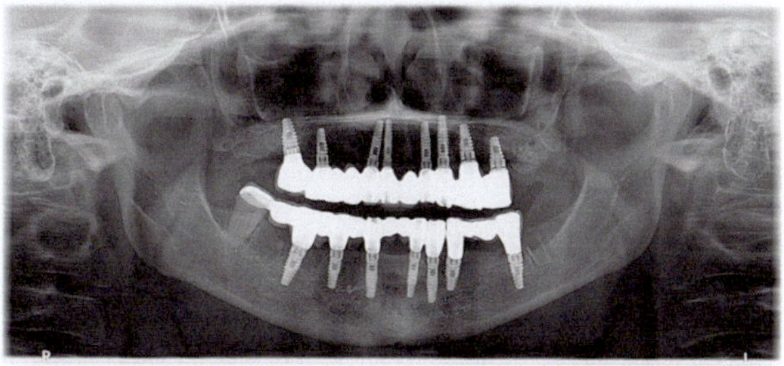

Fig. 8.31 Postoperative radiograph

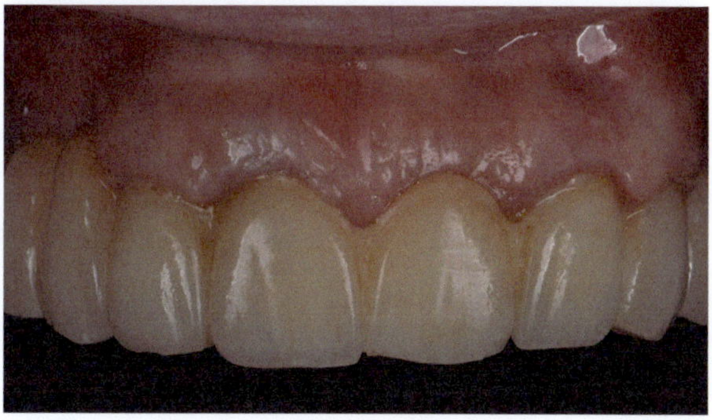

Fig. 8.32 1 year postoperative view displaying good tissue contours and adequate keratinized tissue in the esthetic zone at the sites treated with PET procedures

Four months after the surgery, a zirconia based screw-retained restoration was fabricated and fixed over the 7 implants (Figs. 8.24, 8.25, 8.26, 8.27, 8.28, 8.29, 8.30, 8.31 and 8.32).

8.6 Conclusion

The most desired outcome for long span and full-arch implant-supported cases is to achieve a definitive prosthesis without any pink ceramics to replace the missing alveolar ridge. This is very rarely possible with conventional implant therapy without extensive hard and soft tissue grafting procedures. Preservation of healthy parts of the roots by performing partial extraction therapies has made it possible for clinicians to accomplish such results without subjecting patients to complex augmentation procedures. One of the greatest benefits of PET procedures for full-arch implant-supported reconstructions is the preservation of the attached keratinized tissue around the implants and pontic sites. The presence of attached keratinized tissue around the implants significantly reduces the possibilities of developing biological complications around the implants in future.

Acknowledgement Case 1 restorative dentistry courtesy: Dr Praveen Advani.

References

1. Pietrokovski J, Starinsky R, Arensburg B, Kaffe I. Morpho-logic characteristics of bony edentulous jaws. J Prosthodont. 2007;16:141–7.
2. Tan WL, Wong TL, Wong MC, Lang NP. A systematic review of post-extractional alveolar hard and soft tissue dimensional changesin humans. Clin Oral Implants Res. 2012;23(Suppl. 5):1–21.
3. De Souza Nunes LS, Bornstein MM, Sendi P, Buser D. Anatomical characteristics and dimensions of edentulous sites in the posterior maxillae of patients referred for implant therapy. Int J Periodontics Restorative Dent. 2013;33:337–45.
4. Sharan A, Madjar D. Maxillary sinus pneumatization following extractions: a radiographic study. Int J Oral Maxillofac Implants. 2008;23:48–56.
5. Buser D. Vestibuloplasty with free mucosal grafts in implants in the edentulous mandible. Surgical method and preliminary results. Schweiz Monatsschr Zahnmed. 1987;97:766–72.
6. Schrott AR, Jimenez M, Hwang J, Fiorellini J, Weber H. Five-year evaluation of the influence of keratinized mucosa on peri-implant soft-tissue health and stability around implants supporting full-arch mandibular fixed prostheses. Clin Oral Implants Res. 2009;20:1170–7.
7. Carinci F, Farina A, Zanetti U, et al. Autologous bone grafts and endosseous implants: complementary techniques. J Oral Maxillofac Surg. 1996;54:486–94.
8. Simons AM, Baima RF. Free gingival grafting and vestibuloplasty with endosseous implant placement: clinical report. Implant Dent. 1994;3:235–8.
9. Babbush CA. Reconstruction of the edentulous mandible. Int Dent J. 1985;35(4):266–76. Review.
10. Roccuzzo M, Ramieri G, Spada MC, Bianchi SD, Berrone S. Vertical alveolar ridge augmentation by means of a titanium mesh and autogenous bone grafts. Clin Oral Implants Res. 2004;15(1):73–81.
11. Steigmann M, Monje A, Chan HL, Wang HL. Emergence profile design based on implant position in the esthetic zone. Int J Periodontics Restorative Dent. 2014;34(4):559–63. https://doi.org/10.11607/prd.2016.
12. Hürzeler MB, Zuhr O, Schupbach P, Rebele SF, Emmanouilidis N, Fickl S. The socket-shield technique: a proof-of-principle report. J Clin Periodontol. 2010;37(9):855–62.
13. Bäumer D, Zuhr O, Rebele S, Schneider D, Schupbach P, Hürzeler M. The socket-shield technique: first histological, clinical, and volumetrical observations after separation of the buccal tooth segment—a pilot study. Clin Implant Dent Relat Res. 2015;17(1):71–82.

14. Gluckman H, Du Toit J, Salama M. The Pontic-shield: partial extraction therapy for ridge preservation and Pontic site development. Int J Periodontics Restorative Dent. 2016;36(3):417–23.
15. Esteve-Pardo G, Esteve-Colomina L. Clinical application of the socket-shield concept in multiple anterior teeth. Case Rep Dent. 2018;2018:9014372.
16. McAllister BS, Haghighat K. Bone augmentation techniques. J Periodontol. 2007;78(3):377–96. Review.
17. Salama M, Ishikawa T, Salama H, Funato A, Garber D. Advantages of the root submergence technique for Pontic site development in esthetic implant therapy. Int J Periodontics Restorative Dent. 2007;27:521–7.
18. Gluckman H, Salama M, Du Toit J. Partial extraction therapies (PET). Part 1: maintaining alveolar ridge contour at pontic and immediate implant sites. Int J Periodontics Restorative Dent. 2016;36:681–7.
19. Gluckman H, Salama M, Du Toit J. Partial extraction therapies (PET) part 2: procedures and technical aspects. Int J Periodontics Restorative Dent. 2007;37(3):377–85.
20. Aslan S. Improved volume and contour stability with thin socket-shield preparation in immediate implant placement and provisionalization in the esthetic zone. Int J Esthet Dent. 2018;13(2):172–83.
21. Gluckman H, Salama M, Du Toit J. A retrospective evaluation of 128 socket-shield cases in the esthetic zone and posterior sites: partial extraction therapy with up to 4 years follow-up. Clin Implant Dent Relat Res. 2018;20(2):122–9. https://doi.org/10.1111/cid.12554. Epub 2017 Nov 26.

Definitive Restorations in Partial Extraction Therapy

9

Ali Tunkiwala

Abstract
This chapter outlines the steps for conversion of a well-made provisional to a definitive restoration in cases where partial extraction therapy is employed. The choice of materials and designing of the final restorations will be discussed in detail with a variety of clinical cases that will help the readers understand the finer aspects of the subject.

9.1 Introduction

Definitive restorations must be designed to be functionally accurate, durable and meet the aesthetic requirements of the patient. Objective criteria have been established to judge the soft tissue aesthetics around an implant [1]. The provisional restoration (Chap. 4) should establish ideal soft tissue contours at the end of the healing phase. Fine adjustments of the provisional restoration or an adjunctive soft tissue procedure should be considered in case of a suboptimal soft tissue profile. Fabrication of the definitive restoration should commence following osseointegration only once satisfactory soft tissue architecture has been achieved.

The key steps in the fabrication of the definitive restoration are as follows:

1. Impressions with customized approach.
2. Jaw relation record (if needed).
3. Bisque trials.
4. Final restorations.

A. Tunkiwala (✉)
Smiles by Design, Mumbai, India

U. Kher, A. Tunkiwala (eds.), *Partial Extraction Therapy in Implant Dentistry*,
https://doi.org/10.1007/978-3-030-33610-3_9

9.2 Technical Considerations

The definitive restorations can be either cement-retained or screw-retained [2]. The advantages and disadvantages of either restorative option have been discussed in Chap. 4 on provisional restorations.

9.2.1 Cement-Retained Restorations

Cement-retained restorations are fabricated in two parts. The first part is the abutment, which may be prefabricated or customized and the second is the final restoration. The final restoration is cemented onto the abutment. The concern of residual cement in the sulcus can be addressed by using customized abutments with well designed margins to allow easy cement clean up. Additionally, an occlusal or lingual vent and pre-extrusion of cement on a duplicate abument will aid in this aspect. A dry retraction cord placed in the sulcus during cementation will aid in excess cement clean up too.

Abutments

Abutment selection depends on soft tissue thickness [3, 4], abutment wall thickness [5], patients' functional needs and the definitive restorative material. A good balance between strength and beauty is required for overall success.

In partial extraction therapy cases the overall contours of the labial and proximal aspect are usually very well maintained from a bone and soft tissue perspective if case selection criteria has been stringently followed. Most pre-fabricated abutments do not have the collar dimensions to match this scalloped architecture and thus the gingival tissues get under or over supported and the restorative margins come to lie too deep into the sulcus.

Lack of support in the critical subgingival area can be detrimental to the health and aesthetics of the peri implant tissues [6]. Thus, it is prudent to fabricate a customized abutment for implant restorations in all such cases where partial extraction therapy such as socket shield or pontic shield has been performed. As clear from the underlying figure, the area of the abutment that is 1 mm subgingival is the critical contour and the area below that and until the implant platform is the subcritical contour [6] (Figs. 9.1 and 9.2). If the provisional restoration is accurately contoured it will establish these zones and the definitive restoration has to mimic these contours and adequately support the gingival tissues for optimum health and aesthetics.

Abutments may be customized to offer following features:

(a) *Customization for Colour.*

In the aesthetic zone, the colour of the underlying abutment may influence the colour of the gingival tissues around the final implant restoration. This is more relevant if the gingival biotype is thin [3, 4]. To overcome this problem, a customized tooth (Dentin) coloured abutment may be chosen over which a metal free restoration can be fabricated. The overall specular reflection of the materials will allow better light transmission and the dentin hue will aid in avoiding the show through of the abutment with thin gingival biotype (Fig. 9.3).

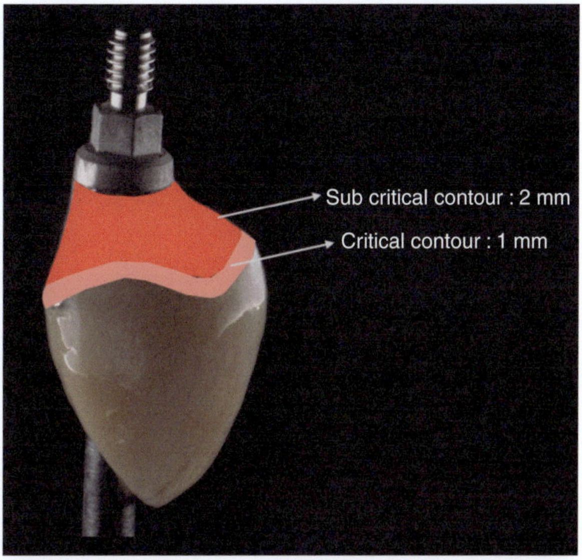

Fig. 9.1 Area of 1 mm subgingival contour is the critical contour of the restoration that has a direct bearing on the health and aesthetics of the soft tissue architecture

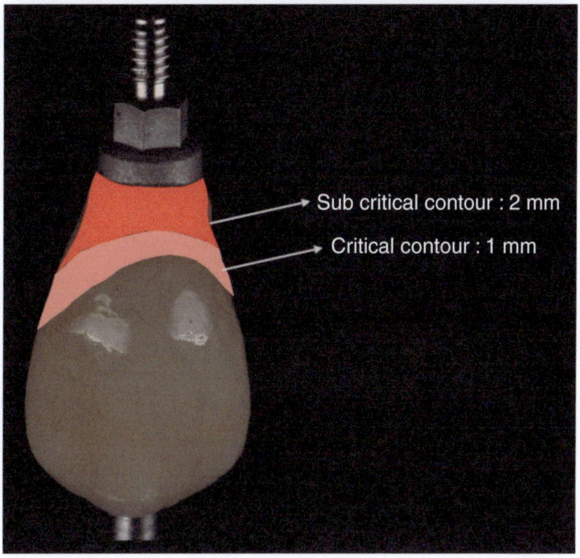

Fig. 9.2 Area that is 2 mm apical from the critical contour is the subcritical contour. This zone can be modified to influence the emergence profile of the restoration

(b) *Customization for Margin Placement.*
A critical factor in designing of abutments for cement-retained restorations is the controlled placement of the restorative margin within the gingival sulcus. A very superficial placement will display the restorative margin-abutment junction and will be aesthetically unacceptable. A deep subgingival margin placement (>1 mm) will lead to difficulty in removal of excess cement [7]. With custom abutments the margins may be designed to be supragingival on the palatal or lingual side and may be no greater than 0.5 mm subgingival on the labial side. This will allow easy clean-up of any residual cement. Thus, customization is paramount for optimum restorative margin placement (Figs. 9.4 and 9.5).

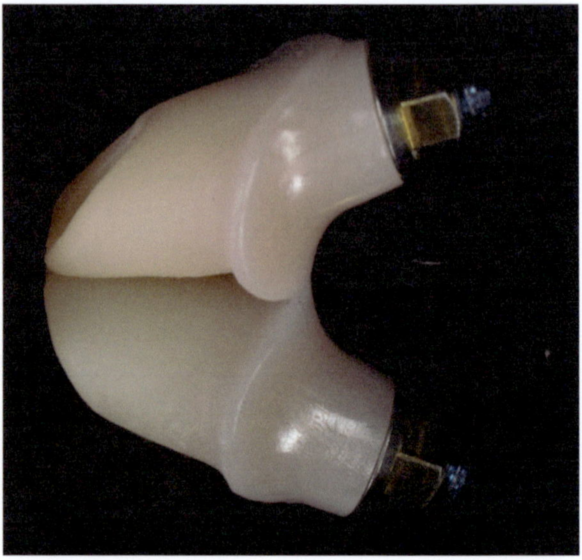

Fig. 9.3 Coloured Zirconia allows better tones for final restorations especially when the gingival biotype is thin

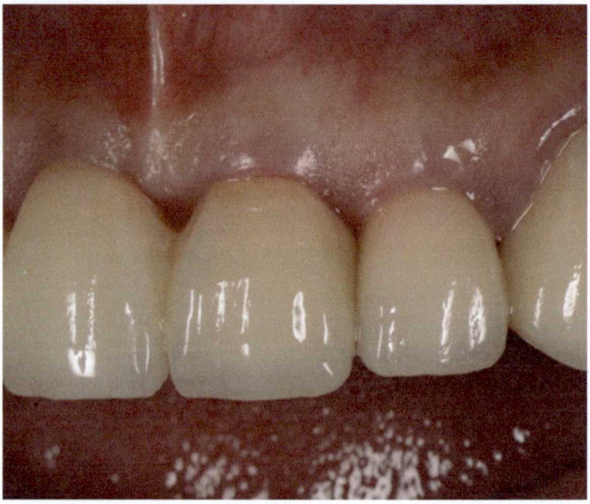

Fig. 9.4 Cement-retained restorations designed to have restorative margin upto 0.5 mm subgingival. This allows for easy cement clean-up and results in good tissue health as seen on this 2-year follow-up

(c) *Customization for Angulation Correction.*
Ideally, an implant in the aesthetic zone must be placed such that its screw access emerges from lingual fossa of the final tooth. This will allow a screw-retained restoration to be made. However, the angulation of the premaxilla presents anatomical difficulties in this type of implant placement with the increased risk of dehiscence or thinning of the labial bone in certain cases. Thus, in such cases if the implant is placed with its trajectory emerging from the incisal edge

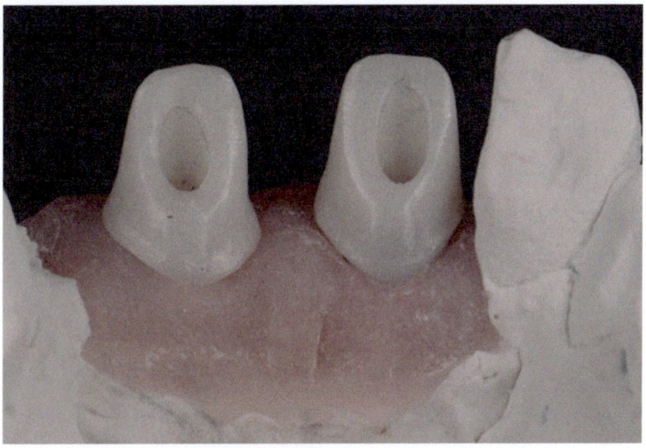

Fig. 9.5 When designing custom abutments, it is prudent to keep the margins for the restorations supragingival on the palatal/lingual side for allowing easy cement clean-up with direct visualization

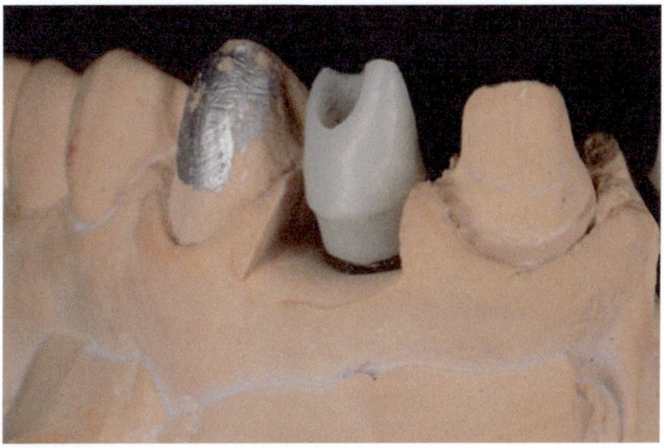

Fig. 9.6 The implant placement in certain cases may get the screw access from the labial/incisal aspect. A custom abutment may be designed in such cases with a cement-retained restoration. In this picture we see the custom abutment on tooth #22

or the labial aspect of the final restoration a cement retained restoration on a well designed custom abutment may be used to mask the labial/incisal screw access (Figs. 9.6 and 9.7).

(d) *Customization for Length.*
Cement-retained restorations need adequate supragingival height on the underlying abutments for adequate resistance form. When the inter arch space is >10 mm, the prefabricated abutments (<6 mm) may be too short to provide resistance form for the final restoration. Customizing the abutments for adequate length will be necessary to achieve adequate retention and resistance form (Fig. 9.8).

When designing the definitive restorations, it is important to give importance not only to the subgingival contour that is responsible for support and stability of the soft tissue but also the supragingival emergence profile which is responsible for protection of the soft tissue and thus its health [8].

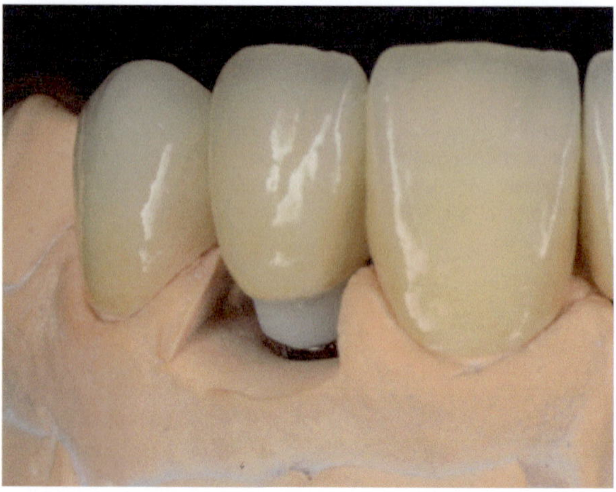

Fig. 9.7 Cement-retained restoration on tooth #22 aids in masking the incisal/labial screw access on the customized abutment

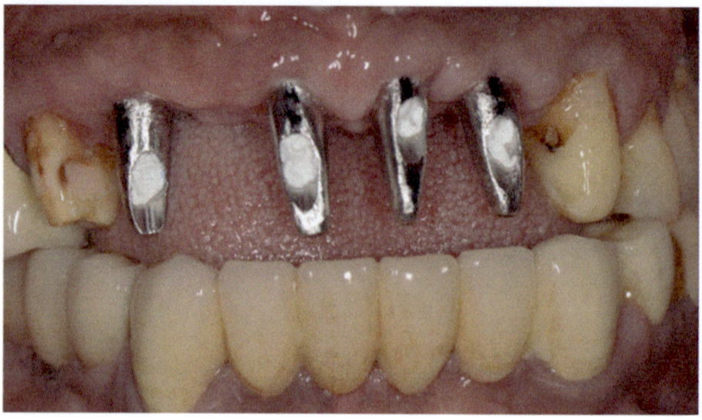

Fig. 9.8 When the available restorative space is too much (>10 mm), the prefabricated abutments for cement-retained restoration will be too short to provide retention form. Thus, customization of the abutment may be done for achieving optimum length

Material Considerations for Custom Abutments

The materials for the customized abutments may be:

1. Metallic (Titanium/Cobalt Chromium).
2. Zirconia.
3. Polymer-based (Bio HPP).

(a) *Titanium abutments* are biocompatible and provide a strong foundation for the restorations. A stable peri-implant mucosa has been shown to be established around titanium abutments. This tissue protects the peri-implant sulcus against bacterial invasion [9].

The grey tint of titanium abutments on the peri-implant mucosa can become a clinically relevant problem [4] due to their show through from underneath thin gingival biotypes, especially in a high lip line patient. The thickness of mucosa has a direct bearing on the colour change. When the mucosa is thicker than 2 mm, the abutment material plays lesser role in this regard [4].

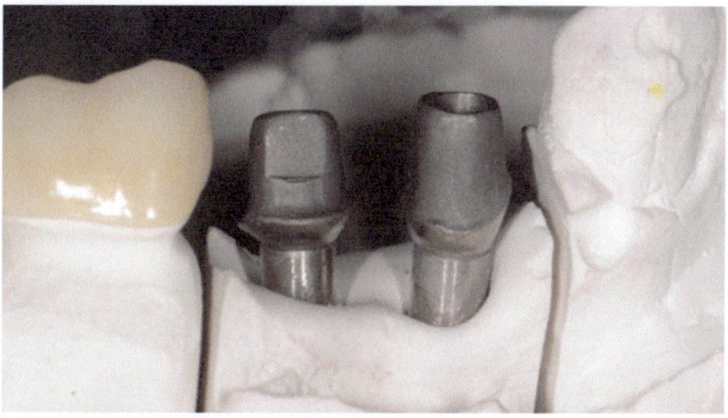

Fig. 9.9 Titanium is the favoured option for customized abutments when the restorative space is restricted

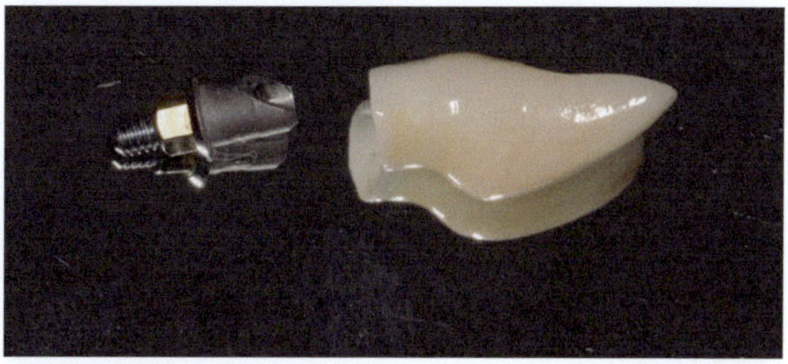

Fig. 9.10 Zirconia substructure to be bonded on hybrid base abutment

In thinner sections and when the restorative space is restricted in mesio-distal and bucco-lingual dimension, titanium is still the material of choice for abutment fabrication as it can provide the necessary strength even in thin cross sections of 0.5 mm (Fig. 9.9).

(b) *Zirconia* is an excellent choice of restorative material and its strength is adequate if minimum wall thickness is 0.5 mm or more. The wall thickness of the abutment depends upon the dual factors of implant position and the implant axis (Figs.9.10, 9.11 and 9.12).

When compared to titanium abutments in terms of biocompatibility and soft tissue response [9, 10], Zirconia abutments have been superior in performance. Research has shown that zirconia abutments also allow less plaque deposition when compared to titanium abutments [11] (Fig. 9.13).

In thin gingival biotypes, zirconia abutments with their white colour offer a distinctive advantage over titanium abutments [12]. The white colour of zirconia can be further modified with veneering ceramics, improving the technician's chances of mimicking the pink hues of the subgingival area and the dentin-coloured hues of the supragingival area [13]. This provides an optimal background for tooth coloured restoration on implants in the aesthetic zone.

(c) PEEK-based materials [14, 15] such as Bio-HPP (Bredent Medical, Germany) provide the same advantages of base colour and biocompatibility that zirconia does. Thus, they can be used as abutment materials with metal-free ceramic restorations over them. Additionally, they have a resiliency similar to bone which dampens the forces on restorations. However, there are no long-term studies on its use as an abutment material and thus caution should be exercised before using these in high stress areas (Figs. 9.14 and 9.15).

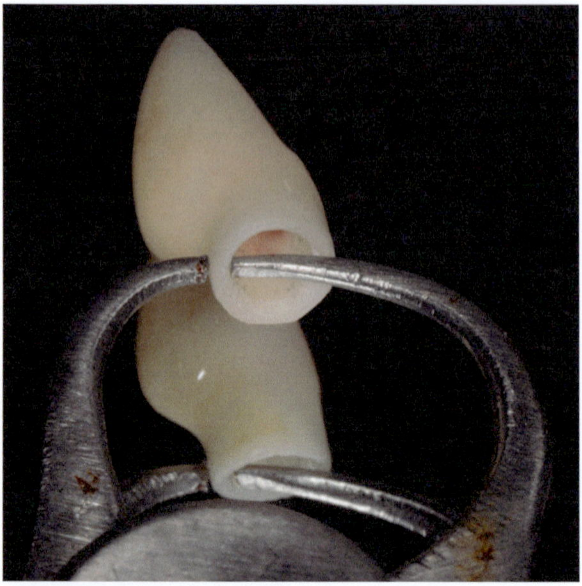

Fig. 9.11 The thickness of the wall of the abutment must be maintained for sufficient strength

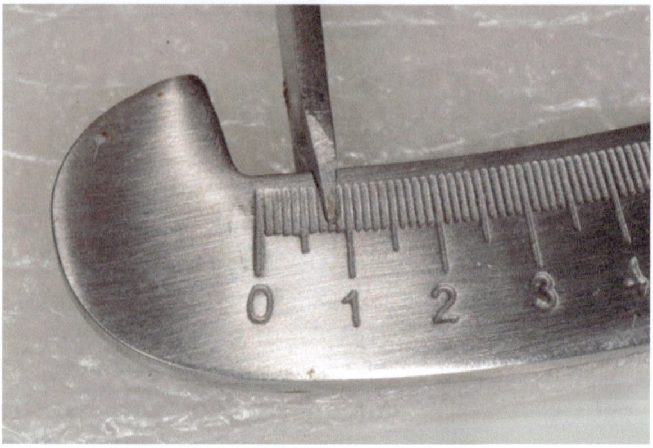

Fig. 9.12 Minimum wall thickness for zirconia abutments must be >0.5 mm

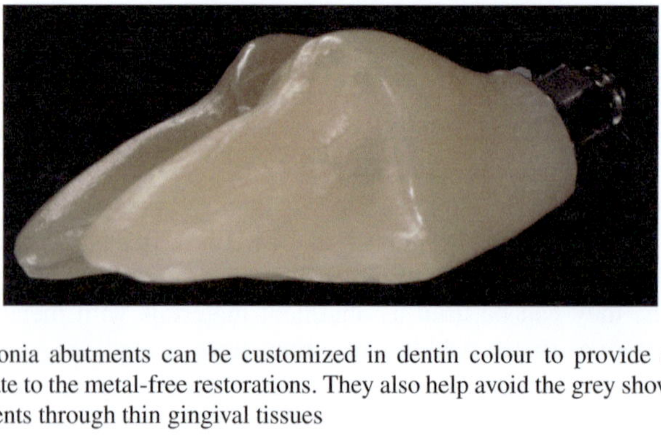

Fig. 9.13 Zirconia abutments can be customized in dentin colour to provide an aesthetically pleasing substrate to the metal-free restorations. They also help avoid the grey show through of the titanium abutments through thin gingival tissues

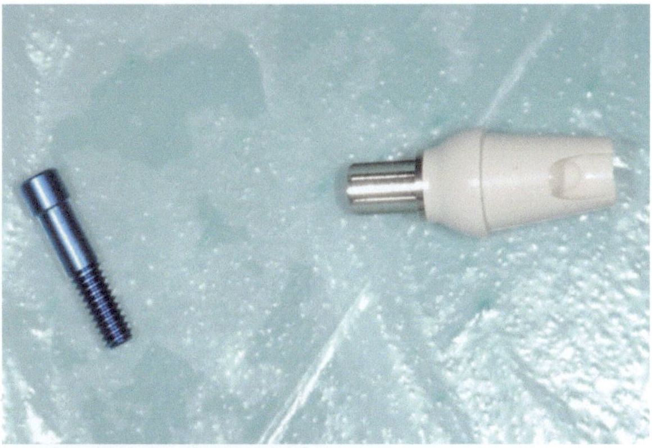

Fig. 9.14 Prefabricated Bio-HPP abutment may be used as a 'one-time' abutment for anterior implants. It can be shaped to fit the requirements of the socket architecture and the tooth being replaced

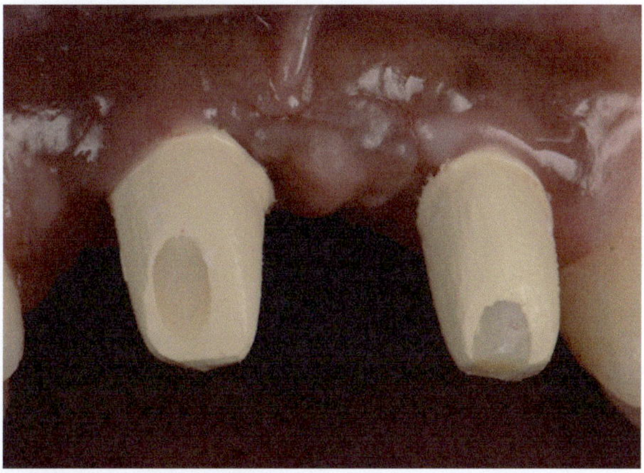

Fig. 9.15 Bio-HPP may be customized, just like zirconia, in a dentin-coloured substrate to create an aesthetically acceptable base for metal-free restorations over it

Clinical Case (Cement-Retained Restoration)

The following case illustrates the use of customized Bio-HPP abutment utilized under lithium disilicate restoration with partial extraction therapy in the form of Socket Shield done for tooth #11 (Figs. 9.16, 9.17, 9.18, 9.19, 9.20, 9.21, 9.22, 9.23, 9.24, 9.25 and 9.26).

9.2.2 Screw-Retained Restorations

Screw-retained restorations are usually preferred over the cement-retained restoration. Their retrievability and lack of residual cement is a distinct advantage. In all cases where the implant trajectory is optimal with the screw access emerging from the lingual fossa of the proposed crown, they may become the restorative design of choice (Figs. 9.27, 9.28 and 9.29).

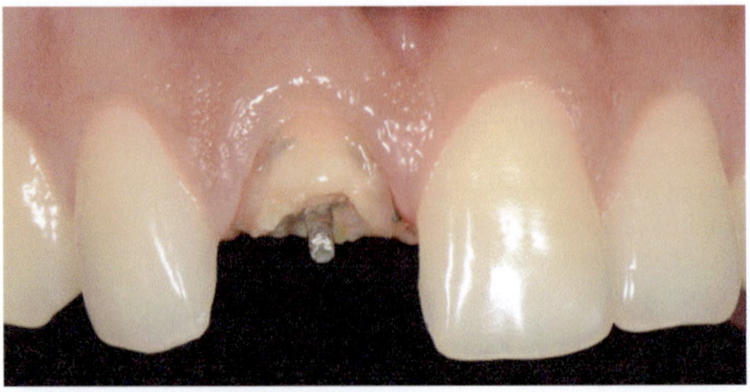

Fig. 9.16 Unrestorable tooth #11

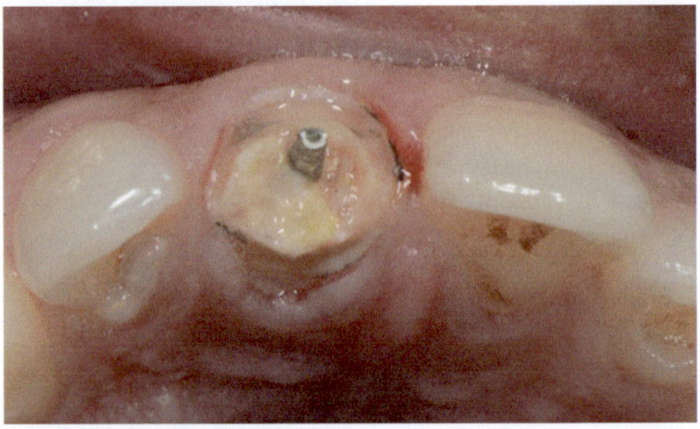

Fig. 9.17 Unrestorable tooth #11

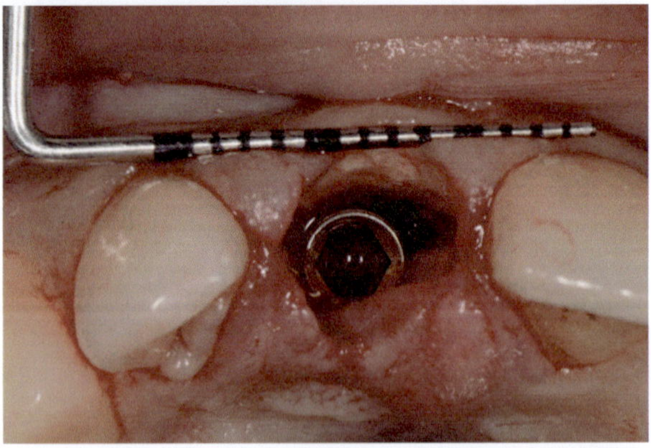

Fig. 9.18 Implant placed in correct 3D position and away from the socket shield

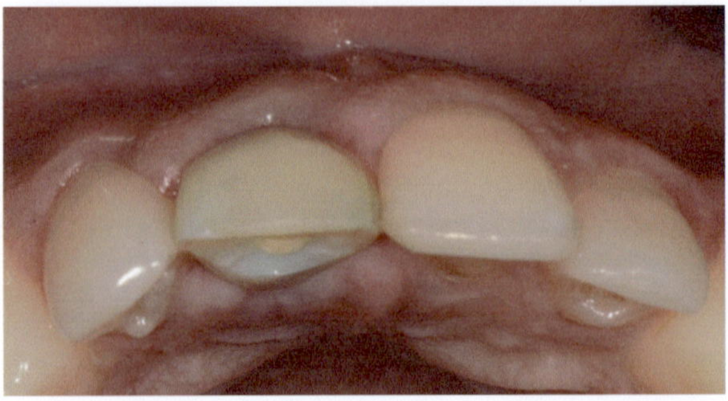

Fig. 9.19 Screw-retained provisional restoration placed over the implant. Note, the well-maintained labial tissue contour of #11 compared to #21

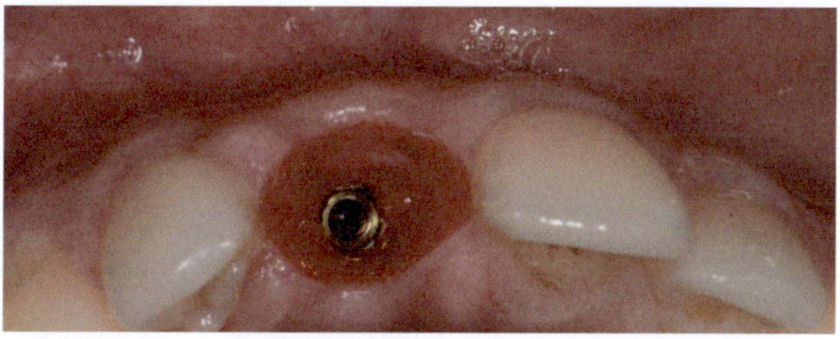

Fig. 9.20 At 4 months, the tissue contours are well maintained. This picture was taken after unscrewing the provisional restoration during impression procedure

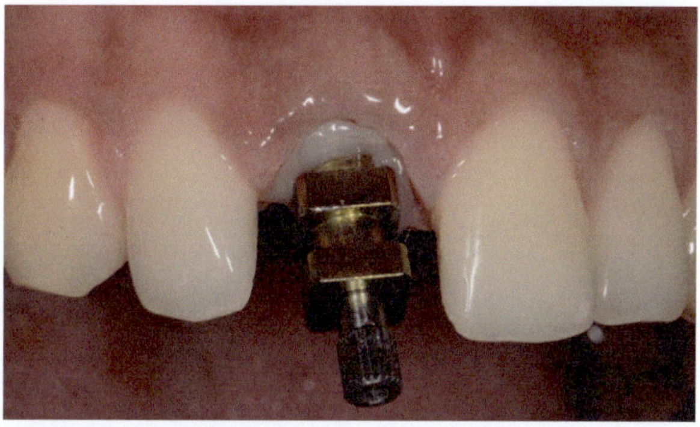

Fig. 9.21 Customized impression coping aids in capturing the anatomically produced morphology of the peri-implant gingival architecture

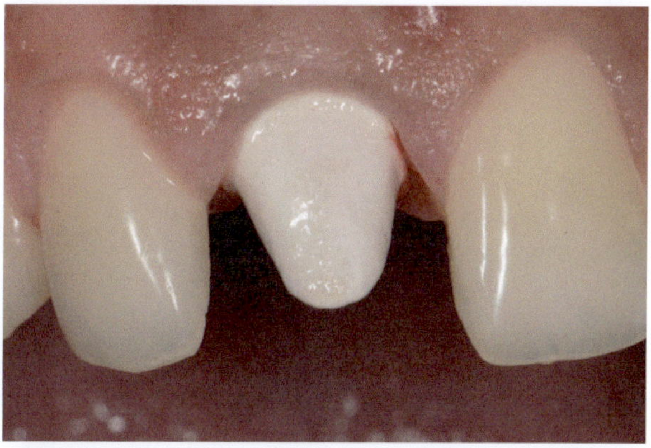

Fig. 9.22 Custom Bio-HPP abutment provides adequate support to the gingival architecture

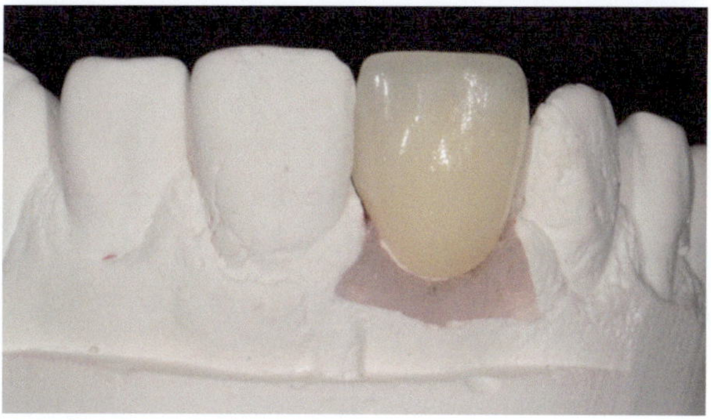

Fig. 9.23 The final lithium disilicate restoration to be cement retained on the custom abutment

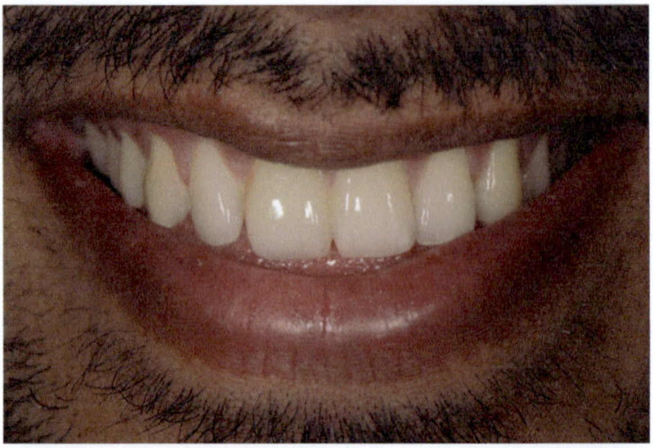

Fig. 9.24 Postoperative smile shows good aesthetic integration of the restoration on #11

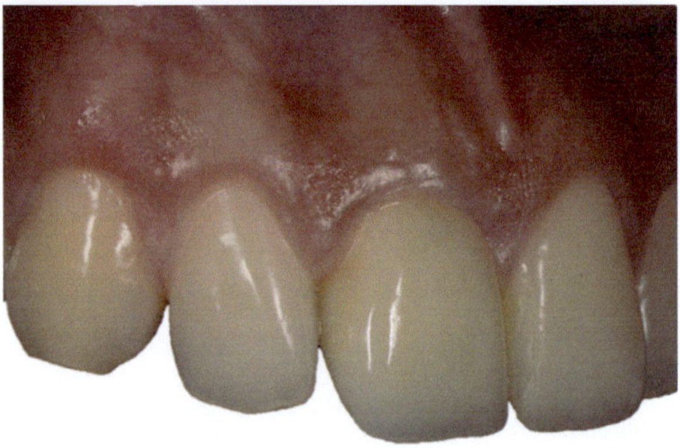

Fig. 9.25 The peri-implant tissue, quantity and quality, with partial extraction therapy and customized abutment is excellent

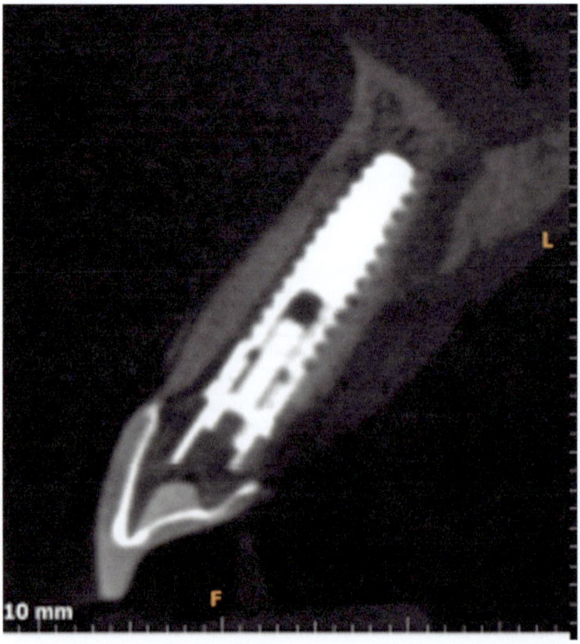

Fig. 9.26 A postoperative scan depicts the overall relation of several elements, such as the shield, the abutment and the implant. This was one of the very early cases that shows the shield not trimmed to the level of crestal bone. In present times, it is considered important that adequate trimming of the shield be done as this could lead to internal exposures. However, as that did not happen in this case, no further action was taken. The case has been followed up for 4 years

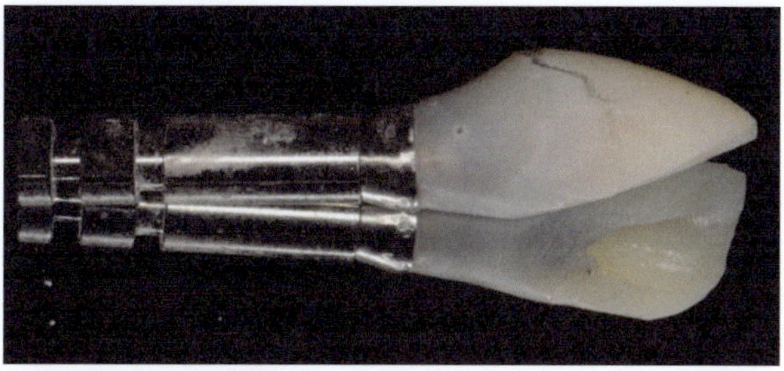

Fig. 9.27 Provisional screw-retained restoration (#12) with screw access from the lingual fossa as ideally recommended

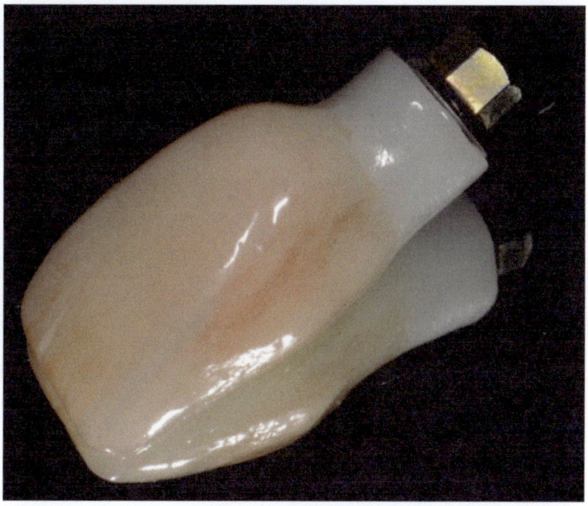

Fig. 9.28 The final screw-retained zirconia restoration (#12) with translucent ceramic veneered to it and stained before glazing

In certain cases, due to the anatomical limitations of the premaxilla and its trajectory, the implant axis may not be located at the lingual fossa in the aesthetic zone. If the implant trajectory emerges from labial or incisal aspect of the restoration, a classic screw-retained restoration may not be possible since the screw access will be visible. In such cases cement-retained restorations are necessary recommended, as discussed in the previous section. However, by using the concept of angulated screw channel (Nobel Biocare India Pvt. Ltd), a screw-retained restoration may now be made even for such a clinical scenario (Fig. 9.30). Angulations up to 25 degrees can be corrected with this concept.

Material Considerations

Screw-retained restorations can be monolithic or layered. If a layered restoration is planned the framework may be metallic or zirconia. The layering material that aids in achieving the final finished restoration in the aesthetic zone is often ceramic.

The materials for definitive restorations (Screw-Retained & Cement-Retained) may be divided as follows:

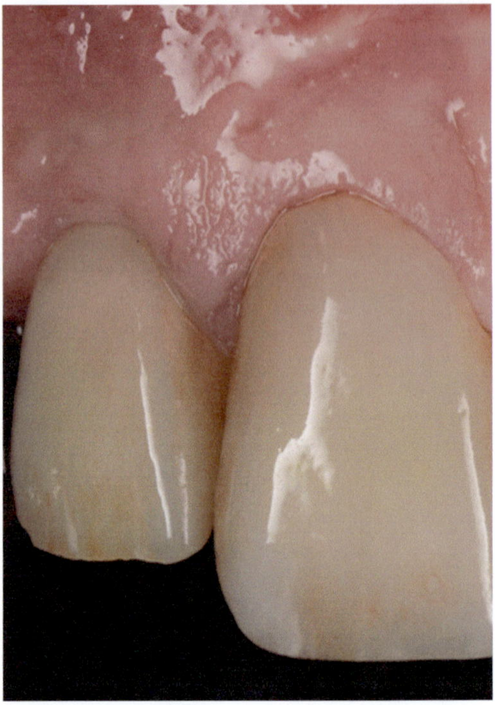

Fig. 9.29 The finalized screw-retained restoration (#12) has the advantage of retrievability and negates the residual cement disadvantage of cement-retained restorations

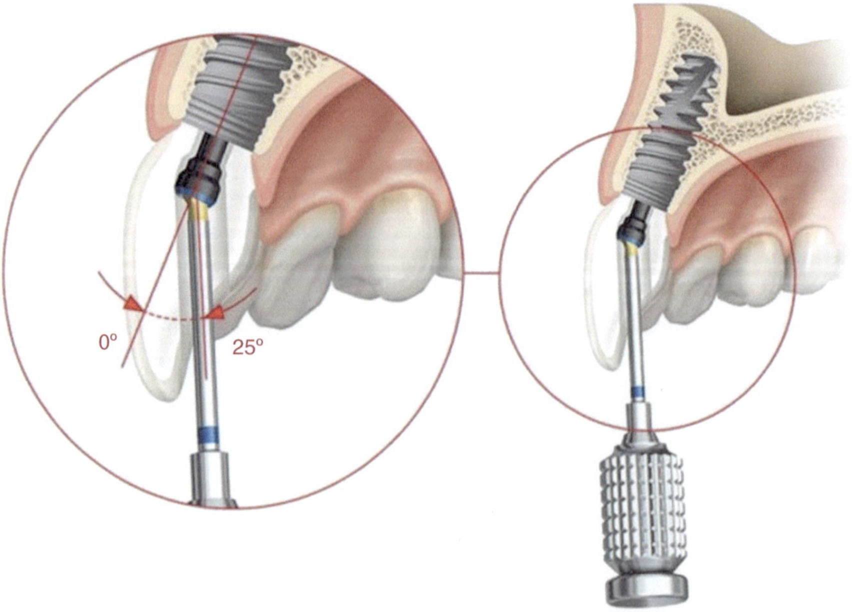

Fig. 9.30 The ASC concept allows screw access to be relocated from labial to the palatal side, thus making it possible to fabricate screw-retained restorations even on implants that have been placed with a labial bias of up to 25°. (Picture from Nobel Biocare India Pvt. Ltd. Prosthetic Catalogue)

1. Porcelain fused to metal.
2. Metal-Free Ceramics (Lithium Disilicate; Zirconia).
3. High-density resins.

(a) *Porcelain fused to metal* has the longest track record, suggested by a number of reviews, with a success rate of 89% for single implant crowns and 80% for implant supported fixed bridges [16, 17]. The strength, durability, aesthetics and biocompatibility of the material are well documented. The main disadvantage of PFM is the metal ions that can leach over a period of time causing discoloration of peri-implant gingival tissues. In restricted restorative spaces, however, this is the material of choice as it can maintain its strength even in thin sections (Fig. 9.31).
(b) *Lithium disilicate* provides excellent aesthetics and biocompatibility and creates a very healthy environment for the peri-implant tissues. However, its strength can be a concern when it is not bonded to the underlying substrate. In natural dentition, once bonded to enamel the strength is sufficient, but in implant dentistry it is prudent to use this material for single anterior restorations or small single pontic bridges, and not in high stress areas [17] (Fig. 9.32).

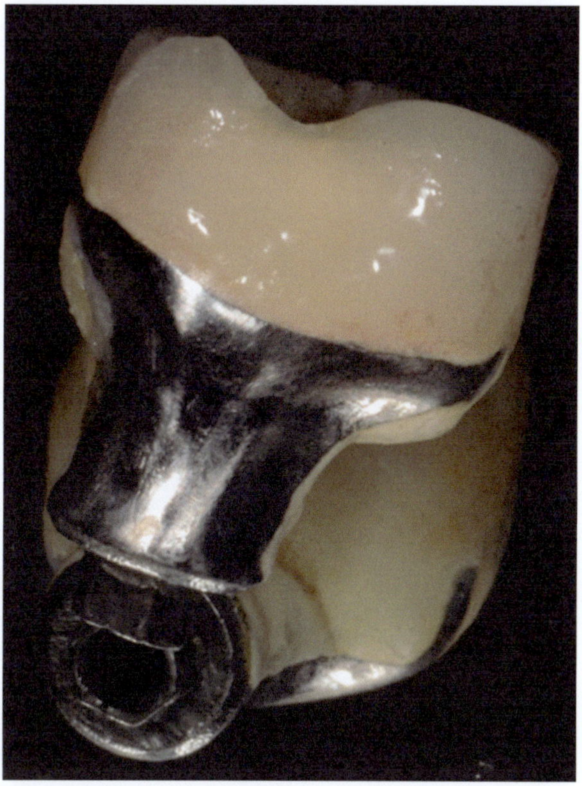

Fig. 9.31 Porcelain fused to metal as a screw-retained restoration may be used in restricted restorative spaces for its strength

(c) *Zirconia,* on the other hand, is very strong and can be minimally layered to provide good aesthetics. For long span implant restorations, zirconia is the favoured material over lithium disilicate. However, there has been a high incidence of chipping of the veneering cermic in long span restorations [18] (Figs. 9.33 and 9.34).

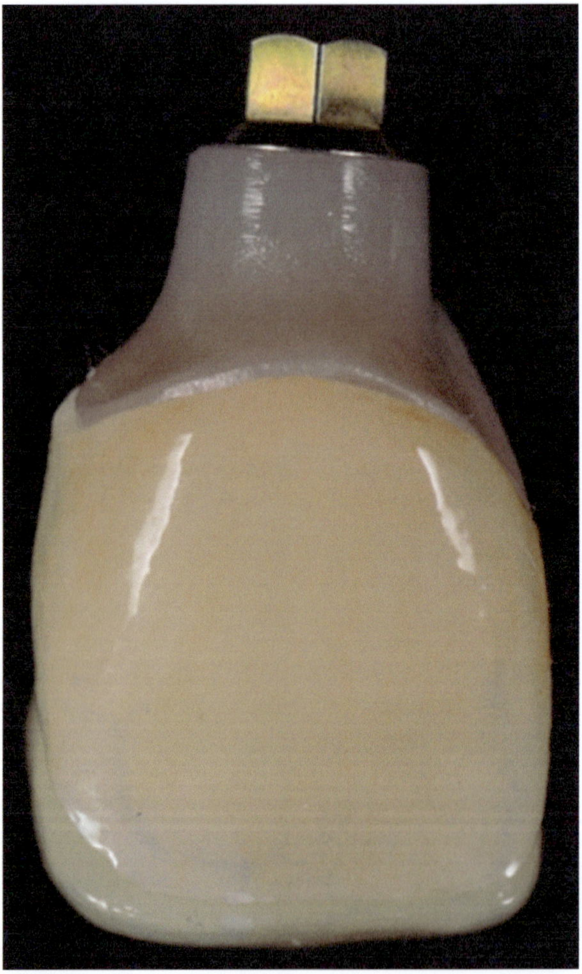

Fig. 9.32 Lithium disilicate can provide excellent aesthetics due to its translucency but has reduced strength when it is not bonded

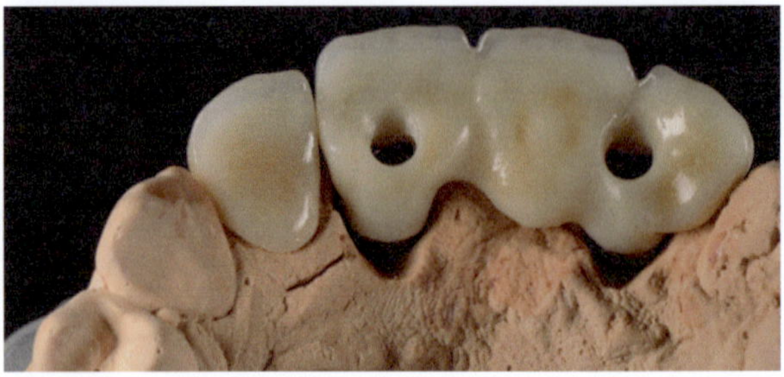

Fig. 9.33 Zirconia can be used as a framework material for screw-retained restorations

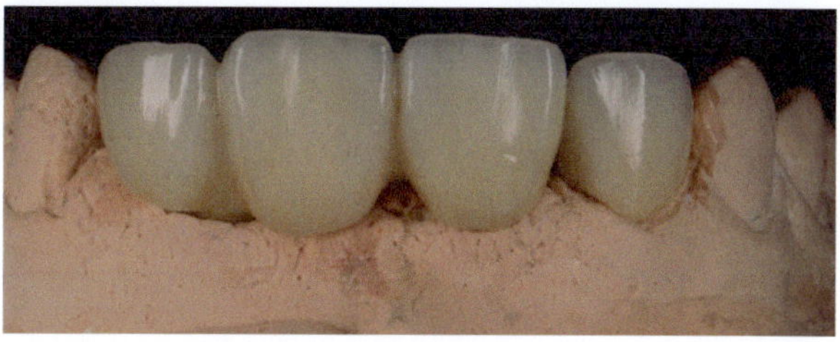

Fig. 9.34 The labial, non-stress bearing, aspect of the zirconia implant bridges may be layered with translucent ceramic

The overall choice of the final restorative material depends on the available restorative space [19]. In cases where the restorative space is restricted, a wrong choice of material will lead to breakages and eventual failure of the restoration. Minimum thickness of material dimensions must be respected to harness its potential for long-term success. The thickness requirements of zirconia change when it is used in the natural dentition, a single implant or a full arch case. The dimensions will change based on location of the restoration in the mouth as the forces will increase significantly on posterior restoration as compared to anterior restorations. Around screw access holes, zirconia, must be at least 2 mm thick. Dimensions for connectors must be 7 mm^2 in anterior area and 9 mm^2 in posterior. Dimensions for inter-pontic connectors must be 12.5 mm^2. It is important that these minimum thickness requirements are met [20, 21].

(d) *High-Density Resins* can be used as long-term provisional restoration in implant cases. However, their wear rate, staining, restorative space requirements and lack of aesthetics make them the last choice as definitive restorative material in the aesthetic implant arena.

9.3 Clinical Considerations for Implant Impressions

The impression of the implants and surrounding soft tissue architecture may be done with conventional techniques or with a Digital Protocol (Fig. 9.35).

9.3.1 Conventional Impression Techniques

Traditional techniques of making impressions for implants remain the same and have been well researched in literature. These techniques have been described in literature in detail [22, 23]. The open tray techniques have been found to be superior in regards to accuracy especially when there are multiple implants [24]. In case of partial extraction therapies, custom impression techniques are recommended, to record the gingival architecture, so that the architecture can be well supported by the critical & the subcritical part of the abutment after fabrication [6].

Once the provisional has been designed with appropriate gingival and subgingival contours, the next step is to make the final impression after an adequate healing period. During impression making, once the provisional restoration is unscrewed

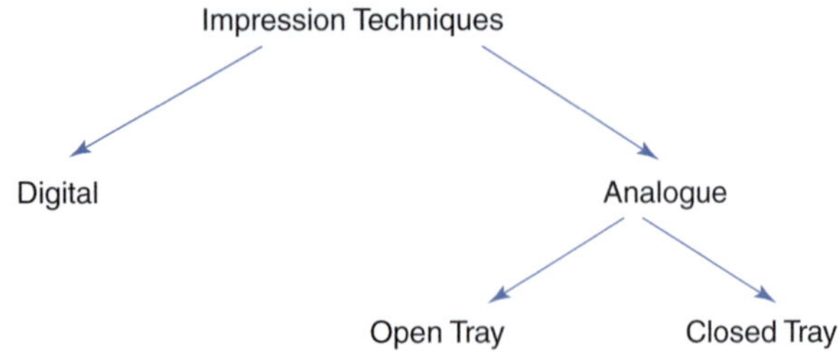

Fig. 9.35 Impression techniques may be conventional or digital

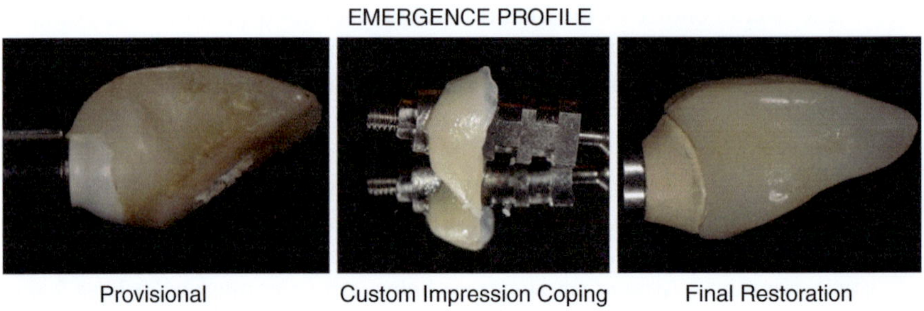

Fig. 9.36 A well-contoured provisional acts as a scaffold for soft tissue healing and creates ideal emergence profile. This is then captured with a customized impression coping and copied in the definitive restoration

from the implant, the gingival architecture begins to collapse and lose its shape. If the final restoration is made with such a gingival architecture, the outcome will be less than optimum. Hence a custom impression coping is needed that will help to transfer the soft tissue information developed by the provisional restoration to a definitive master cast [24, 25] on which the final restoration will be made. The concept, thus, is to make a well-contoured provisional restoration that creates a perfect tissue profile for ideal emergence of the implant restoration. This is then captured with a custom impression coping and transferred to the laboratory setting where a definitive restoration is fabricated with the ideal emergence profile (Fig. 9.36).

The technique for customizing an impression coping is as follows (Figs. 9.37, 9.38, 9.39, 9.40, 9.41, 9.42, 9.43, 9.44, 9.45, 9.46, 9.47 and 9.48):

(a) The well-adjusted, aesthetically acceptable provisional restoration that has a good emergence profile is removed.
(b) It is then fixed to an implant replica after thorough rinsing.
(c) The putty silicone is then mixed and formed into a shape of a ball that is placed on a glass slab. Before the putty sets, the implant analogue is placed into it in such a way that the cervical part of the provisional restoration gets embedded in the putty.

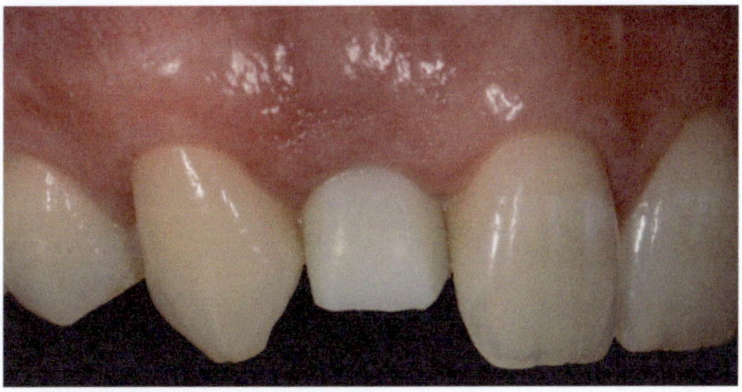

Fig. 9.37 Healed site with provisional restoration for tooth 12

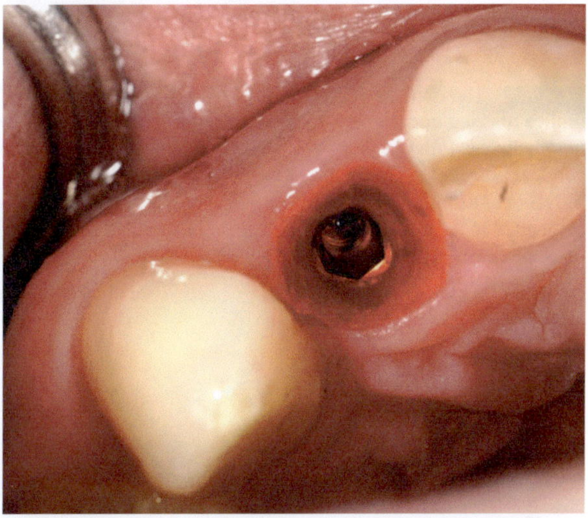

Fig. 9.38 Appearance of gingival architecture after removal of provisional restoration

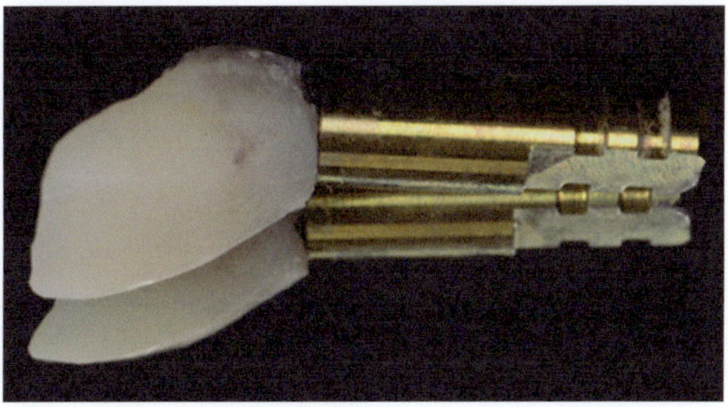

Fig. 9.39 The provisional restoration is attached to the implant replica

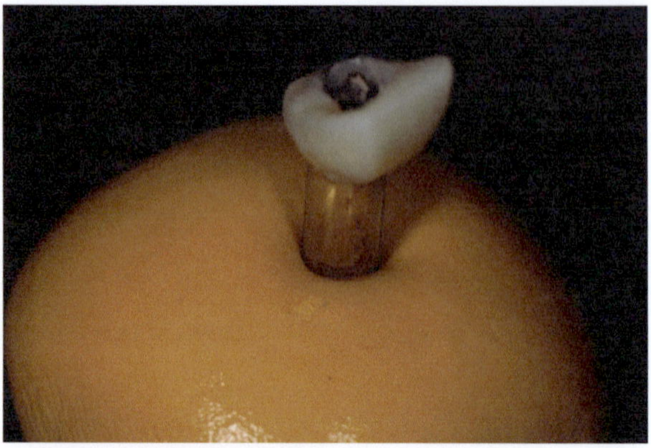

Fig. 9.40 The implant replica being inserted into the putty silicone

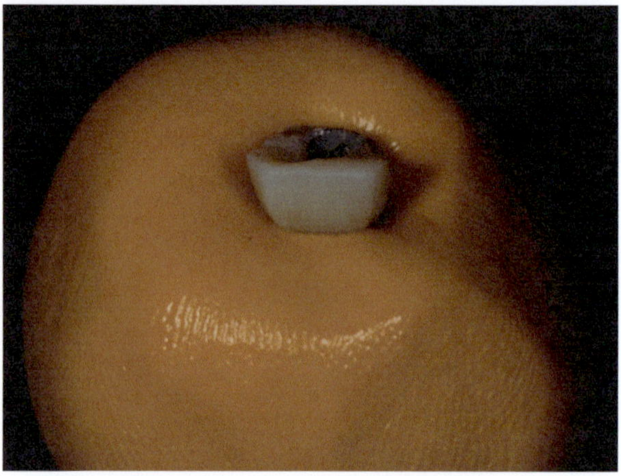

Fig. 9.41 The implant replica inserted into the putty silicone with the cervical aspect of provisional restoration embedded in the putty matrix

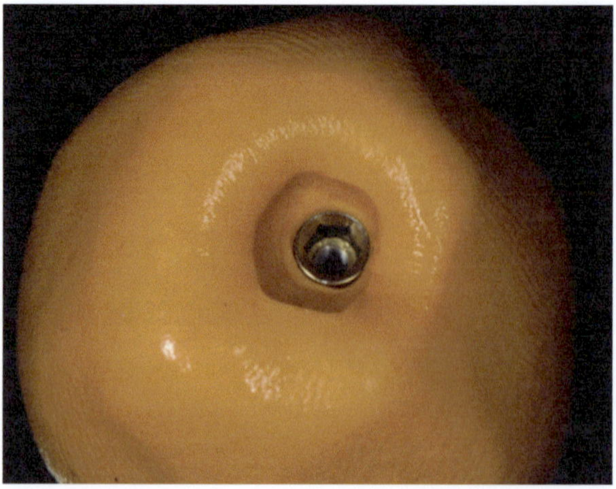

Fig. 9.42 The provisional restoration is removed from the implant replica. The gingival architecture created by the provisional is now clearly demarcated in putty silicone

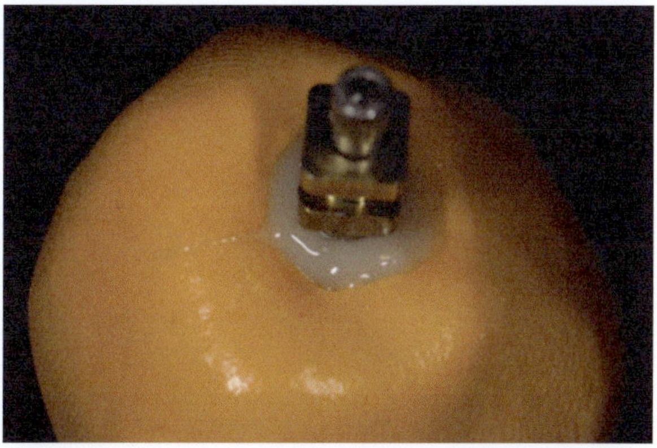

Fig. 9.43 An open tray impression coping is attached to the implant replica and flowable light cured composite used to capture the shape of the gingival architecture

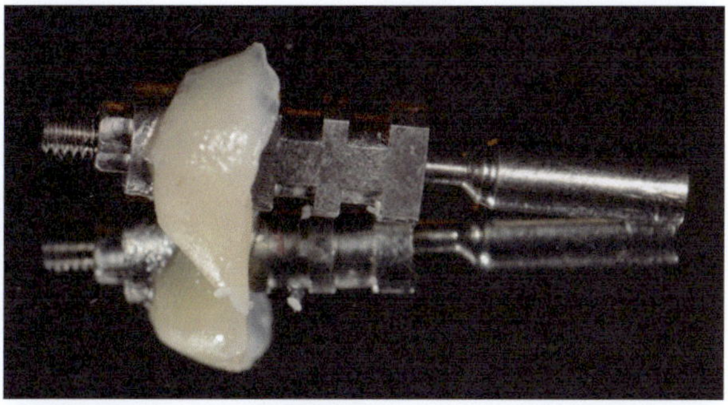

Fig. 9.44 The shape of the customized impression coping depicting the shape of the cervical part of the approved provisional restoration

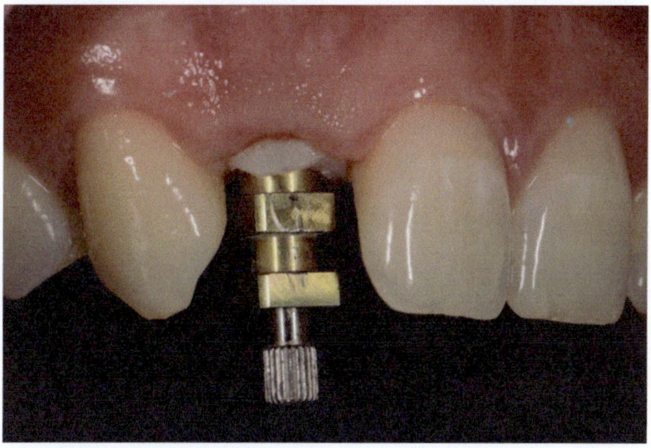

Fig. 9.45 The customized impression coping screwed onto the implant

(d) Once the material has set, the provisional restoration is unscrewed from the implant replica.
(e) The outline of the provisional and its relation to the implant replica will now be clearly visible.
(f) A closed or an open tray impression coping is then placed on the implant analogue.
(g) In the space between the coping and the walls of the putty, the flowable composite is syringed and light cured.

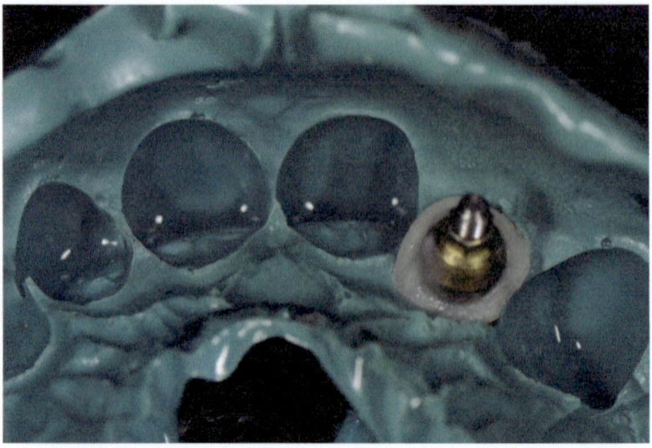

Fig. 9.46 The customized open tray impression coping captured within the final impression

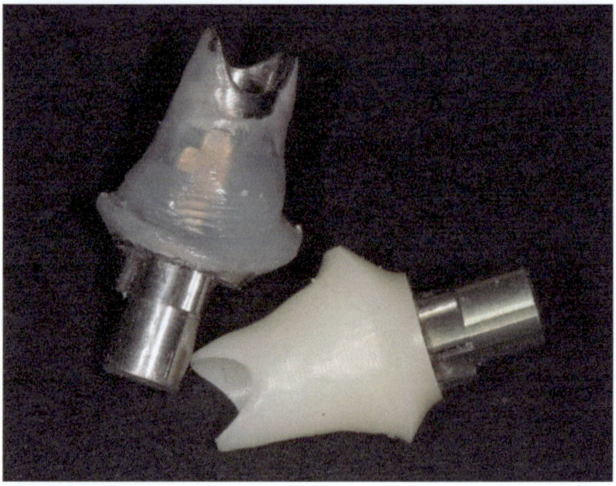

Fig. 9.47 Final customized zirconia abutment fabricated by copy milling the wax design

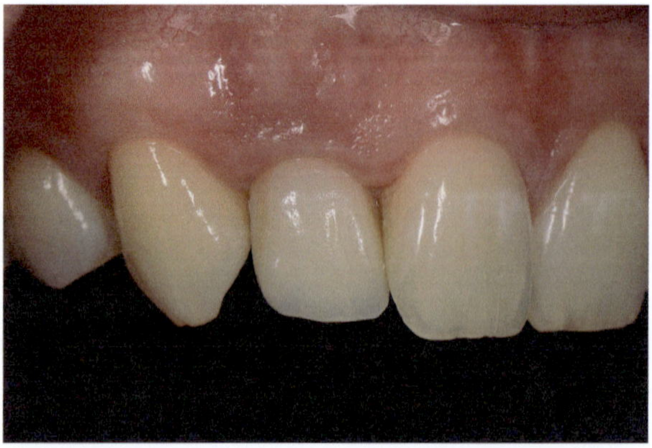

Fig. 9.48 The final restoration depicts an ideal emergence profile for #12

(h) The impression coping is then unscrewed from the implant replica. At this point flowable resin is attached to the impression coping thereby providing the information of the cervical contours of the provisional restoration. This impression coping is now a customized impression coping.
(i) The customized impression coping is then placed on the implant. It will push and support the gingival aspect of the peri-implant tissues in the same way as was done by the provisional restoration.
(j) The impression is then taken using this customized coping as it would be done for a regular implant. A stone cast with a soft tissue mask is fabricated to now mimic the soft tissue architecture that was conditioned by the provisional restoration.

Once the stone cast has been finalized with contours of the gingival architecture, the final abutment or the screw-retained restoration can be designed to support the tissues optimally.

9.3.2 Digital Impressions

Digital impressions are gaining in popularity and this is due to their proven accuracy. The digital workflow involves an intraoral scan and transfer of .stl files to the dental technician. The process needs to be clearly understood and every virtual component selected correctly to avoid mismatch. Any new technology requires learning and application to become a part of regular practice. Each implant system comes with its own, unique scan body that is to be used intraorally. The peri-implant gingival architecture has to be captured along with the implant position. In addition, the accurate capture of the opposing dentition and the interocclusal record is mandatory (Fig. 9.49).

The intraoral scanning procedure involves several key steps. Apart from capturing the position of the implant in relation to other teeth, even the soft tissue architecture (Fig. 9.50) as created by the provisional restoration must be digitally acquired.

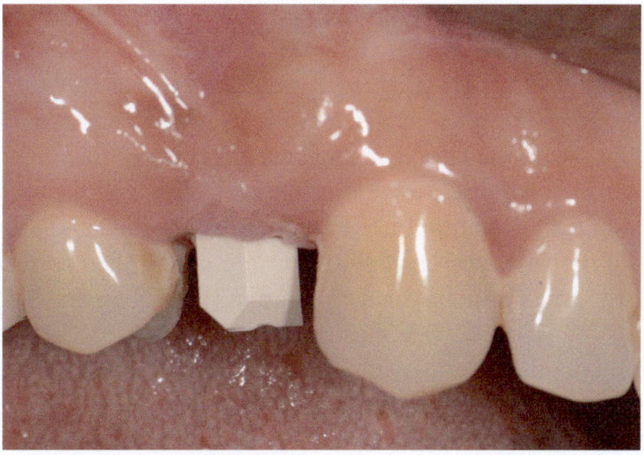

Fig. 9.49 Intraoral scan body, as shown here, allows intraoral digital impressions to be done and is a key component in the digital workflow

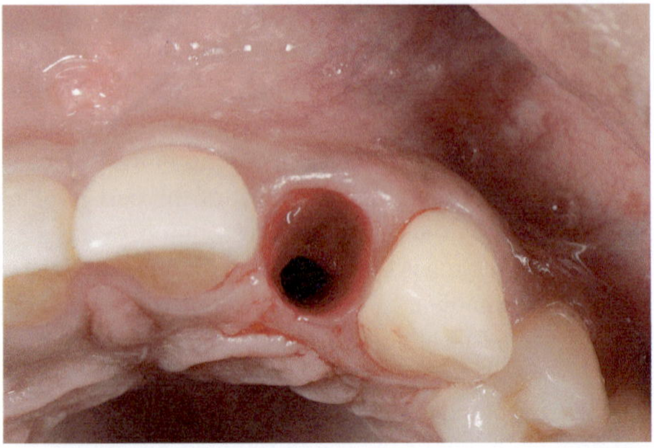

Fig. 9.50 Soft tissue architecture created with a well-designed provisional restoration enables an ideal emergence profile of the final restoration

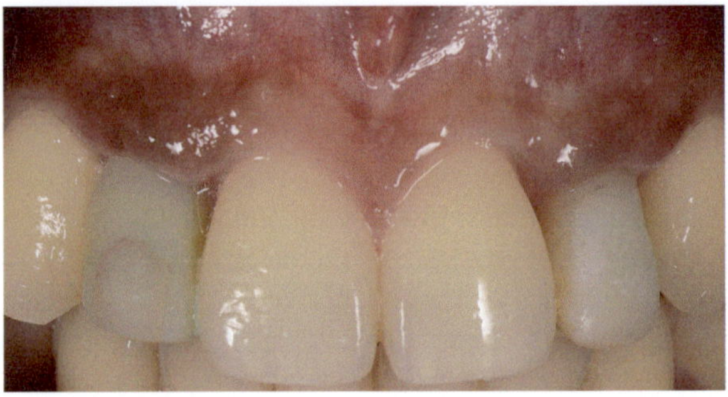

Fig. 9.51 The approved provisional restorations on tooth numbers 12 and 22 are digitally scanned as the first step

Before removal of the approved provisional restoration, an intraoral scan is done to capture its overall morphology and its relation to adjacent teeth and gingiva (Figs. 9.51 and 9.52). The dental technician later uses this scan as a template to design the emergence profile of the final restoration.

After scanning, the provisional restoration is unscrewed from the underlying implant. Like all digital implant impressions, the entire soft tissue architecture and the adjacent teeth are scanned (Fig. 9.53). The intraoral scan body is then placed and captured digitally (Figs. 9.54 and 9.55). In this way the implant position and its surrounding gingival architecture is digitally acquired. The opposing dentition too, along with the bite, is scanned at this stage.

Once the digital intraoral impression is completed, the provisional restorations are attached extra-orally to the implant replica and scanned individually. This will aid the laboratory technician in mimicking the cervical contour of the provisional restoration onto the final restoration (Figs. 9.56 and 9.57).

The scanned files are saved as .stl and .ply or any other equivalent formats and sent to the dental technician . The dental technician will open these files in

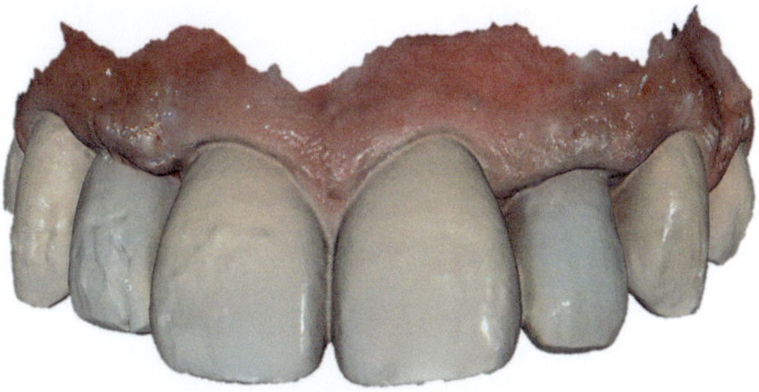

Fig. 9.52 The digital output file of the approved provisional restoration

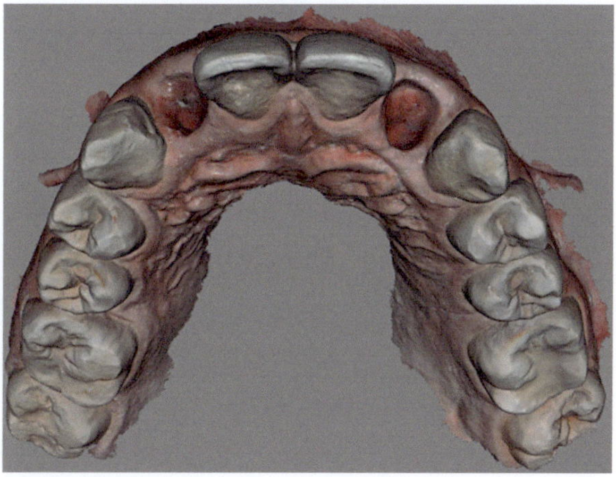

Fig. 9.53 The soft tissue architecture and adjacent teeth are digitally captured as the first step

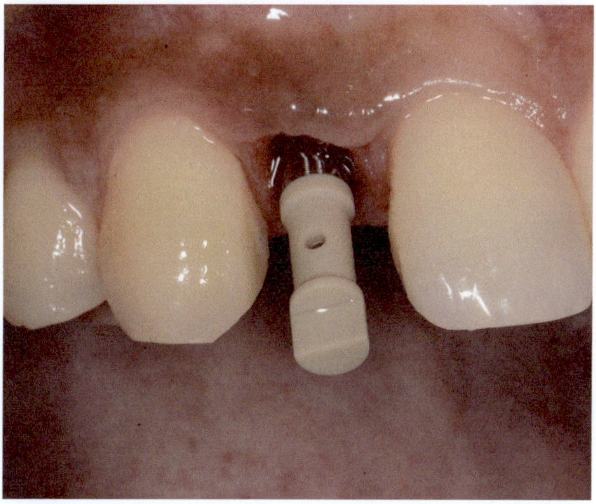

Fig. 9.54 Intraoral scan body aids in digitally acquiring the implant position is relation to adjacent teeth and soft tissue

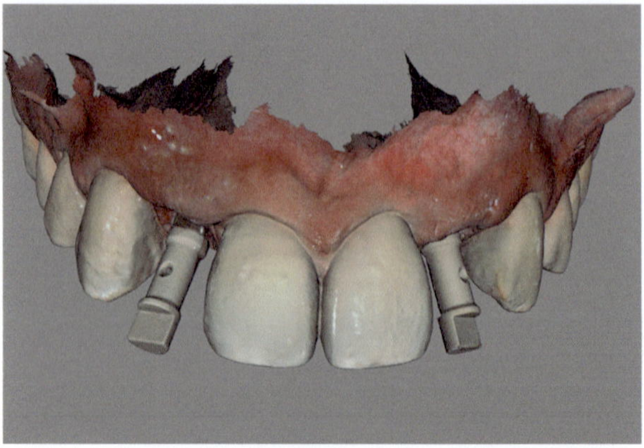

Fig. 9.55 The digital rendition of the teeth along with the intraoral scan bodies

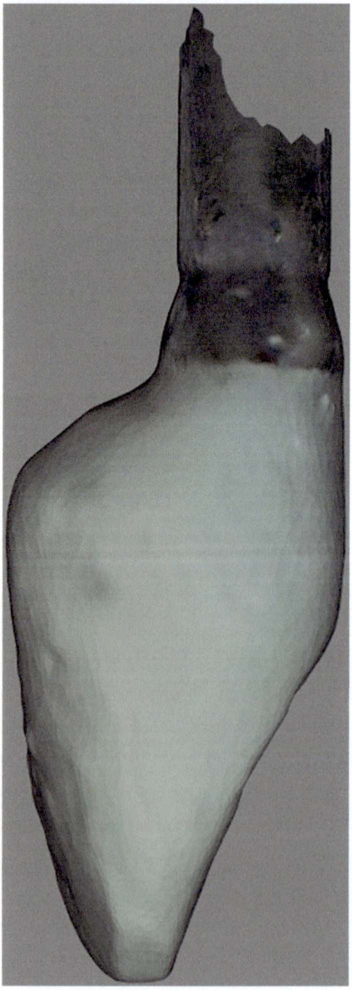

Fig. 9.56 Scans of the approved provisional restorations done extra-orally to help mimic its cervical contours and emergence

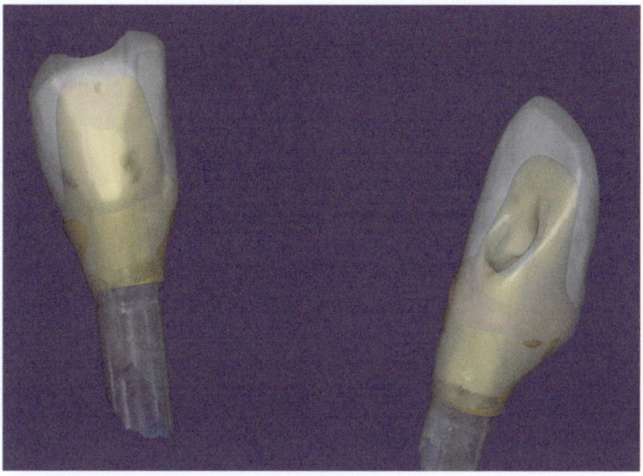

Fig. 9.57 The design of the abutment is retrofitted within the confines of the approved provisional restorations

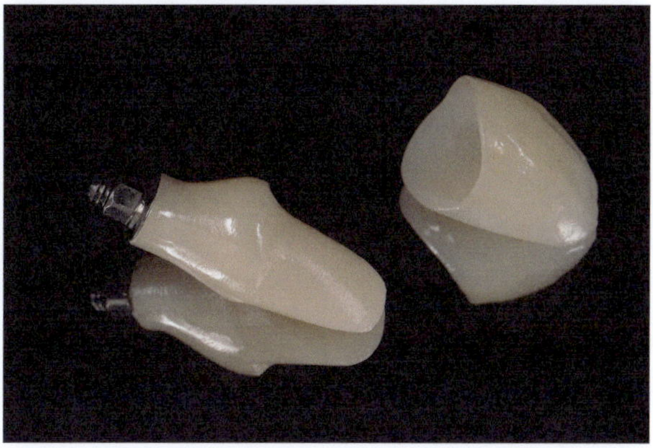

Fig. 9.58 The final abutment mimics the cervical contours and emergence of the provisional restoration

designing software (ExoCad) and the scan body is matched to the specific implant. A virtual model is then generated with the implant replica that has the surrounding, customized, gingival architecture well captured. A virtual abutment can then be designed to support or modify the gingival architecture and emergence. The final abutment (Figs. 9.58 and 9.59) or restoration can be milled from any of the materials discussed in the start in this chapter.

The final restoration (Fig. 9.60) is then delivered as per conventional implantology norms.

9.3.3 Direct Impressions with 'One–Time' Abutment Concept

Frequent disconnection and reconnection of healing abutments and final abutments may lead to disruption of the mucosal barrier around implants and can cause clinically relevant mucosal recession [26]. It has been shown that when the final

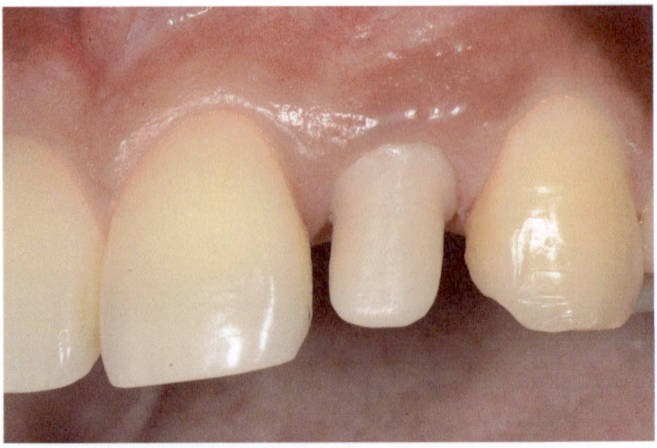

Fig. 9.59 The customized zirconia abutment is fixed to the implant intraorally

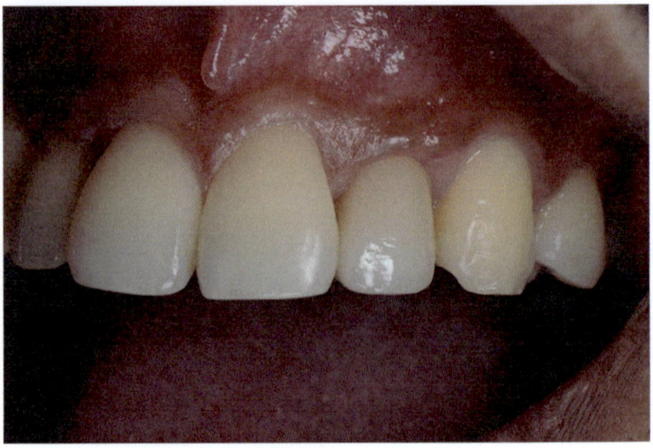

Fig. 9.60 The final restoration in place depicts excellent tissue health and contours. The key factors for success are a well-designed provisional restoration, the acquisition of the gingival architecture with analogue or digital methods, followed by a well-designed custom abutment/restoration

abutment is screwed onto the implant once and then not disconnected again it can minimize bone loss and mucosal recession [27].

In this protocol, immediately after implant placement or after second stage, definitive (final) abutment selection is done. The abutment is modified to achieve correct margin placement and optimal height to accommodate a restoration. All modifications of the abutments must be carried out extra-orally to avoid heat from friction. On this abutment a temporary cement-retained provisional restoration is fixed. Extreme caution is exercised during cementation of the provisional restoration to prevent any residual cement in the peri-implant sulcus. It is incumbent upon the clinician to make sure that the restorative margin placement on the abutment is no deeper than 0.5 mm subgingival. A deep margin will make residual cement difficult to clean. Any cement residue will lead to peri-implant tissue-related healing problems and may even result in failure of osseointegration.

After a suitable healing period of 3–4 months, the provisional restoration is removed from the underlying abutment and the gingival health and architecture is evaluated. If all clinical parameters are satisfactory, a gingival retraction procedure is carried out. A dry knitted cord is placed in the sulcus without undue pressure avoiding any damage to the junctional epithelium attached to the abutment. If margin placement is equigingival or 0.5 mm subgingival, and accessible to digital capture, a digital impression may be taken. In cases where the abutment margins are deeper or difficult to digitally capture, a conventional impression may be chosen. Addition silicones may be used as a two-step technique to capture the abutment contours along with rest of the dentition. The final prostheses can be fabricated on a laboratory fabricated cast from this impression as it would be done for routine crown and bridge cases.

Figures 9.61, 9.62, 9.63, 9.64, 9.65, 9.66, 9.67 and 9.68 show the making of such a restoration for a missing tooth 21 case with onetime abutment concept.

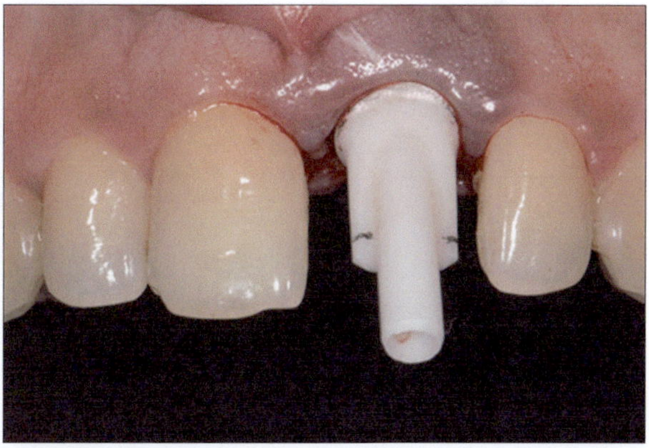

Fig. 9.61 Final zirconia abutment being tried at the time of implant placement

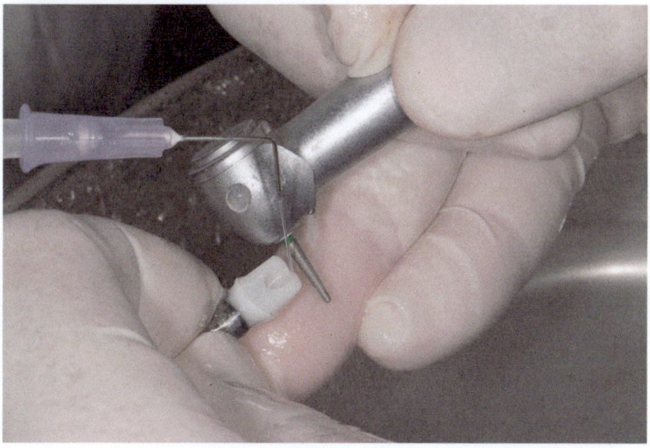

Fig. 9.62 The height of prefabricated abutment adjusted to allow enough room for a definitive cement-retained restoration later

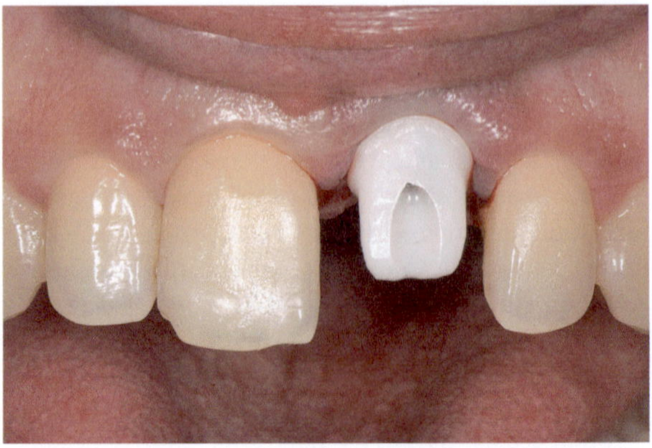

Fig. 9.63 The finalized prefabricated zirconia abutment with equigingival margins

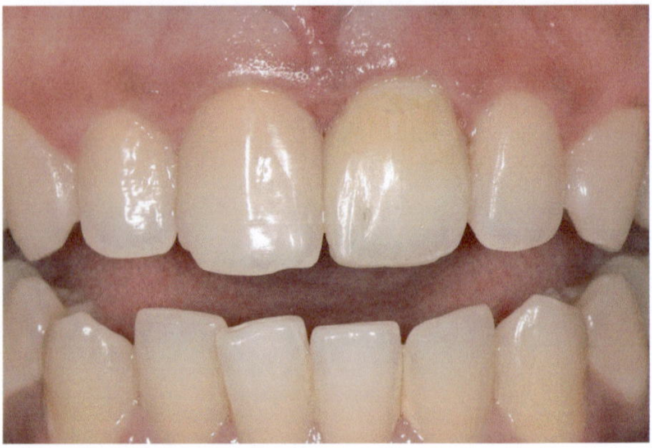

Fig. 9.64 The provisional restoration cemented onto the abutment with temporary cement

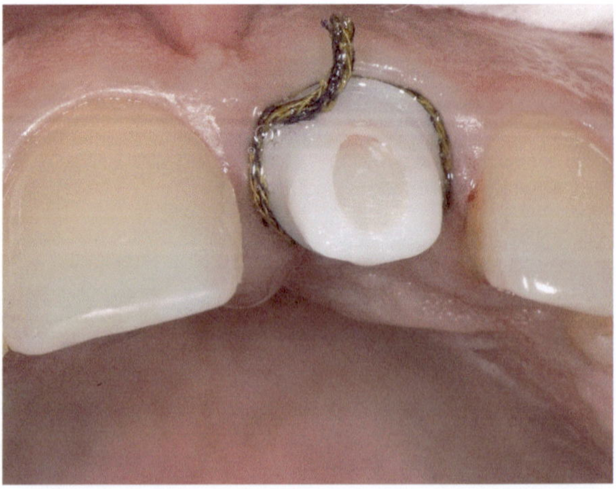

Fig. 9.65 At 4 months, the provisional restoration is removed and a retraction cord placed for an impression

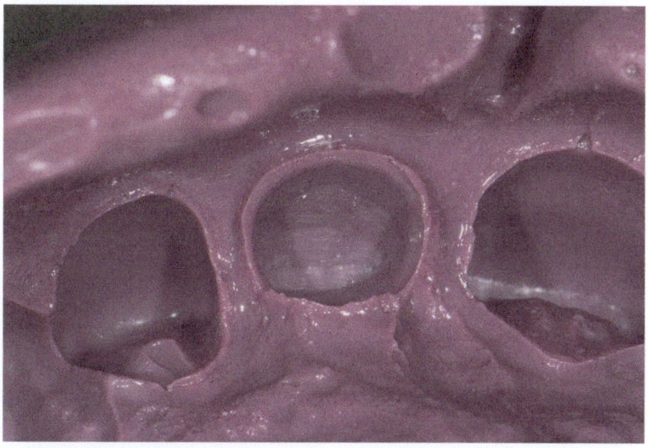

Fig. 9.66 The final impression of the 'One-time Abutment'

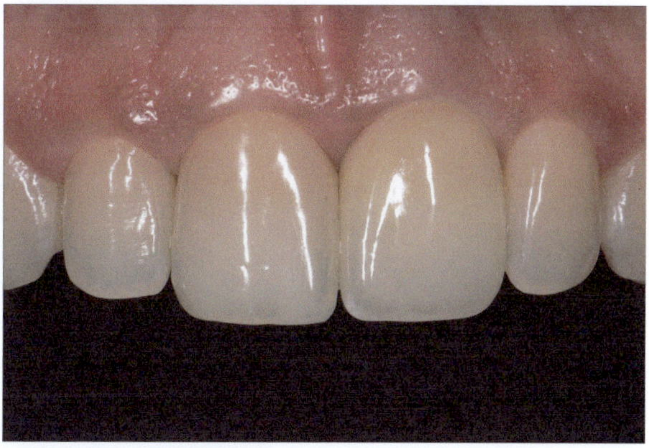

Fig. 9.67 The final restoration made from lithium disilicate cemented onto the one time zirconia abutment

9.4 Fast Tracking Protocol for Implants in the Aesthetic Zone

In certain cases, a provisional restoration on an anterior implant has been in long-term clinical use and is functionally satisfactory and meets the patients' aesthetic requirements. In this scenario a novel technique can be used to fast track the capture of gingival architecture and implant position simultaneously. This protocol is adapted from a similar technique of fast tracking for fully edentulous cases [28]. In the conventional prosthetic protocol, all the steps of impression making, pouring a stone cast, making wax-ups and final restorations tend to incorporate some errors that get built up leading to less than optimal fit and aesthetics of the final restoration. Several trials are needed to allow the clinician to overcome these errors.

Figures 9.69, 9.70, 9.71, 9.72, 9.73, 9.74, 9.75, 9.76 and 9.77 show the fast-tracking technique in detail*. The first step is to unscrew the provisional restoration and check implant integration. Next, the same provisional restoration is fixed back on the implant, replacing the original abutment screw with a long screw of an open tray coping. Polyether adhesive is applied on the abutment and an impression is

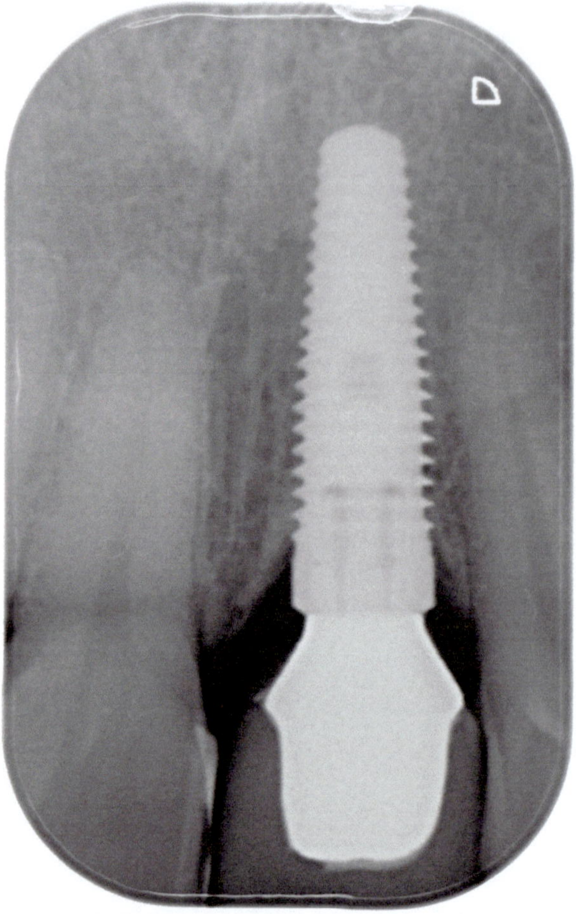

Fig. 9.68 Post-operative radiograph of the final restoration

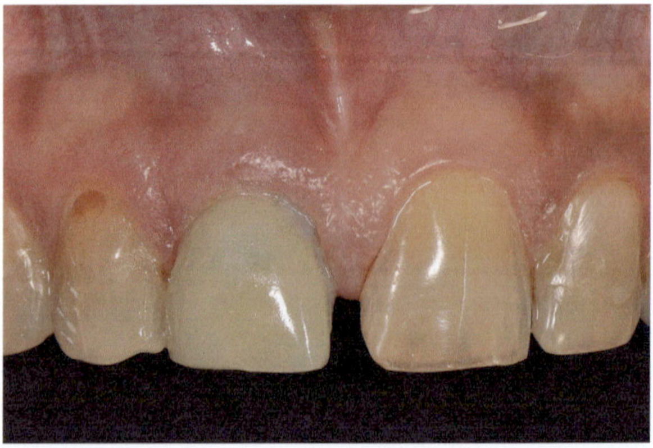

Fig. 9.69 Screw-retained provisional crown

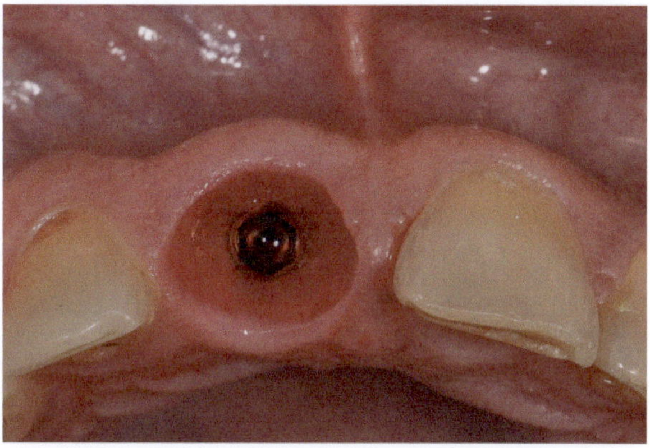

Fig. 9.70 Good soft tissue contours seen after removal of the provisional crown

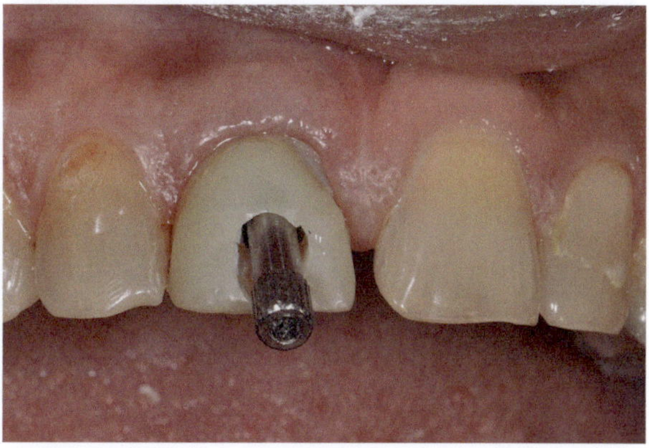

Fig. 9.71 Using long screw of the open tray impression coping to engage the provisional restoration to the implant

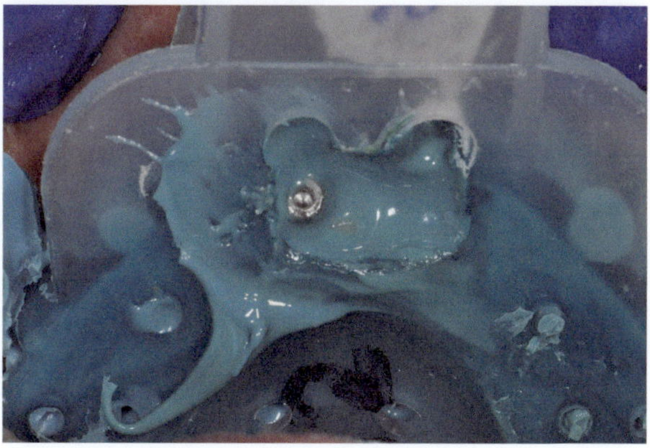

Fig. 9.72 Open tray impression

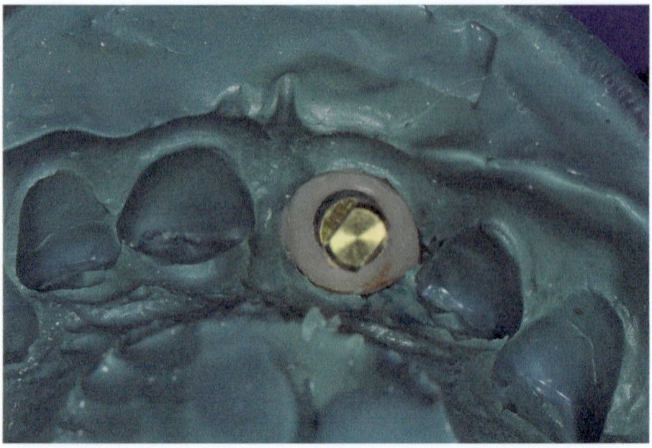

Fig. 9.73 Attaching the implant replica

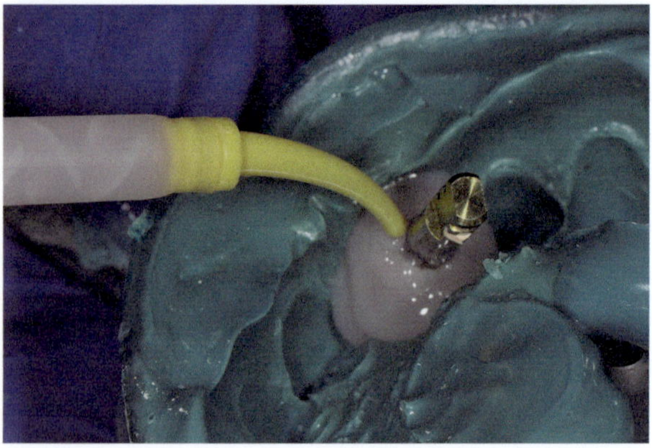

Fig. 9.74 Gingival mask is placed around the implant replica after applying a seperating medium on the impression material

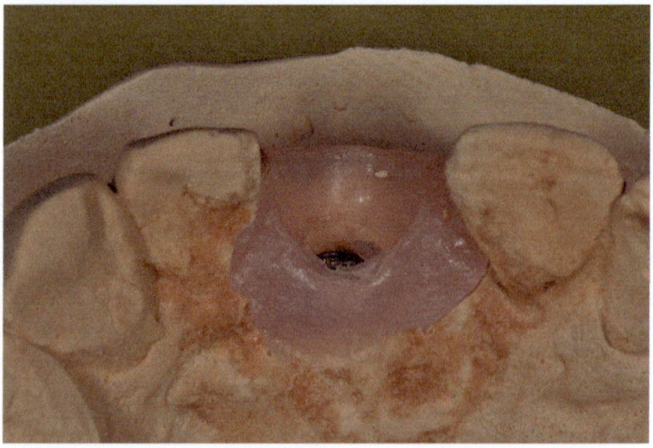

Fig. 9.75 Accurate reproduction of soft tissue contours on the stone cast with gingival mask material

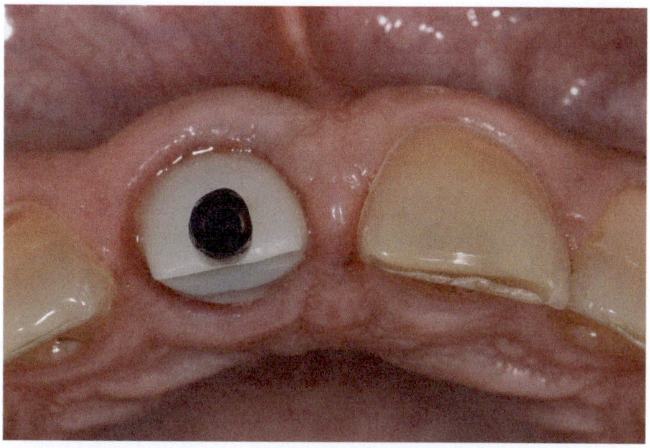

Fig. 9.76 Zirconia abutment on implant. Veneer preparation on #21

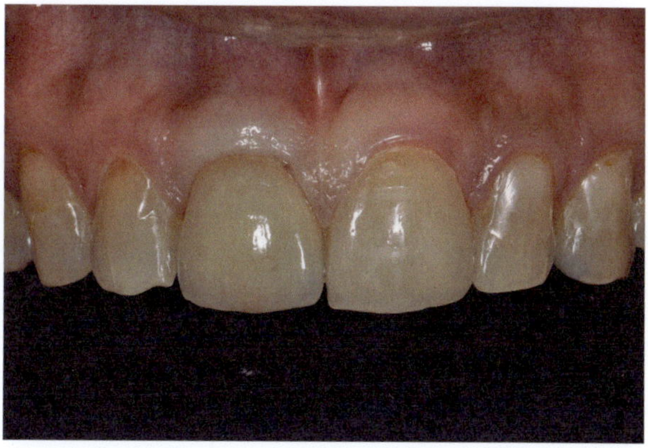

Fig. 9.77 Definitive lithium disilicate crown

taken similar to an open tray impression. On retrieval of the set material, the provisional restoration comes out as a part of the impression. It carries with it a reproduction of the well-contoured gingival architecture that provides good aesthetics and an ideal emergence. A stone cast is generated from this impression and a definitive abutment or restoration is fabricated on this stone cast copying the outline of the gingival architecture.

The advantage of this fast tracking procedure is that it allows the clinician to circumvent several conventional prosthodontic steps that may cause minor inaccuracies and may require multiple checks at each step to produce an acceptable, well-fitted restoration.

9.5 Conclusion

The definitive restorations may be made with different designs based on the mode of retention. Cement-retained restorations bring the disadvantage of the residual cement and lack of retrievability while the screw-retained restorations negate these. Various factors that govern the choice have been discussed. The materials used to make the definitive restorations play a crucial role in long-term health and function of the implant cases. Various impression protocols are possible for minimizing errors and maximizing aesthetics. These have been discussed and the clinician must choose the techniques that may produce the best clinical outcomes.

Acknowledgment Illustrations by: Udatta Kher.
Lab Work on all cases (except Section 9.4): Adaro Dental Lab, Mumbai
Section 9.4 Lab Work: Katara Dental, Pune
*Case Courtesy: Dr Udatta Kher

References

1. Furhauser R, Florescu D, Benesch T, Haas R, Mailath G, Watzek G. Evaluation of soft tissue around single-tooth implant crowns: the pink esthetic score. Clin Oral Implants Res. 2005;16-6:639–44.
2. Chee W, Jivraj S. Screw versus cemented implant supported restorations. Br Dent J. 2006;201:501–7.
3. Linkevicius T, Vaitelis J. The effect of zirconia or titanium as abutment material on soft peri-implant tissues. A systematic review and meta-analysis. Clin Oral Implants Res. 2015;26(suppl 11):139–47.
4. Jung RE, Sailer I, Hammerle CH, Attin T, Schmidlin P. In vitro colour changes of soft tissues caused by restorative materials. Int J Periodontics Restorative Dent. 2007;27:251–7.
5. Foong JK, Judge RB, Palamara JE. Swain MV. Fracture resistance of titanium and zirconia abutments: an in vitro study. J Prosthet Dent. 2013;109:304–12.
6. Su H, González-Martín O, Weisgold A, Lee E. Considerations of implant abutment and crown contour: critical contour and subcritical contour. Int J Periodontics Restorative Dent. 2010;30(4):335–43.
7. Linkevicius T, Vindasiute E, Puisys A, Linkeviciene L, Maslova N, Puriene A. The influence of the cementation margin position on the amount of undetected cement. A prospective clinical study. Clin Oral Implants Res. 2013;24:71–6.
8. Ingelese S. Emergence Profile. Relation between morphology, Biology & Esthetics. Quintessence Dent Technol. 2018:228–41.
9. Abrahamsson I, Berglundh T, Glantz PO, Lindhe J. The mucosal attachments at different abutments. An experimental study in dogs. J Clin. Periodontology. 1998;25:721.
10. Nakamura K, Kanno T, Milleding P, Ortengren U. Zirconia as a dental implant abutment material. A systematic review. Int J Prosthodont. 2010;23:299–309.
11. Scarano A, Piatelli M, Caputi S, Favero GA, Piatelli A. Bacterial adhesion on commercially pure titanium and zirconium oxide disks: an in vivo human study. J Periodontol. 2004;75:292–6.
12. Sailer I, Zembic A, Jung RE, Hammerle CH, Mattiola A. Single tooth implant reconstructions: esthetic factors influencing the decision between titanium and zirconia abutments in anterior regions. Eur J Esthet Dent. 2007;2:296–310.
13. Happe A, Schulte-Mattler V, Strassert C, Naumann M, Stimmelmayr M, Zoller JE, Rothamel D. In vitro colour changes of soft tissues caused by dyed fluorescent zirconia and non dyed, non fluorescent zirconia in thin mucosa. Int J Periodontics Restorative Dent. 2013;33:e1–8.

14. Bechir ES, Bechir A, Cherana G. The advantages of BioHPP polymer as superstructure material in Oral Implantology. Mater Plast. 2016;53(3)
15. Wiesli MG, Öesl M. High performance polymers and their potential application as medical and oral implant materials: a review. Implant Dent. 2015;24(4):448–57.
16. Jung RE, Zembic A, Pjetursson BE, Zwahlen M, Thoma DS. Systemic review of survival rate and incidence of biological, technical and aesthetic complications of single crowns on implants reported in longitudinal studies with mean follow up of 5 years. Clin Oral Implants Res. 2012;23(6):2–21.
17. Pjetusson BE, Bragger U, Lang NP, Zwalen M. Comparision of survival and complication rates of tooth supported fixed dental prostheses and implant- supported fixed dental prostheses and single crowns. Clin Oral Implants Res. 2007;18(Suppl 3):97–113.
18. Papaspyridakos P, Lal K. Computer assisted design/ computer assisted manufacturing zirconia implant fixed complete prostheses: clinical results and technical complications upto 4 years of function. Clin Oral Implants Res. 2013;24:659–65.
19. Tunkiwala A, Kher U, Bijlani P. Numerical guidelines for selection of implant supported prostheses for completely edentulous patients. Quintessence India. 2017;1:46–53.
20. Larsson C, Holm L, Lovgren N, Kokubo Y, Vult von Steyern P. Fracture strength of four-unit Y-TZP FPD cores designed with varying connector diameter. An in vitro study. J Oral Rehabil. 2007;34:702–9.
21. Sasse M, Kern M. Survival of anterior cantilevered all ceramic resin bonded fixed dental prostheses made from zirconia ceramic. J Dent. 2014;42:660–3.
22. Lee H, So JS, Hochstedler JL, Ercoli C. The accuracy of implant impressions: a systemic review. J Prosthet Dent. 2008;100:285–91.
23. Lee YJ, Heo SJ, Koak JY, Kim SK. Accuracy of direct impression techniques for internal connection implants. Int J Oral Maxillofac Implants. 2009;24:823–30.
24. Chappuis V, Martin W. Implant therapy in the esthetic zone. ITI treatment guide Vol. 10. Berlin: Quintessence Publishing; 2017.
25. Patras M, Martin W. Simplified custom impression post for implant supported restorations. J Prosthet Dent. 2016;115(5):556–9.
26. Abrahamsson I, Berglundh T, Lindhe J. The mucosal barrier following abutment dis/reconnection. An experimental study in dogs. J Clin Periodontol. 1997;24:568–72.
27. Rodriguez X, Vela X, Mendez V, Segala M, Calvo-Guirado JL, Tarnow DP. The effect of abutment dis/reconnections on per implant bone resorption: a radiologic study of platform -switched and non platform-switched implants placed in animals. Clin Oral Implants Res. 2013;24:305–11.
28. Kher U, Tunkiwala A, Bijlani P. Fast-tracking the implant Prosthodontic workflow for full-arch restorations: case series. Compend Contin Educ Dent. 2018;39(7):e5–8.

Errors and Complications in Partial Extraction Therapy

10

Sudhindra Kulkarni, Tarun Kumar, T. V. Narayan, and Ali Tunkiwala

Abstract

Partial extraction therapies have gained popularity in the past few years. They aid in preserving hard and soft tissues by retaining a part of the buccal aspect of the root during implant placement. As with any procedure which is technique sensitive, one needs to exercise caution while performing these surgeries. Complications are to be expected during the course of such procedures. Most of the complications occur due to inappropriate case selection and few occur during the execution. This chapter deals with the prevention and management of such complications associated with PET procedures.

10.1 Introduction

Cascades of biologic events follow tooth extraction. To a clinician, the most relevant amongst these is the bone remodeling which results in loss of buccal contour leading to horizontal and vertical soft tissue loss [1–3]. Multitudes of procedures have been carried out to prevent the resorption of the residual ridge with variable success rates. All these techniques are aimed at maintenance of the labial contour, which will

S. Kulkarni
Department of Implantology, SDM Dental College, Sri Dharmasthala Manjunatheshwara University, Dharwad, Karnataka, India

Private Practice, Hubli, Karnataka, India

T. Kumar
Department of Implantology, Bapuji Dental College, Davanagere, Karnataka, India

T. V. Narayan
Private Practice, Bengaluru, Karnataka, India

A. Tunkiwala (✉)
Smiles by Design, Mumbai, India

U. Kher, A. Tunkiwala (eds.), *Partial Extraction Therapy in Implant Dentistry*,
https://doi.org/10.1007/978-3-030-33610-3_10

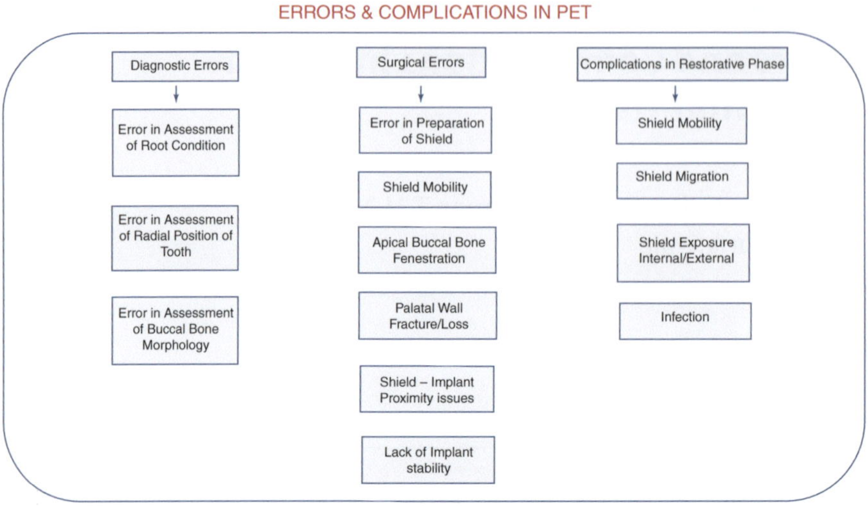

Fig. 10.1 Classifications of errors and complications in partial extraction therapies

provide a satisfactory emergence profile for the final restoration [4, 5]. The socket shield technique (SS) is a recent addition to these procedures that help to preserve bone ridge contour [6, 7]. Gluckman et al. coined the term partial extraction therapies (PET) [8–10]. The scope of these involve socket shield, pontic shield, and root submergence. All these techniques have been described in various previous chapters.

Since these are newer treatment modalities, their exact guidelines are in a process of evolution. The procedures are technique sensitive, the learning curve to perform them with exactitude is steep, due to which errors and complications may occur. Case selection criteria and contraindication of the procedures are described in Chap. 3.

The errors and complications that are likely to occur during the PET procedures are categorized into the following (summarized in Fig. 10.1):

1. Diagnostic errors.
2. Surgical errors.
3. Complications in restorative phase.

10.2 Diagnostic Errors

10.2.1 Errors in Assessment of Root Condition

As all partial extraction therapies (PET) deal with preparation of the radicular portion of the tooth, it is of utmost importance that the clinician evaluates the root status clinically as well as radiographically. A healthy root is a prerequisite for long-term success of the PET procedure. Assessment of the root condition, its radial position, and the surrounding bone with any accompanying lesions is paramount [11]. This

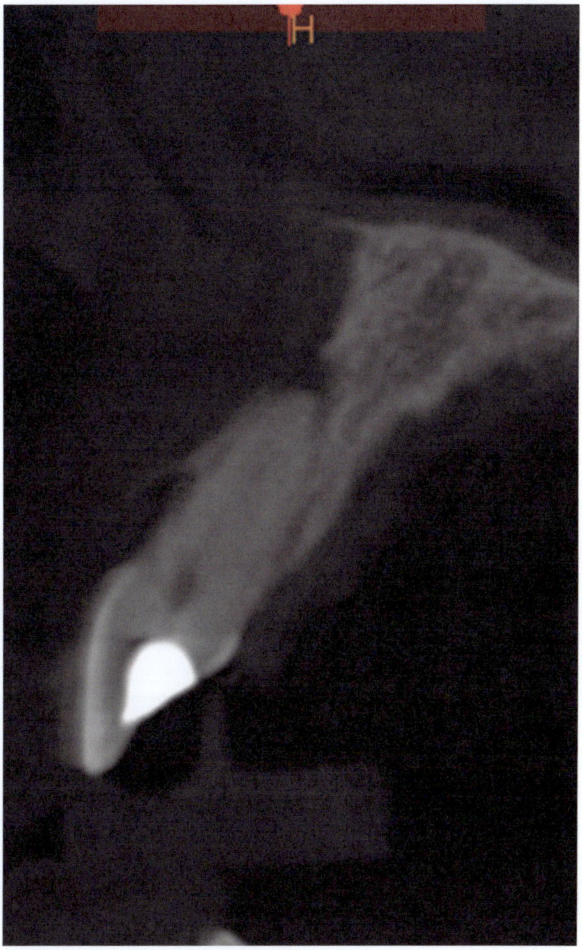

Fig. 10.2 In cases such as these, apical fenestration in the bone and inadequate palatal bone width will make this case a poor choice for a socket shield procedure

will aid in minimizing intraoperative and postoperative complications. The following aspects with respect to the root should be evaluated preoperatively (Fig. 10.2).

Root Length

If the length of the root is inadequate the chances of shield mobility during preparation will increase (Fig. 10.3). If the shield is too long, it will become difficult to extract the apical portion.

The maxillary cuspid has the longest root amongst all the teeth in the mouth [12]. This can pose a higher degree of difficulty during the surgical execution, especially while removing the apex (Fig. 10.4).

Caries Status

Root caries is usually supra-crestal. Therefore, it can be excavated and cleaned thoroughly during the PET procedure [13]. Heavily decayed roots are not an

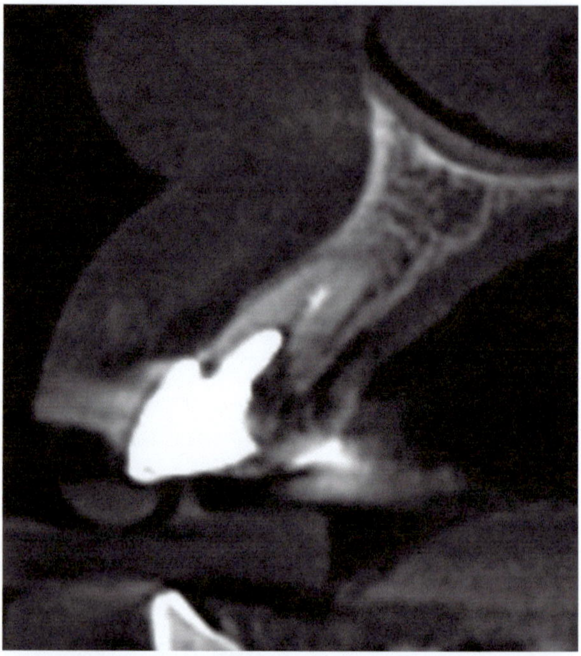

Fig. 10.3 The length of the root in the following case is short. After decoronation and removal of apex, inadequate length of the shield will remain, which may lead to an unstable shield. Such teeth can become mobile during the procedure

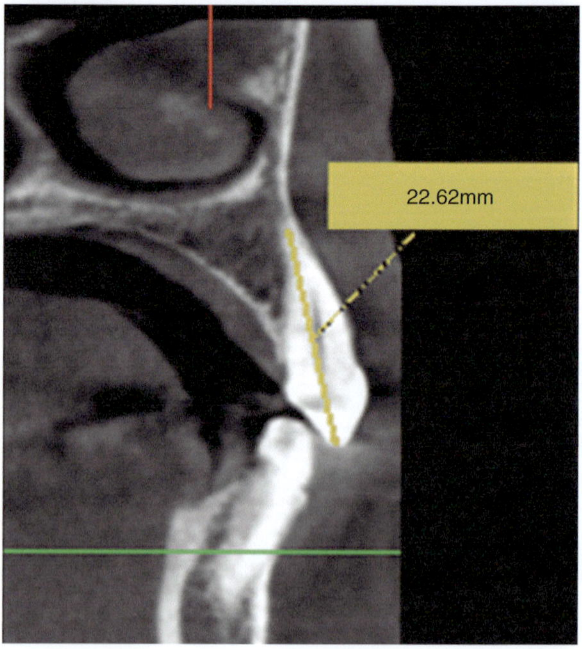

Fig. 10.4 Maxillary cuspids have the longest root. This makes removal of the apex challenging

ideal choice as they can lead to short/long-term complications. Such roots are difficult to section and may fracture at unfavorable points during the preparation of the shield. Thus, they should be avoided for PET procedures (Figs. 10.5 and 10.6).

As illustrated in the following case, when a grossly carious root is selected for a PET procedure, complications may arise. At the time of prosthetic phase, shield mobility was noted adjacent to an osseointegrated implant (Figs. 10.7, 10.8, 10.9, 10.10, 10.11, 10.12, 10.13 and 10.14). The shield was removed and the buccal dehiscence caused due to its removal was grafted using guided bone regeneration (GBR) principles. Sticky bone, created out of a xenograft and i-PRF, was used to graft the defect [14]. This was then layered with a PRF membrane and a collagen membrane followed by complete closure of the surgical site [15–17].

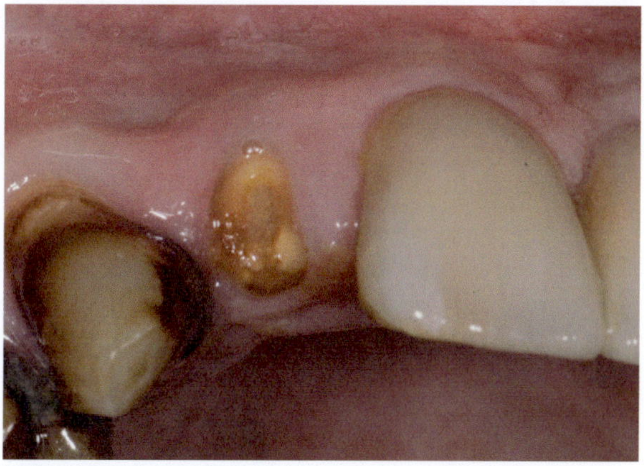

Fig. 10.5 Ideal teeth for PET are unrestorable teeth with no decay

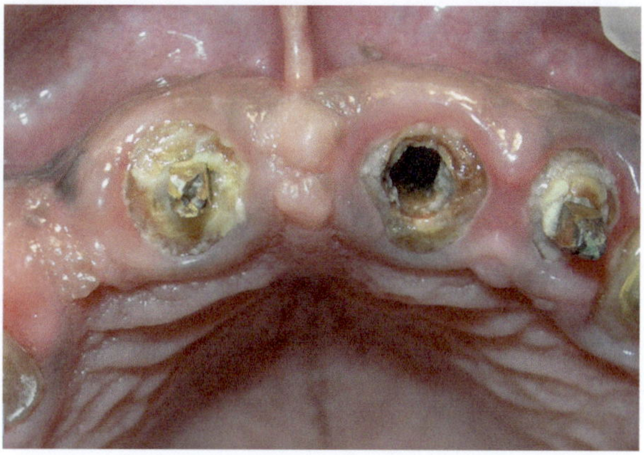

Fig. 10.6 Root on tooth 21 showing extensive caries affecting a large depth of the root

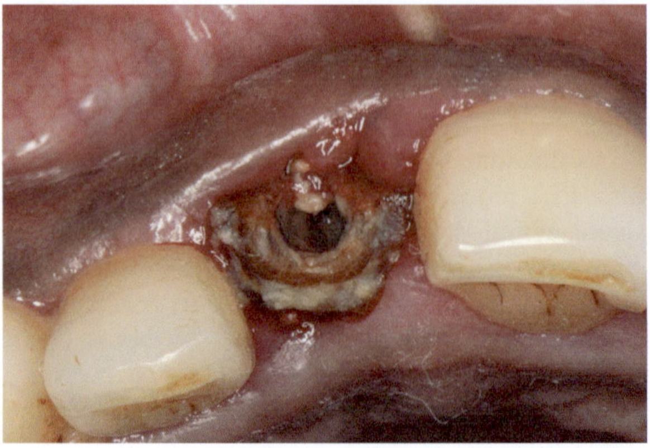

Fig. 10.7 Grossly carious root (11)

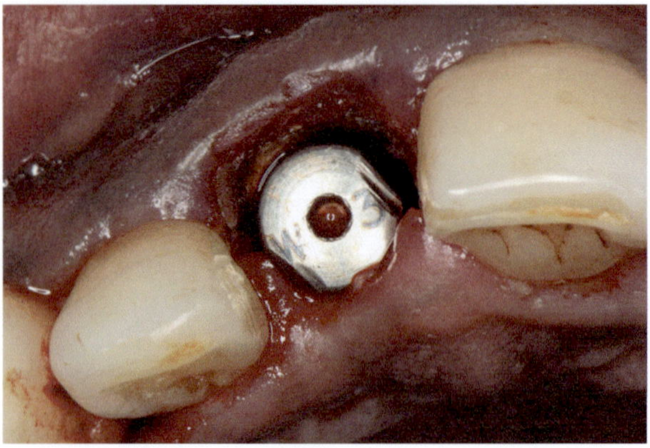

Fig. 10.8 Infection detected around the shield during the prosthetic phase of the treatment

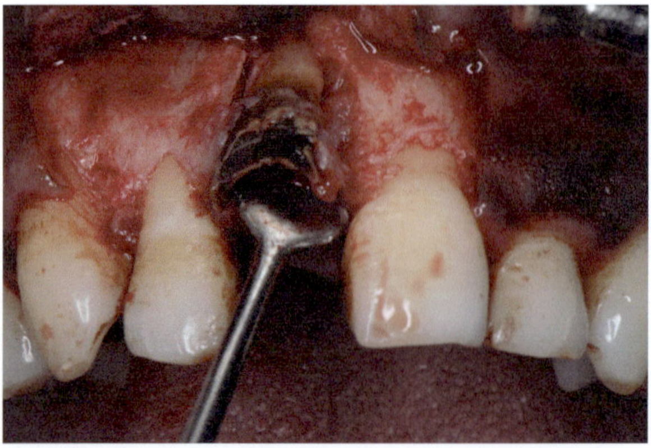

Fig. 10.9 Shield mobility was detected. This case was not suitable for PET procedure due to presence of deep root caries

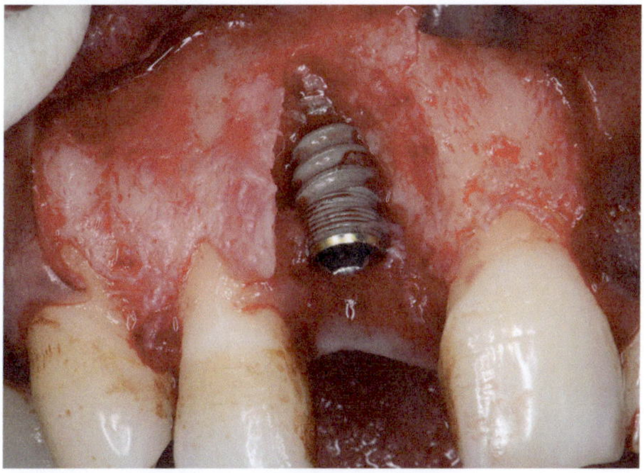

Fig. 10.10 Buccal dehiscence seen after the removal of the shield

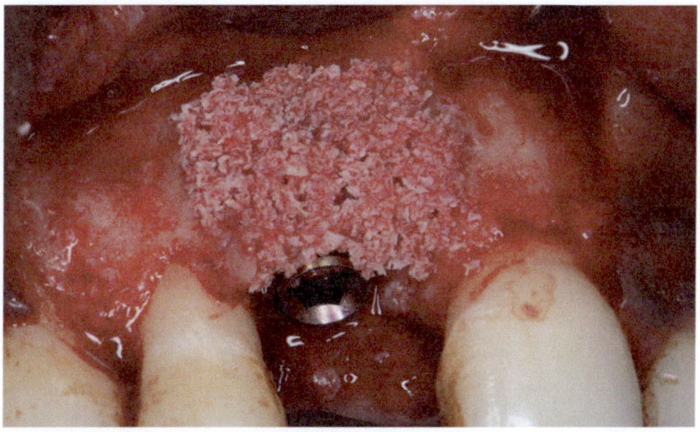

Fig. 10.11 GBR (guided bone regeneration) done using xenograft

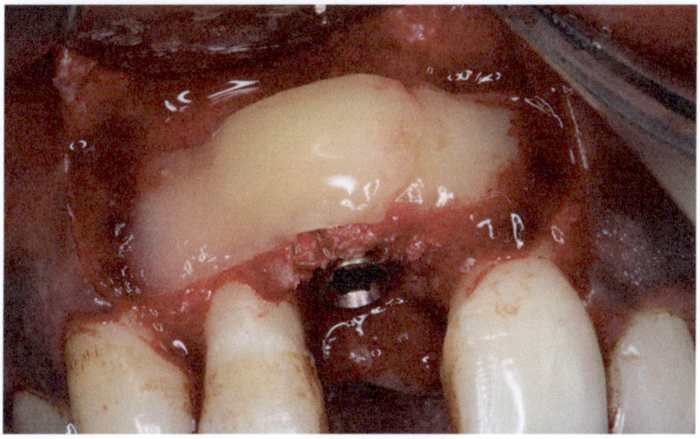

Fig. 10.12 PRF membranes placed over the graft

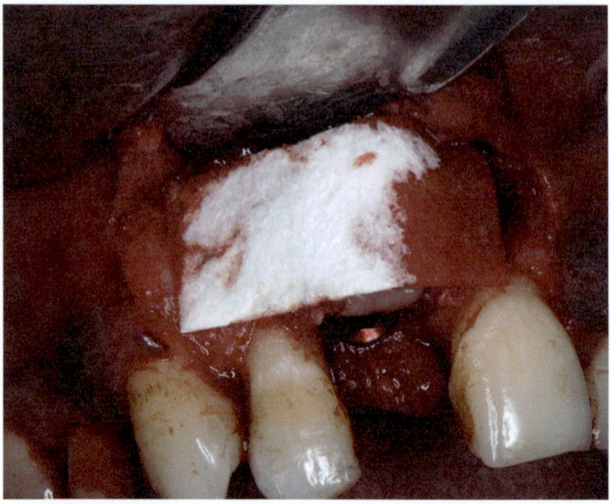

Fig. 10.13 Collagen membrane placed and secured

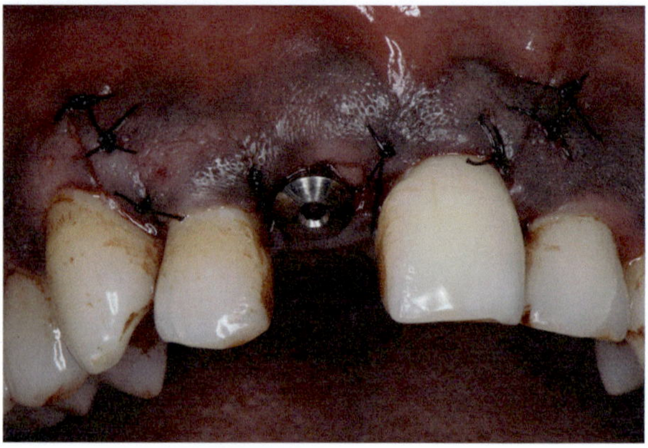

Fig. 10.14 Flap sutured. Since the implant was already osseointegrated, the healing abutment was placed

Periodontal Status

Periodontal disease that has led to bone loss around the tooth can cause mobility of the shield and ultimately failure of the procedure (Figs. 10.15a, b and 10.16). Teeth with periodontal disease are a contra-indication for PET [18].

Infection in Existing Teeth

Implant placement is contraindicated in the presence of an acute infection [19]. The infection should resolve before attempting any PET as chances of developing post-operative complications will be higher in such cases (Fig. 10.16).

External Resorption

External resorption that perforates the buccal bone is a contraindication for PET (Fig. 10.17).

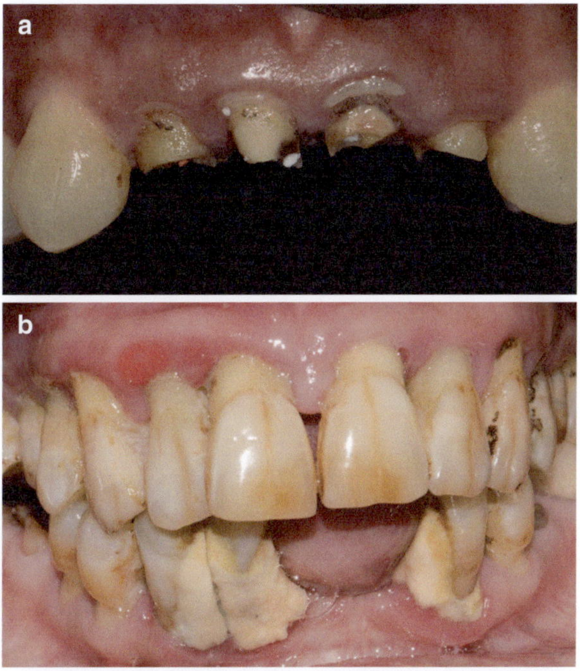

Fig. 10.15 (**a**) Teeth that are unrestorable but are periodontally sound are good candidates for PET procedures. (**b**) Periodontally compromised mobile teeth are contraindicated for PET

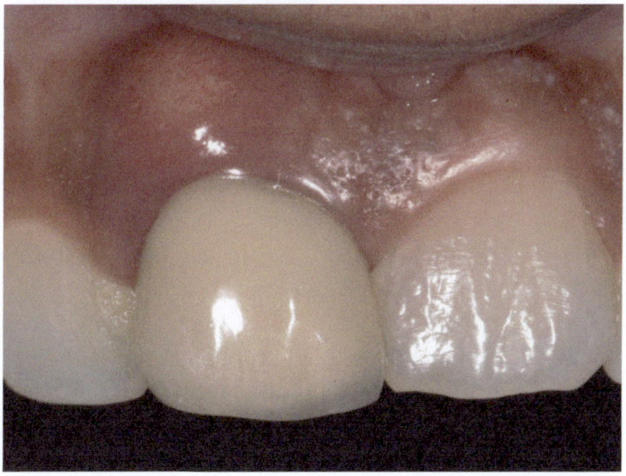

Fig. 10.16 Tooth 11 has acute infection in periapical area and hence is not a good candidate for PET

Vertical/Oblique Fracture

Root fractures may compromise the position of the root after the shield preparation. Socket shield procedures should be avoided if fractures are detected or suspected [7].

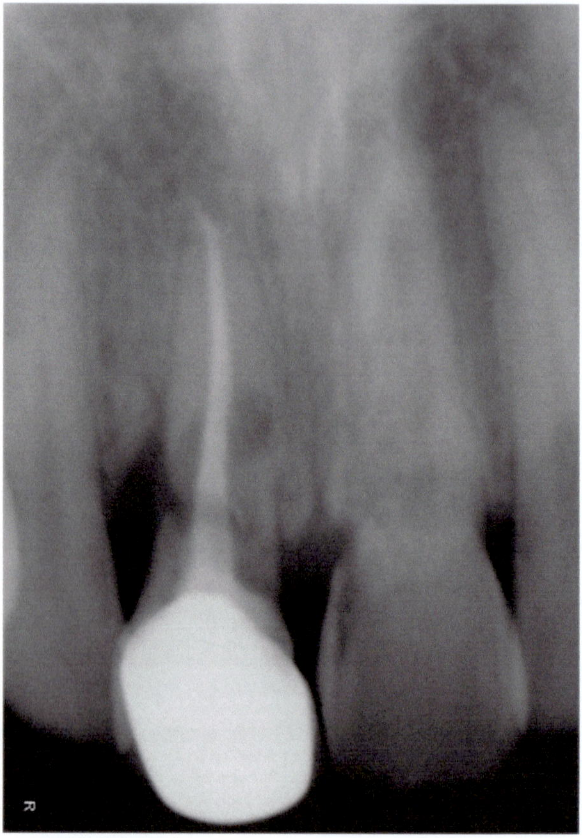

Fig. 10.17 Both incisors showing internal and external resorption. Such teeth are ruled out for PET if the resorption has perforated the tooth and affected the buccal bone. The extent of resorption must be ascertained on preoperative radiographs

10.2.2 Errors in Assessment of the Radial Position of the Tooth

The radial position of the tooth in its socket and the trajectory of the root in its alveolar housing will have a direct bearing during the surgical phase of PET. The amount of palatal bone and apical bone has to be adequate to engage the planned implant [20]. Gluckman et al. published the various graphical illustrations of the radial tooth positions and highlighted the importance of identifying these planes during PET procedures (Chap. 3) [11]. Errors in identifying these trajectories based on available bone may lead to iatrogenic complications during implant placement (Figs. 10.18 and 10.19).

10.2.3 Errors in Assessment of Buccal Bone Morphology

Fenestrations and Dehiscences:

For partial extraction therapies, it is mandatory to have a CBCT that displays the available buccal and palatal bone morphology (Figs. 10.20 and 10.21).

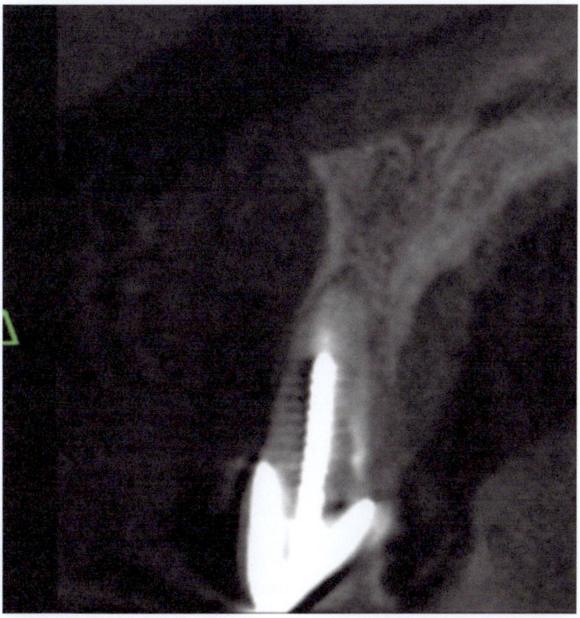

Fig. 10.18 The absence of adequate bone palatal to the designated implant position, makes this case unfavorable for socket shield with immediate placement of implant

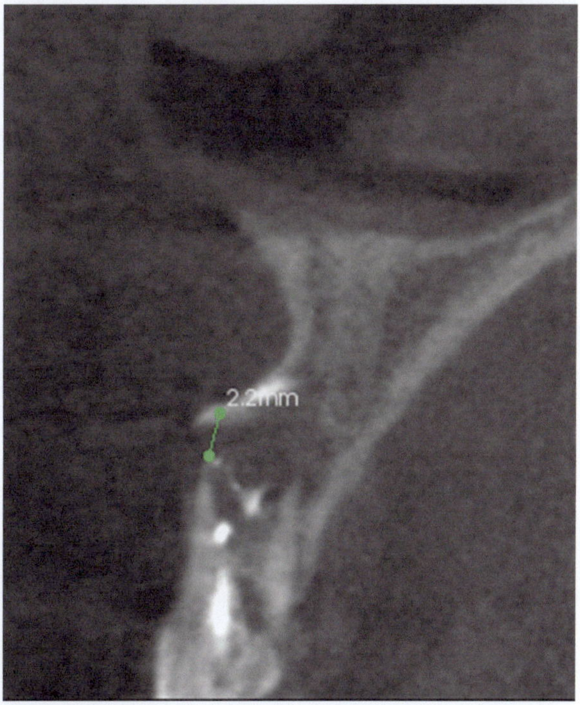

Fig. 10.19 Alveolus with very little palatal bone and an infected socket with a perforated labial plate. This is a contraindication for PET

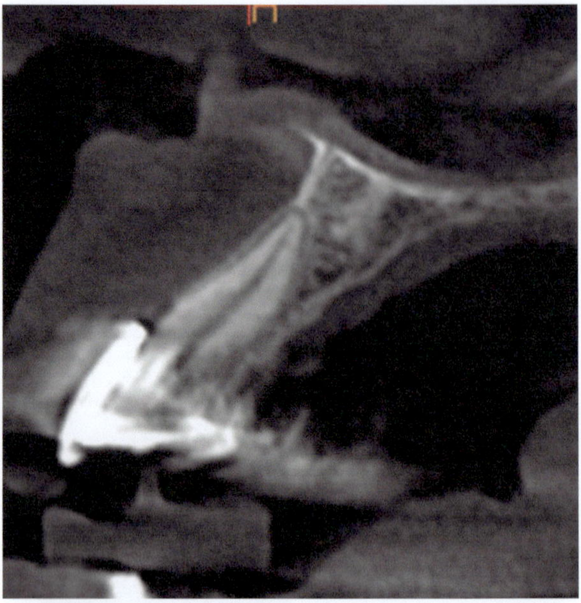

Fig. 10.20 An intact buccal plate and adequate palatal bone is a prerequisite for PET

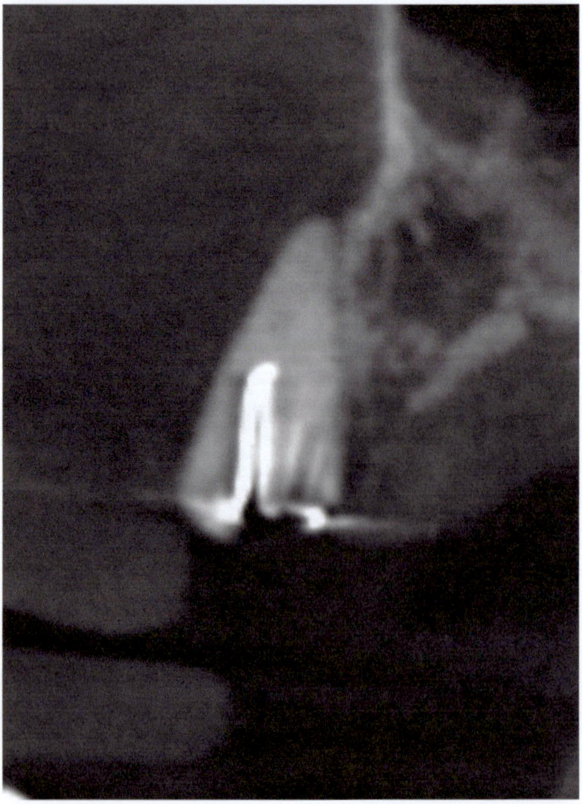

Fig. 10.21 Absence of labial cortical plate is an absolute contraindication for PET

Fenestrations can be managed during shield preparation with the help of a remote semilunar incision (Chap. 6) [21, 22]. A dehiscence, however, may lead to complications such as shield mobility or migration and should not be chosen for PET.

10.3 Surgical Errors/Complications

10.3.1 Errors in Shield Preparation

Shield Thickness

Guidelines for the optimum thickness of the shield (Fig. 10.22) have been discussed in Chap. 2 [23, 24]. If the shield is prepared too thin (Fig. 10.23), it will not have enough remaining structure to allow a stable attachment to the bundle bone which

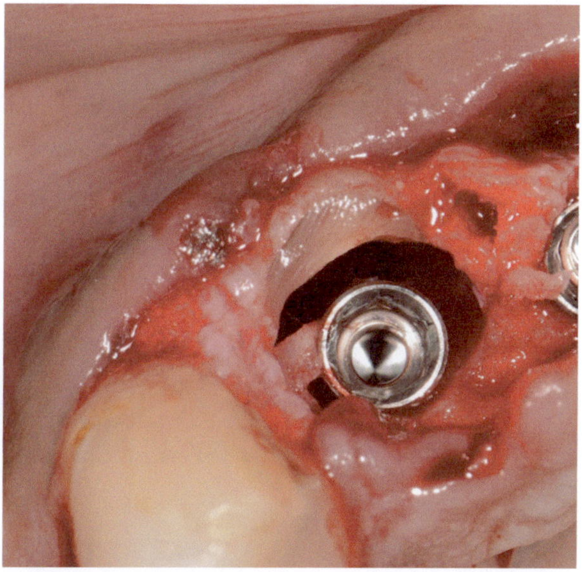

Fig. 10.22 Optimum shield thickness of 1.5 mm. The implant diameter chosen should allow for a space of at least 1 mm between the implant and the shield

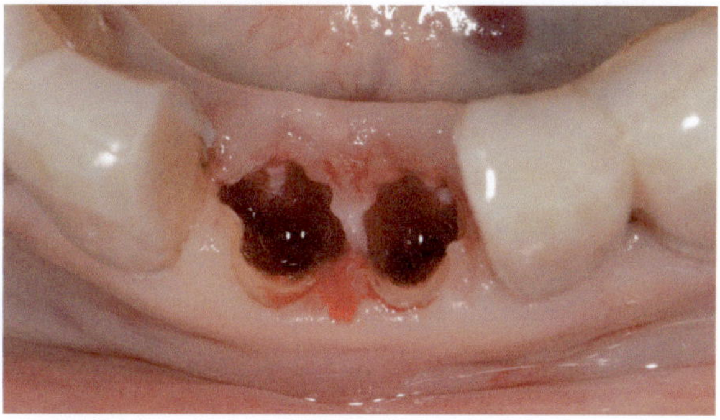

Fig. 10.23 Thin shields may be prone to dislodgement and need extreme care while handling them

lines the socket. On the other hand, a very thick shield will limit the space available for the implant within the socket. This may lead to the shield and the implant being in close proximity. A thick shield also compromises the space required for the emergence of the provisional and permanent restorations [10, 25]. Figure 10.24 depicts a situation in which the shield is thicker than desired.

For larger diameter teeth such as the cuspids, the bicuspids, and the central incisors, a shield thickness of 1.5 mm is optimum. For maxillary lateral incisors and mandibular incisors, the optimal thickness is 1–1.2 mm. In case the socket dimensions are such that this optimum thickness cannot be achieved, the clinician must re-evaluate the possibility of the PET procedure (Fig. 10.25).

Inadequate Length of the Shield

The shield must be of sufficient length to maintain its integrity without any mobility [24]. The optimum length should be 8 mm or 2/3rds the length of the root;

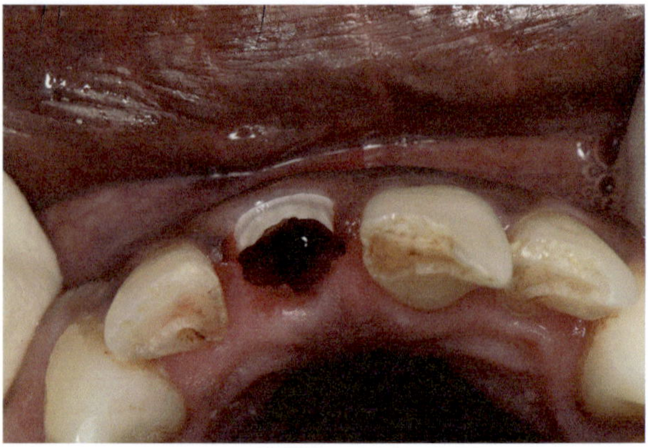

Fig. 10.24 Thick shield reduces room for the implant

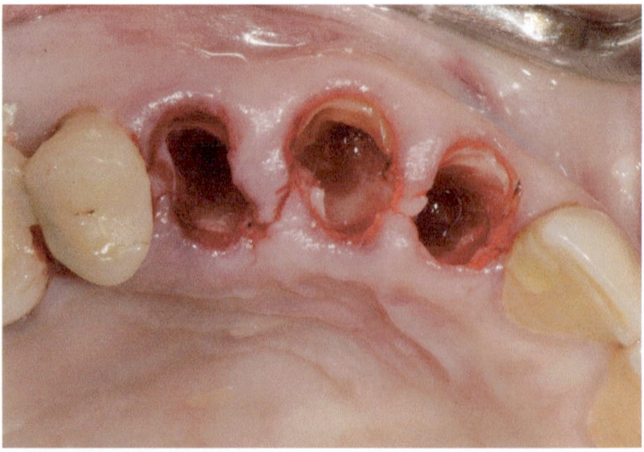

Fig. 10.25 The shield thickness will vary with the anatomical limitations of the socket. Note thicker shield (1.5mm) for the cuspid compared to a thinner shield (1mm) for the lateral incisor

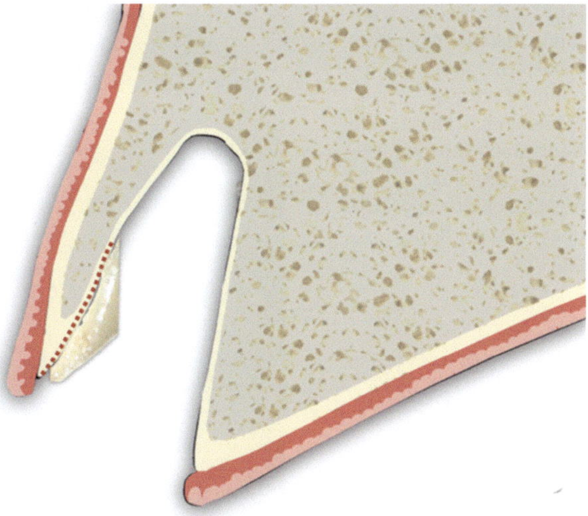

Fig. 10.26 A shorter shield maybe prone to dislodgement or mobility

whichever is more. A shield shorter than 8 mm may perform its function of maintaining the buccal bone only as long as it is stable (Fig. 10.26).

Root Apex Left Behind

The success of socket shield and pontic shield procedures depends on the removal of all endodontic filling material and the apex of the root (Figs. 10.27 and 10.28) [9]. If the apex has not been removed, the residual infection in the implant site will lead to postoperative infection. To ensure complete removal of the canal contents and the root apex, an intraoral periapical xray should be taken after shield preparation. In long roots such as the cuspids, it may not be easy to extract the apex of the root since the length of the drill is inadequate (Chap. 6).

Incorrect Shield Shape

The desired shape of the shield has undergone some variations in the recent past. The goal of the shield is to encompass approximately 150° of the socket diameter (Fig. 10.29), to prevent labial bone loss [24]. The C-shaped shield described in Chap. 6 covers more area by extending into the interproximal space (Fig. 10.30). Whilst this is advantageous when it comes to preservation of the interdental papilla, there is a greater risk of contacting the implant [26, 27]. This may limit the vascular supply to the peri-implant area and may affect the process of osseointegration. The clinician should weigh the benefits of the C-shaped design before making a decision. It is important to understand that if the shield is not shaped adequately to cover sufficient circumference of the socket it may become loose and be eventually lost.

Damage to Proximal Bone Walls During Shield Preparation

The mesio-distal sectioning of the root should be carried out carefully. An overzealous shield preparation may cause a lot of damage to the lateral walls of the socket

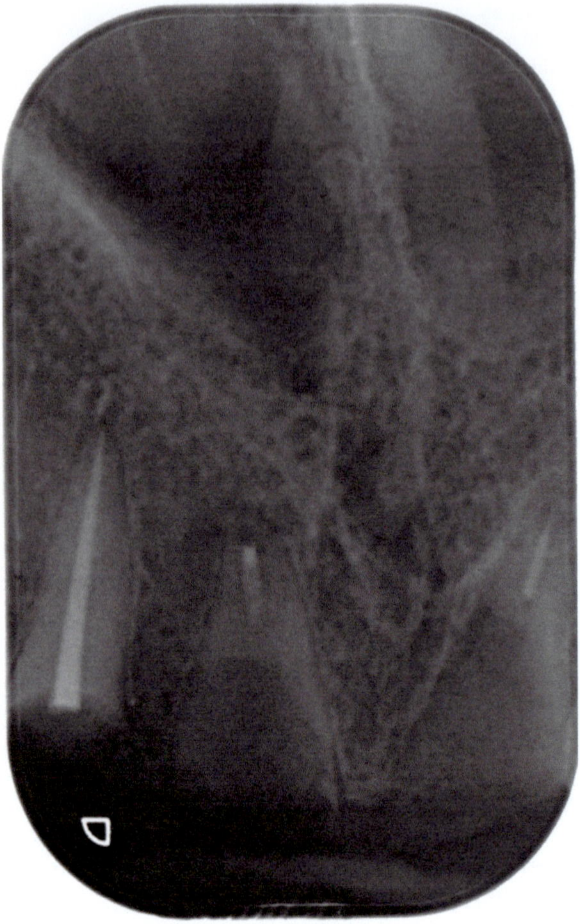

Fig. 10.27 Endodontic filling material from the canal space should be removed prior to preparation of the shield. Radiograph showing inadequate shield preparation due to presence of endodontic filling material

and result in achieving inadequate stability for the implant. If the damage is extensive, and complicates the implant placement, the procedure may need to be abandoned (Fig. 10.31).

10.3.2 Shield Mobility

Cause: The main causes for shield mobility are

- Mobile tooth (not indicated for PET).
- Vibration from the bur during sectioning of the root.
- Inadequate shield thickness and length.

A common cause for the shield mobility is the incorrect use of the elevator for extracting the palatal root. The elevator should never be inserted in between the gap created by the mesio-distal sectioning. The ideal position of the elevator should be between the palatal root and palatal bone.

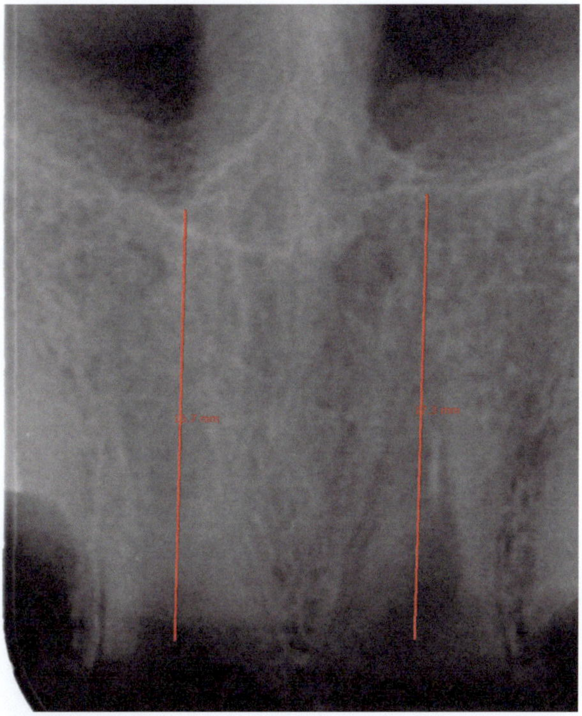

Fig. 10.28 The residual endodontic filling material visible in tooth 21 must be removed

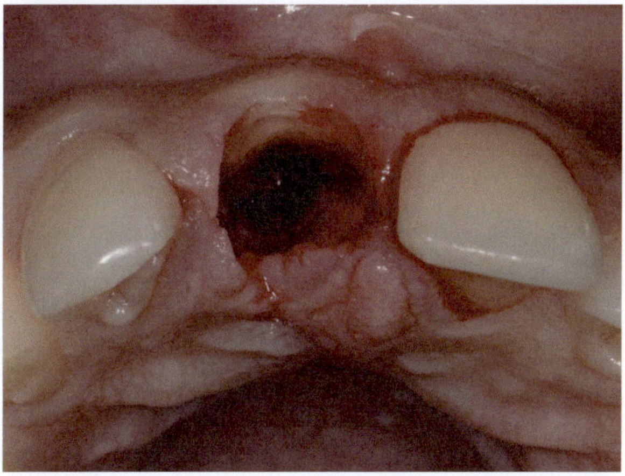

Fig. 10.29 Conventional shield preparation is made from mesio-labial to disto-labial line angle

Prevention: The shield mobility can be prevented by selecting cases with firm teeth without large periapical lesions. Also, the drill must be used at high speed to avoid chatter and vibration. Dull, worn out drills should not be used. Copious amount of irrigant will help in debridement and prevent of burs.

Management: If the shield becomes mobile during preparation, it is necessary to remove the shield and discard it [28]. The clinician must then proceed with conventional post-extraction implant placement. Implant placement and bone grafting protocols like the dual-zone therapeutic concept should be considered [5]. It is important

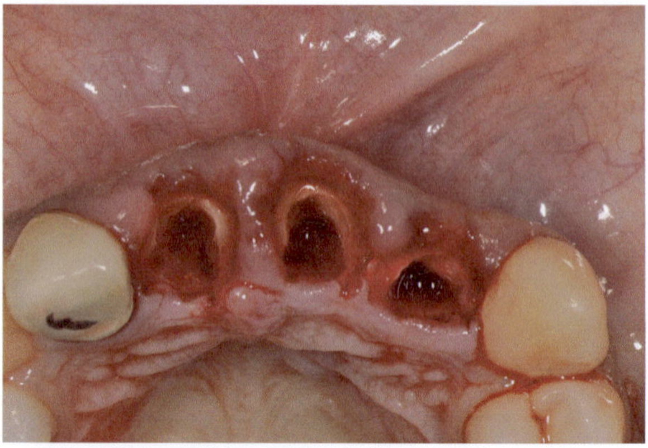

Fig. 10.30 C-shaped socket shields

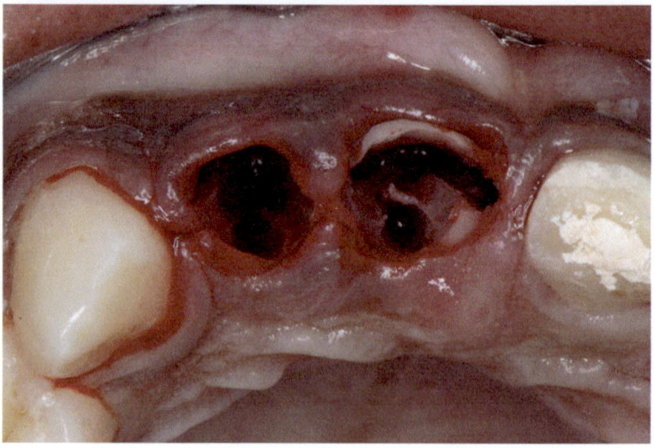

Fig. 10.31 The lateral walls of the socket have been accidentally drilled during the shield preparation. This may result in lack of primary stability for the implant

to emphasize that a mobile shield will not serve any biologic purpose and no attempt must be made to secure the shield or place it back in the socket.

10.3.3 Apical Fenestration

Cause: An existing periapical lesion that has perforated the apical buccal bone or such a apical fenestration may be caused iatrogenically (Fig. 10.32).

Prevention: Case selection criteria for PET clearly describes the need for preoperative radiographic evaluation of the socket for any pathology in the apical region [19]. The best way to prevent the apical bone fenestration is to evaluate the radiographs thoroughly and not choose cases with large periapical lesions. Also, cases in which the radial tooth position is such that the shield preparation may lead to an apical fenestration must be avoided [11].

Management: In case, a fenestration is observed on the scans or the operator has inadvertently created one, shield preparation followed by an esthetic buccal flap to graft the site of bone fenestration should be performed (Figs. 10.33, 10.34, 10.35 and 10.36) [21, 29]. In cases of large fenestrations, the implant placement maybe deferred at this stage. A staged implant placement after complete socket healing maybe considered.

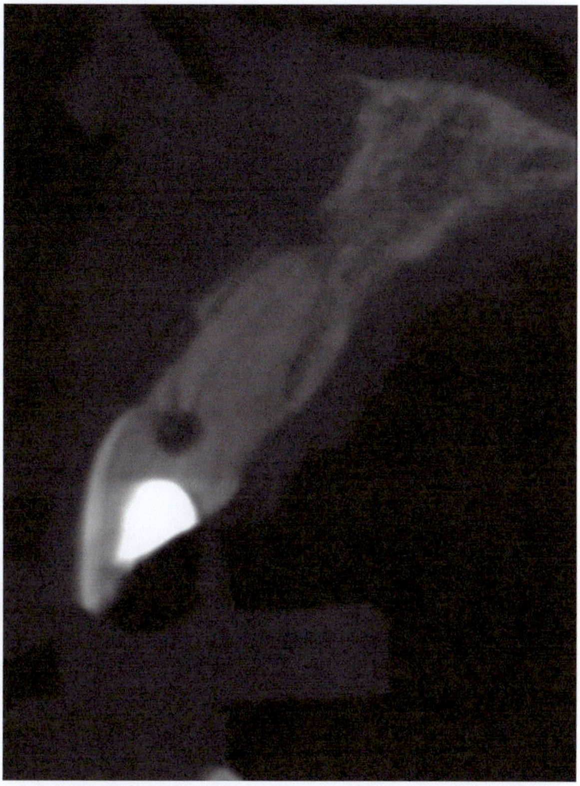

Fig. 10.32 Preoperative identification of the apical bone fenestration

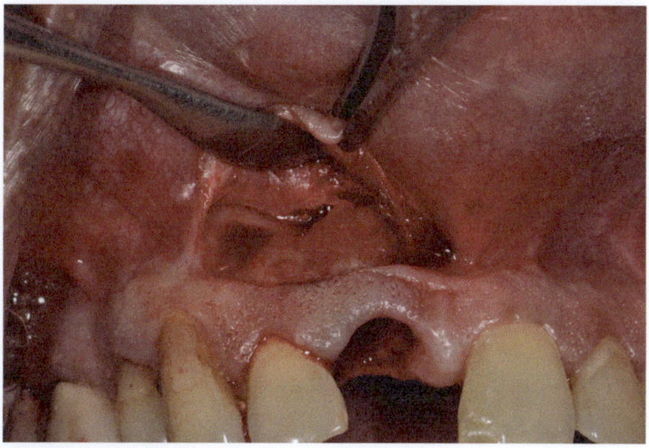

Fig. 10.33 Apical fenestration caused due to the wrong angulation of the drill

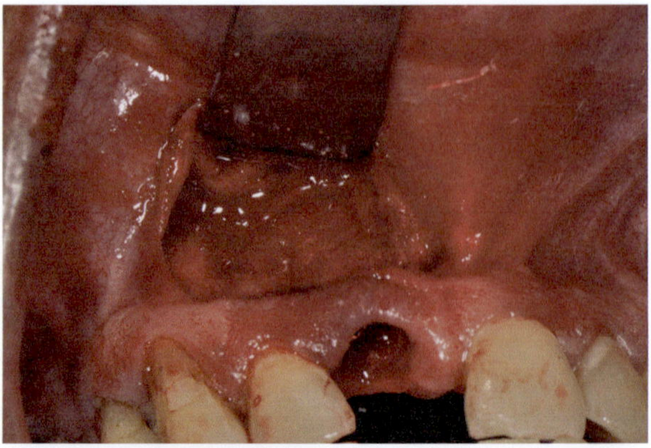

Fig. 10.34 Apical defect grafted using a bone substitute material and a collagen membrane

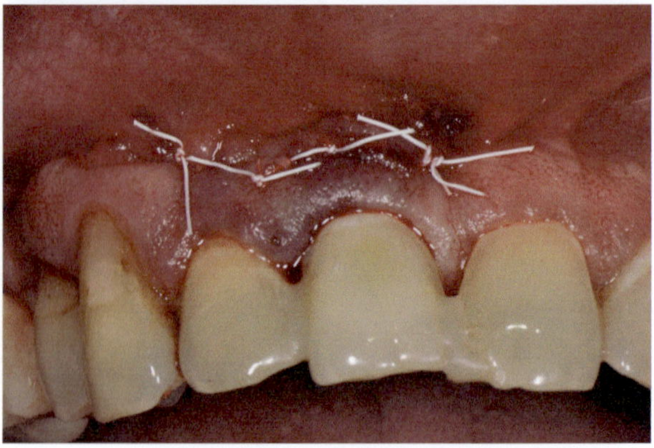

Fig. 10.35 Defect closed using PTFE sutures

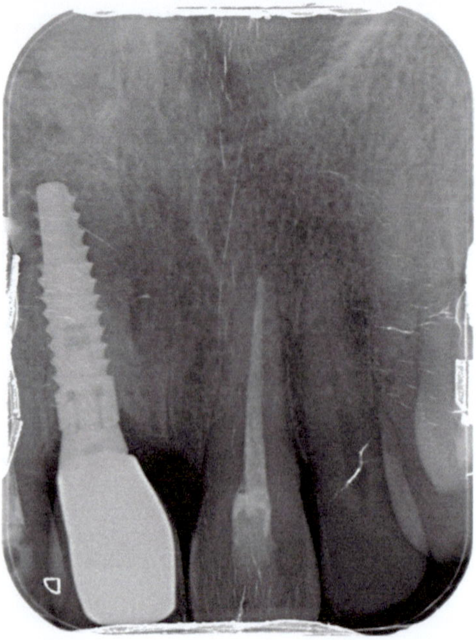

Fig. 10.36 Radiograph after final restoration

10.3.4 Palatal Wall fracture

The palatal wall of the socket is an important anatomical structure necessary for a successful immediate post-extraction implant placement. Since the palatal wall takes the entire brunt of supporting the implant, its integrity needs to be ascertained. Absence of the palatal bone can have serious implications during the osteotomy procedure for the implant placement [11].

Cause:

1. Excessive pressure from the root elevators during removal of the palatal portion of the root.
2. Pressure during insertion of the implant: An over-prepared palatal plate may break down if excessive torque is exerted during implant placement.

Prevention: Preoperative assessment of the palatal bone must be done to ascertain adequate volume of bone prior to surgery. The partial root extraction should be carried out very gently. The implant should be placed under controlled torque.

Management: In case of fracture of the palatal wall, it is necessary to evaluate if sufficient bone has remained to allow the implant to be inserted with adequate primary stability.

In case of a large fracture, it may be necessary to abort the implant placement (Fig. 10.37).

Augmentation of the lost bone will be necessary to compensate for the destroyed palatal bone. This augmentation maybe carried out using a combination of autogenous bone and a suitable bone substitute material [30].

Management of the Perforated Palatal Wall

The following case describes the occurrence and management of the perforation of the palatal wall. Extraction and implant placement for teeth #21 and #11 were

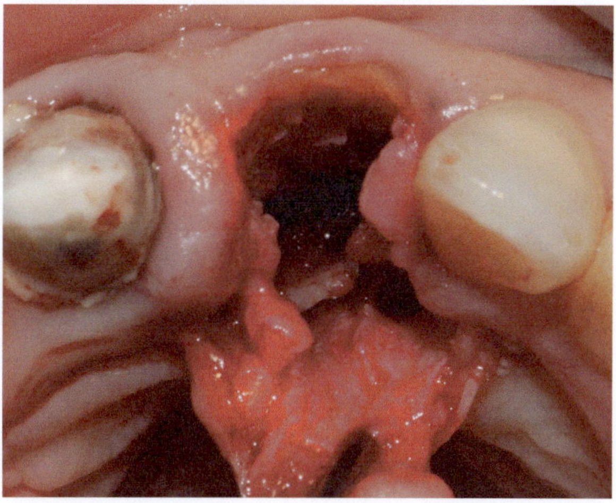

Fig. 10.37 The shield in tooth #21 is well prepared, however the palatal bone is fractured and will not facilitate implant placement

planned. The plan was to start with tooth #21 and use tooth #11 to support a temporary cantilevered restoration, and once the implant in the tooth #21 is integrated, extract tooth #11 and repeat a similar procedure.

At the initial surgical appointment, the shield was prepared for tooth #21 and while preparation of the osteotomy, the palatal wall accidentally perforated. The site was covered with soft tissue rotated from the palate and left to heal. Three months later, the site was re-entered and it was found that, the socket was filled with soft tissue. No bone formed in the socket due to the lack of osteogenic potential from the palatal side. Three-months later when the flap was reflected, the site was augmented with a combination of autogenous bone and a xenogenic graft material. The palatal wall was supported with a titanium mesh. Implant placement was carried out after 3-months for sites #11 and #21. Both implants were immediately restored with provisional crowns. The final restorations were made after 4-months (Figs. 10.38, 10.39, 10.40, 10.41, 10.42, 10.43, 10.44, 10.45, 10.46, 10.47, 10.48, 10.49, 10.50, 10.51 and 10.52).

10.3.5 Shield-Implant Proximity

There should be no contact between the shield and the implant [8, 24, 25]. And there should not be a very large gap between the two.

Shield and Implant are in Physical Contact

Inadequate space between shield and the implant will lead to reduced area for the blood clot to fill in and thus reduced bone between the implant and the shield. Due to the presence of the shield one osseous wall is less in SS sites as compared to a conventional immediate post-extraction socket. Thus, it is preferable to have adequate gap of at least 1 mm between the implant and the shield.

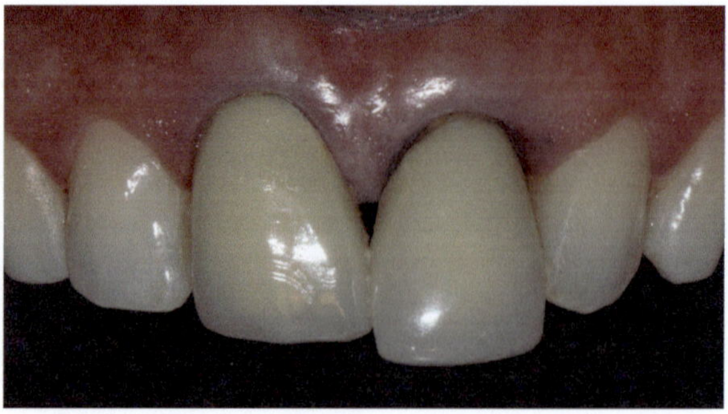

Fig. 10.38 Preoperative view: Teeth #11 and #21 were indicated for extraction

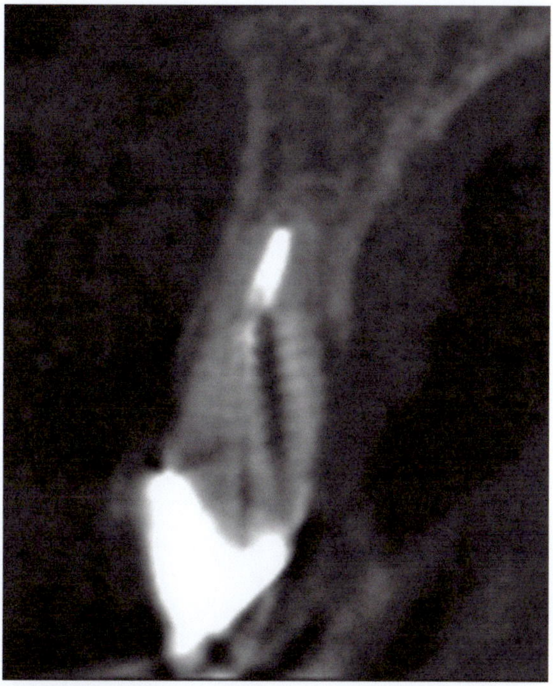

Fig. 10.39 Radiograph showing the position of the root and the alveolus. Note the thin alveolar width and minimal amount of bone available on the palatal side

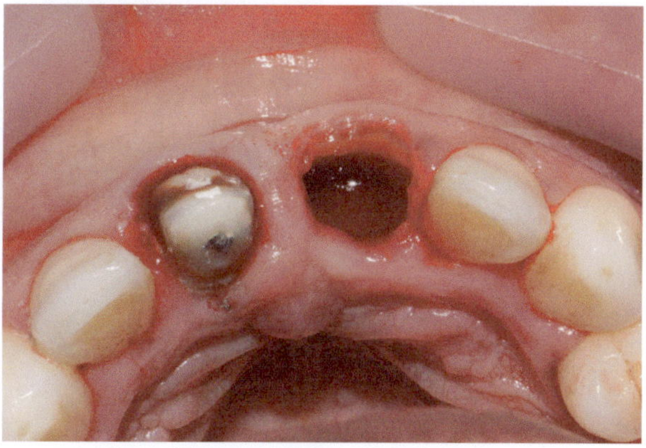

Fig. 10.40 Shield prepared with #21

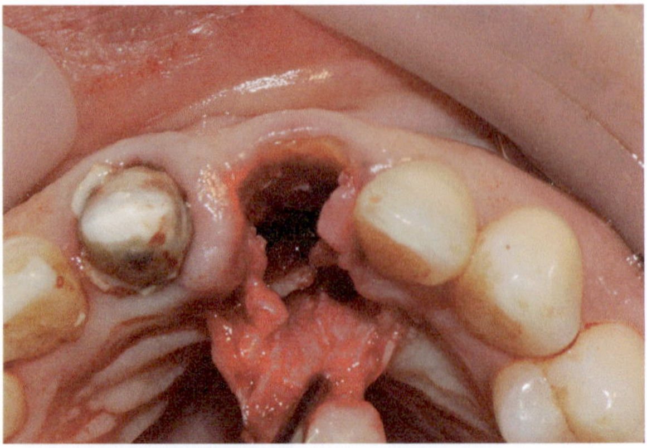

Fig. 10.41 Note the loss of palatal wall and the intact shield

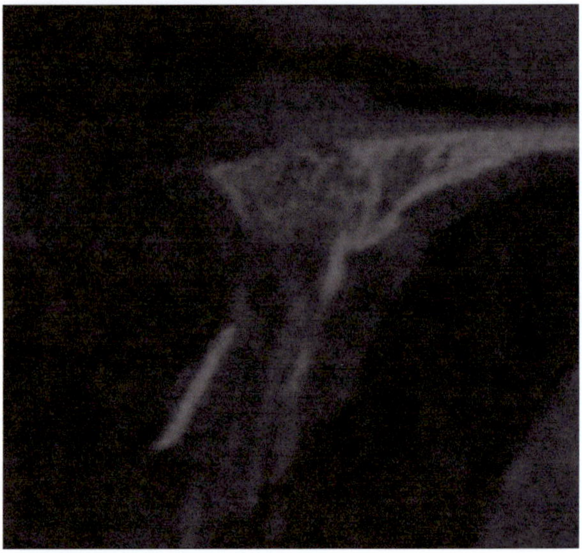

Fig. 10.42 Intraoperative CBCT image showing the intact shield but absence of palatal wall

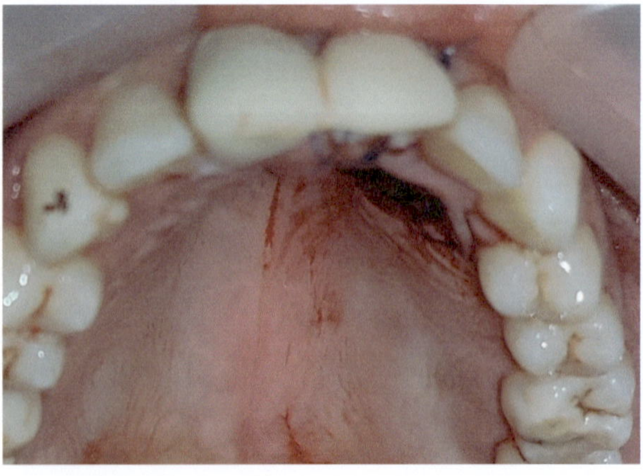

Fig. 10.43 The palatal tissue was mobilized to cover the socket and left to heal

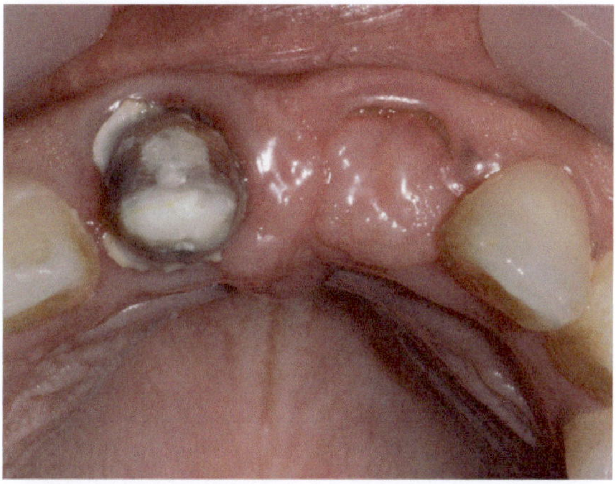

Fig. 10.44 3-months postoperative view showing that the site was re-entered. Note shield exposure at the crest

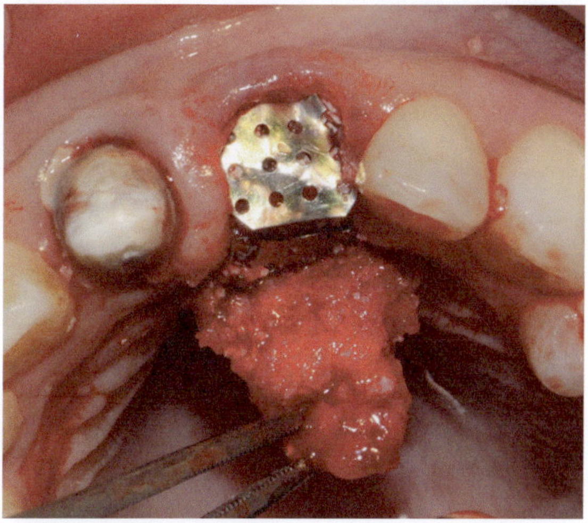

Fig. 10.45 The site was re-entered and a titanium mesh was adapted after shaping to cover the defect to form the new palatal wall

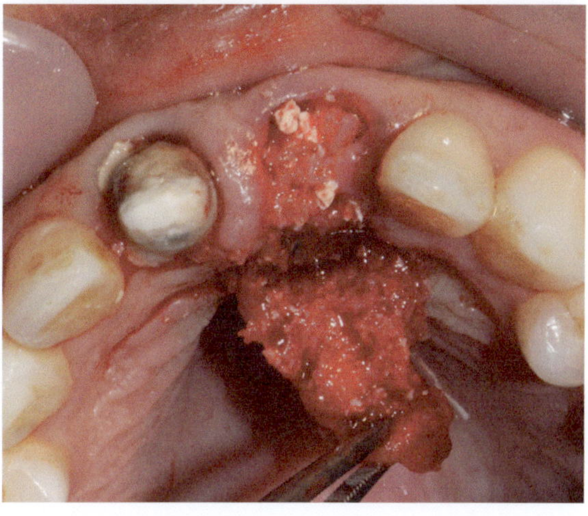

Fig. 10.46 The site was grafted with particulate autogenous and xenogenic bone graft

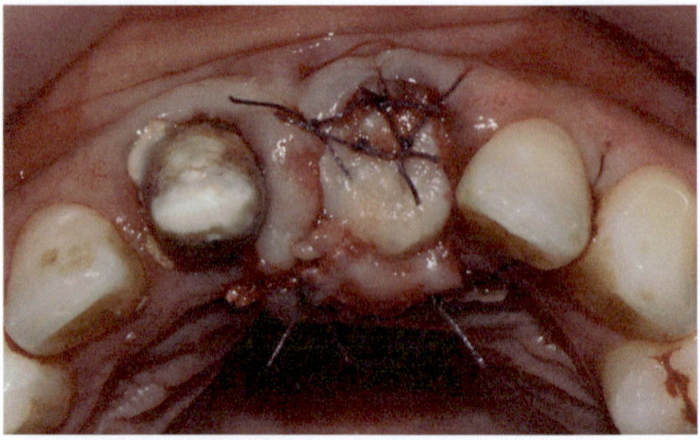

Fig. 10.47 The palatal defect was covered after mobilizing the flap

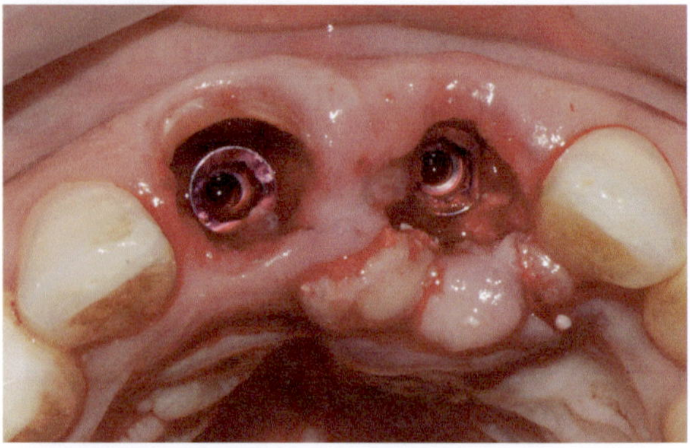

Fig. 10.48 3 months after the augmentation procedure, the site was re-entered and the implants were placed

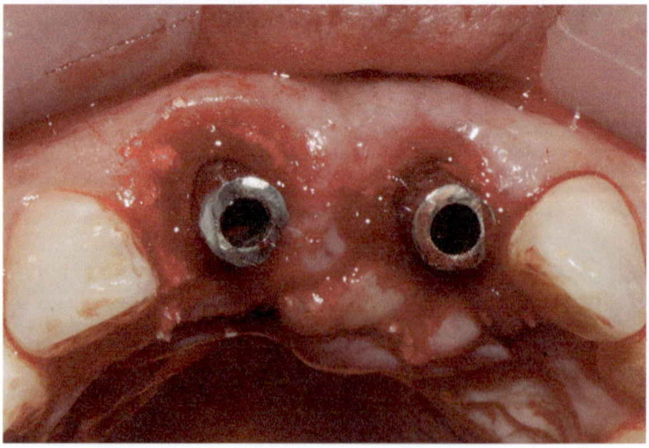

Fig. 10.49 Abutments were connected and chairside immediate temporary restorations were fabricated

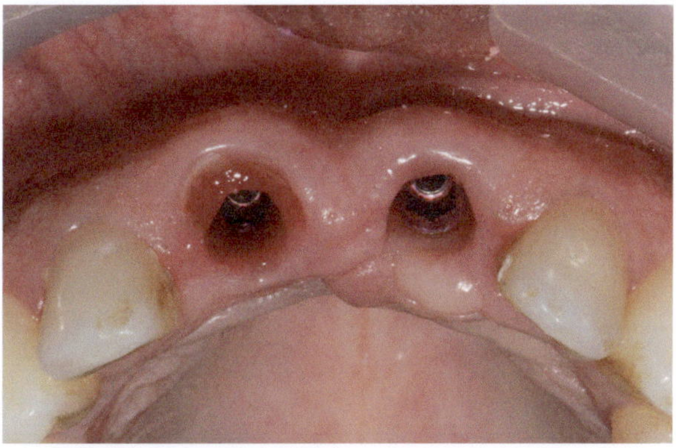

Fig. 10.50 The sites in tooth #11 and tooth #21 were ready to receive the final restorations at 3-months after the implant placement. The internal shield exposure with site #21 was corrected by trimming the shield down to the bone crest

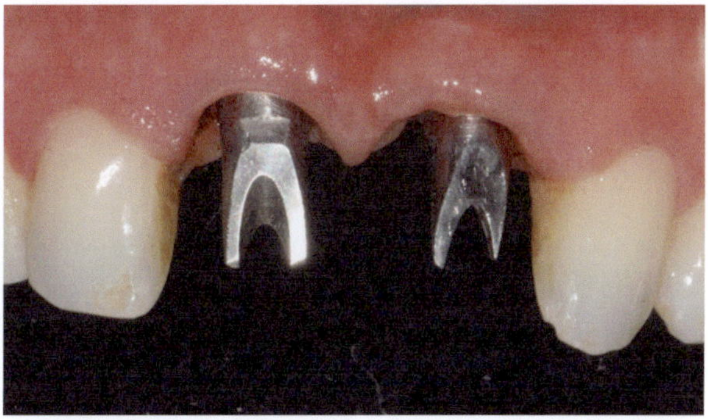

Fig. 10.51 Final abutments in situ

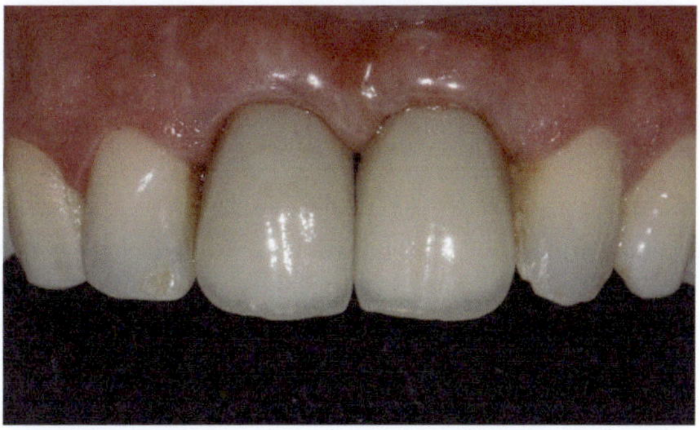

Fig. 10.52 Final restorations. The keratinized gingival width as well as health and tissue contours appear acceptable

Cause: This may occur if the shield is too thick or the implant diameter is too large. It may also occur if the implant is placed with an incorrect bucco-lingual trajectory. A buccally inclined implant is very likely to come close to the shield or even contact it (Figs. 10.53 and 10.54).

Prevention: The coronal aspect of the shield should be thinned out to provide sufficient space for the provisional restorative material. This aspect was discussed in detail in the chapter on provisional restorations [31]. It is likely that there may be no contact of the shield and implant in the coronal aspect but

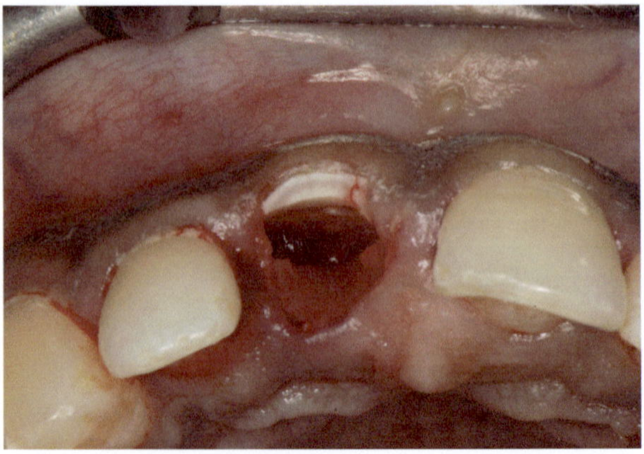

Fig. 10.53 The shield is prepared in tooth #11 area to receive an implant

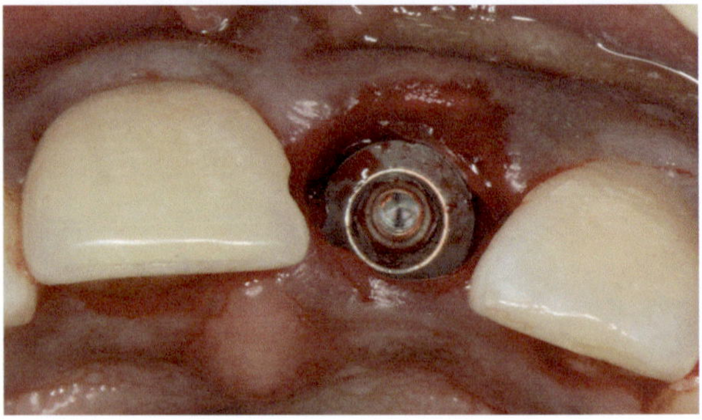

Fig. 10.54 Very little gap between the shield in #21 and the implant. Incorrect implant diameter selection or a very thick shield can lead to this complication

at an apical level there may be some light contact between the two. In the human histology studies reported so far, such a contact does not have any detrimental effect, provided there is no pressure from the implant on the shield [32, 33].

Management: If contact between the implant and the shield is noticed then, it is prudent to explant and trim the shield further and place the implant back.

There is a Very Large Gap Between the Shield and the Implant

Cause:

- Shield too thin or implant diameter very small.
- Socket diameter is too large; as it would be for cuspids and multirooted teeth.

Prevention: Optimal shield thickness must be achieved and the implant diameter chosen to adequately fit in the socket without obliterating it and without contacting the shield (Fig. 10.55). Ideally there should be a gap of about 1–1.5 mm between the shield and the implants.

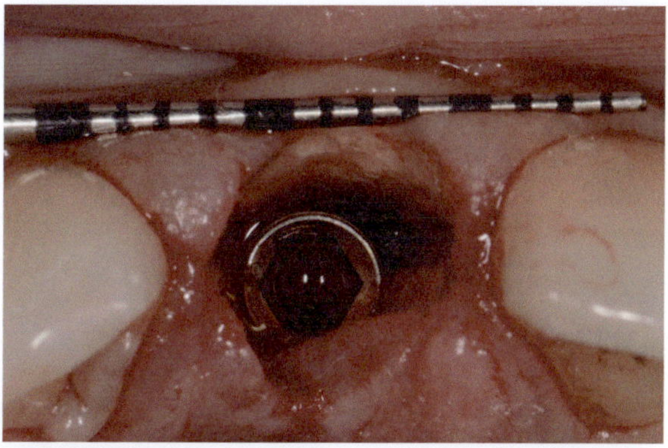

Fig. 10.55 Optimum gap between the shield and the implant

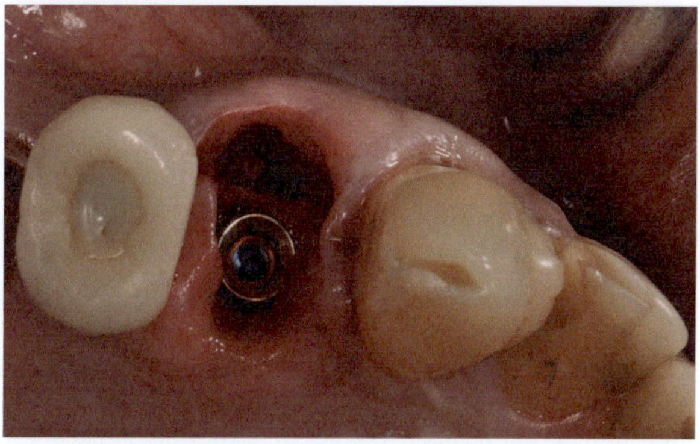

Fig. 10.56 Large gap between implant and labial shield

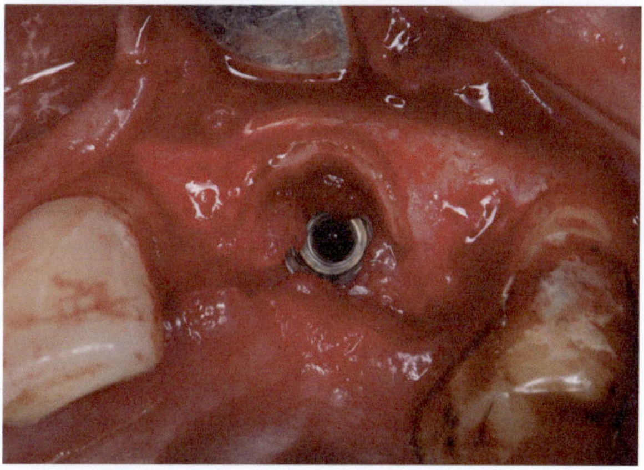

Fig. 10.57 Soft tissue invagination during second stage between shield and Implant

Management: In cases where the gap is large between the implant and the shield, soft tissue invagination may occur (Fig. 10.56).

The amount of invasion will vary. At times it may be restricted to the coronal few of threads of the implant or could invaginate to the full length of the implant (Figs. 10.57 and 10.58). Soft tissue invagination into the sites of PET in the space

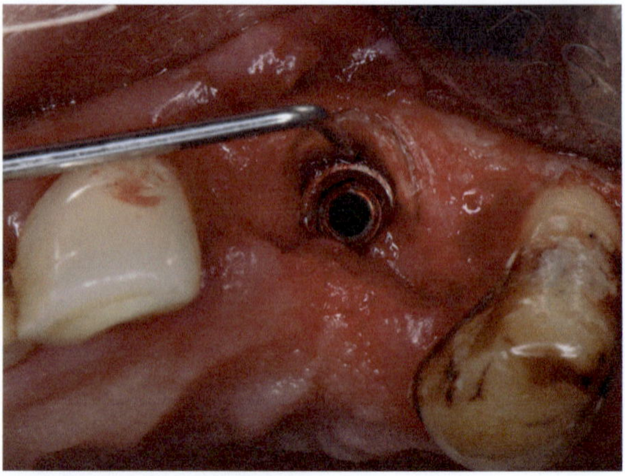

Fig. 10.58 Increased probing depth between shield and implant

between shield and implant has been observed by the authors especially in cases where the gap more than 2 mm has not been grafted with a bone material and also in sites without immediate fixed provisional restorations on the implants. Gluckman et al. suggested if space is present between the shield and implant, it should be grafted [8]. In contrast Mitsias et al., who refer to this technique as "root membrane" (RM), do not recommend the same since according to them, preservation of periodontal ligament and the associated vascular contribution is more crucial [33]. The authors have also experienced situations where no graft was placed in the gap and an immediate temporary restoration was placed, the soft tissue invagination had not occurred. It is thus opined that if one is unable to graft, then at least a fixed temporary restoration or a customized healing abutment should be placed on the implant in PET sites [31, 34].

When the primary stability of the implant is inadequate to support a provisional restoration, the gap has to be grafted and a submerged healing protocol is recommended. In situations wherein adequate primary stability of the implant has not been attained, a modification of the Glocker's technique is suggested, i.e., delayed implant placement with grafting of the space during surgical phase [35].

Soft tissue invaginations are observed more in Glocker's technique sites. It is suggested that the socket be grafted with fast resorbing graft like cancellous allograft or alloplastic graft material to avoid soft tissue invagination into the site. Implant placement in such cases is staged and can be planned a few months after the grafting procedure. If large gaps are left in SS cases, a higher possibility of soft tissue ingress is noticed. It is therefore recommended to augment the sockets in Glocker's technique to ensure adequate bone formation in the sites.

10.3.6 Lack of Implant Stability

Cause:

- Improper osteotomy preparation.

- Poor quality of bone.
- Bone damaged during shield preparation.

Prevention: Adequate precautions taken during shield preparation and correct surgical protocols should be followed during implant placement.

Management: If the primary stability is inadequate, it is advisable to remove the implant and replace it with a larger diameter one, if the socket morphology allows it. If that option is not possible, it may be necessary to abort the implant placement and graft the site keeping the shield in place. Re-entry after a suitable healing period may be attempted.

Soft Tissue Invagination into a Staged Socket Shield Site

The following is a case of soft tissue invagination into a site prepared by Glocker's technique (Figs. 10.59, 10.60, 10.61, 10.62, 10.63, 10.64, 10.65, 10.66 and 10.67). Tooth 11 was indicated for extraction. The root being non-carious, firm and of adequate dimension, a PET approach was planned. However, as the site did not offer adequate implant stability, the implant placement was deferred and the

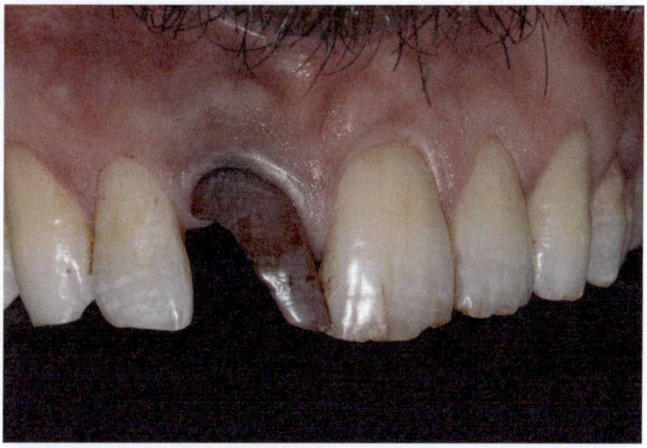

Fig. 10.59 Preoperative status showing highly discolored tooth 11

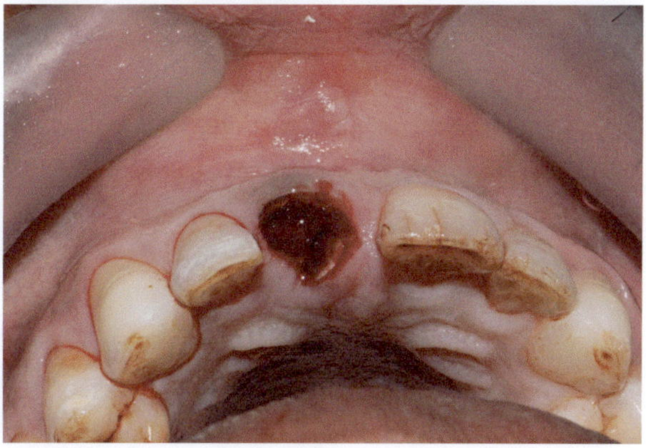

Fig. 10.60 Shield prepared but implant not placed

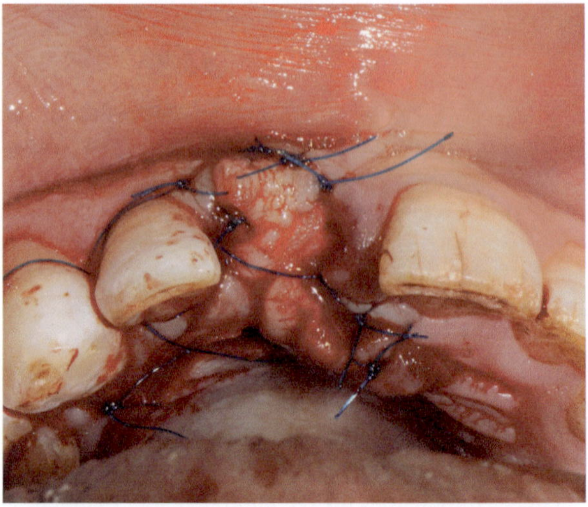

Fig. 10.61 Rotated palatal pedicled flap for closure of the socket. No graft was placed

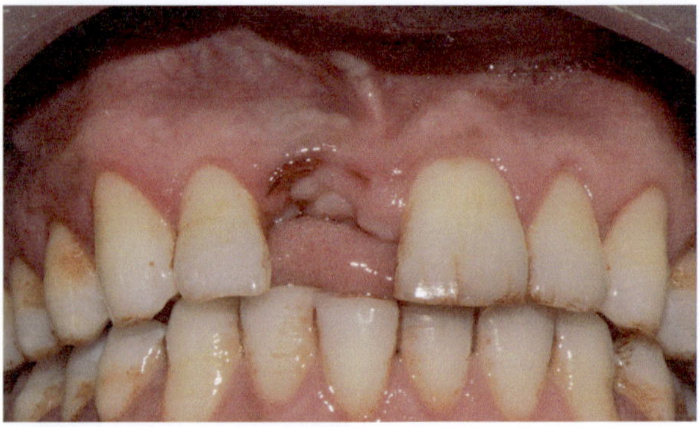

Fig. 10.62 Soft tissue invagination into the socket

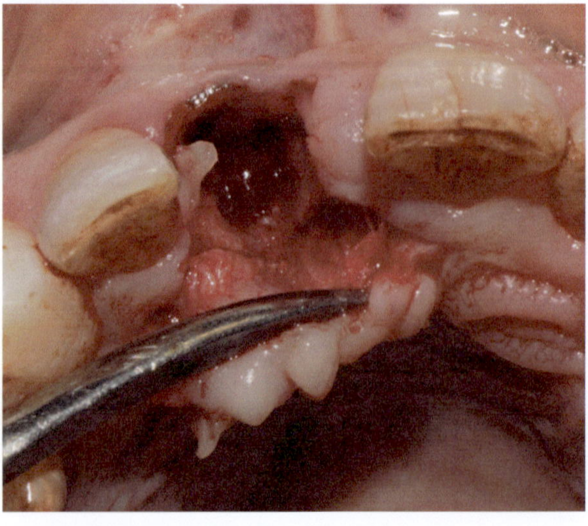

Fig. 10.63 No bone in the socket

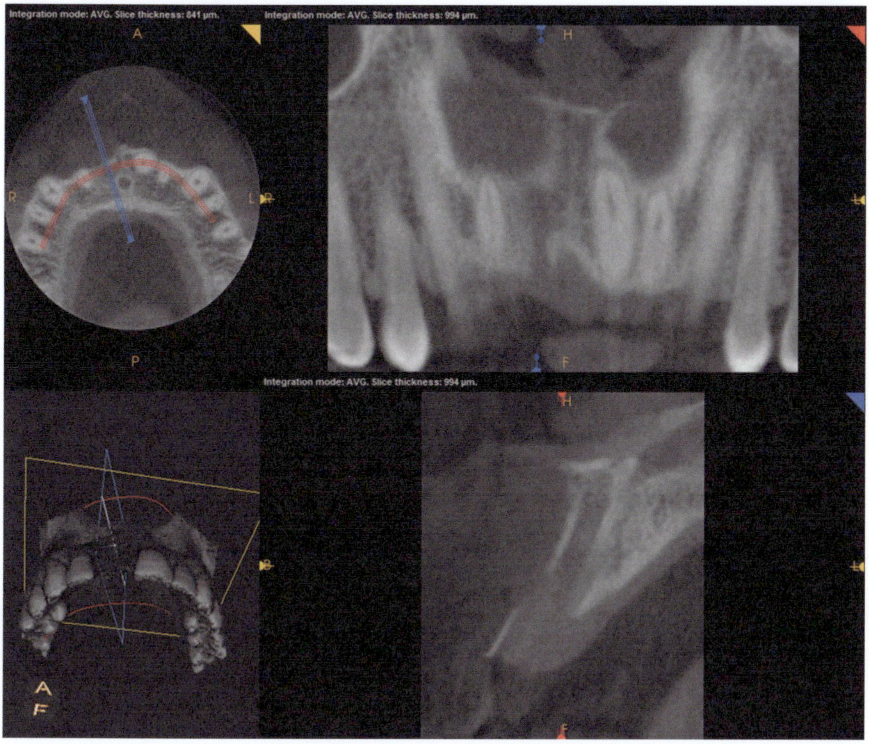

Fig. 10.64 CBCT image showing absence of bone in the socket, but the shield is intact

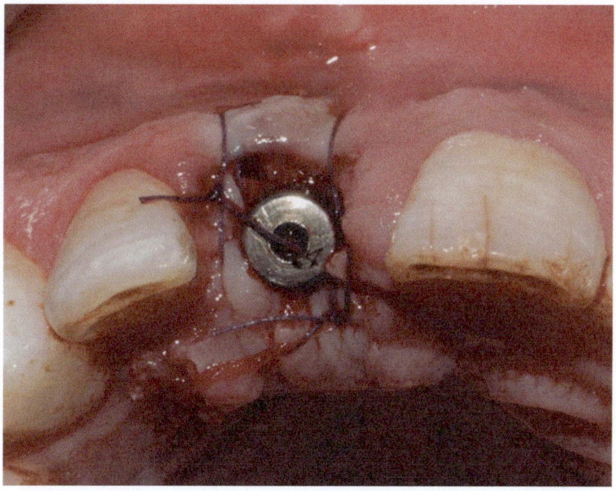

Fig. 10.65 A longer implant extending beyond the apex was placed and the rest of the site was grafted

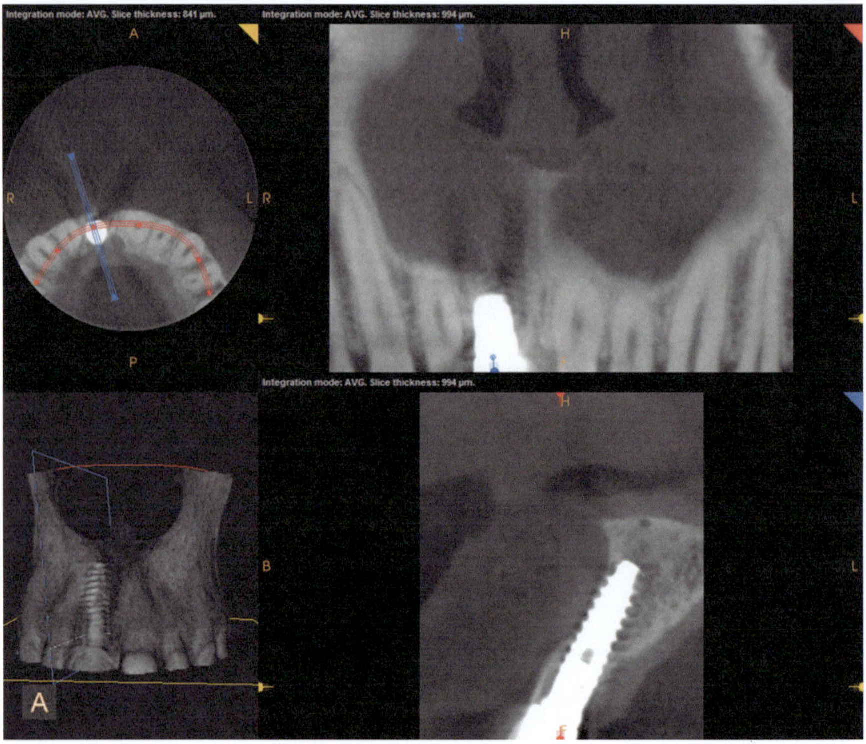

Fig. 10.66 Final restoration on #11

Fig. 10.67 Final restoration in situ

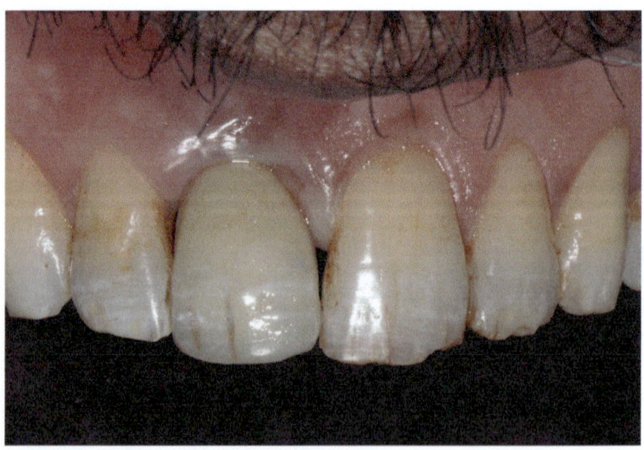

socket opening was closed with a palatal pedicled flap. After a period of 3 months, it was observed that soft tissue had infiltrated into the site. However, some bone had generated in the apical areas which helped in providing adequate stability for the implant. The implant was loaded after 3 months of healing.

10.4 Complications in Restorative Phase

These complications may occur in the healing phase before restorative work is carried out or in the post-restorative phase after delivery of the final restorations.

10.4.1 Shield Mobility

Cause:

Shield mobility may occur in the following situations:

- Tooth with grade-1 mobility prior to the procedure.
- Vibrations from the drill due to chatter during shield preparation.
- Thin shield.
- Contact of the shield with implant during placement.
- Absence of buccal bone.
- Faulty extraction technique.

Prevention: Accurate case selection criteria will avoid cases with mobile teeth or with absence of buccal bone. The shield preparation guidelines as discussed must be deployed to prevent the shield from becoming too thin. The implant size and placement must avoid any contact with the shield. During the extraction procedure, it must be confirmed that the palatal root portion is totally separated from the buccal portion before the elevation of the root is carried out. If the fragments are united, mobilization of palatal root will lead to mobility of the buccal shield too.

Management: In cases where the shield has become mobile, it must be removed and the surgery for implant placement may be carried out using conventional post-extraction immediate placement protocols. Bone augmentation may be needed to maintain contour [5] (Figs. 10.68 and 10.69).

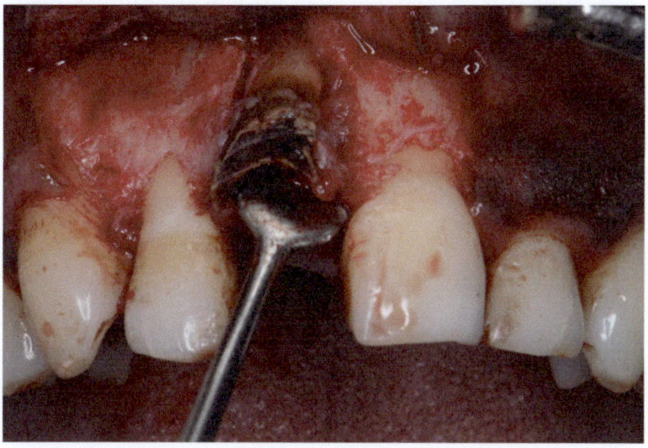

Fig. 10.68 Dehisced, carious and mobile shield

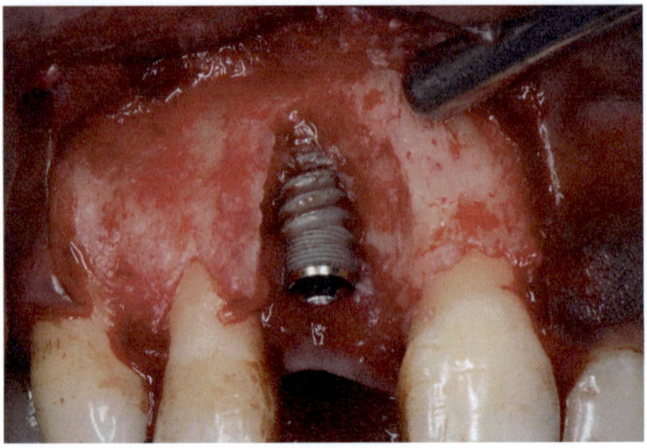

Fig. 10.69 Buccal dehiscence after removal of mobile shield

10.4.2 Shield Migration

Migration of the shield is its bodily movement in any direction [13]

Cause:

- This happens if there is minor shield mobility that has gone undetected during the surgical phase. The loose root fragment may then migrate during the healing phase.
- The pressure from the contacting implant during placement may lead to some pressure on the shield leading to migration.
- The pressure from the provisional as well as the definitive restoration can lead to the shield being thrust away and lead to its migration.

Prevention: There must be no contact between the shield and the implant to prevent this complication. Moreover, after the implant site is prepared it is prudent to check the integrity of the shield along with its firmness to ensure that there is no mobility in the shield and thus no chance of future migration. The restorations must be designed with a concave subcritical contour as discussed in the chapter on provisional restorations.

Management: A mobile shield should be removed and the resultant defect caused by the loss of the shield should be grafted using guided bone regeneration principles.

10.4.3 Shield Exposure

Gluckman et al. 2017 reported that 16 out of 128 sites had developed a shield exposure; citing it as one of the most frequent complication [13, 36].

Shield exposure may be internal or external in nature. Internal shield exposure is defined as extrusion of a portion of the shield between the implant and the restoration, usually the provisional restoration. External exposure is defined as extrusion of part of the shield through the gingival tissues toward the oral vestibule. Thus, the exposure of the shield can be internal (Figs. 10.70 and 10.71), i.e., toward the restoration or external (Fig. 10.72), i.e., toward the oral cavity.

Cause:

Internal shield exposure may be caused due to

- A shield which has been left supra-crestal.
- The provisional restoration has a bulky emergence and hence not enough space is left for the soft tissue between the under surface of the provisional restoration and the shield.

External shield exposure may be due to

- Shield mobility/migration in the buccal direction.
- Thin tissue biotype.

Gluckman and group observed association between shield exposures and sites deficient in buccal bone like lower anterior or teeth with previous orthodontic treatments [13].

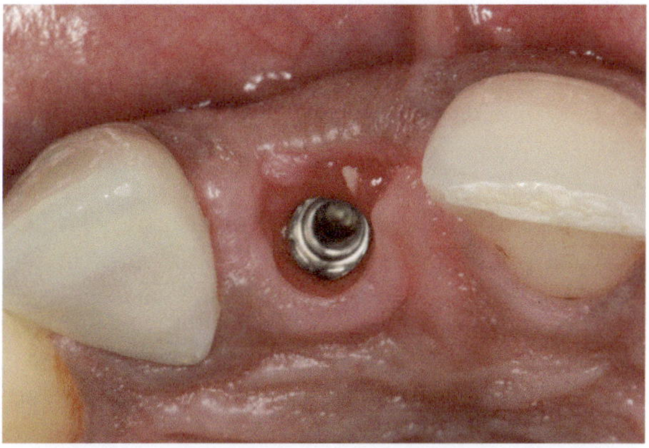

Fig. 10.70 SS performed for tooth 12#. The shield is exposed toward the implant, i.e., internal exposure. This was observed after the removal of the provisional restoration. Note a sharp spicule of the root shield which has resulted in the subsequent exposure

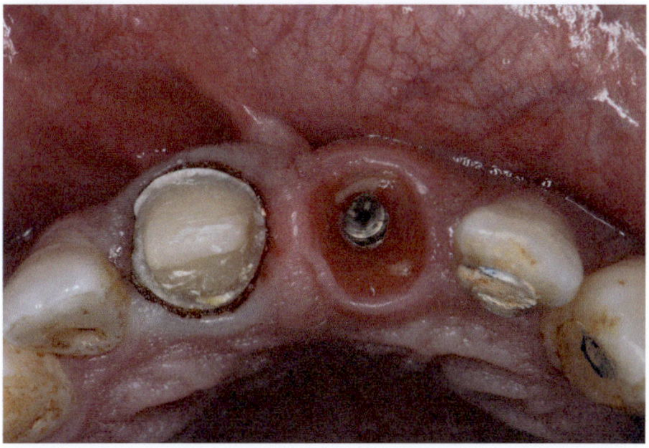

Fig. 10.71 Case depicting the internally exposed parts of the shield in the tooth #21 region

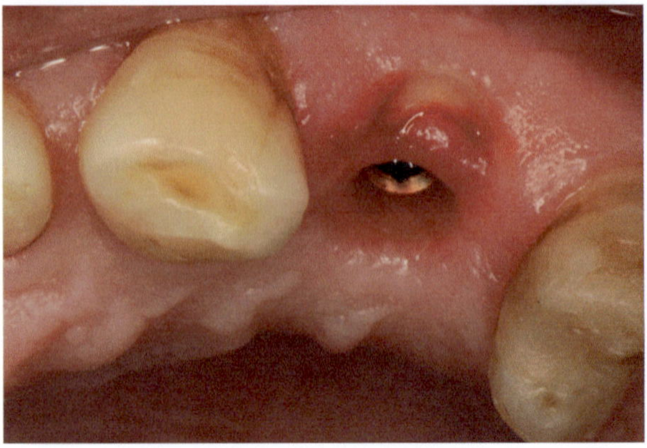

Fig. 10.72 Case showing the external exposure of the shield associated with tooth #24

Prevention: Internal shield exposure can be avoided by trimming the shield to the level of crestal bone and making sure that the provisional restoration has a concave subcritical contour to allow at least 1.5 mm space between the restoration and the shield Chap. 4 [10, 13, 37].

Beveling of the internal coronal portion of the shield is required to create the space [10, 24, 31].

External shield exposure can be prevented by ensuring that there is no contact or pressure on the shield from the implant or the restoration.

Management of Shield Exposures: The illustrative troubleshooting diagram below depicts an overview of the management of the clinical complication of socket shield exposures (Fig. 10.73).

Internal Shield Exposure Management with Connective Tissue Graft (CTG)

The case illustration here discusses internal exposure observed during the healing. The exposure was trimmed using a high-speed drill. The maxillary tuberosity was used as a donor site for harvesting the CTG. The harvested tissue covered the exposed shield (Figs. 10.74, 10.75, 10.76 and 10.77).

Management of External Shield Exposure

A maxillary second premolar site was prepared for a PET procedure. During shield preparation, a sharp edge was inadvertently generated and went unnoticed. Following implant placement, the socket was filled with sticky bone graft (prepared with Perioglas (0.5 g, bioactive synthetic alloplastic graft, Nova Bone products, LLC) + Injectable Platelet rich fibrin (i-Prf)) [14–17, 38, 39]. The socket was secured with collagen plug and cross mattress.

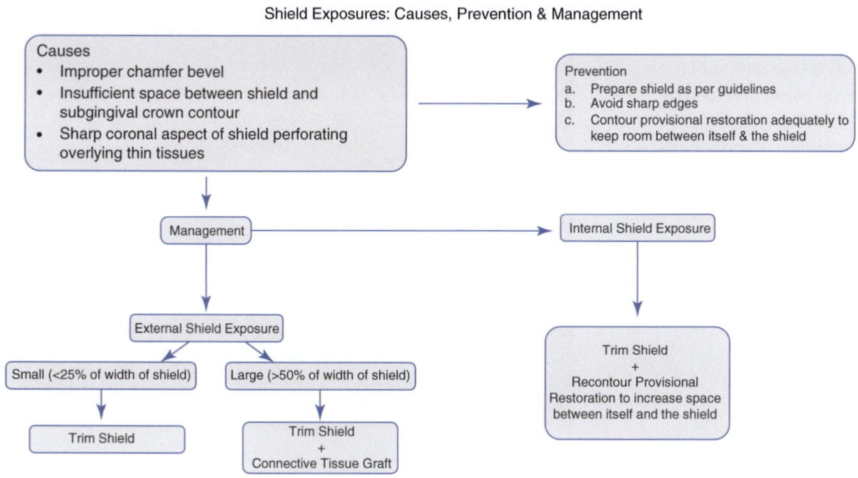

Fig. 10.73 Flowchart for shield exposure management

Fig. 10.74 Internal exposure noticed at 2nd stage procedure

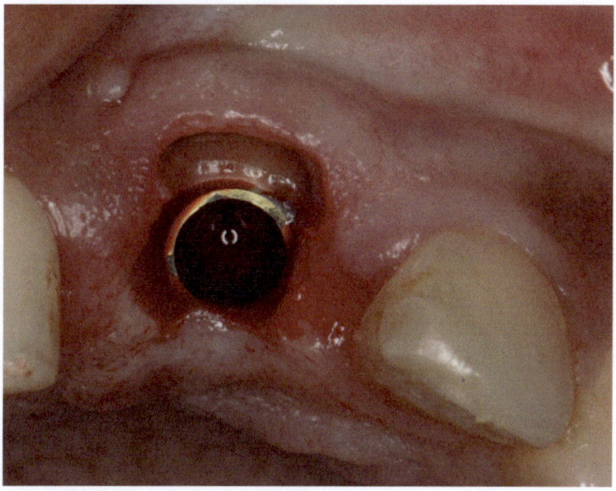

However, during prosthetic phase, external exposure was observed, which could be attributed to improper bevel and due to the sharp edge generated during shield preparation. The exposure was trimmed with high-speed handpiece and diamond bur (Figs. 10.78, 10.79, 10.80, 10.81, 10.82 and 10.83). Soft tissue healed above the trimmed shield over a period of 2 weeks (Fig. 10.84).

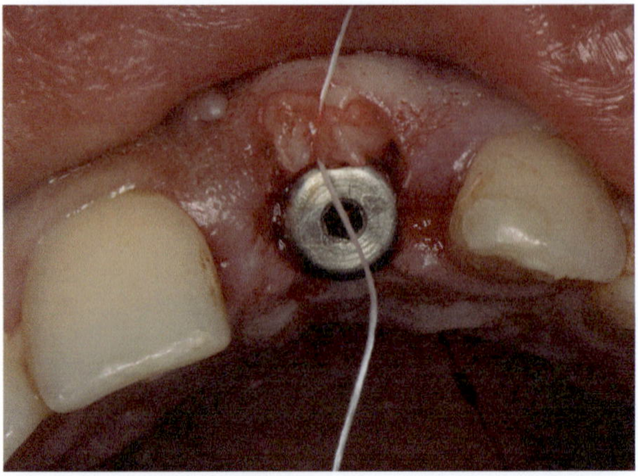

Fig. 10.75 Trimming of exposed shield followed by soft tissue augmentation done using connective tissue harvested from maxillary tuberosity to cover the exposed shield

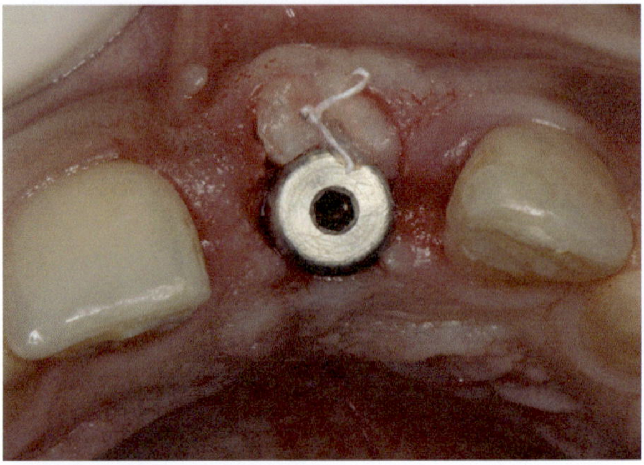

Fig. 10.76 Connective tissue graft sutured at the site

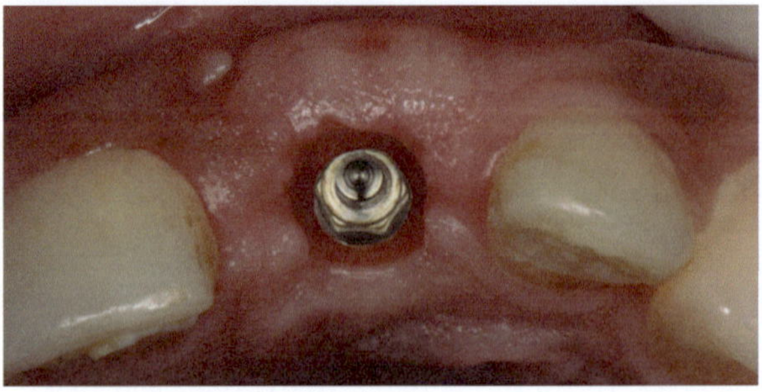

Fig. 10.77 Favourable soft tissue profile after the healing. Note the stippling indicating optimal tissue health

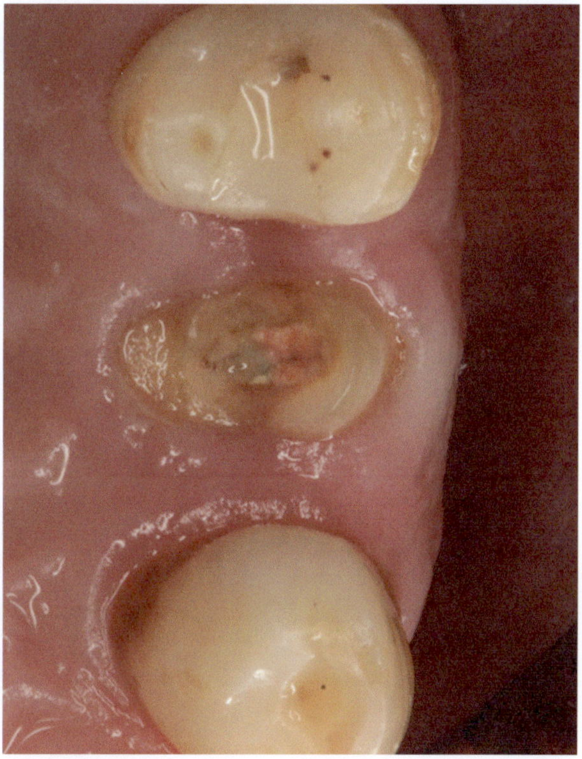

Fig. 10.78 Tooth #24 indicated for post-extraction implant placement

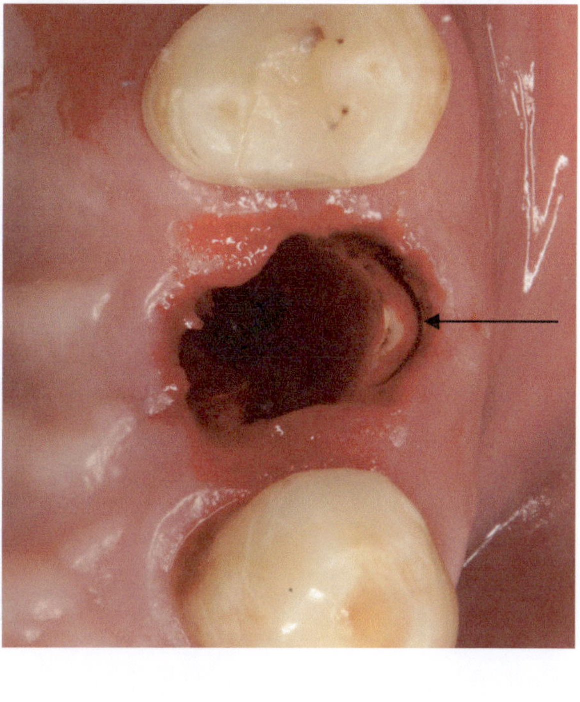

Fig. 10.79 Socket shield preparation. Note the sharp external edge accidentally generated

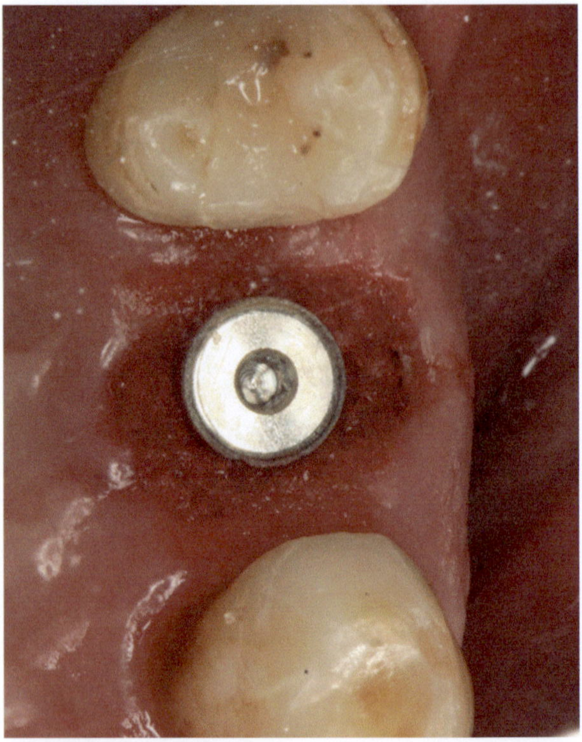

Fig. 10.80 Implant placement followed by grafting in the gap

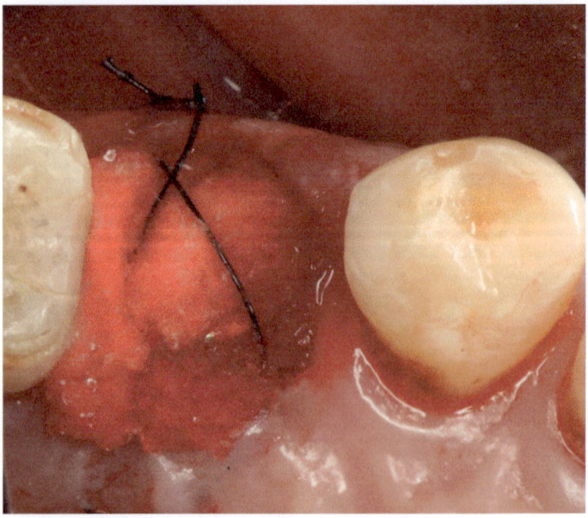

Fig. 10.81 Graft secured with collagen plug and cross mattress suture

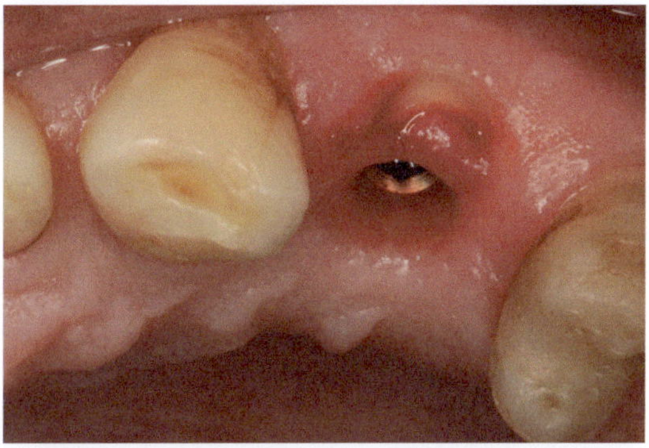

Fig. 10.82 External exposure seen during prosthetic phase

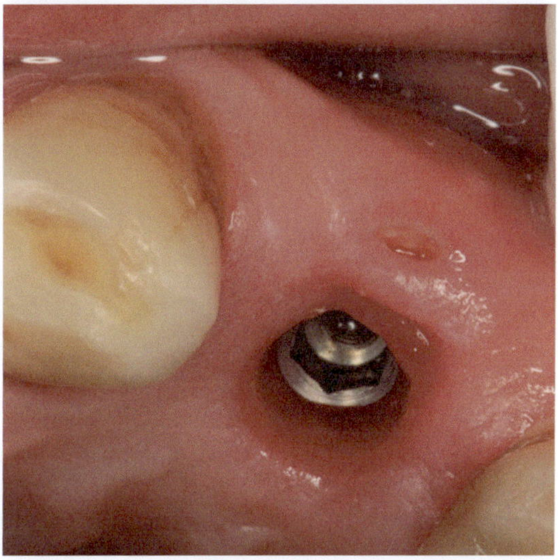

Fig. 10.83 External Shield exposure trimmed gradually till soft tissue closure is achieved

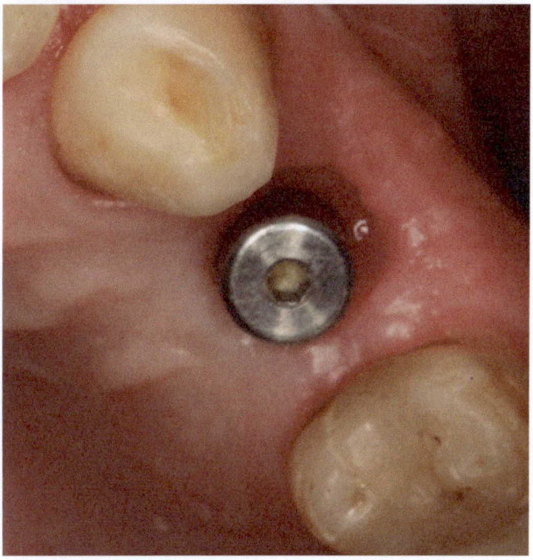

Fig. 10.84 Complete coverage of the shield after trimming

Management of External Shield Exposure in Lower Cuspid and Bicuspid

The case below* describes external shield exposure that was observed at 2nd stage procedure (Figs. 10.85, 10.86, 10.87, 10.88, 10.89, 10.90, 10.91, 10.92, 10.93, 10.94, 10.95, 10.96, 10.97, 10.98, 10.99, 10.100, 10.101, 10.102, 10.103 and 10.104). During second-stage surgery, the implants were uncovered and the shields trimmed to the level of bone crest on the buccal aspect. A connective tissue graft was harvested and inserted between the buccal flap and the shield to augment the soft tissue dimensions in the area and prevent any further shield exposure*.

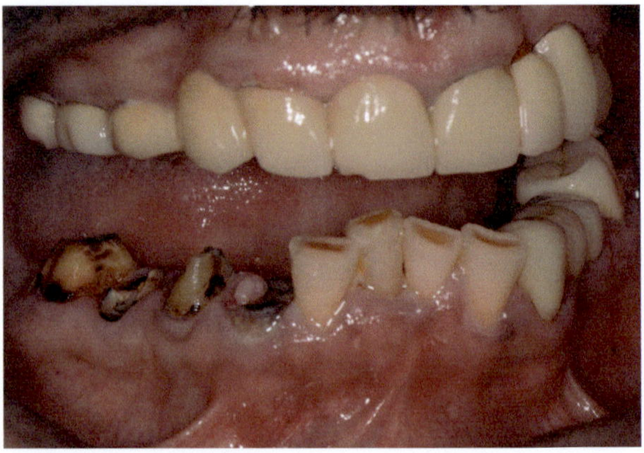

Fig. 10.85 #43 to #47 structurally failed and needed extractions

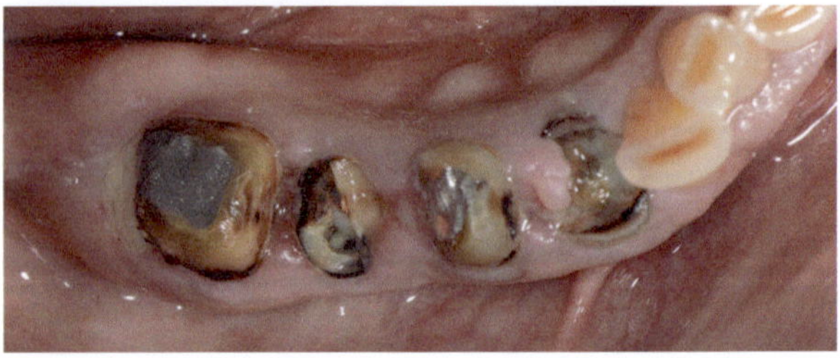

Fig. 10.86 Occlusal view showing the teeth destroyed by decay

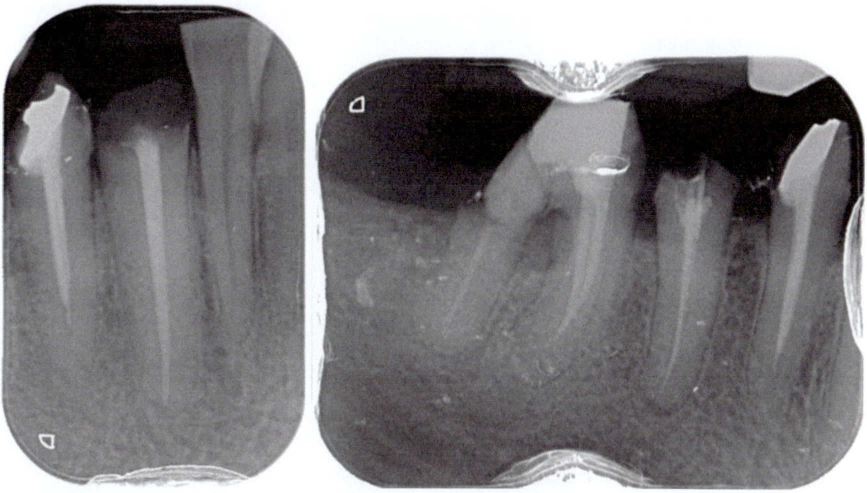

Fig. 10.87 Preoperative radiographs showing tooth #46 structurally poor

Fig. 10.88 Cross section of #43 showing adequate bone dimensions on apical and lingual aspect of the tooth

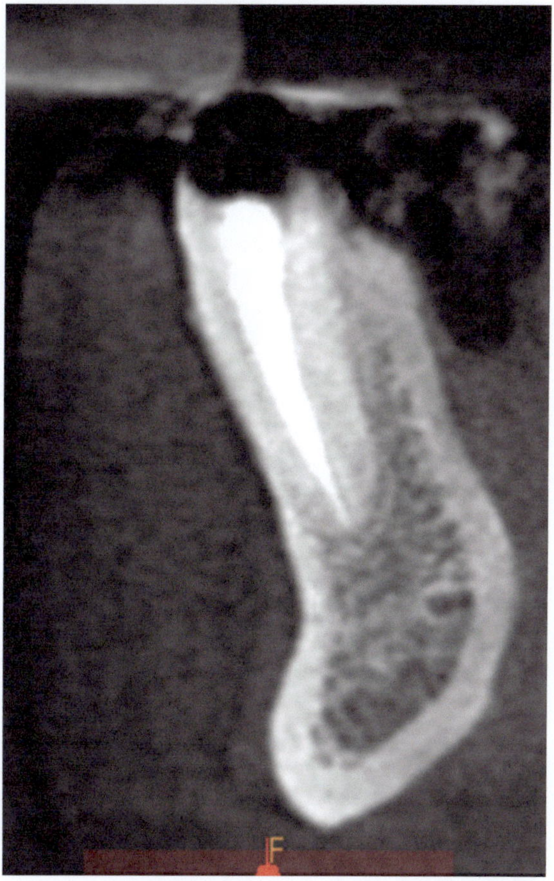

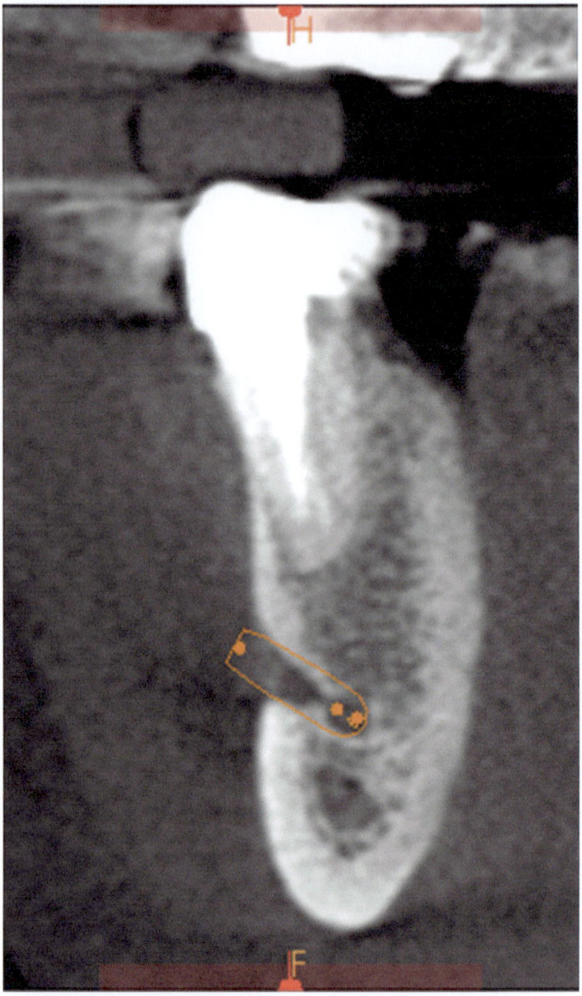

Fig. 10.89 Cross section of #45 showing adequate bone dimensions on apical and lingual aspect of the tooth

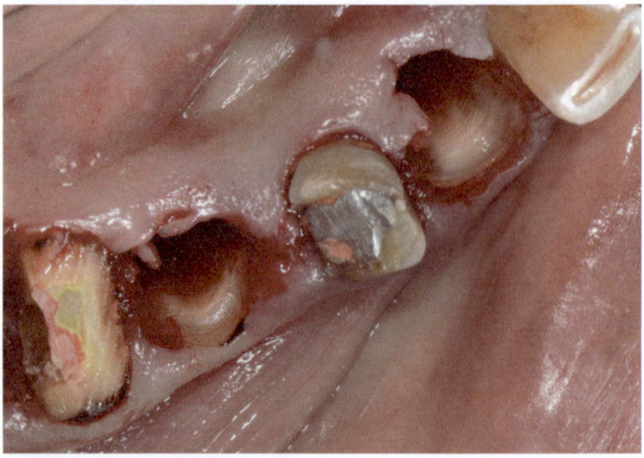

Fig. 10.90 Shields prepared for #43, #45. #44 was saved and will be restored as it had sufficient wall thickness

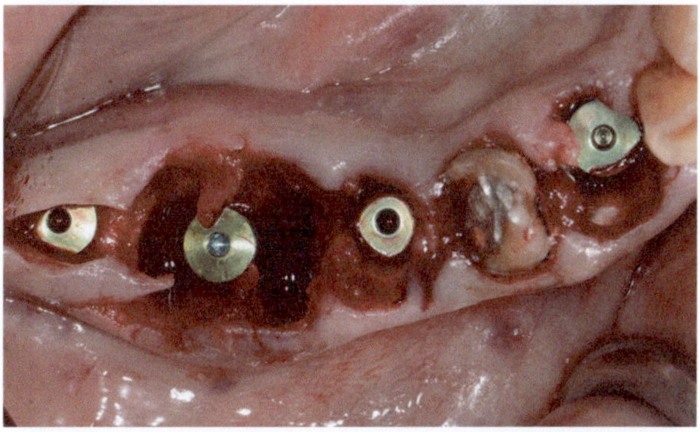

Fig. 10.91 Implants placed in correct 3D positions

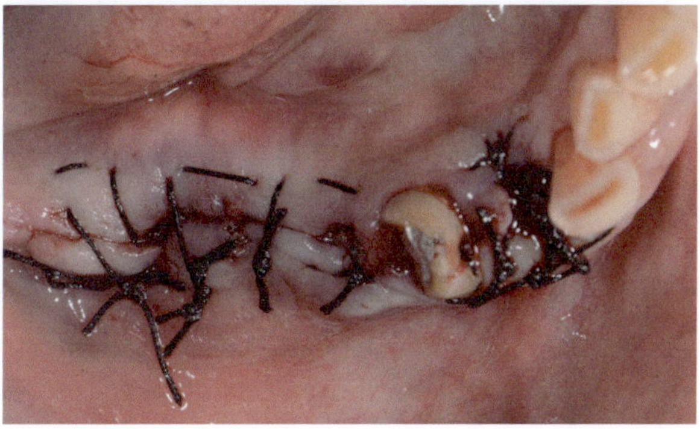

Fig. 10.92 Site sutured to allow submerged healing protocol

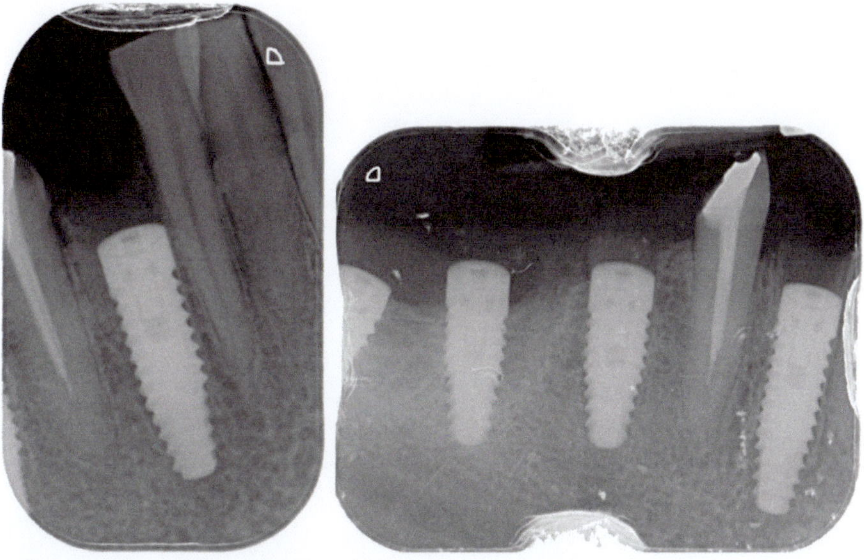

Fig. 10.93 Postsurgical radiographs

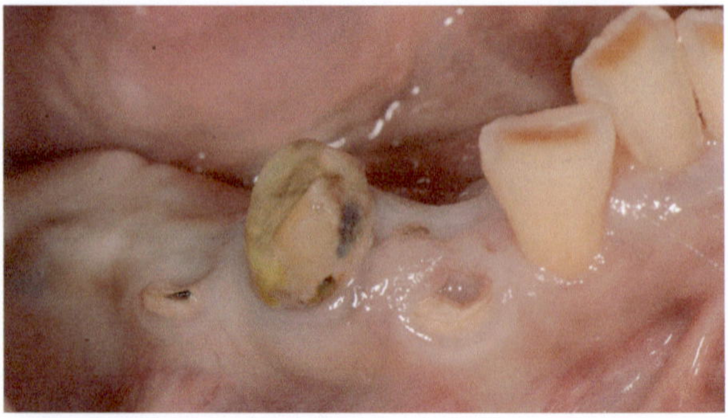

Fig. 10.94 Healed site with external shield exposures in sites #43 and #45 at 3-months

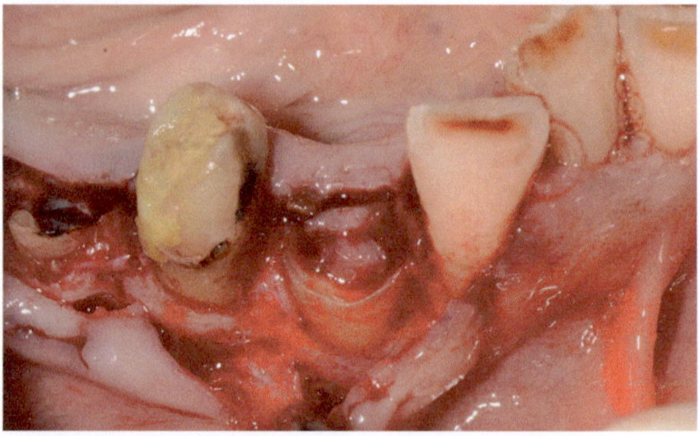

Fig. 10.95 Sites opened to gain access to the implants for second stage surgery. Shield exposed to be trimmed

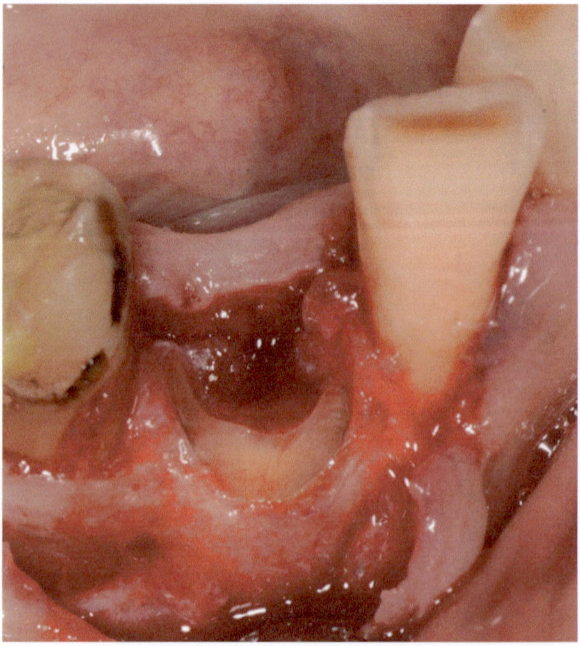

Fig. 10.96 Shield trimmed to bone level in #43

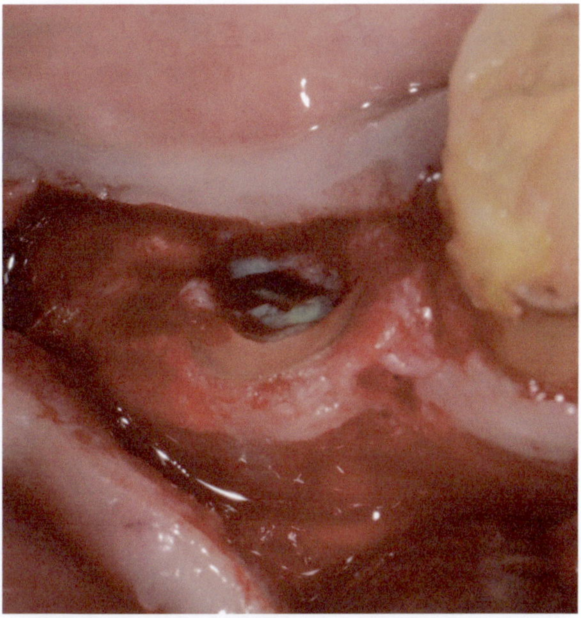

Fig. 10.97 Shield in #45 trimmed to level of bone

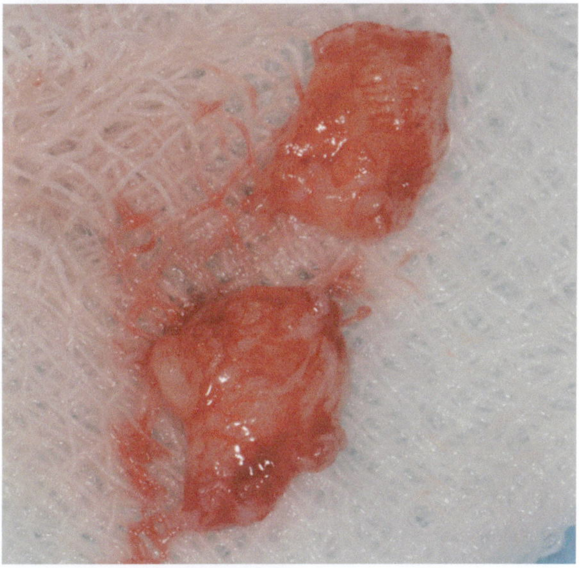

Fig. 10.98 Connective tissue graft harvested from palate to augment the soft tissue thickness in the area*

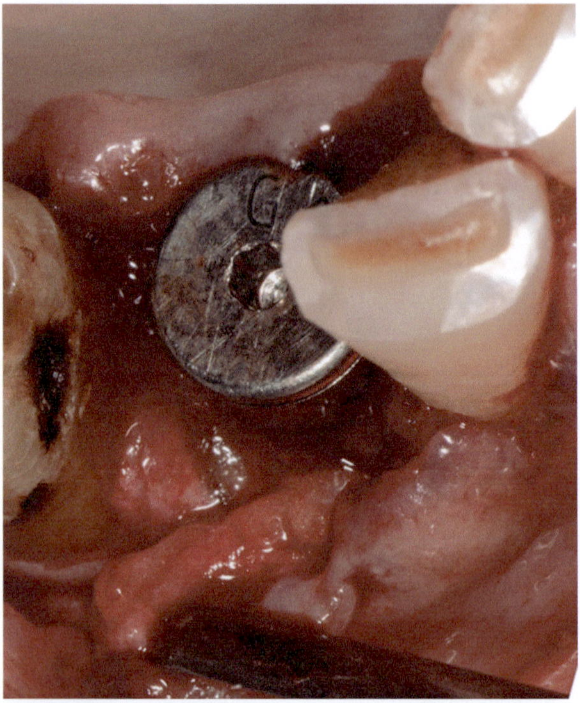

Fig. 10.99 CT graft in place to cover the shield and healing abutments placed on the implants

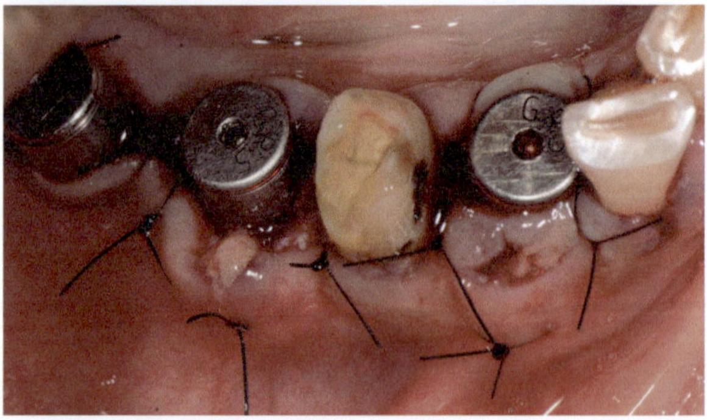

Fig. 10.100 The buccal flap sutured over the sites with soft tissue augmentation

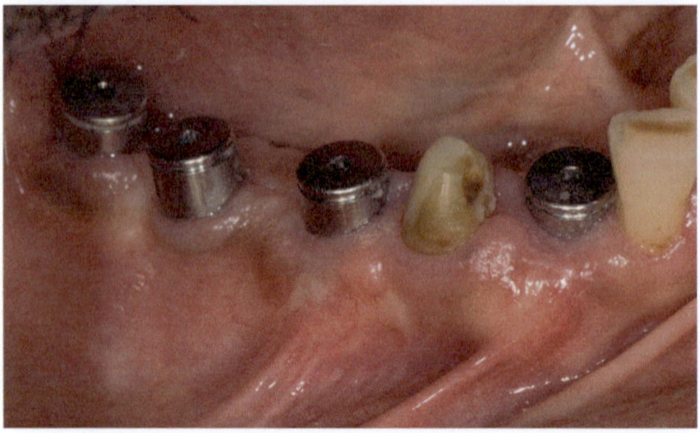

Fig. 10.101 Healed sites after soft tissue augmentation showing healthy peri-implant tissues

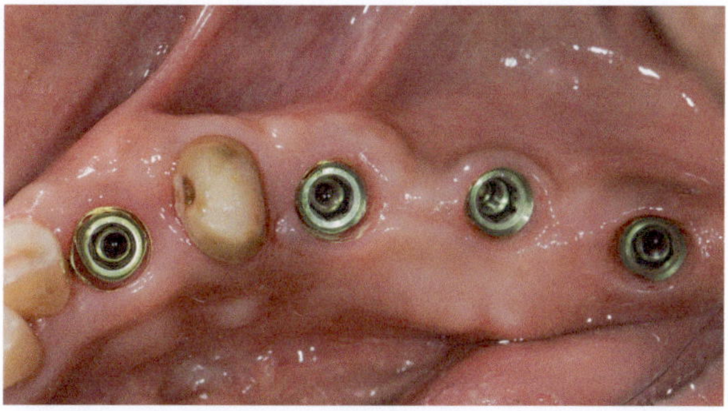

Fig. 10.102 Healed sites. The volume and contour of tissues in #43 and #45 implant region with socket shields present can be fully appreciated

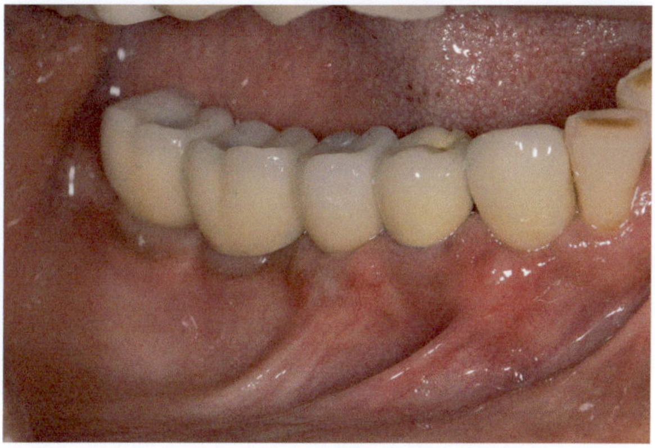

Fig. 10.103 Final restorations on all lower posterior teeth. The contours of #43 and #45 maintained with the socket shield technique

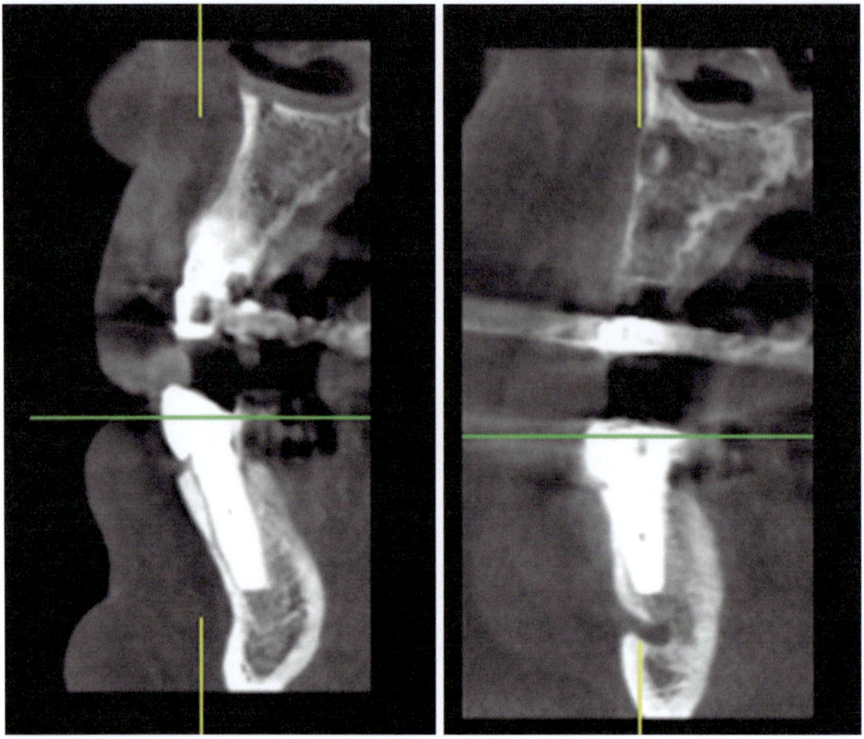

Fig. 10.104 Final CBCT data of #43 and #45 showing excellent maintenance of buccal bone contour where the shields have been done

10.4.4 Infection

Causes:

Postsurgical infection specific to PET procedures are as follows:

- Residual endodontic filling material.
- Mobile shield.
- Implant in close proximity with shield [32, 40].
- Incomplete removal of the root apex.
- Large gap between the implant and the shield.
- Large periapical lesion that has not been curetted out.
- Inadequate wound closure.

Prevention: Ensuring that the apex and all the residual endodontic filling material have been removed is paramount to the success of the procedure. Any peri-apical lesion must be removed with thorough curettage and copious irrigation [19].

Management: In case the peri-implant site has got infected, it is necessary to remove the implant, debride, and allow the site to heal. No socket grafting should be attempted at this stage because of the presence of local infection. In such cases, if the shield is intact, firm and is not the cause of the infection it may be left in place to maintain the labial contour.

Implant Failures in SS

An implant may fail to integrate in PET sites [13]. In such cases, if the shield and implant are found to be mobile, then both should be removed; else only implant is removed leaving the intact shield behind (Figs. 10.105 and 10.106).

In case the shield is not mobile, but only the implant has failed to integrate the shield can be left behind and a new implant can be placed at the same site at a later date.

Implant Failure and Shield Removal

The following case demonstrates an implant failure associated with a shield in the mandibular incisor area. The teeth #32 and #42 were extracted and socket shield done. Implants were placed and temporary restorations were made. At 3-months, the implant in the #42 site failed to integrate and had to be removed. The shield with tooth #42 was also mobile and was removed. The site was then allowed to heal. After 3-months tooth #42 site received a new implant and was subsequently restored (Figs. 10.107, 10.108, 10.109, 10.110, 10.111, 10.112, 10.113, 10.114, 10.115, 10.116, 10.117, 10.118, 10.119, 10.120, 10.121 and 10.122).

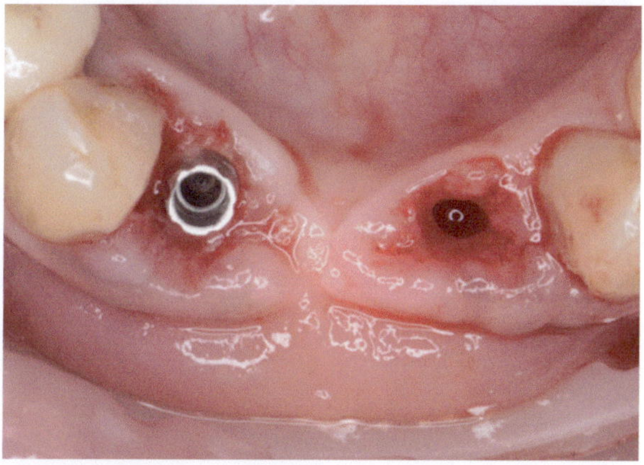

Fig. 10.105 Implant failed to osseointegrate in tooth 42 site

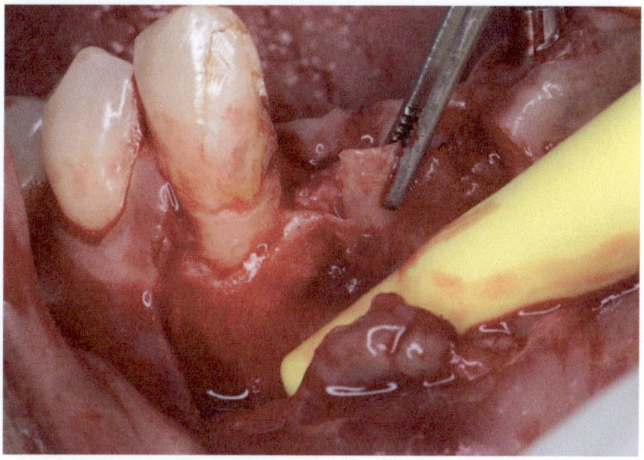

Fig. 10.106 Shield being removed in the #42 site

Fig. 10.107 Preoperative situation in relation to teeth #31 and #42

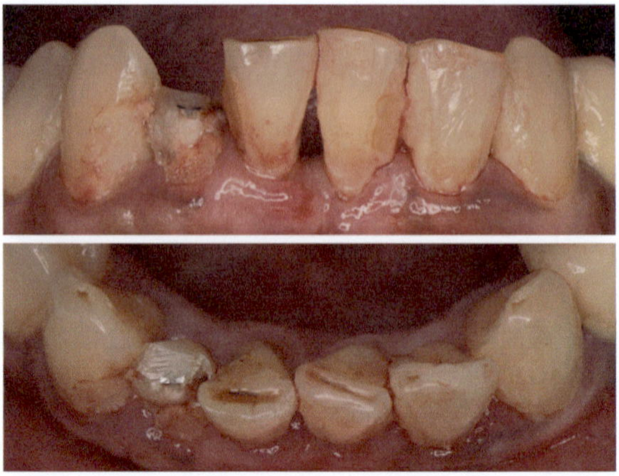

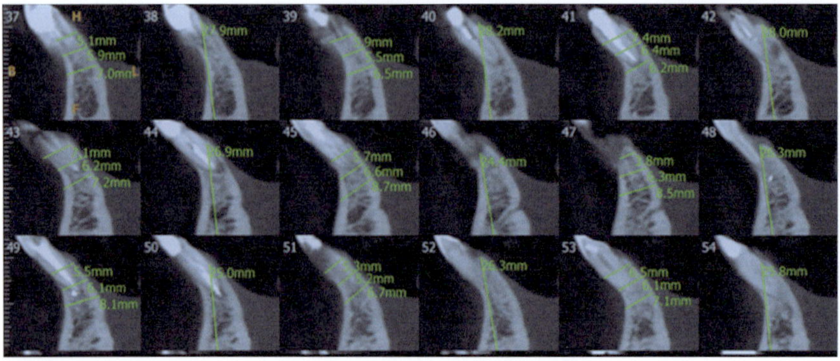

Fig. 10.108 CBCT axial sections used for planning the procedure

Fig. 10.109 Socket shield preparation and implant placement

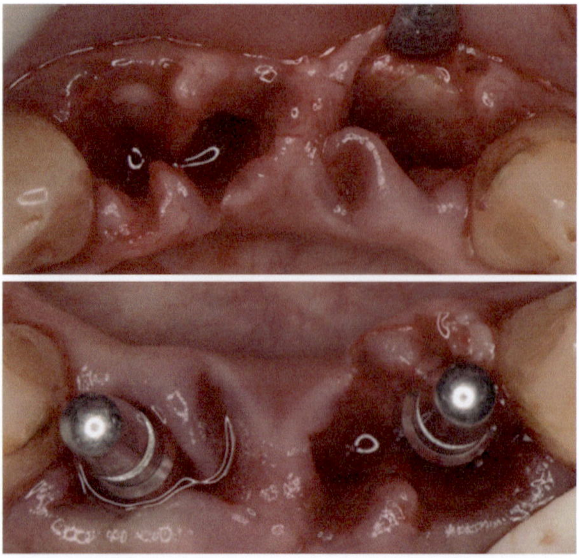

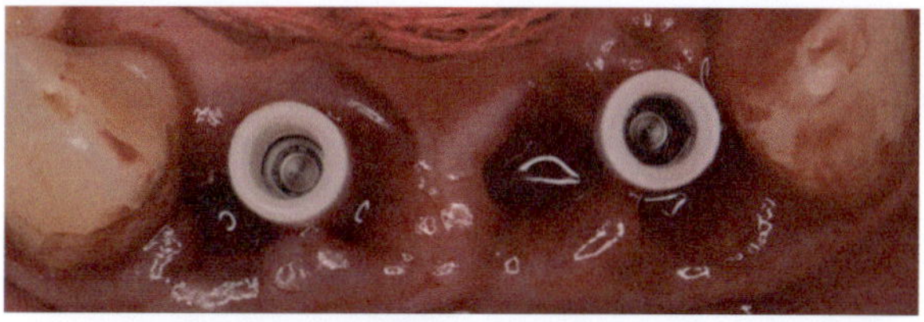

Fig. 10.110 Implant placed in teeth 32 and 42 regions

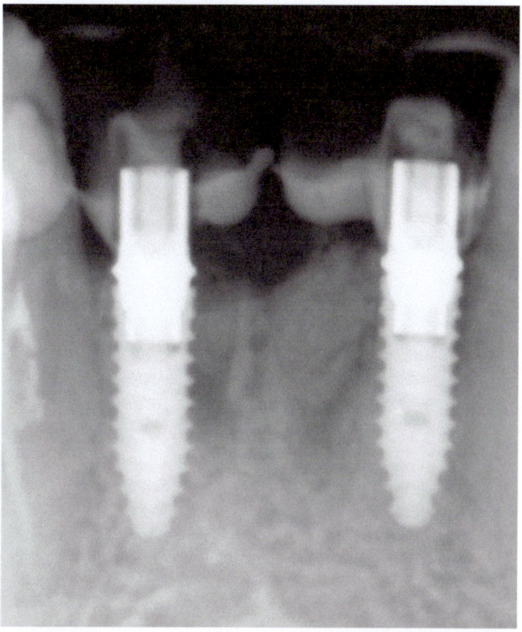

Fig. 10.111 Periapical radiograph depicting implant placement along with provisional restoration

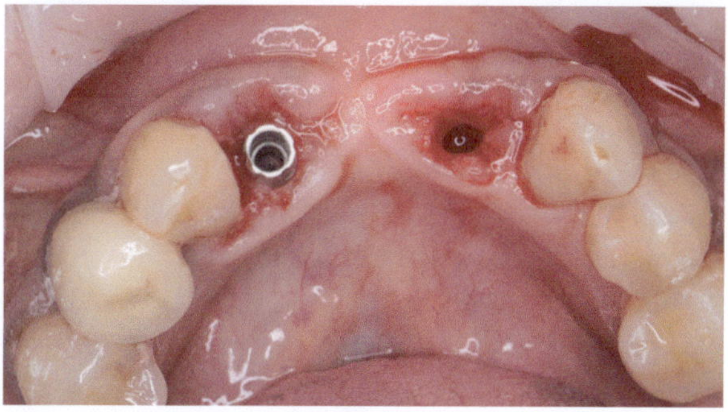

Fig. 10.112 Failure of the implant noted at the time of final restorative stage

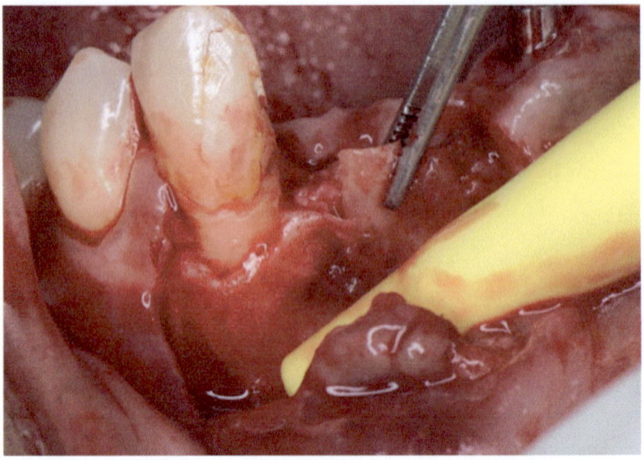

Fig. 10.113 The shield in relation to the failed implant was mobile and was removed

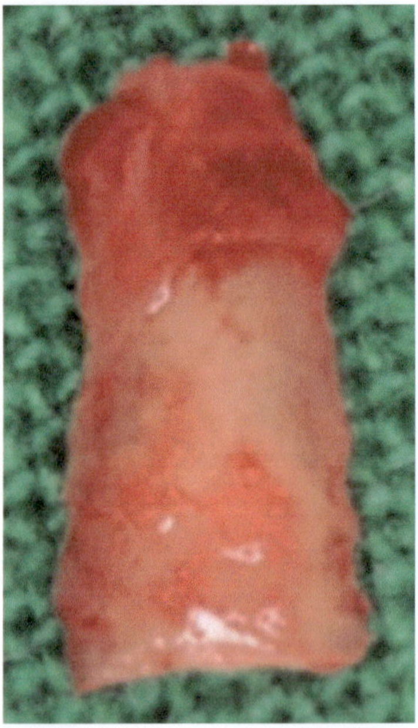

Fig. 10.114 Extracted shield

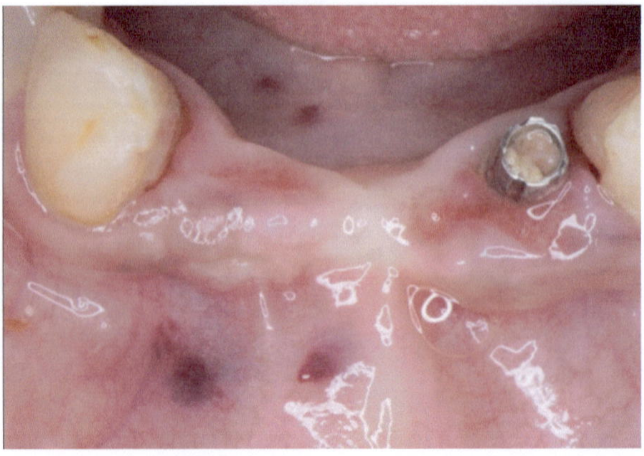

Fig. 10.115 The site was allowed to heal for a period of 3-months

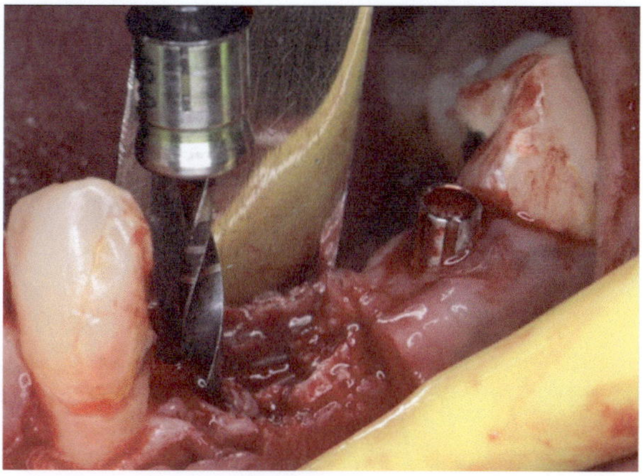

Fig. 10.116 Conventional osteotomy preparation was done

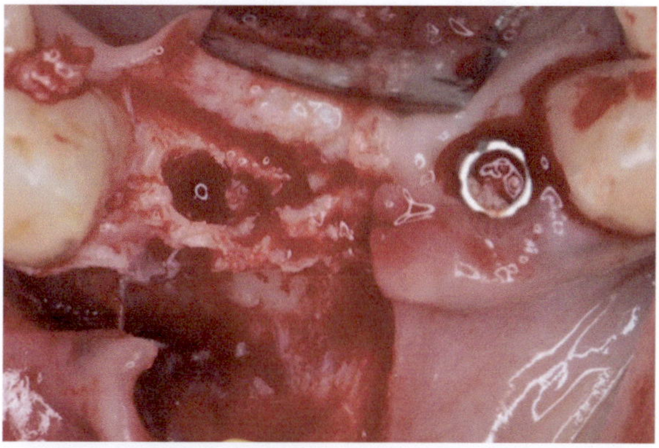

Fig. 10.117 The site is prepared to receive an implant

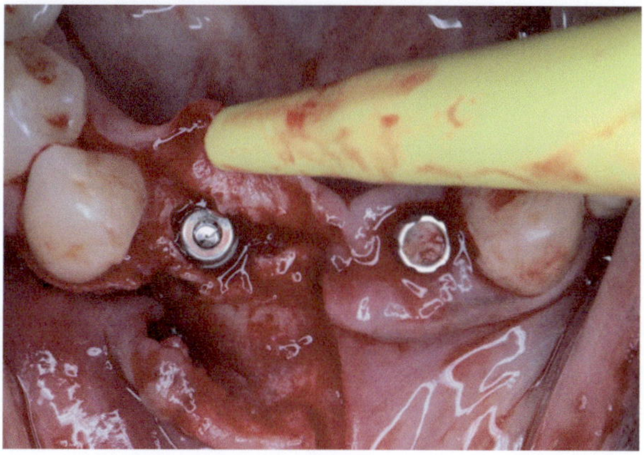

Fig. 10.118 New implant placed in the tooth #42 area

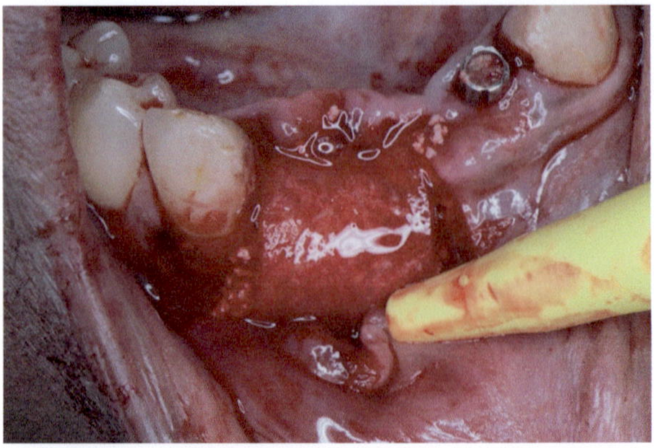

Fig. 10.119 Guided bone regeneration done for the site after implant placement

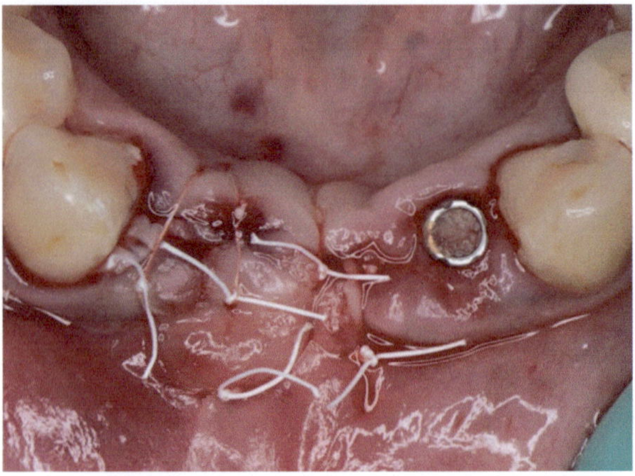

Fig. 10.120 Primary closure was attained as the implant did not have adequate primary stability and was allowed a submerged healing

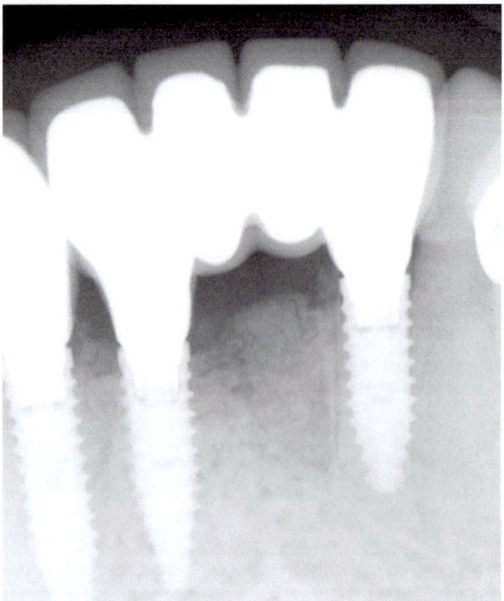

Fig. 10.121 Radiograph at 4-year recall

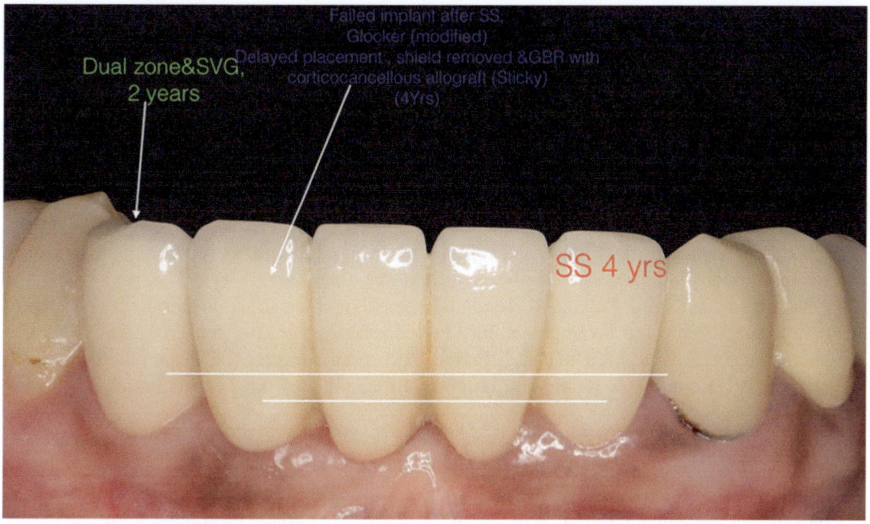

Fig. 10.122 Final restoration at the 4-year follow-up showing satisfactory tissue contours on a SS site and the site with a conventional implant placement

10.5 Conclusion

Socket shield and pontic shield techniques aid in hard and soft tissue preservation by maintaining buccal bone. Since the procedure has a steep learning curve, complications are bound to occur. However, the complications associated with the technique are manageable by taking simple corrective steps. The postoperative morbidity in spite of complications is very low. The treatment procedures to treat these complications are easy to perform and are very predictable. Like any surgical procedure, errors and the ensuing complications can be prevented by thorough preoperative evaluation, precise surgical execution, and well-designed provisional restorations.

Acknowledgment Illustrations by: Udatta Kher.
*Case Courtesy: Dr Ali Tunkiwala; Connective Tissue Graft by Dr Bhakti Tunkiwala

References

1. Araújo MG, Lindhe J. Dimensional ridge alterations following tooth extraction. An experimental study in the dog. J Clin Periodontol. 2005;32:212–8.
2. Schropp L, Wenzel A, Kostopoulos L, Karring T. Bone healing and soft tissue contour changes following single tooth extraction: a clinical and radiographic 12-month prospective study. Int J Periodontics Restorative Dent. 2003;23:313–23.
3. Araujo M, Sukekava F, Wennstrom J, Lindhe J. Ridge alterations following implant placement in fresh extraction sockets: an experimental study in the dog. J Clin Periodontol. 2006;32:645–65.

4. Fickl S, Zuhr O, Wachtel H, Stappert C, Stein J, Hurzeler MB. Dimensional changes of the alveolar ridge contour after different socket preservation techniques. J Clin Periodontol. 2008;35:906–13.
5. Chu SJ, Salama MA, Salama H, Garber DA, Saito H, Sarnachiaro GO, Tarnow DP. The dual-zone therapeutic concept of managing immediate implant placement and provisional restoration in anterior extraction sockets. Compend Contin Educ Dent. 2012;33(7):524–32, 534
6. Hürzeler MB, Zuhr O, Schupbach P, Rebele SF, Emmanouilidis N, Fickl S. The socket-shield technique: a proof-of principle report. J Clin Periodontol. 2010;37:855–62.
7. Bäumer D, Zuhr O, Rebele S, Schneider D, Schupbach P, Hürzeler M. The socket-shield technique: first histological, clinical, and volumetrical observations after separation of the buccal tooth segment—a pilot study. Clin Implant Dent Relat Res. 2015;17(1):71–82.
8. Gluckman H, Du Toit J, Salama M. The Pontic-shield: partial extraction therapy for ridge preservation and Pontic site development. Int J Periodontics Restorative Dent. 2016;36(3):417–23.
9. Gluckman H, Salama M, Du Toit J. Partial extraction therapies (PET) part 1: maintaining alveolar ridge contour at pontic and immediate implant sites. Int J Periodontics Restorative Dent. 2016;36(5):681–7.
10. Gluckman H, Salama M, Du Toit J. Partial extraction therapies (PET) part 2: procedures and technical aspects. Int J Periodontics Restorative Dent. 2017;37(3):377–85.
11. Gluckman H, Pontes CC, Du Toit J. Radial plane tooth position and bone wall dimensions in the anterior maxilla: a CBCT classification for immediate implant placement. J Prosthet Dent. 2018;120(1):50–6.
12. Ash MM, Nelson SJ. The permanent canines: maxillary and mandibular. In: Wheeler's dental anatomy, physiology, and occlusion. 8th ed. St. Louis, Mo: Elsevier; 2007. p. 191–214.
13. Gluckman H, Salama M, Du Toit J. A retrospective evaluation of 128 socket-shield cases in the esthetic zone and posterior sites: partial extraction therapy with up to 4 years follow-up. Clin Implant Dent Relat Res. 2018;20(2):122–9.
14. Choukroun J, Diss A, Simonpieri A, Girard MO, Schoeffler C, Dohan SL, Dohan AJ, Mouhyi J, Dohan DM. Platelet-rich fibrin (PRF): a second-generation platelet concentrate. Part IV: clinical effects on tissue healing. Oral Surg Oral Med Oral Pathol Oral Radiol Endod. 2006;101(3):e56–60.
15. Jin K. Utilization of autologous concentrated growth factors (CGF) enriched bone graft matrix (sticky bone) and CGF-enriched fibrin membrane in implant dentistry. J Implant Adv Clin Dent. 2015;7:11–29.
16. Dohan DM, Choukroun J, Diss A, Dohan SL, Dohan AJ, Mouhyi J, et al. Platelet-rich fibrin (PRF): a second-generation platelet concentrate. Part II: platelet-related biologic features. Oral Surg Oral Med Oral Pathol Oral Radiol Endod. 2006;101(3):45–50.
17. Choukroun J, Diss A, Simonpieri A, Girard MO, Schoeffler C, Dohan SL, Dohan AJ, Mouhyi J, Dohan DM. Platelet-rich fibrin (PRF): a second-generation platelet concentrate. Part V: histologic evaluations of PRF effects on bone allograft maturation in sinus lift. Oral Surg Oral Med Oral Pathol Oral Radiol Endod. 2006;101(3):299–303.
18. Mitsias ME, Siormpas KD, Kotsakis GA, Ganz SD, Mangano C, Iezzi G. The root membrane technique: human histologic evidence after five years of function. Biomed Res Int. 2017;2017:7269467.
19. Zhao D, Wu Y, Xu C, Zhang F. Immediate dental implant placement into infected vs. non-infected sockets: a meta-analysis. Clin Oral Implants Res. 2016;27:1290–6.
20. Kan JY, Roe P, Rungcharassaeng K, Patel RD, Waki T, et al. Classification of sagittal root position in relation to the anterior maxillary osseous housing for immediate implant placement: a cone beam computed tomography study. Int J Oral Maxillofac Implants. 2011;26:873–6.
21. Grandi C, Pacifici L. The ratio in choosing access flap for surgical endodontics: a review. Oral Implantol (Rome). 2009;2(1):37–52.
22. Gluckman H, du Toit J, Salama M. Guided bone regeneration of a fenestration complication at immediate implant placement simultaneous to the socket-shield technique. Int Dent. 2015;5:58–66.

23. Mitsias ME, Siormpas KD, Prasad H, Garber D, Kotsakis GA. A step-by-step description of PDL-mediated ridge preservation for immediate implant rehabilitation in the esthetic region. Int J Periodontics Restorative Dent. 2015;35:835–41.
24. Kumar PR, Kher U. Shield the socket: procedure, case report and classification. J Indian Soc Periodontol. 2018;22(3):266–72.
25. Mitsias ME, Ganz SD, Tawil I. The root membrane concept: in the zone with the "triangle of bone". Contin Educ. 2017;36(10):80.
26. Cherel F, Etienne D. Papilla preservation between two implants: a modified socket-shield technique to maintain the scalloped anatomy? A case report. Quintessence Int. 2014;45(1):23–30.
27. Kan JY, Rungcharassaeng K. Proximal socket shield for interimplant papilla preservation in the esthetic zone. Int J Periodontics Restorative Dent. 2013;33:e24–31.
28. Gluckman H, Du Toit J, Salama M. The socket-shield technique to support buccofacial tissues at immediate implant placement: a case report and review of the literature. Int Dent Africa Ed. 2015;5:1–7.
29. Gutmann JL. Surgical endodontics: past, present, and future. Endod Top. 2014;30(1):29–43.
30. Vignoletti F, Matesanz P, Rodrigo D, et al. Surgical protocols for ridge preservation after tooth extraction: a systematic review. Clin Oral Implants Res. 2012;23:22–38.
31. Gluckman H, Nagy K, Du Toit J. Prosthetic management of implants placed with the socket-shield technique. J Prosthet Dent. 2019;121(4):581–5.
32. Schwimer C, Pette GA, Gluckman H, Salama M, Du Toit J. Human histologic evidence of new bone formation and osseointegration between root dentin (unplanned socket-shield) and dental implant: case report. Int J Oral Maxillofac Implants. 2018;33:e19–23.
33. Mitsias ME, Siormpas KD, Kotsakis GA, Ganz SD, Mangano C, Iezzi G. The RootMembrane technique: human histologic evidence after five years of function. Biomed Res Int. 2017;2017:7269467.
34. Ruales-Carrera E, Pauletto P, Apaza-Bedoya K, Volpato CAM, Özcan M, Benfatti CAM. Peri-implant tissue management after immediate implant placement using a customized healing abutment. J Esthet Restor Dent. 2019:1–9.
35. Glocker M, Attin T, Schmidlin P. Ridge preservation with modified "socket-shield" technique: a methodological case series. Dent J. 2014;2(1):11–21.
36. Gharpure AS, Bhatavadekar NB. Current evidence on the socket-shield technique: a systematic review. J Oral Implantol. 2017;43:395–403.
37. Han CH, Park KB, Mangano FG. The modified socket shield technique. J Craniofac Surg. 2018;29(8):2247–54.
38. Peck MT, Marnewick J, Stephan LX, Singh A, Patel N, Majeed A. The use of leucocyte- and platelet-rich fibrin (L-PRF) to facilitate implant placement in bone-deficient sites: a report of two cases. SADJ. 2012;67(2):54–49.
39. Lee JW, Kim SG, Kim JY, Lee YC, Choi JY, Draqos R, et al. Restoration of a peri-implant defect by platelet-rich fibrin. Oral Surg Oral Med Oral Pathol Oral Radiol Endod. 2012;113(4):459–63.
40. Langer L, Langer B, Salem D. Unintentional root fragment retention in proximity to dental implants: a series of six human case reports. Int J Periodontics Restorative Dent. 2015;35(3):305–13.

11 Visual Essays of Clinical Cases

Udatta Kher and Ali Tunkiwala

Abstract

Various treatment modalities of partial extraction therapies have been described in the previous chapters. Step-by-step techniques of the surgical and restorative procedures have been explained in great detail. This chapter is a culmination of all the partial extraction therapy philosophies illustrated through case reports. These include cases ranging from implant-supported restoration of a single tooth to multiple teeth requiring rehabilitation. The chapter will exemplify the PET treatment concepts and workflow through a plethora of cases. The cases include socket shield, pontic shield, and root submergence techniques for single teeth and multiple teeth.

11.1 Introduction

The previous chapters have discussed in great details the philosophy of PET, step-by-step techniques, case selection criteria, and management of complications in an organized manner. Solutions for a wide range of clinical situations, utilizing PET procedures, are demonstrated in this chapter in the form of short case reports. The objective of this chapter was to bring together all aspects of diagnosis, treatment planning, surgical procedures, and fabrication of the restorations through visual essays.

U. Kher
Only Smiles Dental Centre, Mumbai, India

A. Tunkiwala (✉)
Smiles by Design, Mumbai, India

U. Kher, A. Tunkiwala (eds.), *Partial Extraction Therapy in Implant Dentistry*,
https://doi.org/10.1007/978-3-030-33610-3_11

11.2 Case 1: Single Upper Incisor with Socket Shield and Immediate Placement

Surgical Dentistry: Dr. Udatta Kher.

Restorative dentistry: Dr. Hetal Kothari.

Lab credits: Dentech Lab, Mumbai.

A 45-year-old lady reported with a mobile tooth 21 which was had a crown. The root canal was calcified and the tooth had a periapical infection. A socket shield procedure was performed with an immediate provisional restoration. The final lithium disilicate screw retained restoration was made after 3 months (Figs. 11.1, 11.2, 11.3, 11.4, 11.5, 11.6, 11.7, 11.8, 11.9, 11.10, 11.11, 11.12, 11.13, 11.14, 11.15, 11.16, 11.17, 11.18 and 11.19).

Challenges:

1. Young patient with high esthetic expectations.
2. Average lipline with display of interdental soft tissue.
3. Thin to medium biotype.

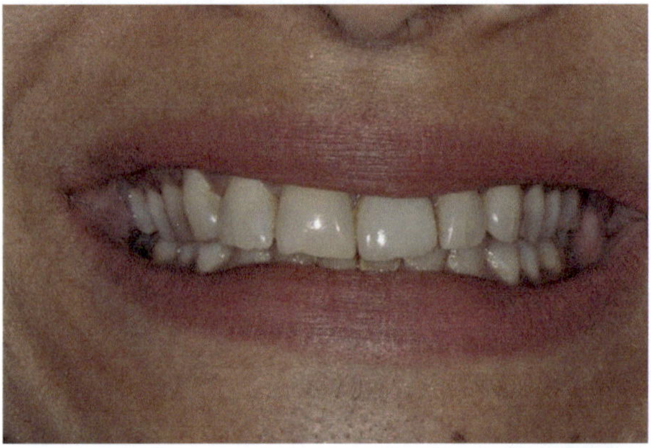

Fig. 11.1 Preoperative smile

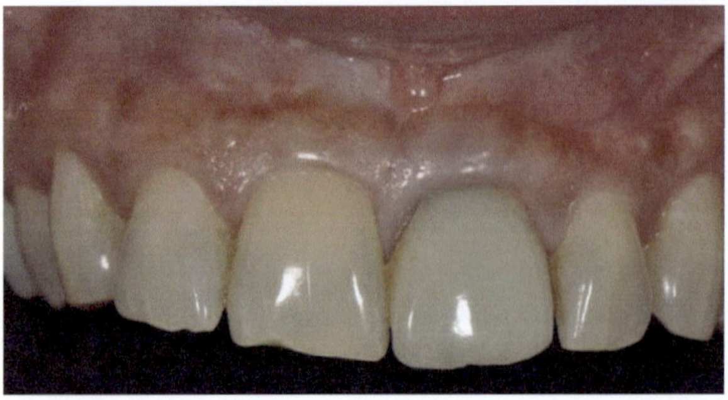

Fig. 11.2 Preoperative situation. Old PFM crown on tooth #21

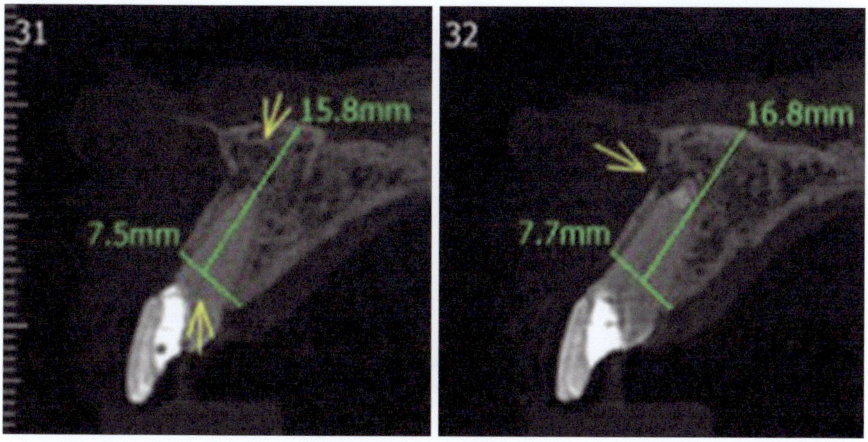

Fig. 11.3 CBCT showing calcified canal in tooth 21 and a periapical infection

Fig. 11.4 Decoronation of tooth 21

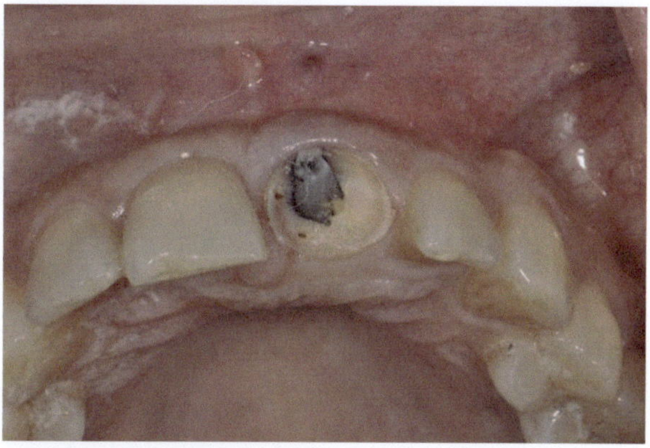

Fig. 11.5 Mesio-distal sectioning of the tooth

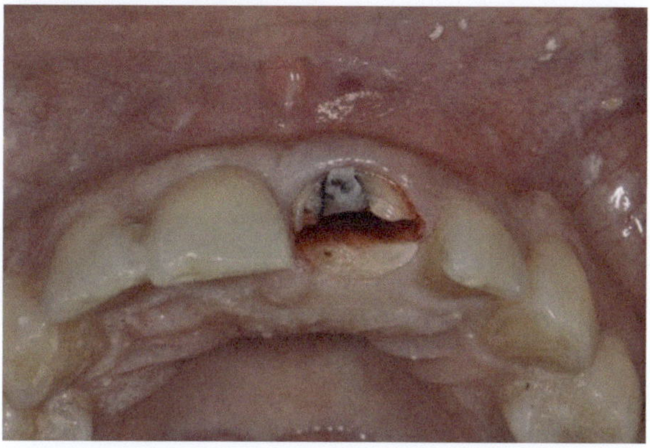

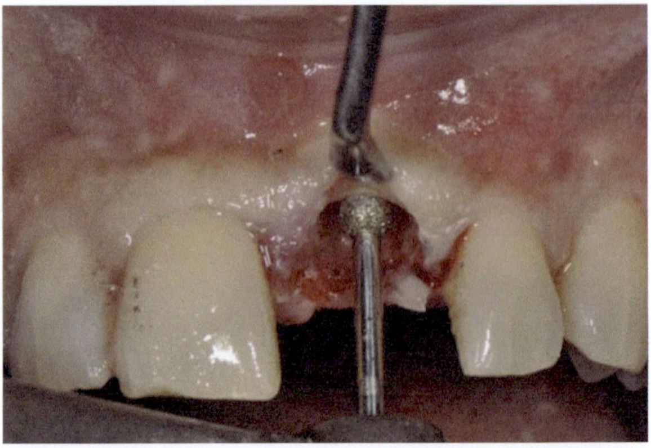

Fig. 11.6 Gingival protection during shield preparation

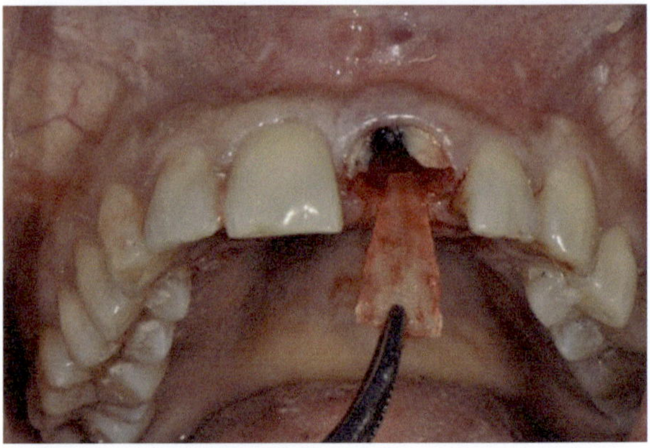

Fig. 11.7 Extraction of the palatal fragment

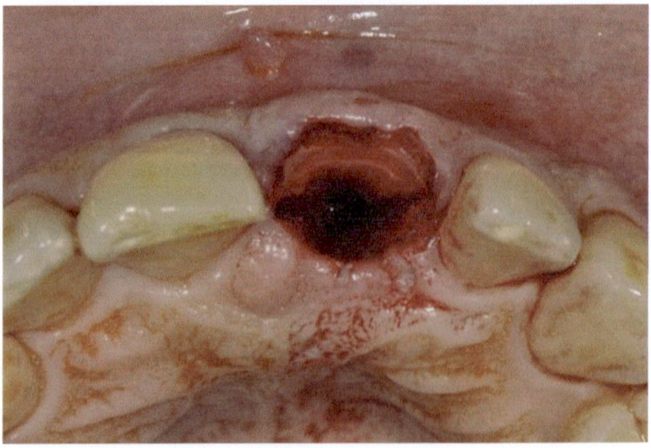

Fig. 11.8 Prepared socket shield

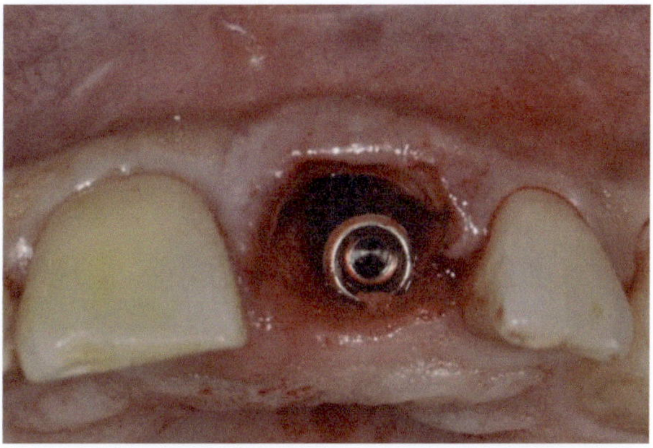

Fig. 11.9 Implant placement done in a prosthetically driven position

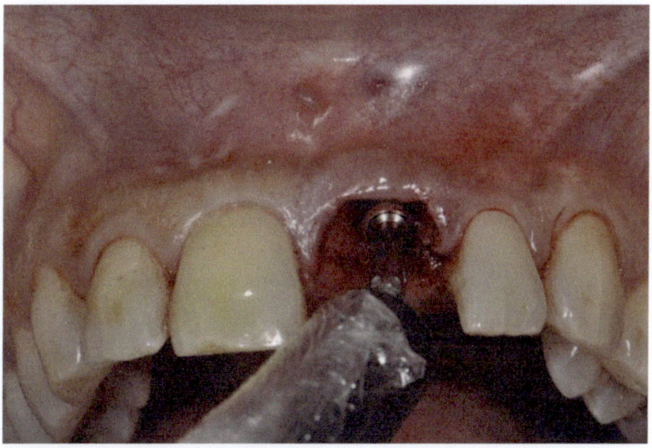

Fig. 11.10 Implant stability measured using ISQ device

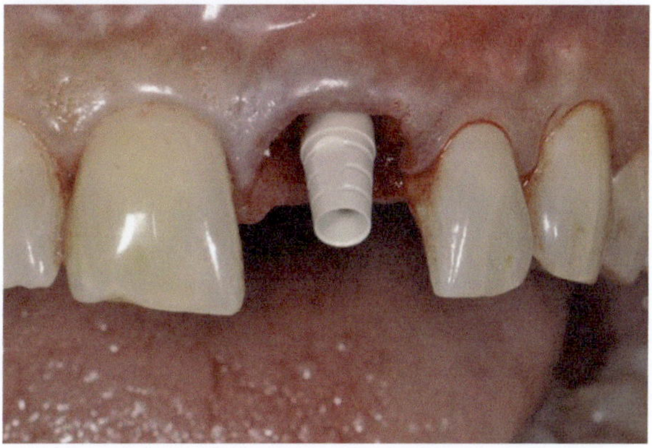

Fig. 11.11 Temporary PEEK abutment

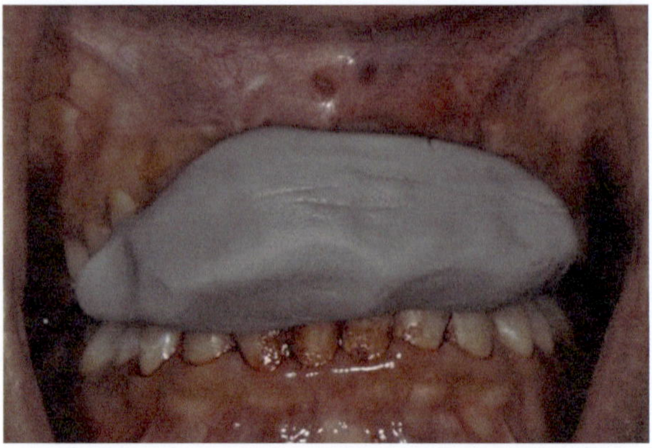

Fig. 11.12 Silicone putty index for fabrication of a chairside provisional restoration

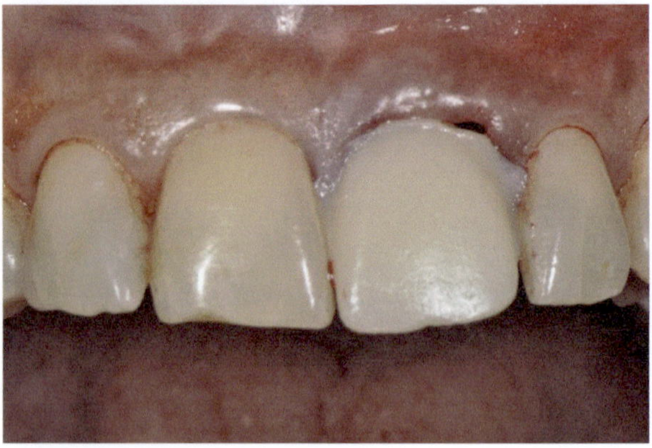

Fig. 11.13 Basic form of the provisional crown fabricated in autopolymerizing composite resin (Protemp 4, 3M Inc., USA)

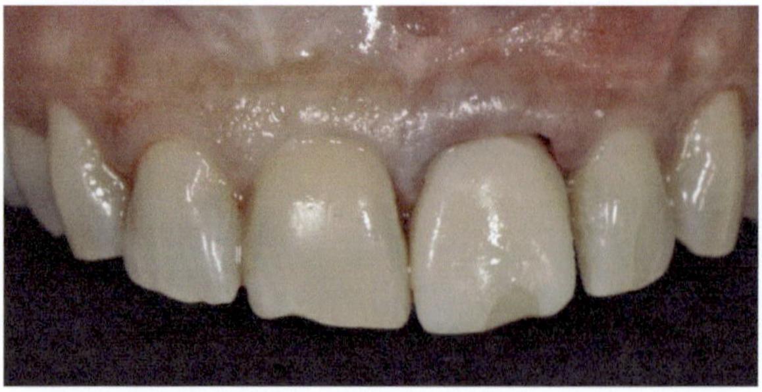

Fig. 11.14 Screw-retained provisional crown

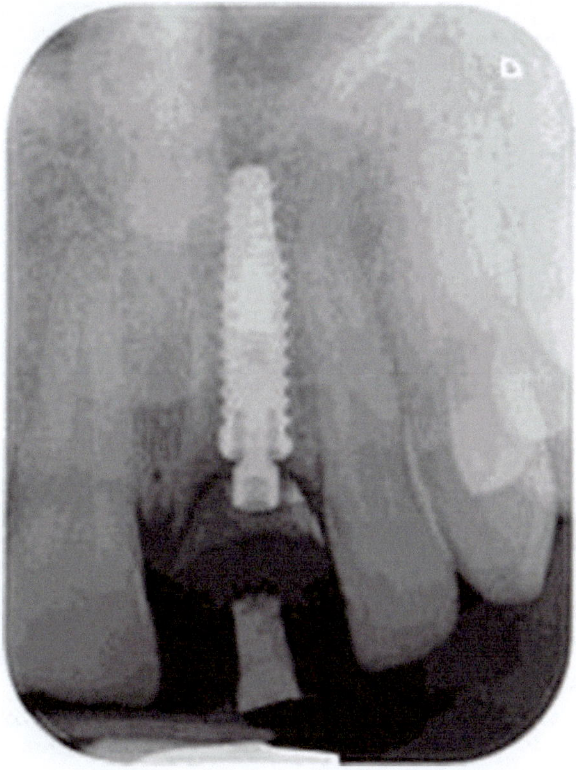

Fig. 11.15 Immediate postoperative radiograph

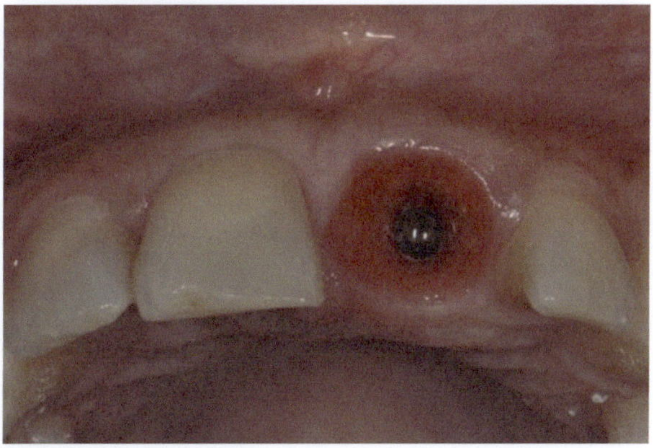

Fig. 11.16 Situation after 3 months on removal of the provisional restoration

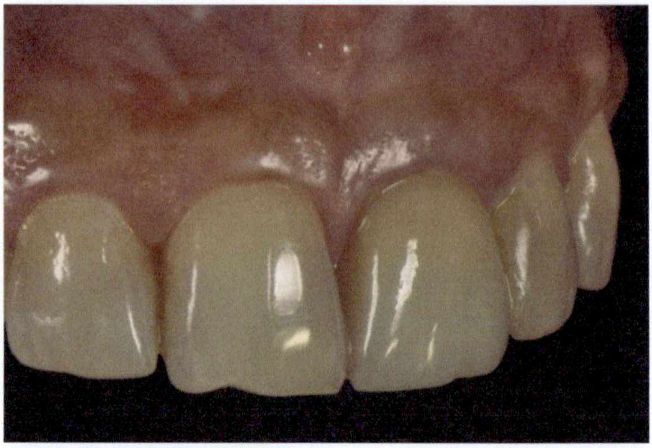

Fig. 11.17 Postoperative view of the definitive lithium disilicate crown on a zirconia abutment

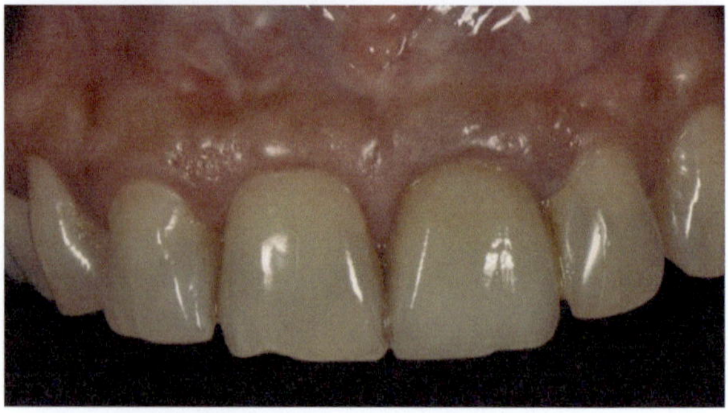

Fig. 11.18 Postoperative view of the definitive crown displaying good soft tissue contours

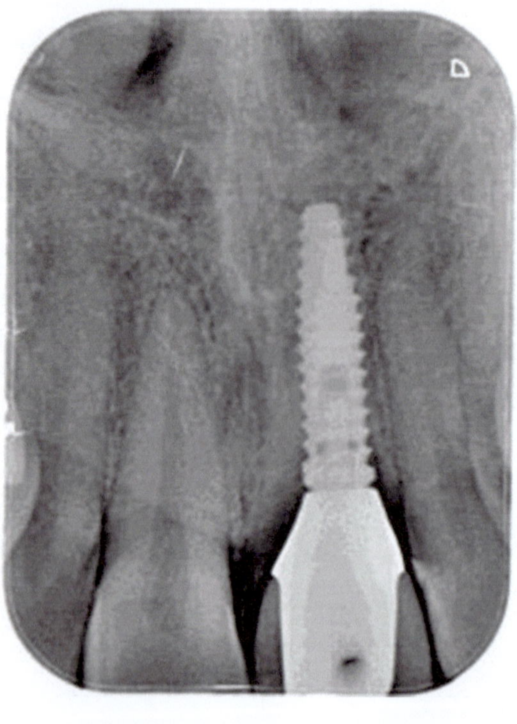

Fig. 11.19 Postoperative radiograph of the implant and definitive crown

11.3 Case 2: Single Lower Incisor with Socket Shield and Immediate Implant Placement

Surgical & Restorative Dentistry: Dr. Udatta Kher.

Lab Credits: Katara Dental, Pune.

A 45-year-old patient reported with a fractured lower left central incisor. The tooth had been endodontically treated 11 years ago and was restored with a post, core, and crown. The tooth was not unrestorable because of lack of ferrule.

Challenges

1. Highly technique sensitive procedure of shield preparation due to the small size of the root of a lower incisor.
2. Minimal margin for error during implant placement.

A socket shield procedure was performed followed by a chairside provisional crown. The definitive screw retained lithium disilicate restoration was made after 3 months (Figs. 11.20, 11.21, 11.22, 11.23, 11.24, 11.25, 11.26, 11.27, 11.28, 11.29 and 11.30).

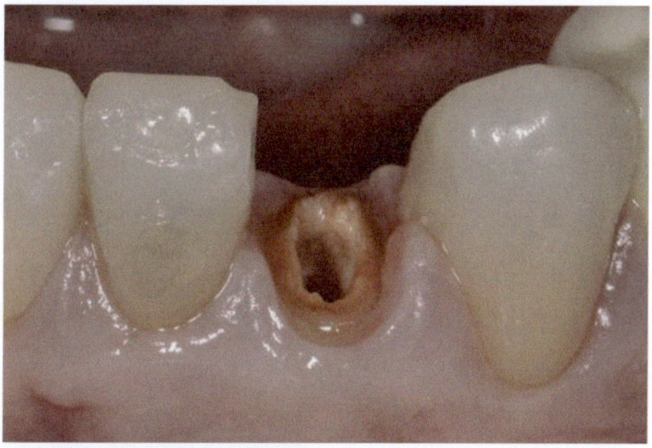

Fig. 11.20 Fractured tooth # 32

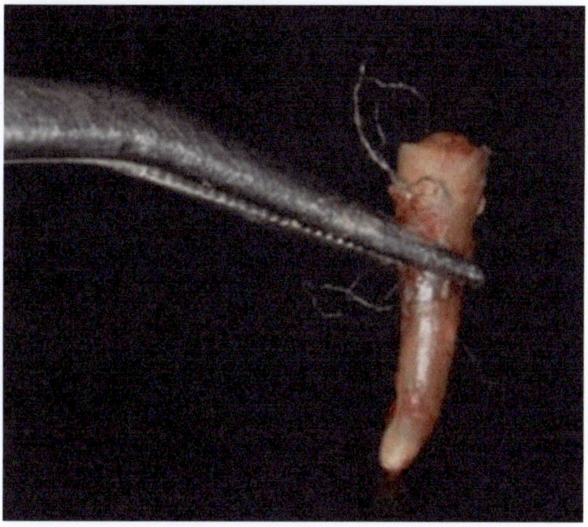

Fig. 11.21 Partial extraction of the lingual and apical portion of the root

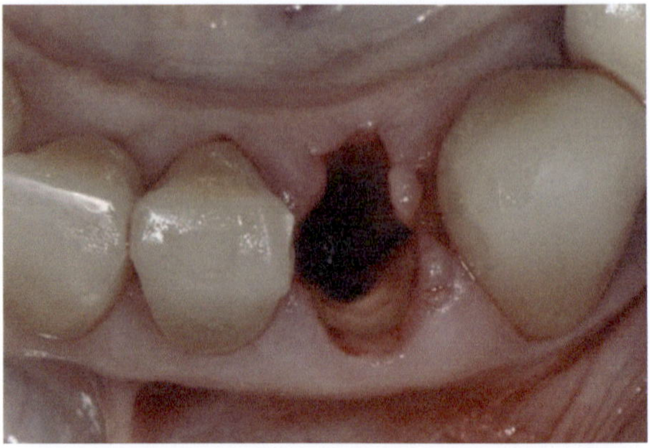

Fig. 11.22 Labial part of the shield preparation

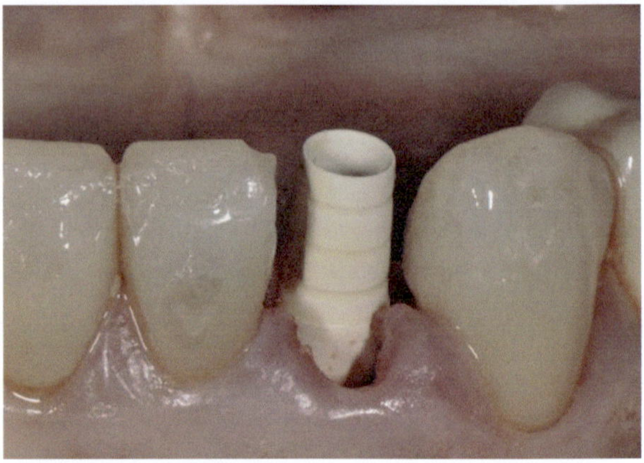

Fig. 11.23 Temporary PEEK abutment

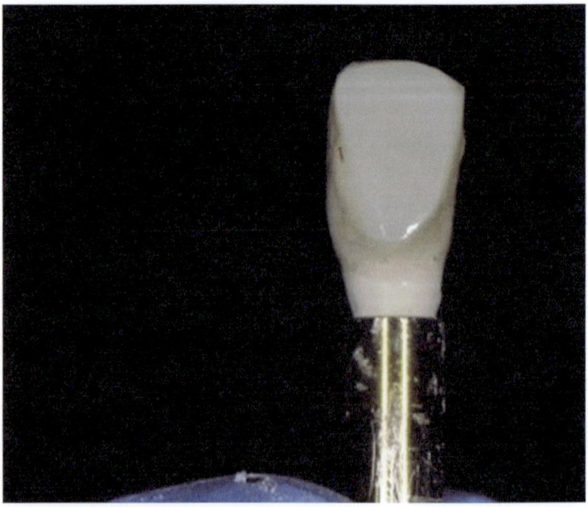

Fig. 11.24 Screw-retained provisional crown

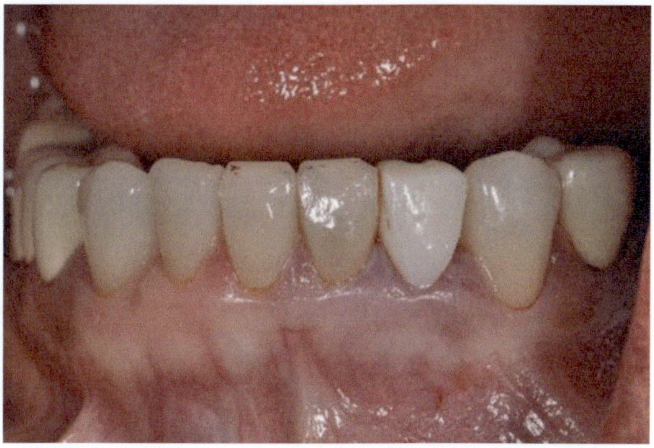

Fig. 11.25 Immediate postoperative view of the screw-retained provisional crown

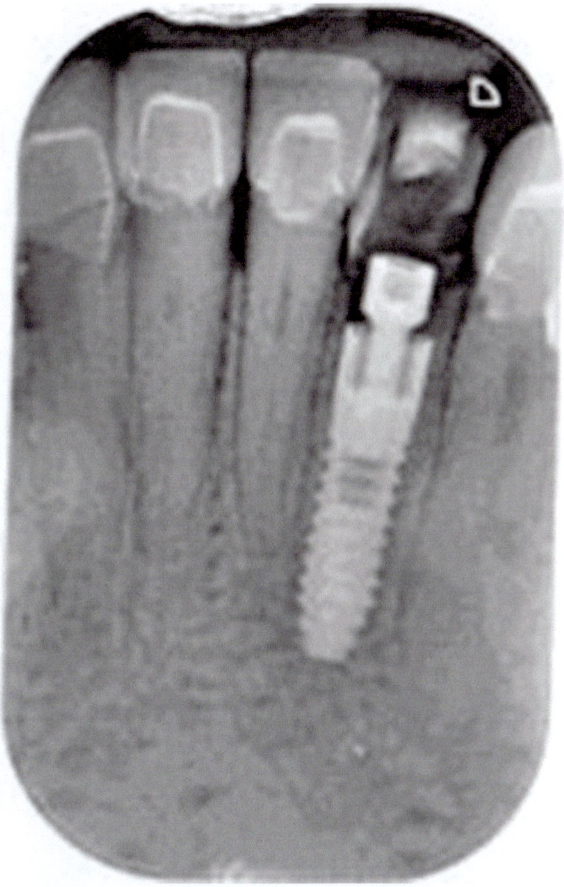

Fig. 11.26 Immediate postoperative view of the implant and screw-retained provisional crown

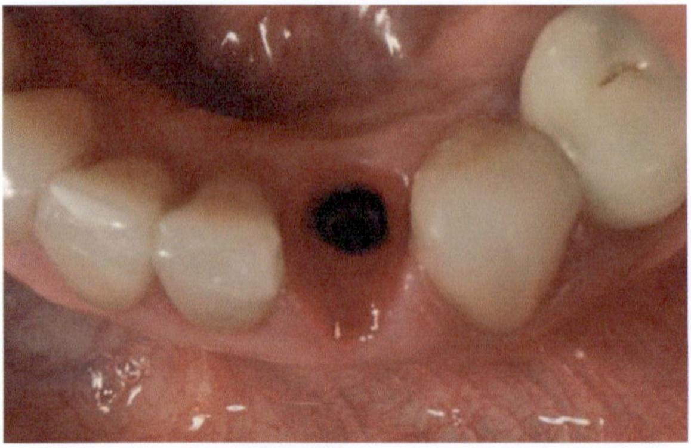

Fig. 11.27 Situation on removal of the provisional crown 3 months after implant placement

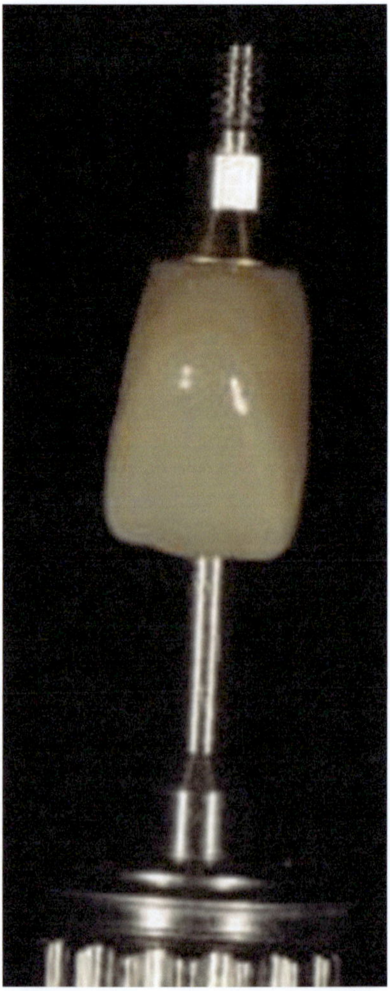

Fig. 11.28 Definitive screw-retained porcelain fused to zirconia restoration

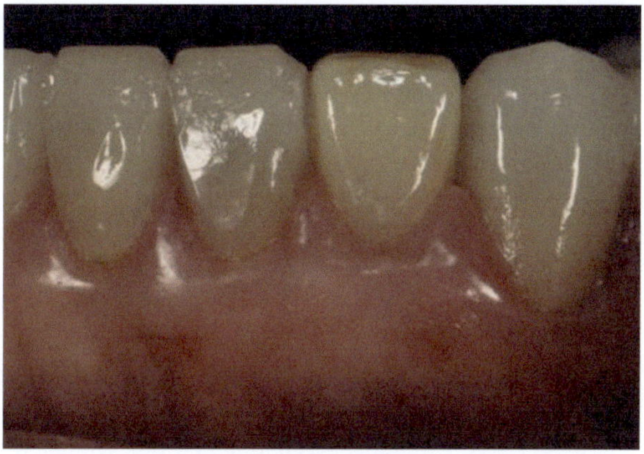

Fig. 11.29 Definitive restoration. Note healthy peri-implant soft tissue

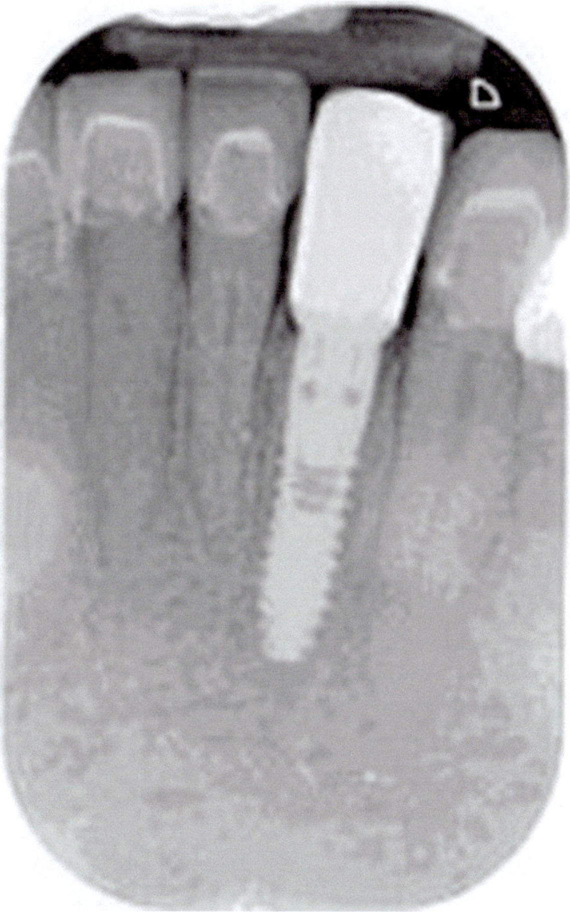

Fig. 11.30 Postoperative radiograph of the final restoration

11.4 Case 3: Single Implant with Mid Treatment Complication and its Management

Surgical & Restorative Dentistry: Dr. Ali Tunkiwala.

Lab Credits: Danesh Vazifdar, Adaro Lab, Mumbai.

Case Details:

A 50-year-old male patient with H/o trauma reported with horizontal fracture of tooth #11. The horizontal fracture was well placed to allow socket shield to be considered. Minor soft tissue edema was present while active infection was absent.

Shield preparation was done and implant placed immediately. The ISQ was 55 and hence the implant was not used to retain a provisional restoration. Bone grafting with Mineross was carried out. Provisional restoration in the form of a Maryland bridge was provided. After 4 months, screw-retained provisional was attached. Two weeks later, when the provisional restoration was removed, there was an internal shield exposure. The exposed area was trimmed and the contours of provisional modified to allow more space for soft tissue ingrowth. The case was finished with a colored zirconia custom abutment and a lithium disilicate crown following a digital impression protocol (Figs. 11.31, 11.32, 11.33, 11.34, 11.35, 11.36, 11.37, 11.38, 11.39, 11.40, 11.41, 11.42, 11.43, 11.44, 11.45, 11.46, 11.47, 11.48, 11.49, 11.50, 11.51, 11.52, 11.53, 11.54, 11.55, 11.56, 11.57, 11.58, 11.59, 11.60, 11.61, 11.62, 11.63, 11.64 and 11.65).

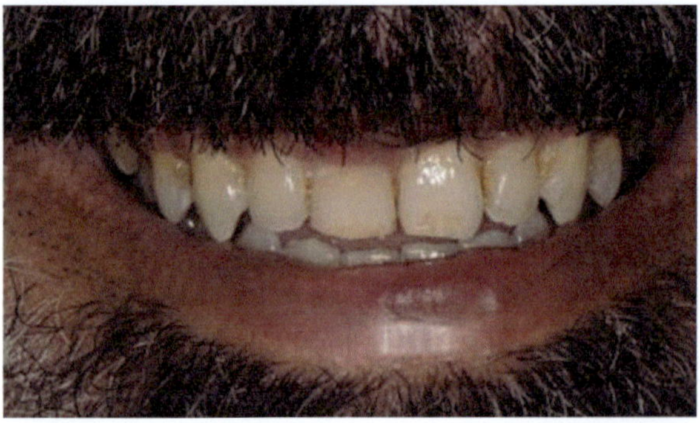

Fig. 11.31 Preoperative smile with fractured #11

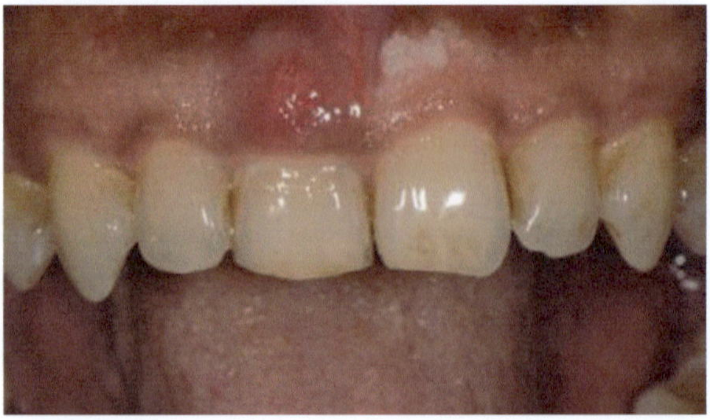

Fig. 11.32 Preoperative close-up view of the offending tooth that had trauma

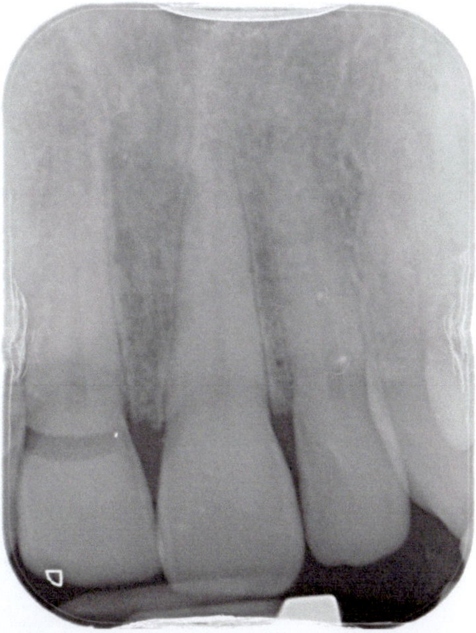

Fig. 11.33 Horizontal fracture in #11 evident

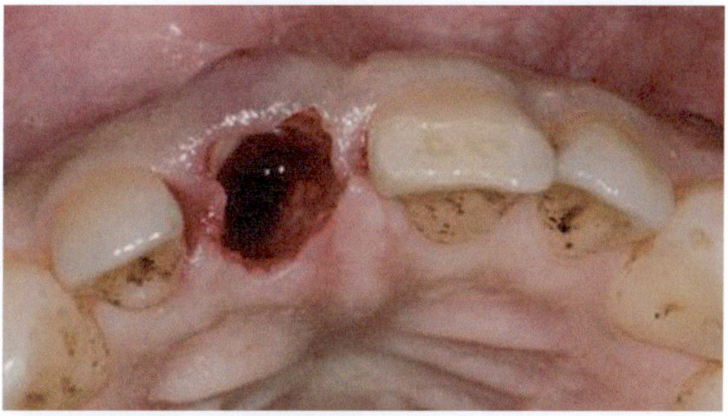

Fig. 11.34 Socket shield prepared

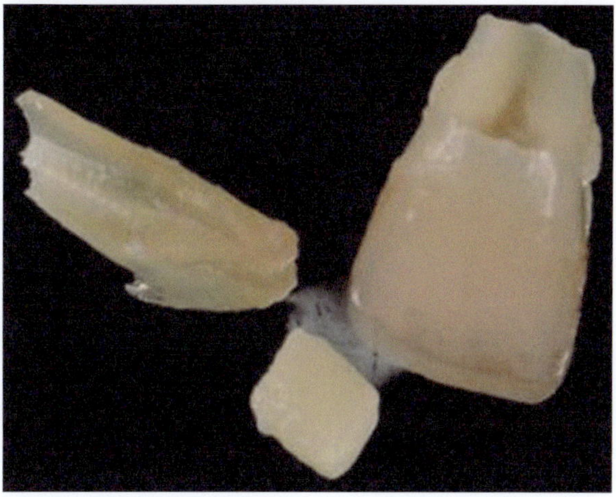

Fig. 11.35 The broken coronal part and the extracted palatal portion with the apex

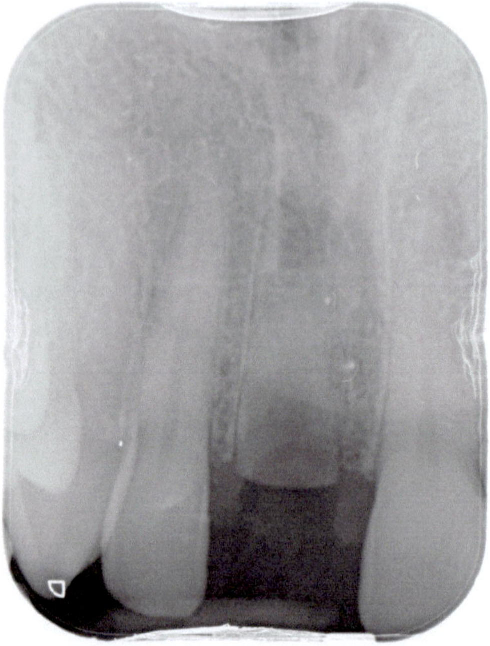

Fig. 11.36 The radiograph showing the prepared shield and verifying the apex removal

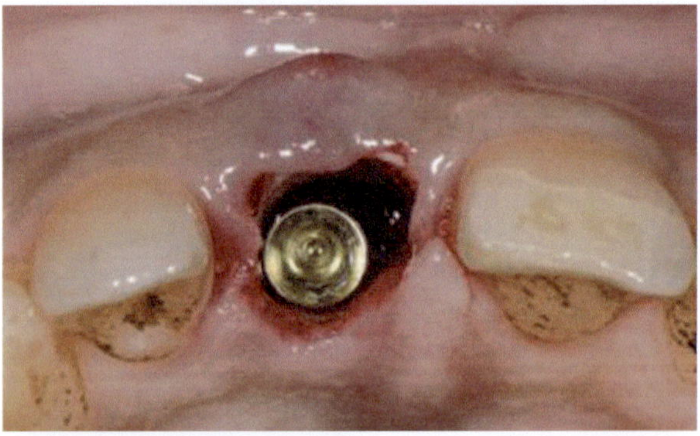

Fig. 11.37 Implant placed with a large gap between the two entities in the socket

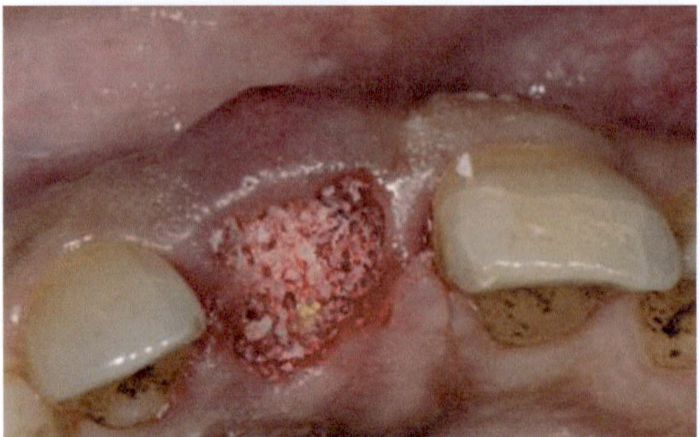

Fig. 11.38 Bone graft added to fill the gap

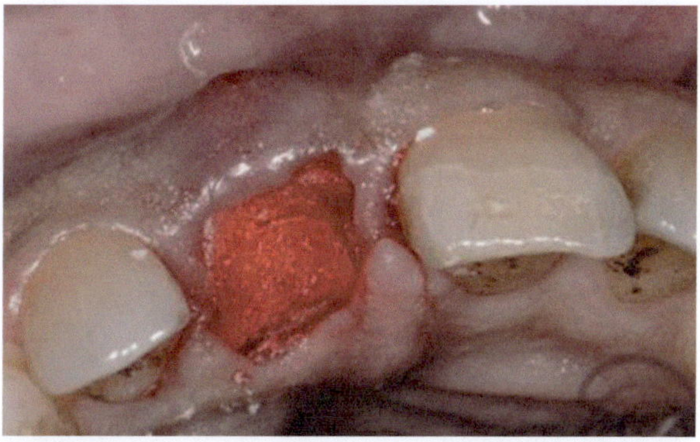

Fig. 11.39 Collagen membrane tucked in to protect the graft

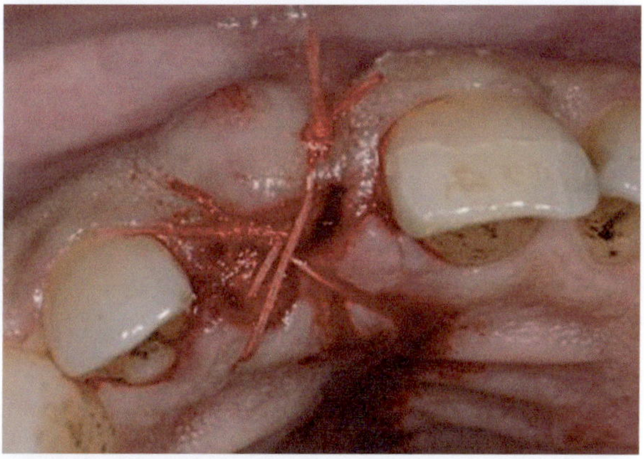

Fig. 11.40 Holding sutures

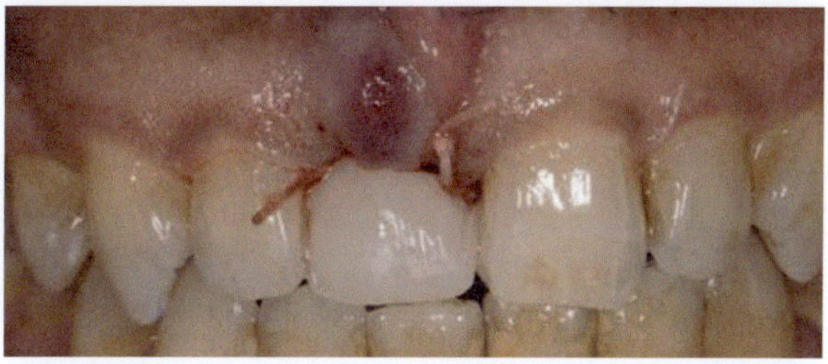

Fig. 11.41 Maryland bridge in situ at 48 h. The patient's low lip line helped in keeping the provisional restoration short at the gingival aspect

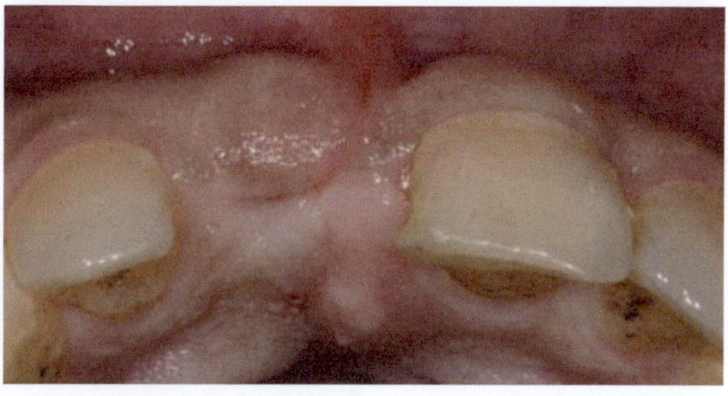

Fig. 11.42 Healed site at 4 months. Observe the excellent tissue contours maintained

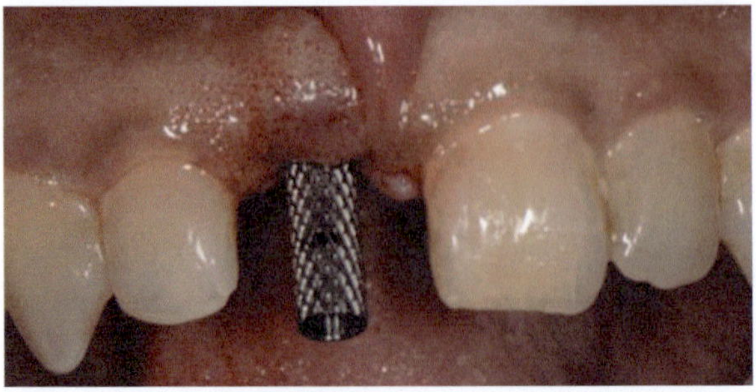

Fig. 11.43 Temporary cylinder attached to support a screw-retained provisional restoration

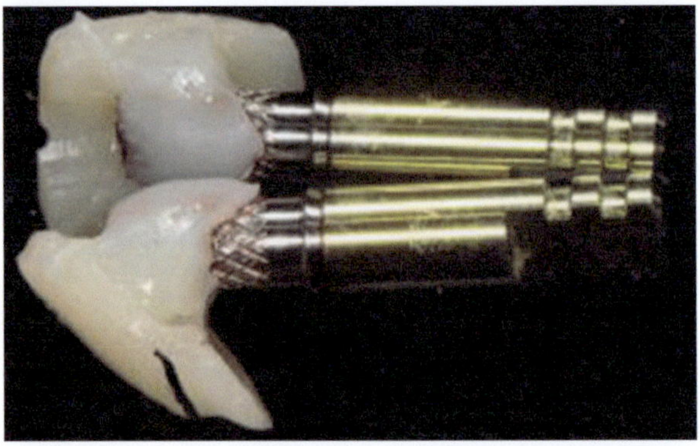

Fig. 11.44 Provisional resin shell attached to the cylinder intraorally

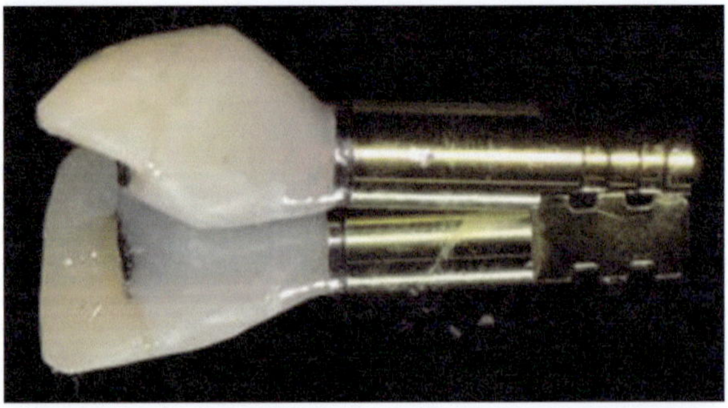

Fig. 11.45 Provisional restoration customized to act as a scaffold for the gingival architecture

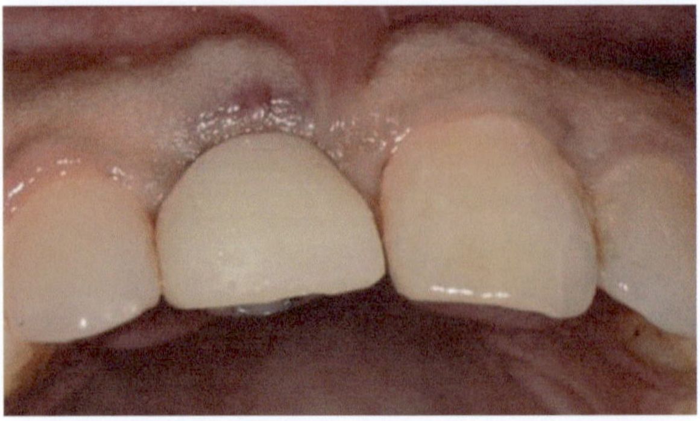

Fig. 11.46 Provisional restoration in situ

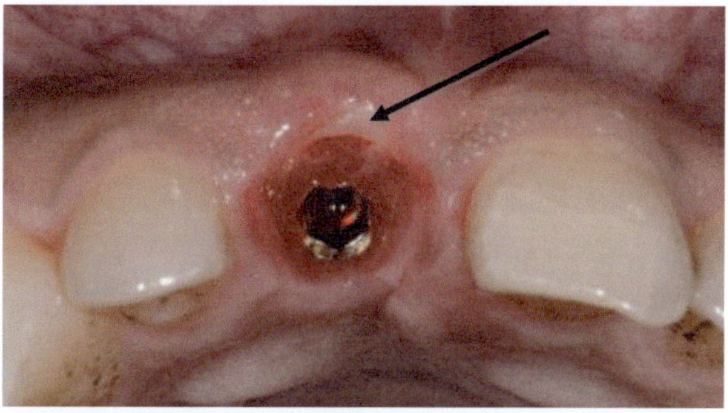

Fig. 11.47 Internal shield exposure evident when provisional restoration was unscrewed at 2 weeks

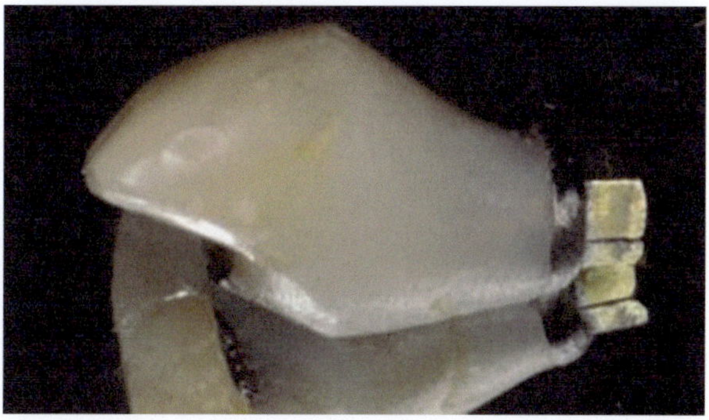

Fig. 11.48 Convex emergence modified into a better S-shaped concave emergence. This will allow the necessary space for the soft tissues

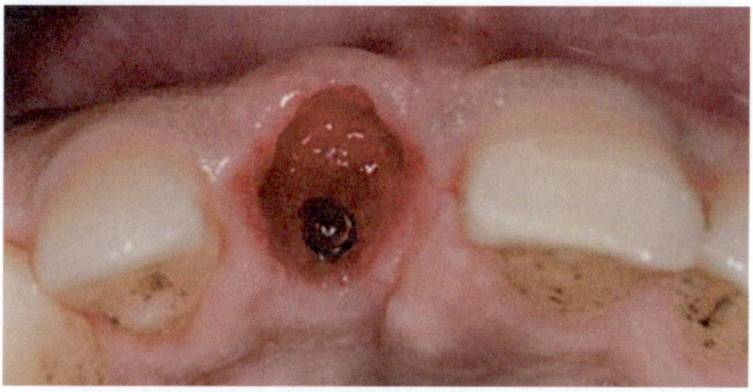

Fig. 11.49 The internal exposure managed with trimming of the shield

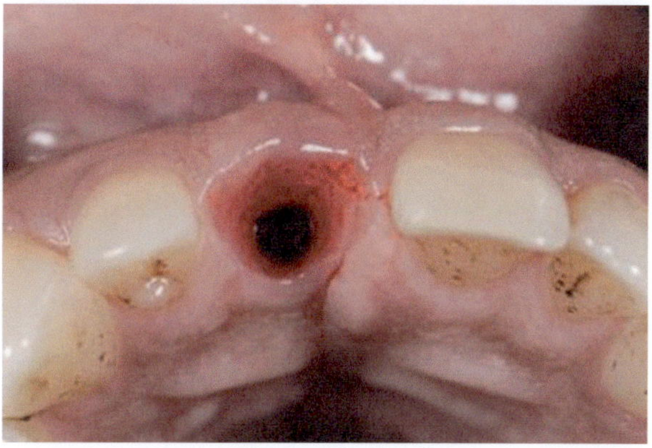

Fig. 11.50 Well healed site at 6 weeks after internal exposure management

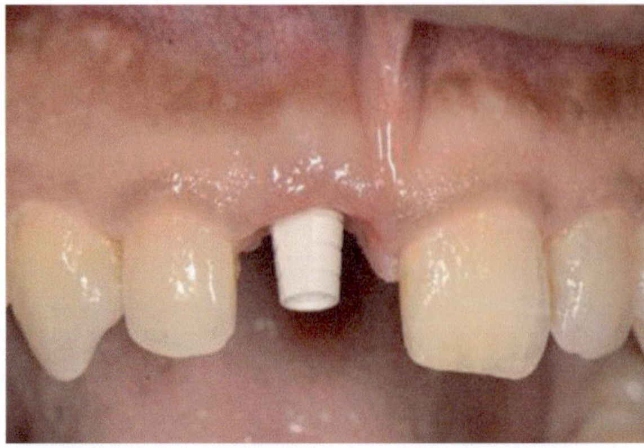

Fig. 11.51 Digital impressions using intraoral scan body

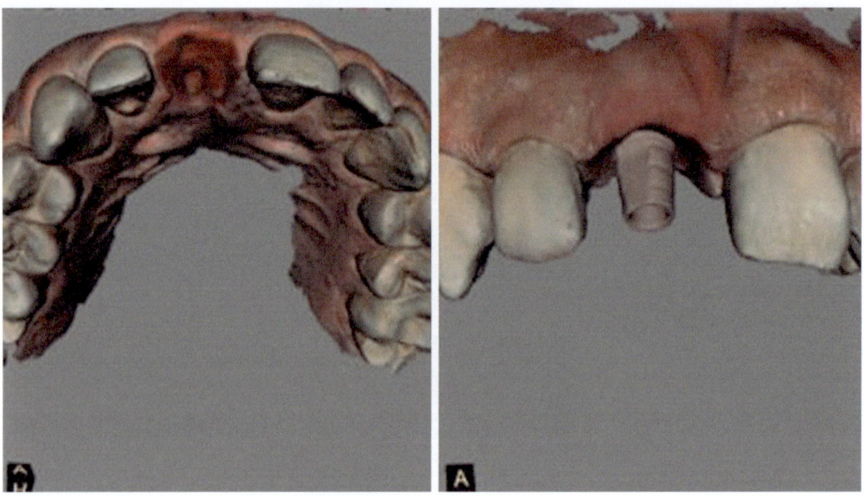

Fig. 11.52 The data of the gingival architecture and the implant position sent to the lab

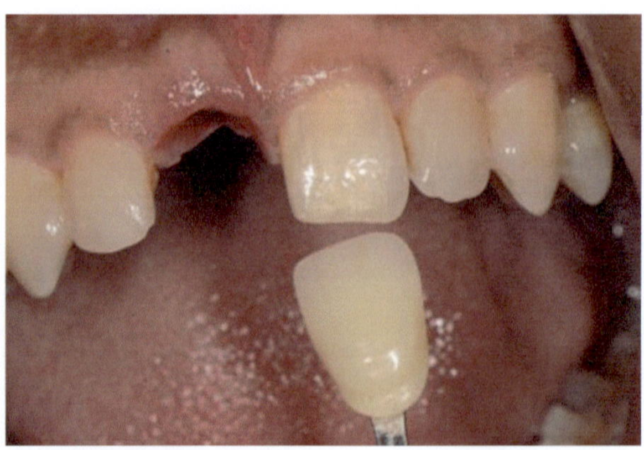

Fig. 11.53 Shade tab picture. Single anterior teeth are the most difficult to match

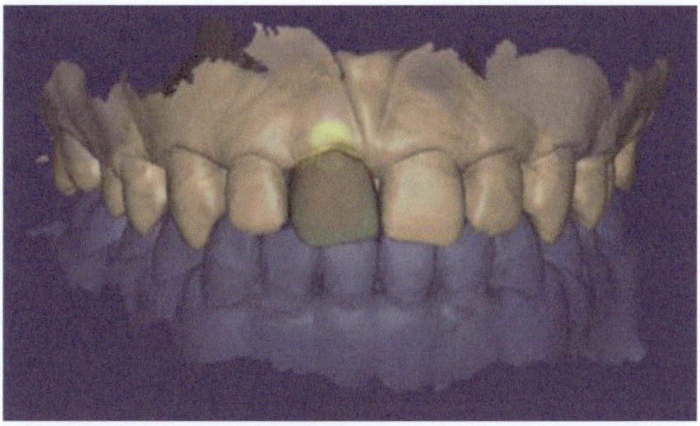

Fig. 11.54 The process of designing the custom abutment and crown

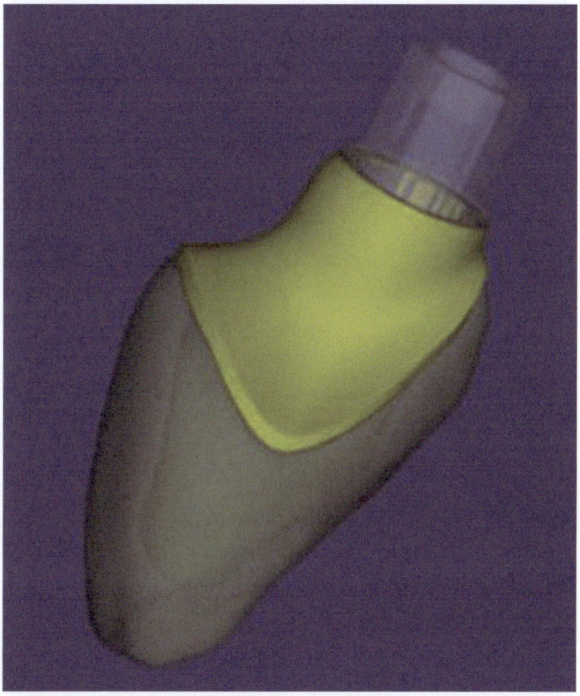

Fig. 11.55 The subgingival contour of the provisional can be copied onto the final abutment design

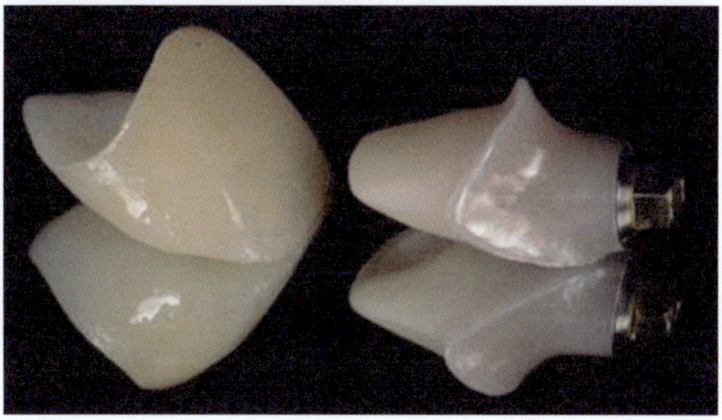

Fig. 11.56 Custom colored zirconia abutment with accurately reproduced critical and subcritical contour

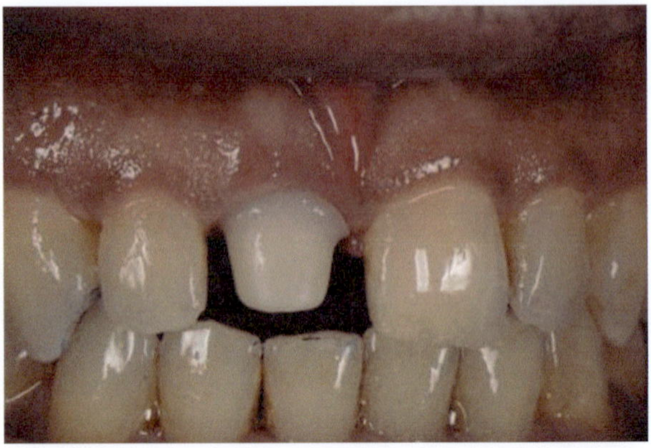

Fig. 11.57 Custom zirconia abutment secured and torqued in place

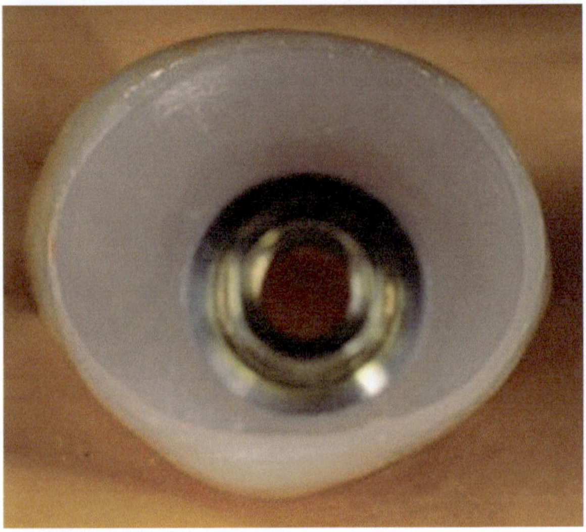

Fig. 11.58 View of abutment and crown from the gingival aspect

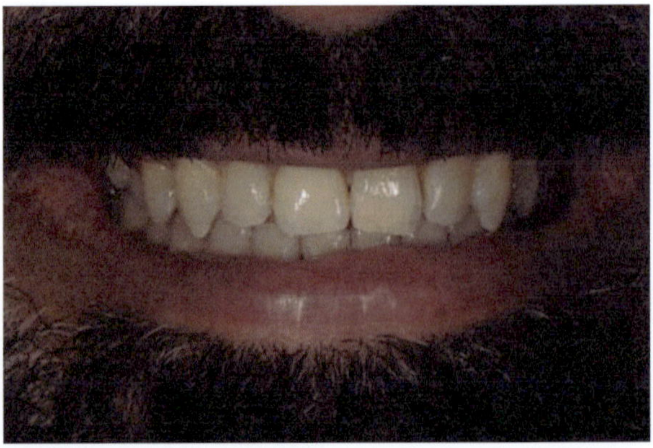

Fig. 11.59 Postoperative smile

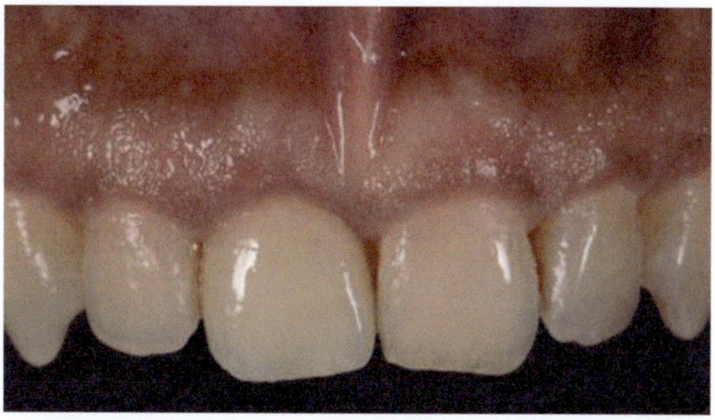

Fig. 11.60 Frontal close-up view

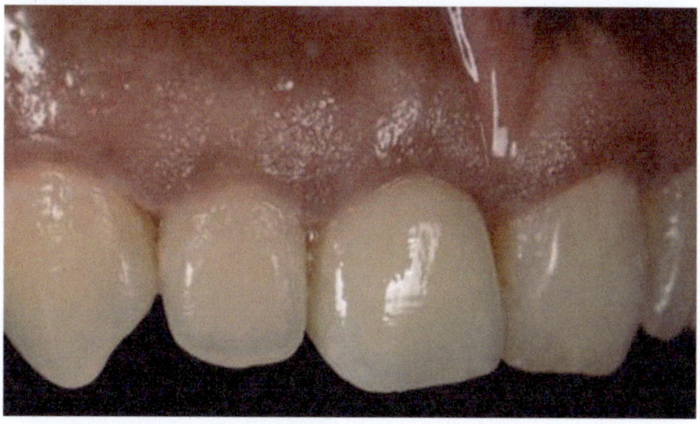

Fig. 11.61 Right close-up view depicts excellent tissue health and contours

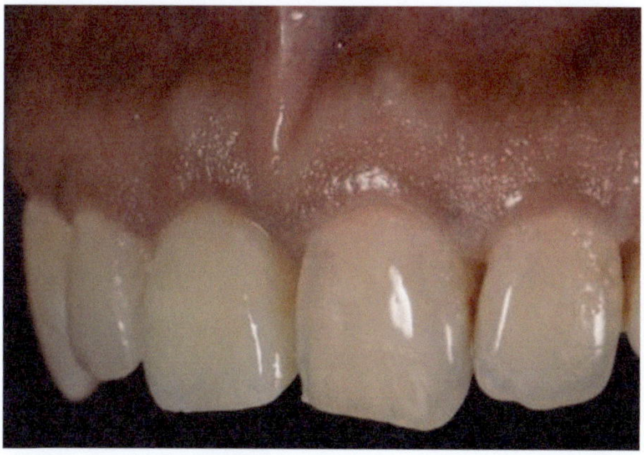

Fig. 11.62 Left close-up view depicts acceptable emergence of #11

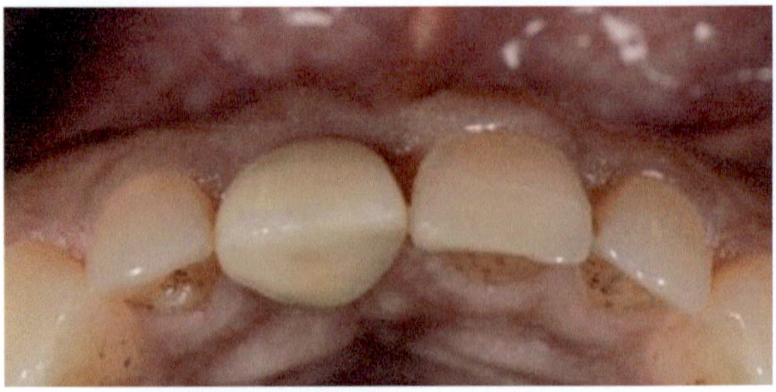

Fig. 11.63 Occlusal view depicts well maintained labial contours at par with adjacent teeth

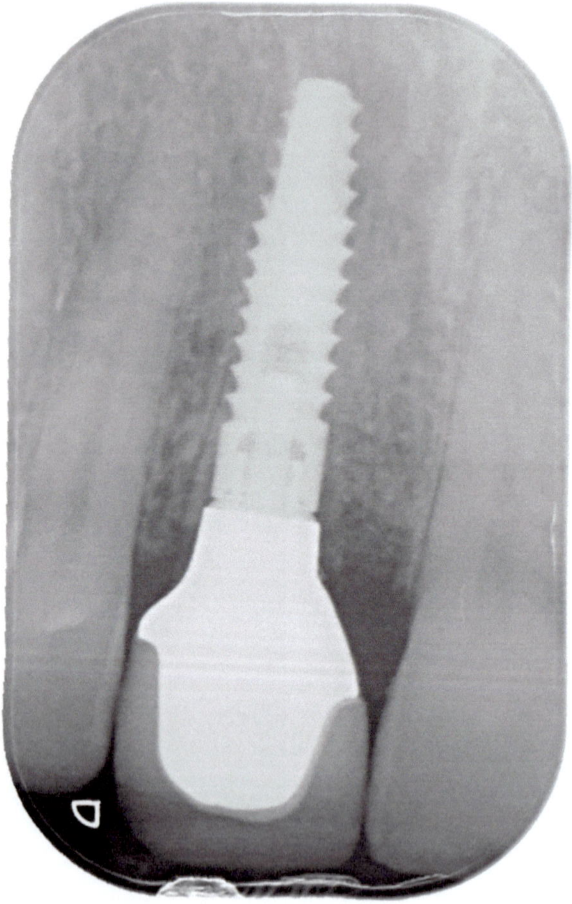

Fig. 11.64 Intraoral radiograph showing excellent bone levels at baseline

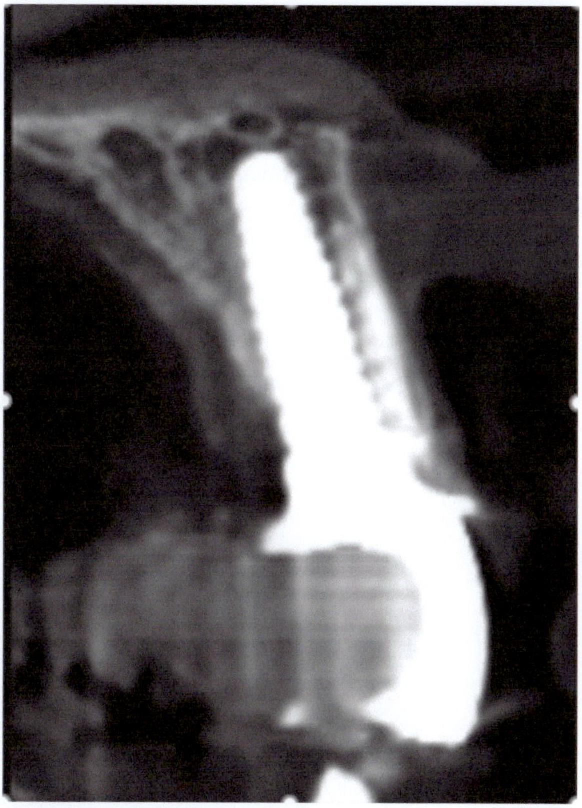

Fig. 11.65 Postoperative CBCT showing the shield and the implant with the contours of the buccal bone intact.

11.5 Case 4: Single Canine in Maxillary Arch. Socket Shield with Immediate Placement

Surgical Dentistry: Dr. Udatta Kher.

Restorative dentistry: Dr. Praveen Advani.

Lab credits: Dentech Lab.

A 32-year-old man reported with a fractured tooth 33. Part of the tooth on the palatal side was fractured subgingivally but above the bone crest.

Challenges

1. The root had an unusual trajectory and was inclined distally.
2. Root trajectory not aligned to ideal implant location.
3. Very long root of the canine.

Since the tooth was unrestorable, a socket shield procedure was done. The challenge in the case was the sectioning of the long canine root and unfavorable implant trajectory. The implant placement trajectory had to be changed during the course of the osteotomy to place the implant in an ideal 3-D position. Since the patient's occlusal scheme was not favorable, an immediate provisional restoration was not made. Instead a healing abutment was placed on the day of the surgery. The definitive porcelain fused to metal crown was made after 3 months of healing (Figs. 11.66, 11.67, 11.68, 11.69, 11.70, 11.71, 11.72, 11.73, 11.74, 11.75, 11.76 and 11.77).

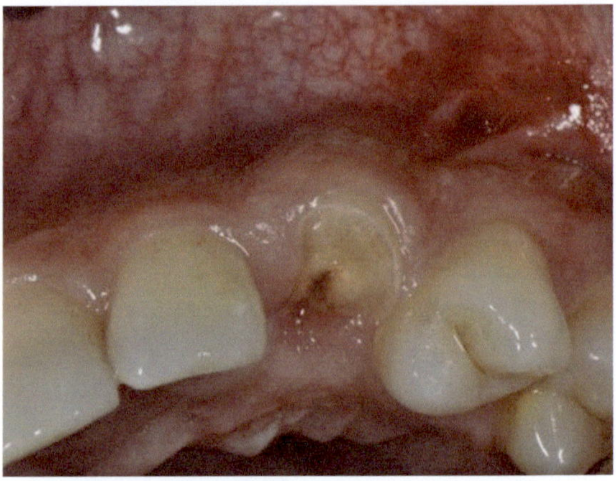

Fig. 11.66 Fractured tooth # 23

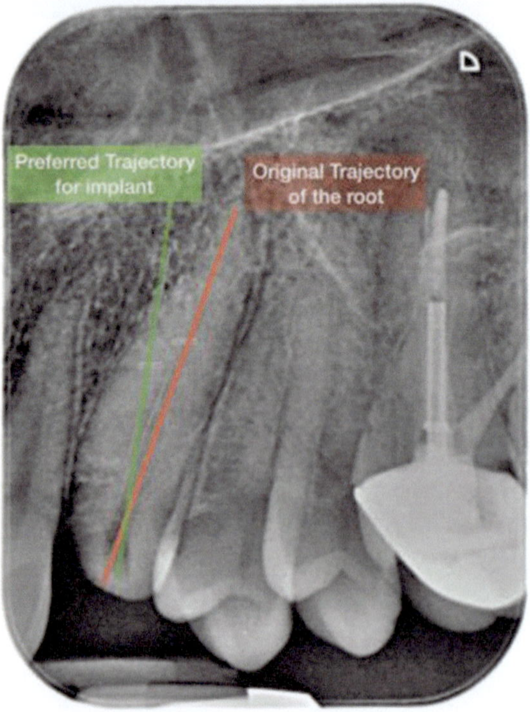

Fig. 11.67 Radiograph of the fractured canine

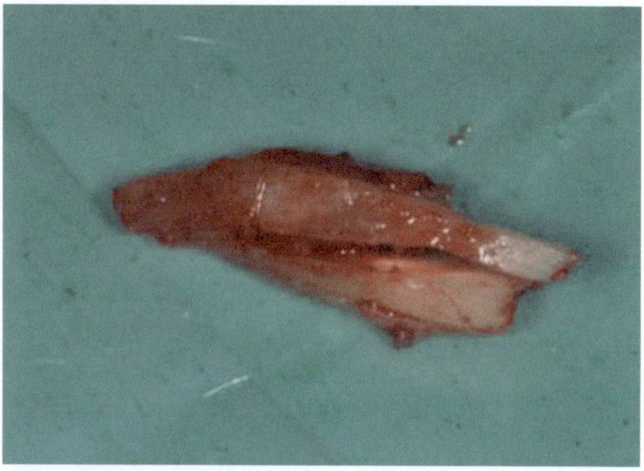

Fig. 11.68 Partial extraction of the long canine root

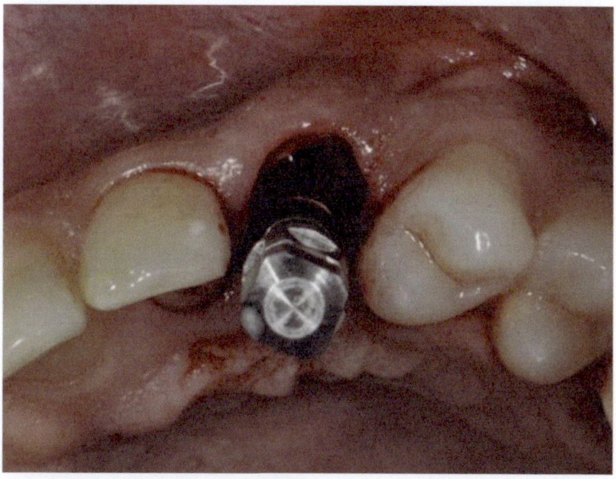

Fig. 11.69 Osteotomy of implant placement in the palatal wall of the extraction socket

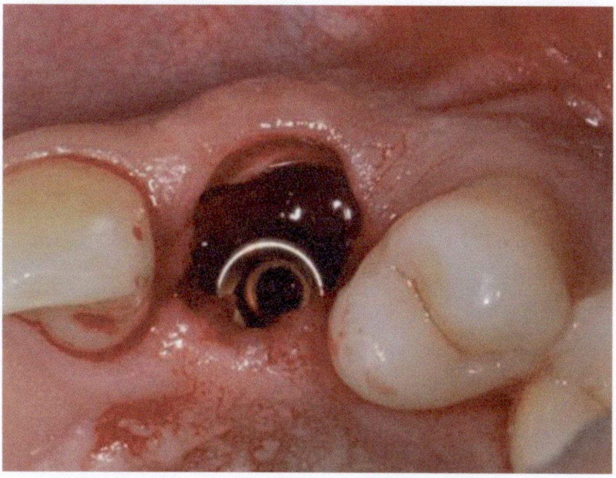

Fig. 11.70 Prosthetically driven implant placement in a three-dimensional position

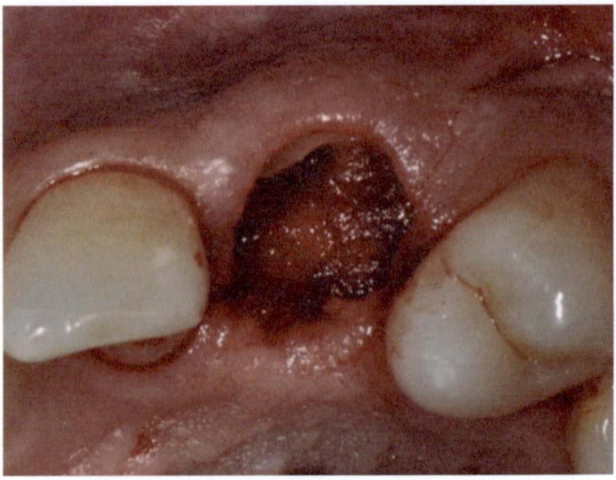

Fig. 11.71 Collagen sponge used to cover the socket and allow secondary intention wound healing

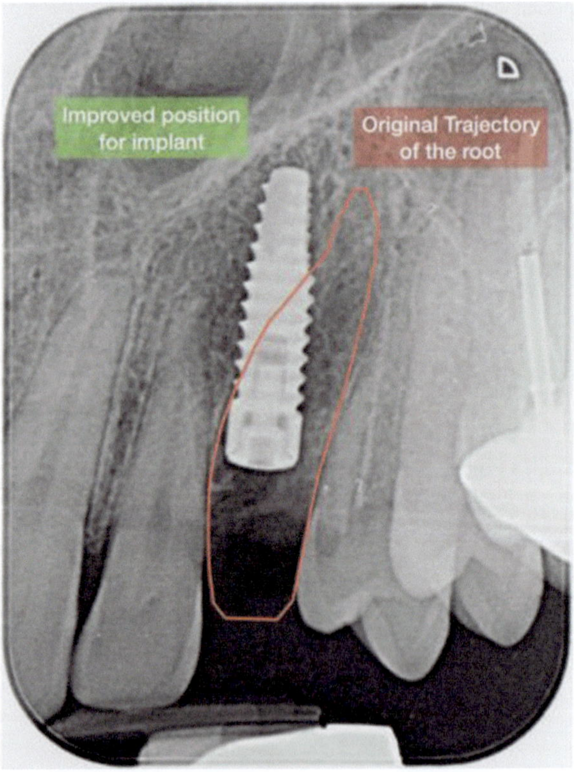

Fig. 11.72 Immediate postoperative radiograph depicting original root trajectory and the corrected implant position

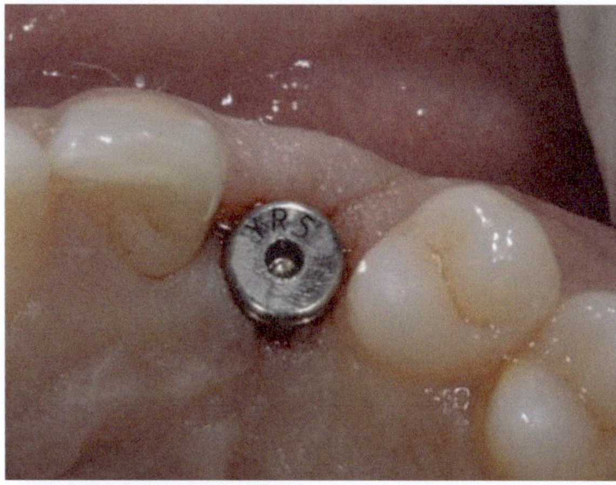

Fig. 11.73 Situation after 3 months with healing abutment

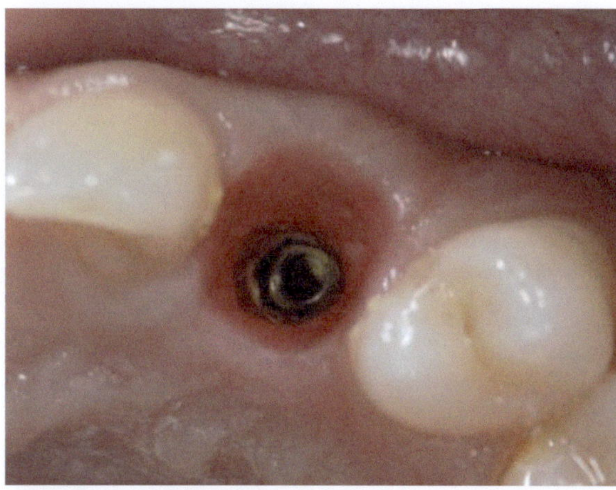

Fig. 11.74 View of the implant and healthy peri-implant tissue on removal of the healing abutment

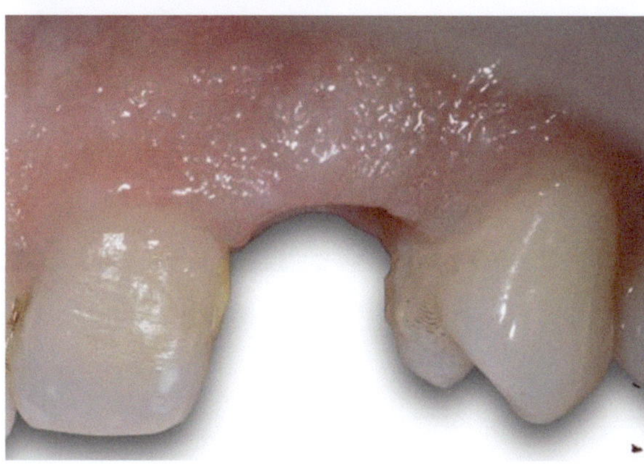

Fig. 11.75 Ideal soft tissue contours

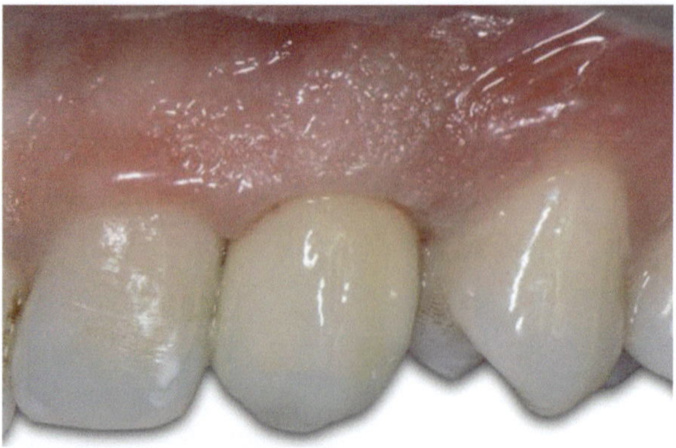

Fig. 11.76 Definitive screw-retained porcelain fused to metal restoration

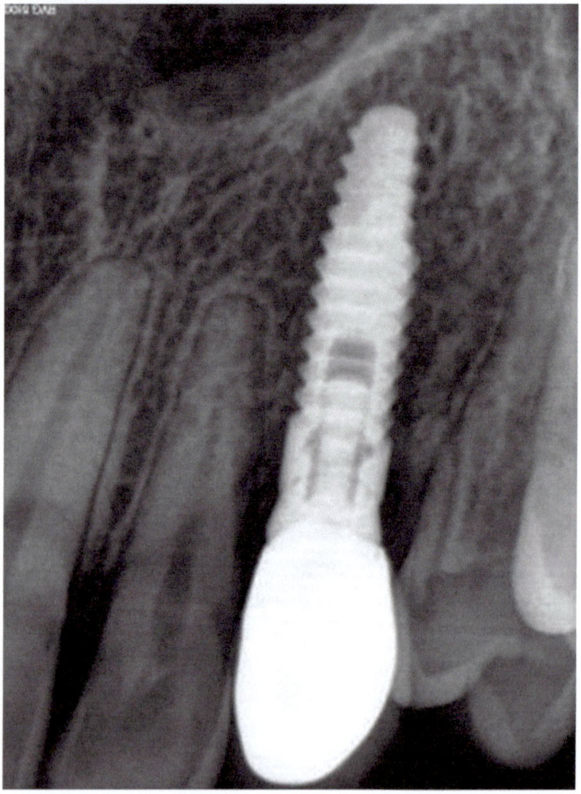

Fig. 11.77 Postoperative radiograph of the restored implant and good crestal bone levels

11.6 Case 5: Single Implant with Socket Shield in Upper Incisor Along with Esthetic Buccal Flap to Remove the Apical Infection

Surgical and restorative Dentistry: Dr. Udatta Kher.

Lab credits: Katara Dental, Pune.

A 38-year-old female reported with fractured 21. Teeth 11 and 21 had old lithium disilicate restorations. Tooth 11 was discolored due to the old endodontic treatment. The discoloration was seen through the translucent lithium disilicate crown.

Challenges

1. Tooth in the esthetic zone with an adjacent tooth that has been previously restored with a crown.
2. Fabrication of a suitable provisional restoration to match the contra lateral restoration.

Since the tooth was badly decayed and was non-restorable, a socket shield procedure was done and an implant was placed in an ideal 3D position. The patient's existing crown was modified and used to fabricate a chairside provisional restoration. The definitive restoration was screw-retained zirconia crown with layered lithium disilicate (Figs. 11.78, 11.79, 11.80, 11.81, 11.82, 11.83, 11.84, 11.85, 11.86, 11.87, 11.88, 11.89, 11.90, 11.91, 11.92, 11.93, 11.94, 11.95, 11.96 and 11.97).

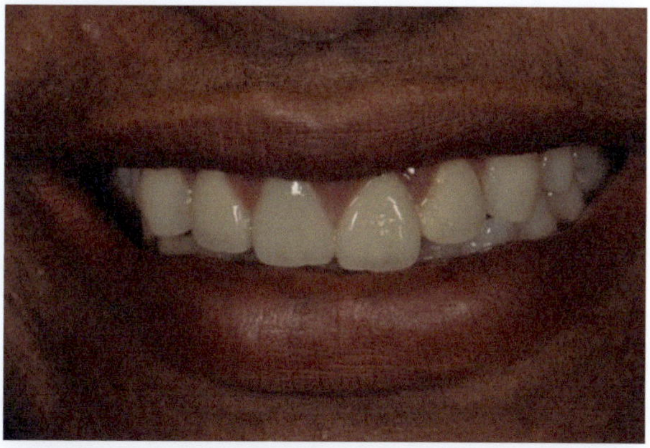

Fig. 11.78 Preoperative smile view

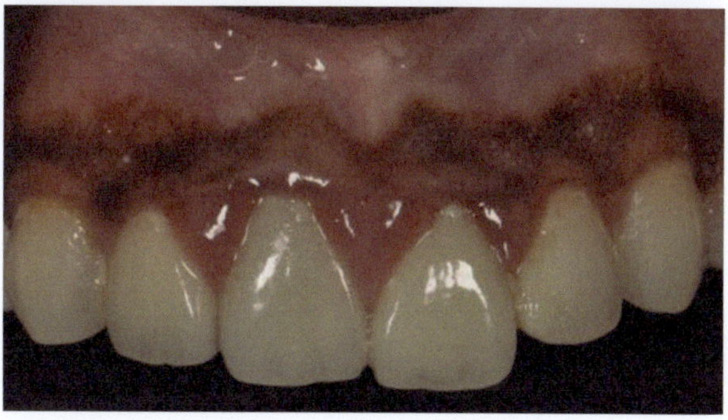

Fig. 11.79 Preoperative view showing crowns on teeth #11 and 21. Tooth #21 was fractured at the cementoenamel junction leading to mobility of the crown

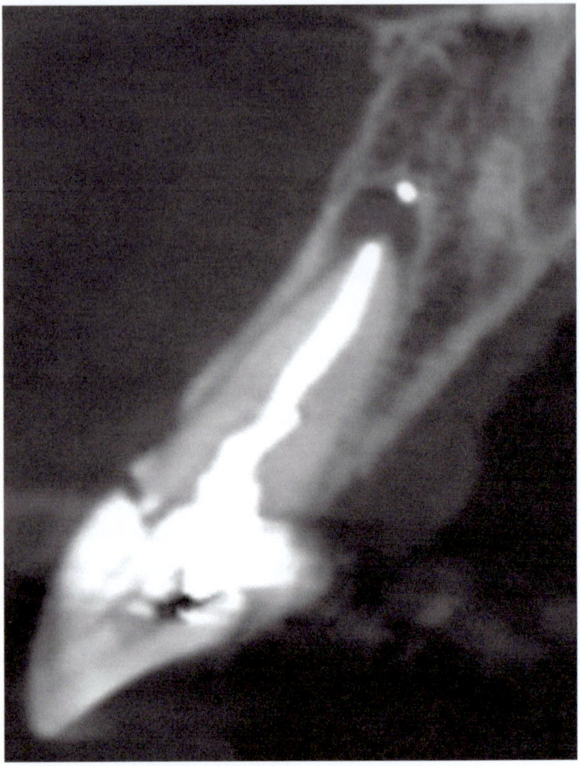

Fig. 11.80 CBCT showing fractured crown of tooth #21 and a periapical lesion

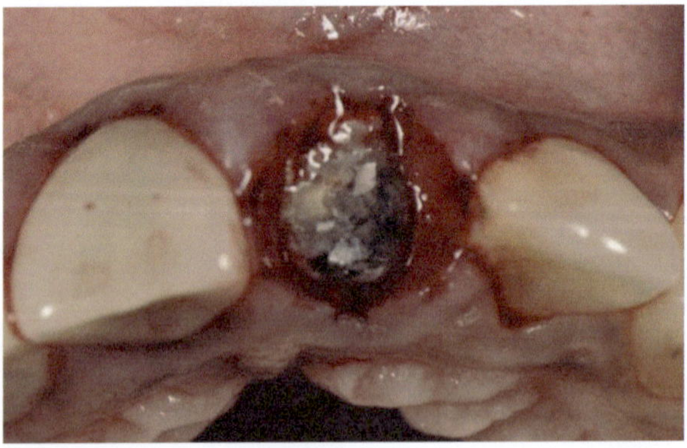

Fig. 11.81 View after removal of the mobile crown. Underlying tooth is extensively decayed

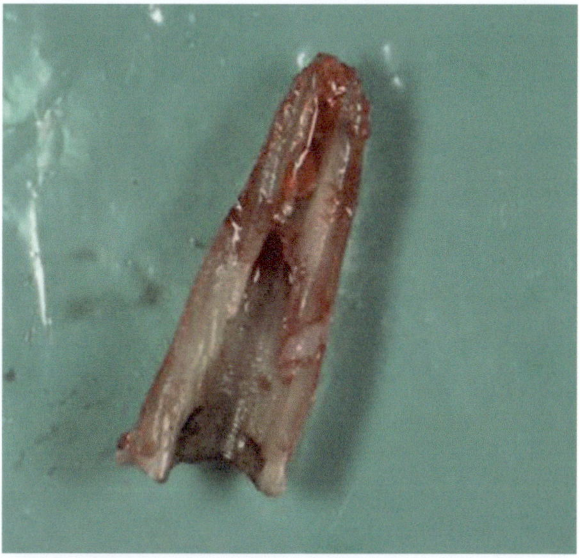

Fig. 11.82 Partial extraction of the root. Note section going through the root canal space and includes the apex of the root

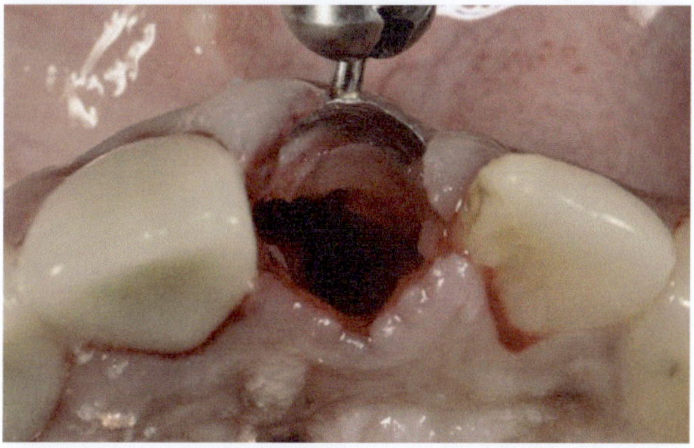

Fig. 11.83 Shield preparation done. Note gingival retractor to prevent damage to soft tissue

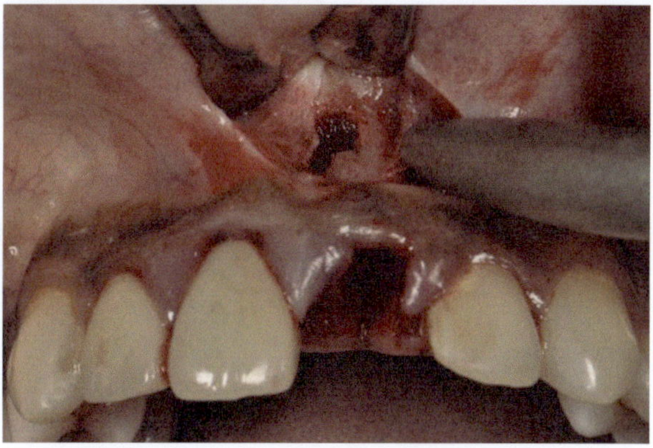

Fig. 11.84 Esthetic buccal flap to access periapical region

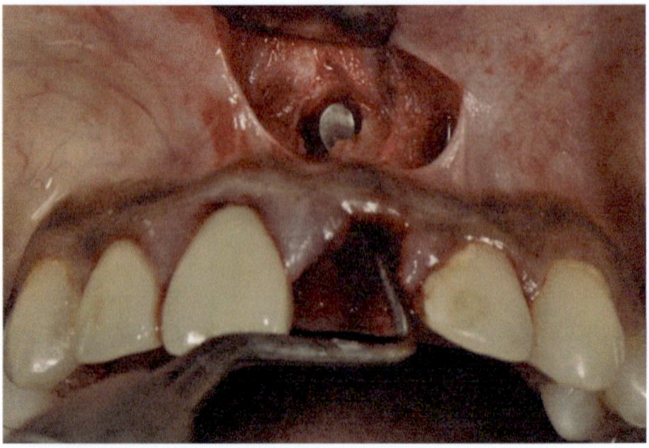

Fig. 11.85 Fenestration defect seen. Thorough curettage done to eliminate periapical pathology

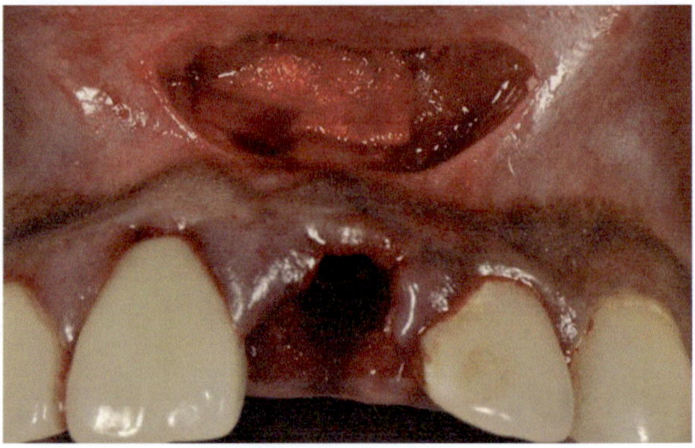

Fig. 11.86 Apical defect grafted with bone substitute material and covered with collagen membrane

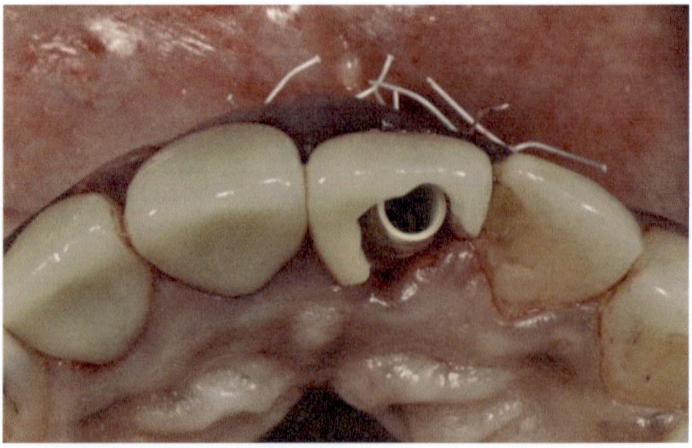

Fig. 11.87 Temporary PEEK abutment for fabrication of a chairside provisional crown. Patient's existing crown used as a veneer for the screw-retained provisional crown

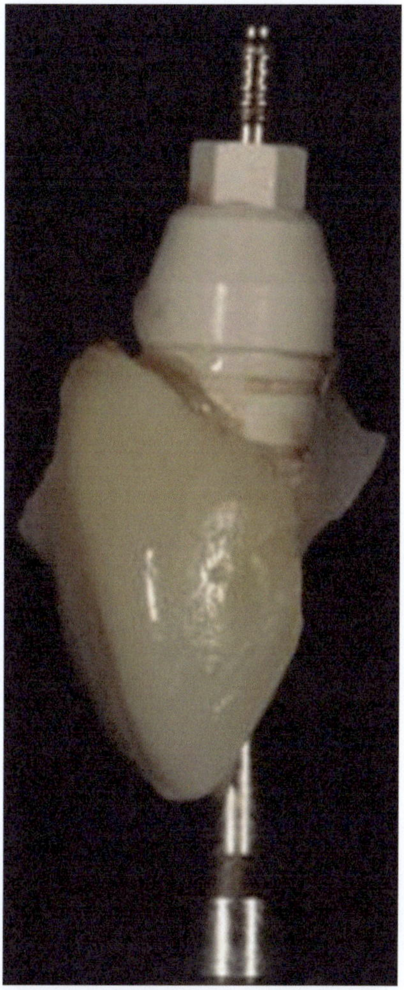

Fig. 11.88 Intra-oral pick up done using flowable composite resin

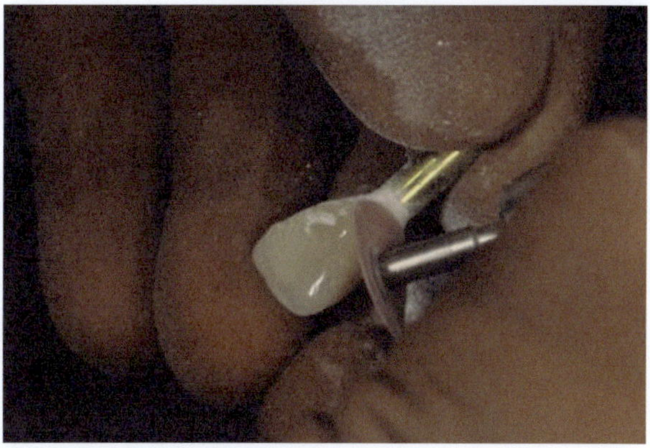

Fig. 11.89 Finishing and polishing of the provisional restoration

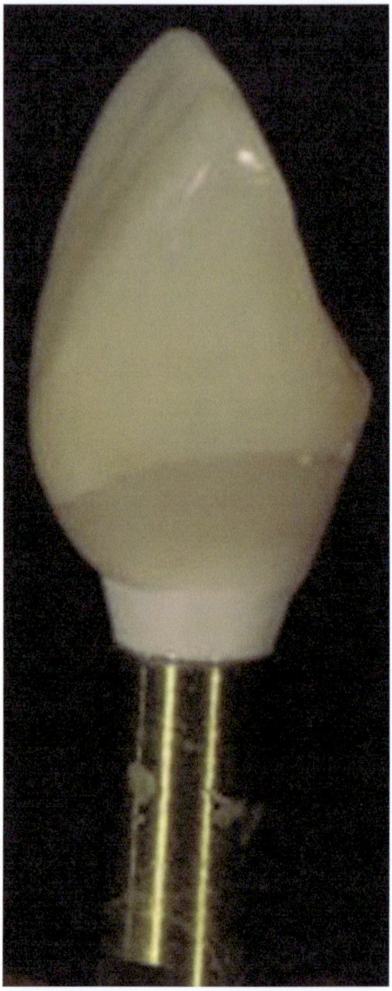

Fig. 11.90 Screw-retained restoration. Patient's existing crown forms the veneer for the provisional crown

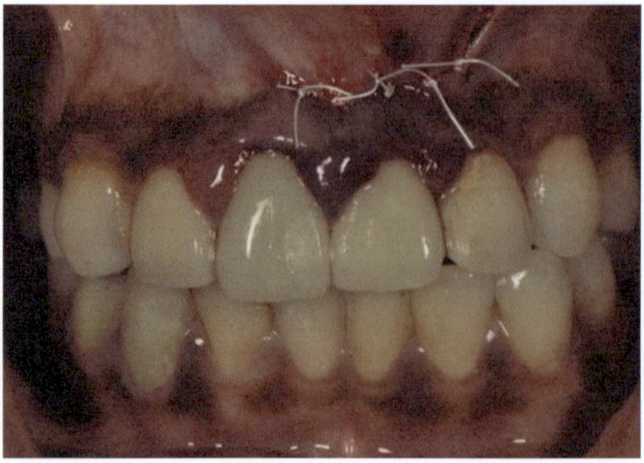

Fig. 11.91 Provisional crown fixed over the implant. Soft tissue closure done to cover apical defect and graft

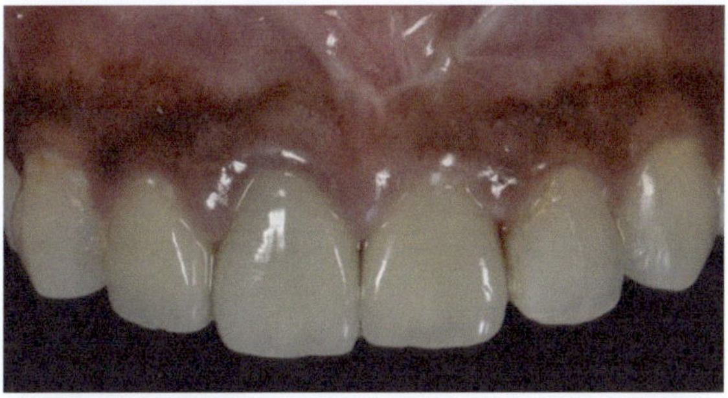

Fig. 11.92 Situation after 3 months. Note excellent soft tissue healing around provisional restoration

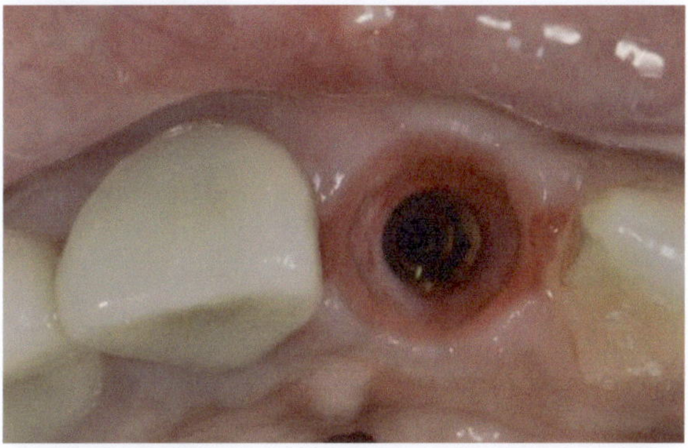

Fig. 11.93 View of peri-implant soft tissue after removal of the provisional restoration. Note healthy cuff of tissue surrounding the osseointegrated implant

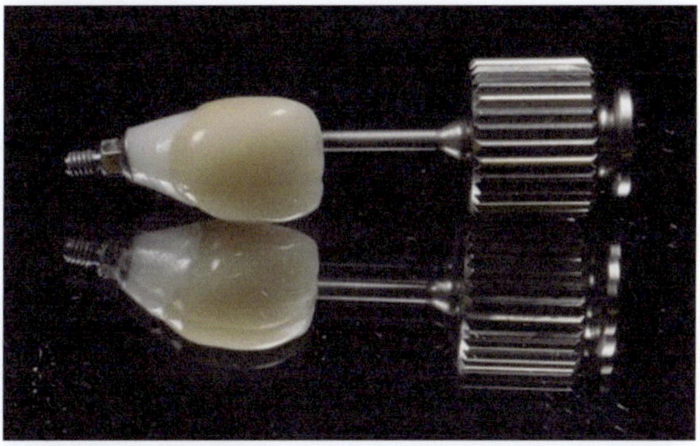

Fig. 11.94 Zirconia-based screw-retained restoration layered with lithium dilsilicate

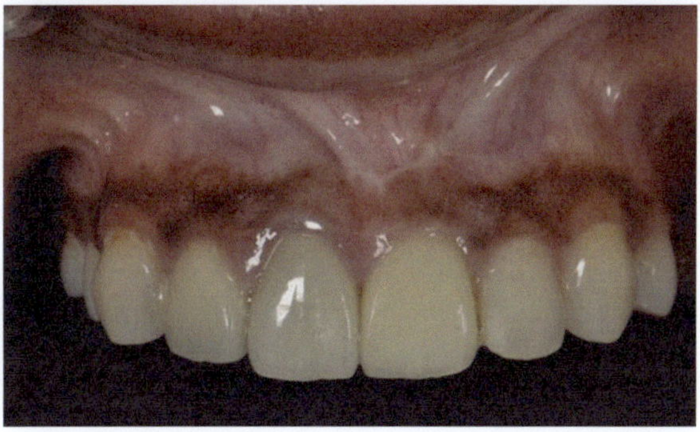

Fig. 11.95 Postoperative view displaying healthy soft tissue around the definitive restoration

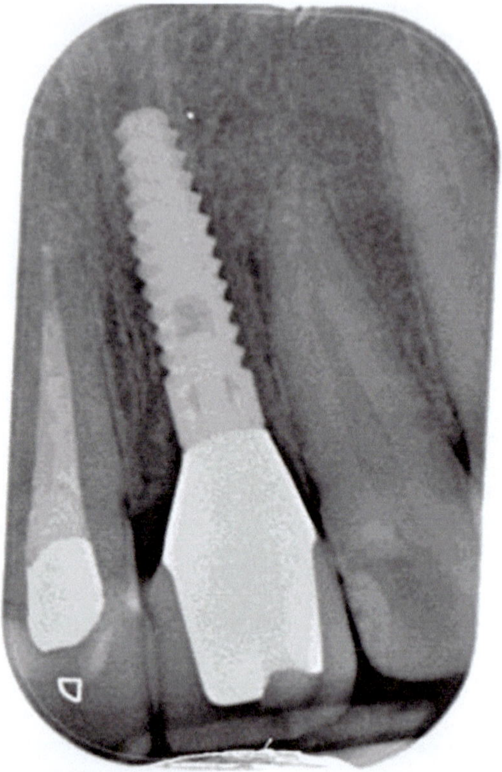

Fig. 11.96 Postoperative radiograph showing maintenance of proximal crestal bone levels

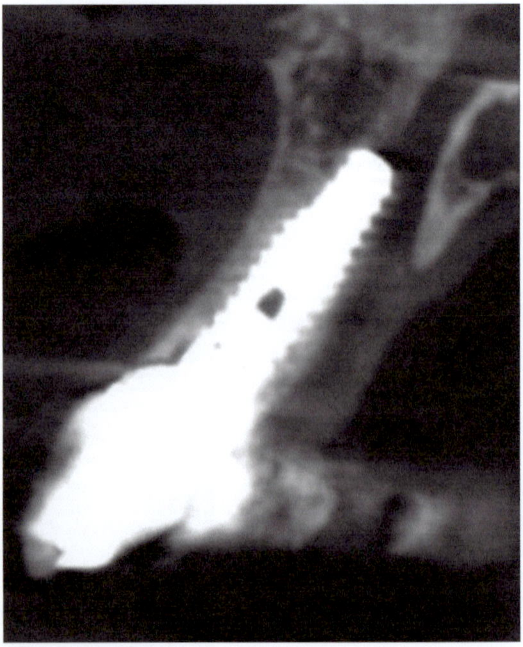

Fig. 11.97 Postoperative CBCT showing complete resolution of the periapical infection, the socket shield, and maintenance of the labial bone

11.7 Adjacent Implants in Aesthetic Zone with Socket Shield

11.7.1 Case 6: Adjacent Incisors PET with Overall Enhancement of Smile

Surgical & Restorative Dentistry: Dr. Ali Tunkiwala.

Lab Credits: Danesh Vazifdar, Adaro Lab, Mumbai.

A 50-year-old healthy female patient reported with non-restorable upper central incisors and upper right lateral incisor. Socket shield was done for centrals and root submergence for right lateral. The greatest challenge in this case was to manage the implants with the rest of the restorations on adjacent teeth and sequencing it all so that the patient gets a well-integrated end result. Veneers and full coverage restorations were made as needed to get the smile designed correctly, encompassing second bicuspids on each side (Figs. 11.98, 11.99, 11.100, 11.101, 11.102, 11.103, 11.104, 11.105, 11.106, 11.107, 11.108, 11.109, 11.110, 11.111, 11.112, 11.113, 11.114, 11.115, 11.116, 11.117, 11.118, 11.119, 11.120, 11.121, 11.122, 11.123, 11.124, 11.125, 11.126, 11.127, 11.128, 11.129, 11.130, 11.131, 11.132, 11.133 and 11.134).

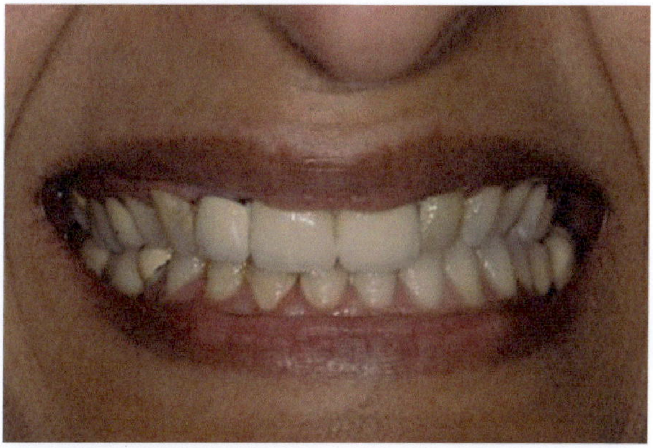

Fig. 11.98 Preoperative smile showing the need for a comprehensive treatment

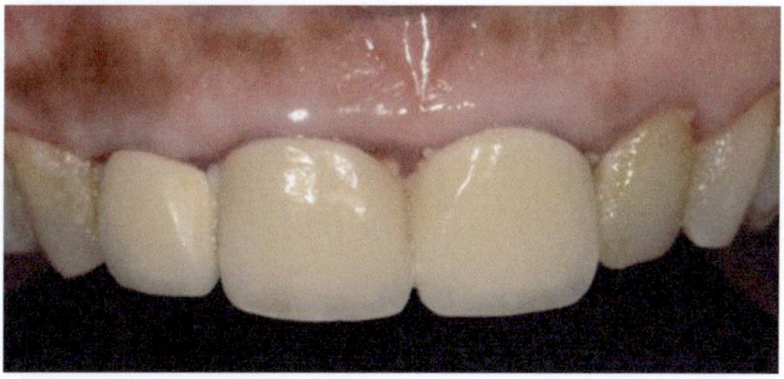

Fig. 11.99 Close up of upper anterior with faulty crowns and leaky margins

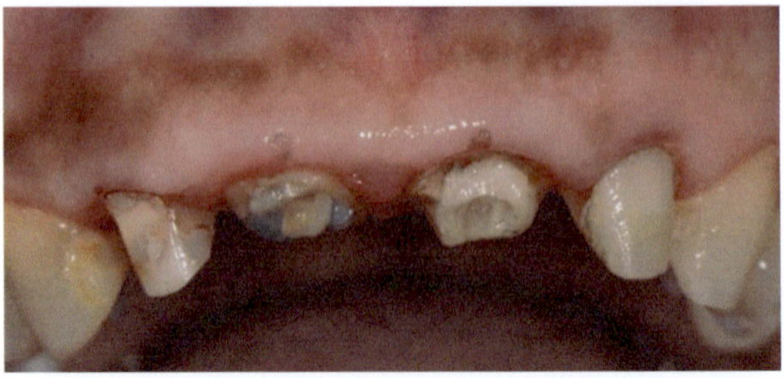

Fig. 11.100 The situation of underlying teeth after removal of old restorations. #11, #21 were planned implant sites with socket shield and #12 was planned root submergence

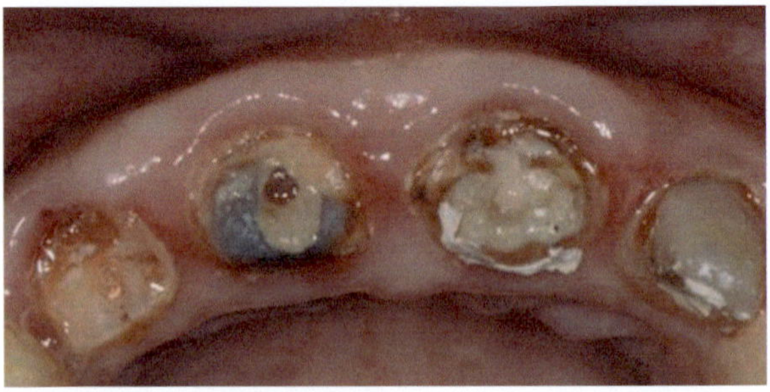

Fig. 11.101 The incisal view of the failing teeth. Observe the convex contours of the labial bone

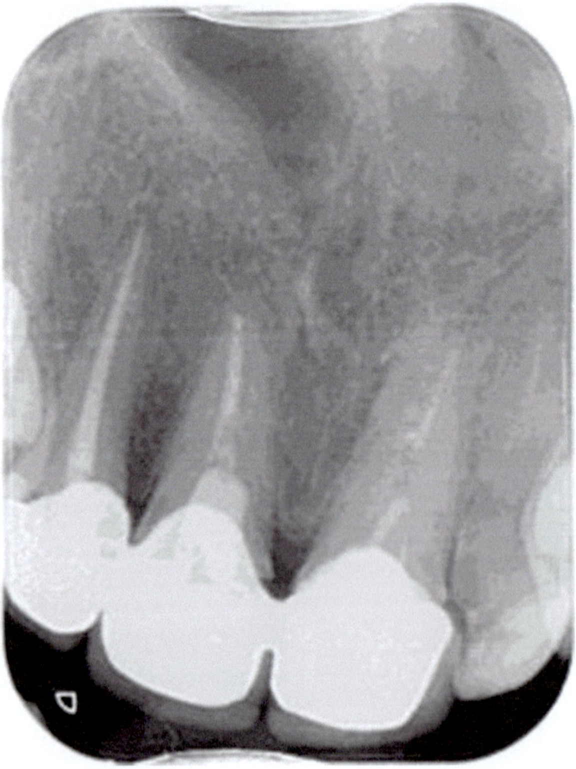

Fig. 11.102 Preoperative radiograph

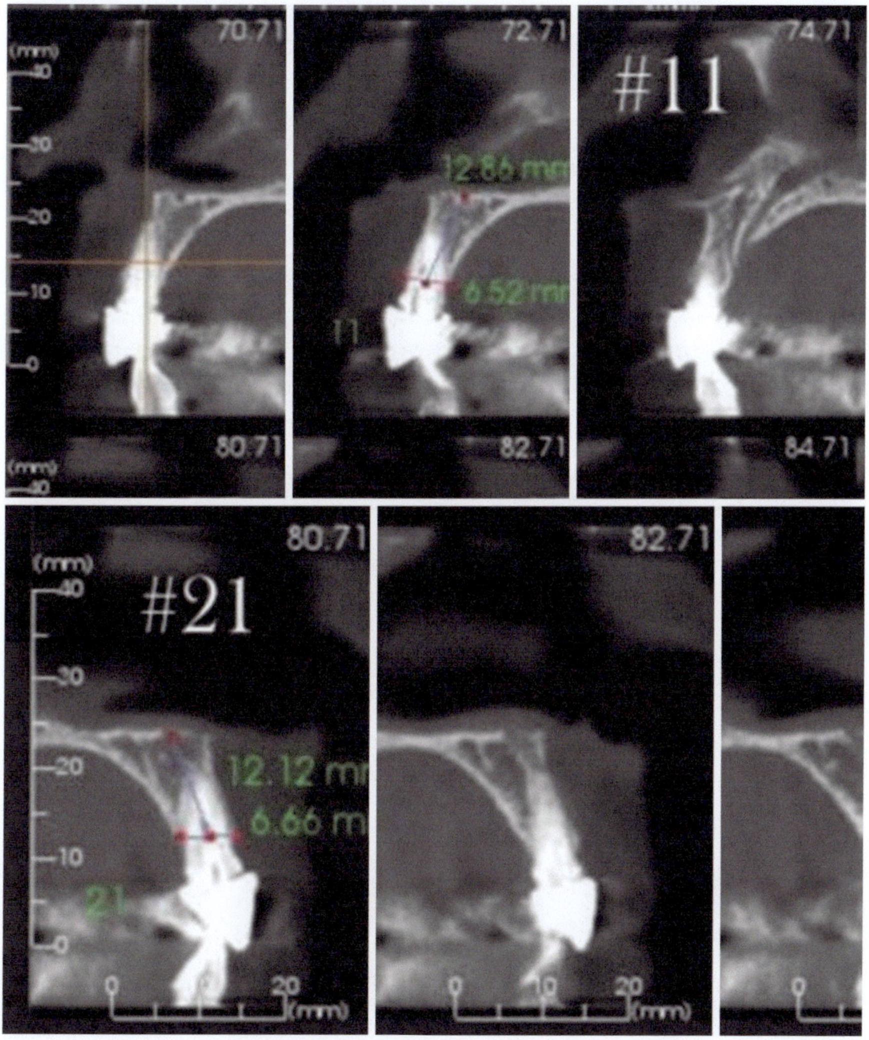

Fig. 11.103 Preoperative CBCT of the anterior maxilla. The radial tooth position shows sufficient available palatal bone to place the implants in the correct 3D position

Fig. 11.104 Wax-up depicting the proposed smile design

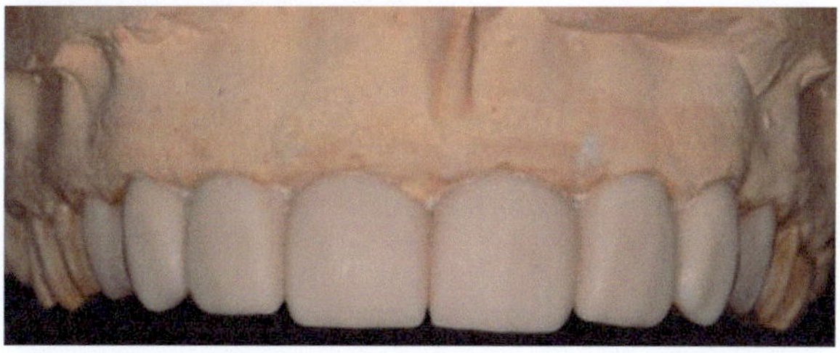

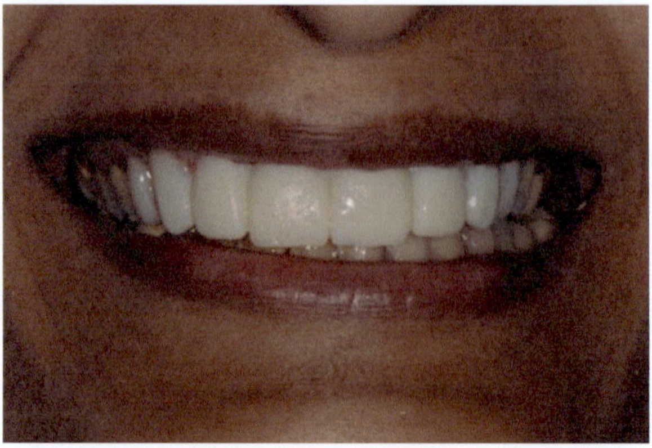

Fig. 11.105 Mock-up done with bonded provisional material to test drive the smile aspects

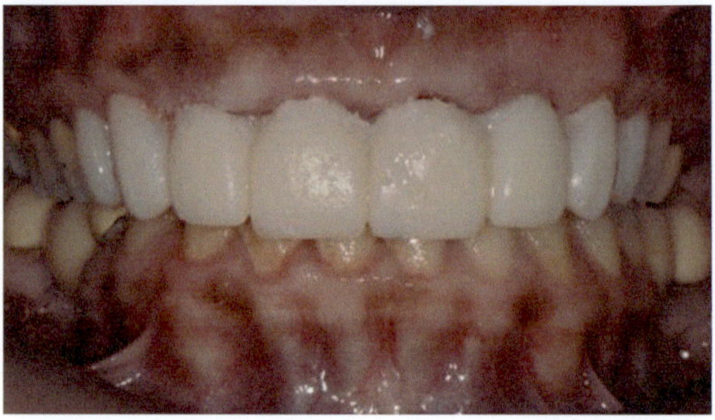

Fig. 11.106 Intraoral view of the first mock-up

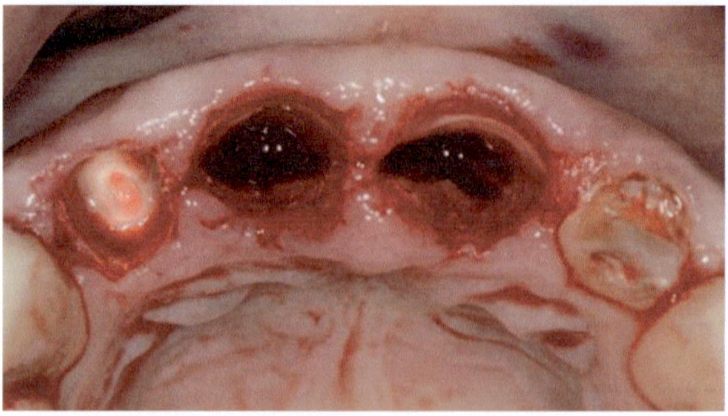

Fig. 11.107 The shields prepared

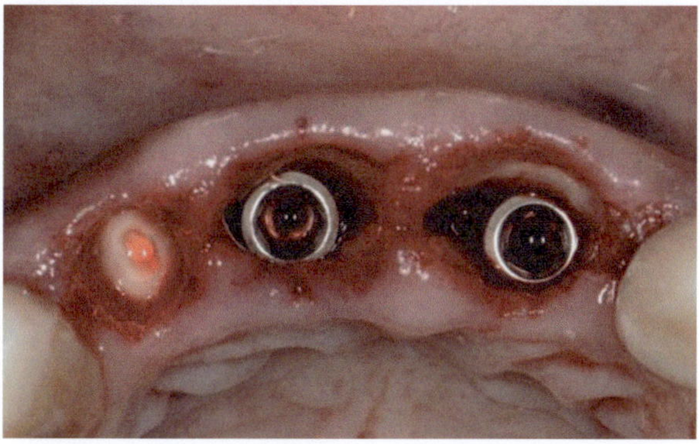

Fig. 11.108 Implants placed in the sockets keeping in mind the principles discussed

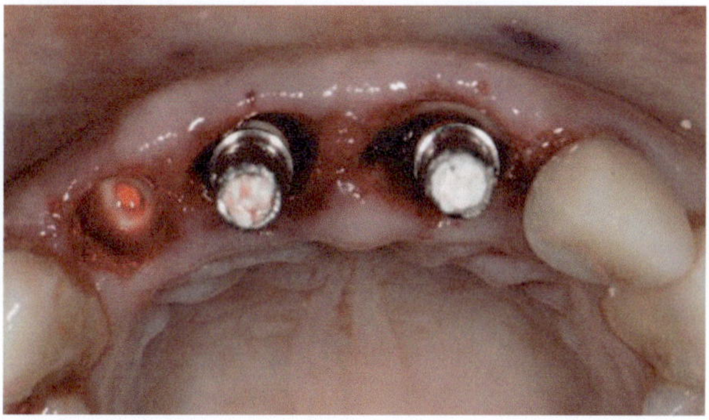

Fig. 11.109 The #12 prepared as root submergence to help maintain the bone contour in that region

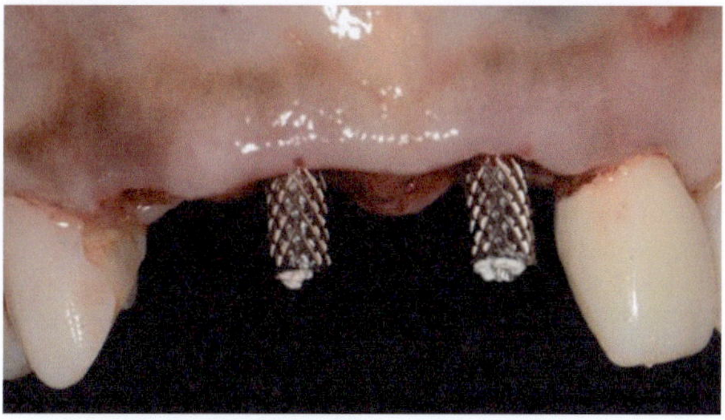

Fig. 11.110 Nonengaging temporary titanium cylinders attached to the implants

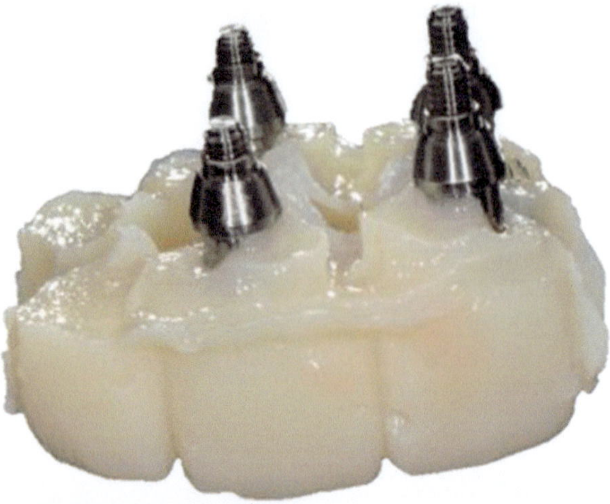

Fig. 11.111 The putty index used with the Bis-GMA resin to initiate the making of a screw-retained immediate provisional restoration

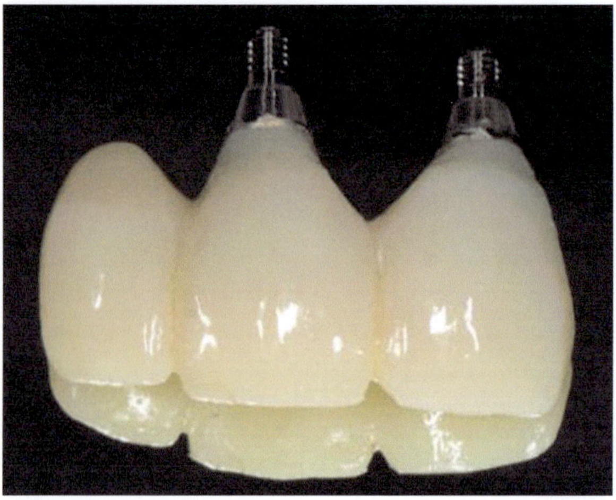

Fig. 11.112 The provisional neatly finished to perform its task of providing an immediate aesthetic replacement while acting as a scaffold to support soft tissues as needed

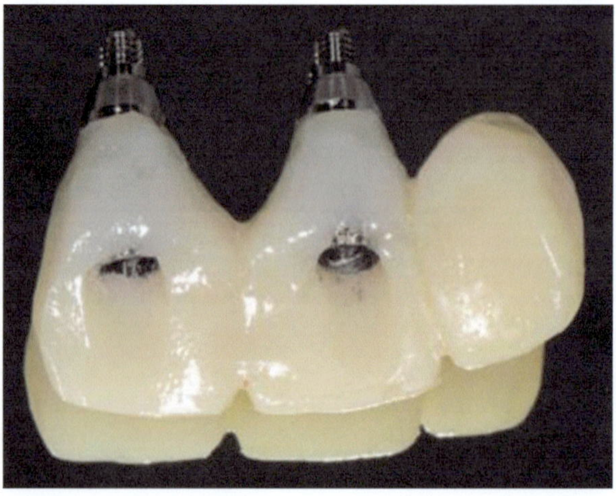

Fig. 11.113 The palatal view of the provisional. Observe the design of the #12 pontic area where root submergence has been done

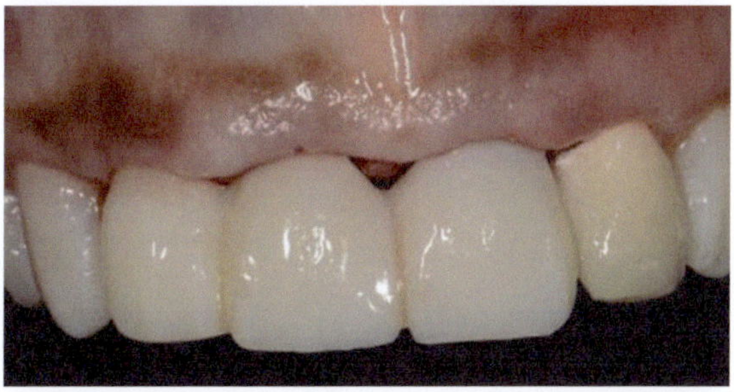

Fig. 11.114 Immediate screw-retained provisional in situ. It should be kept out of all centric and eccentric contacts

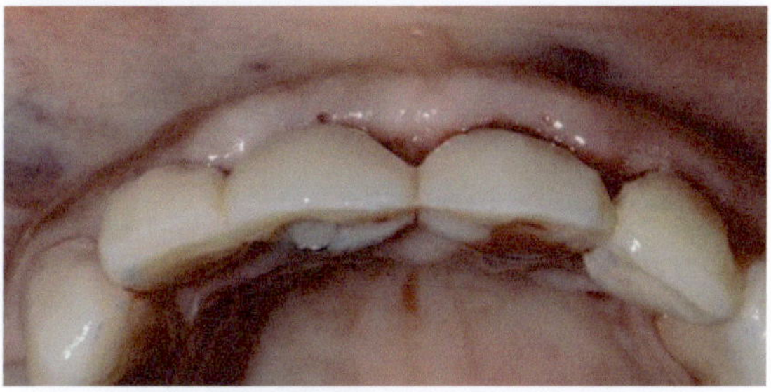

Fig. 11.115 At the end of the procedure the labial contours are well preserved

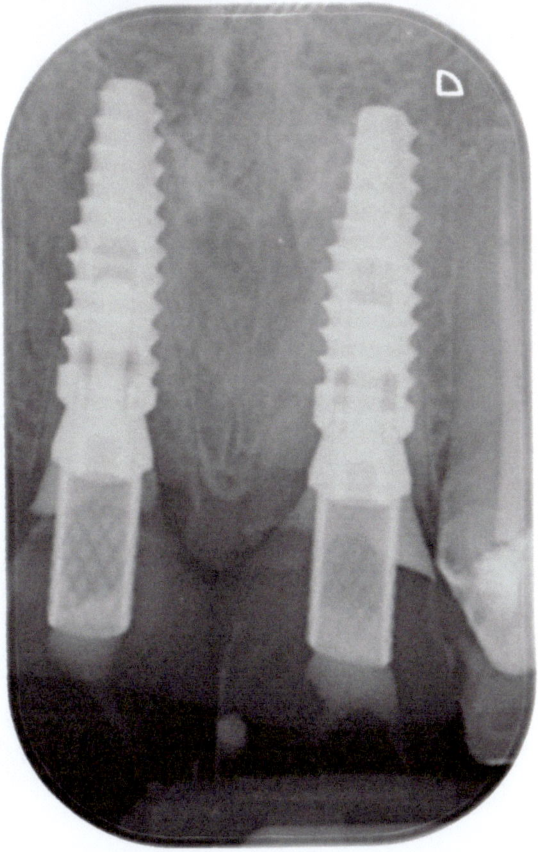

Fig. 11.116 Radiograph after implants and provisional restorations

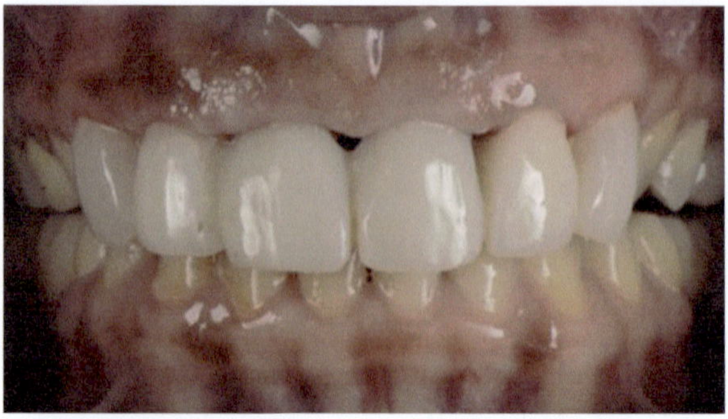

Fig. 11.117 The smile at 4 months after implant placement

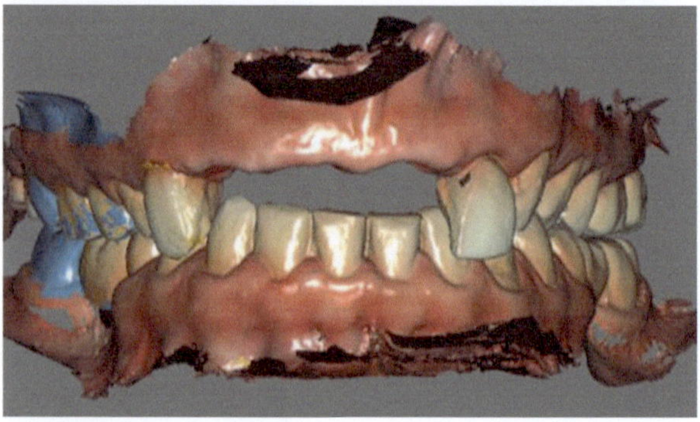

Fig. 11.118 Digital impressions for the gingival architecture of the implant sites

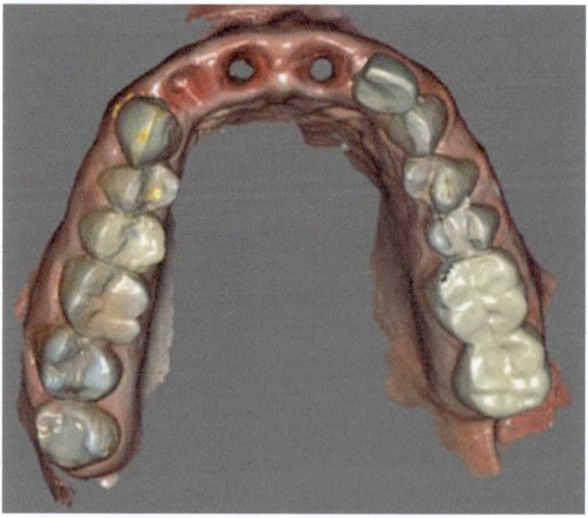

Fig. 11.119 It is important to record all structures completely

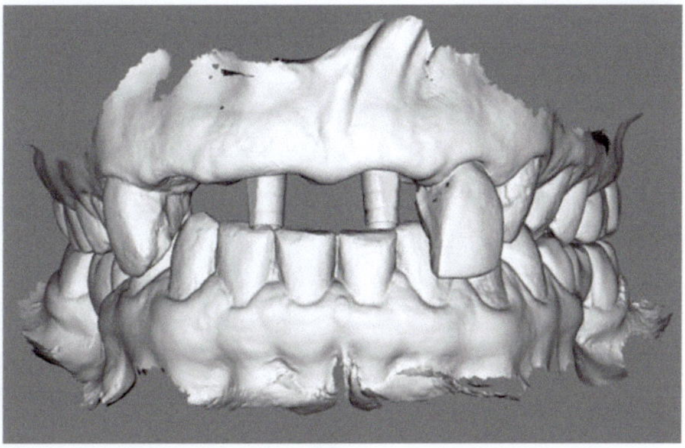

Fig. 11.120 The STL file with the scan post sent to the labs

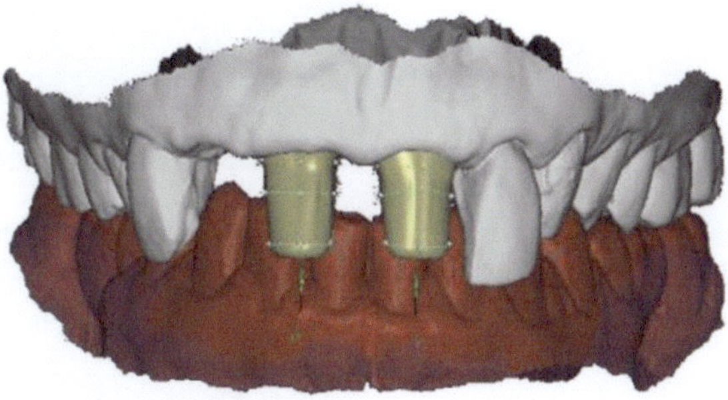

Fig. 11.121 The designing of the custom abutments in zirconia for #11 and #21

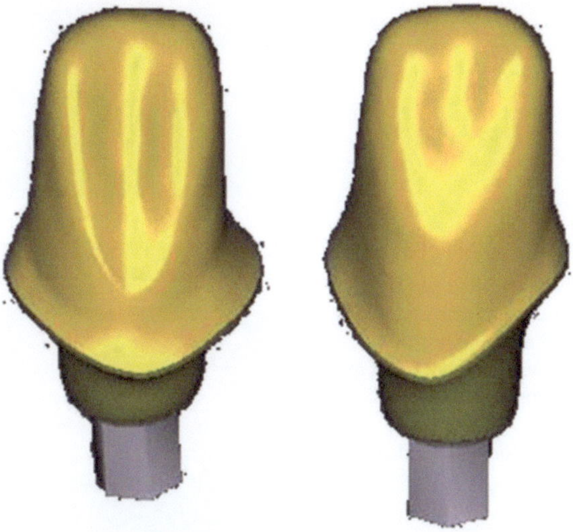

Fig. 11.122 The final design of the zirconia abutments to receive cement retained lithium disilicate crowns

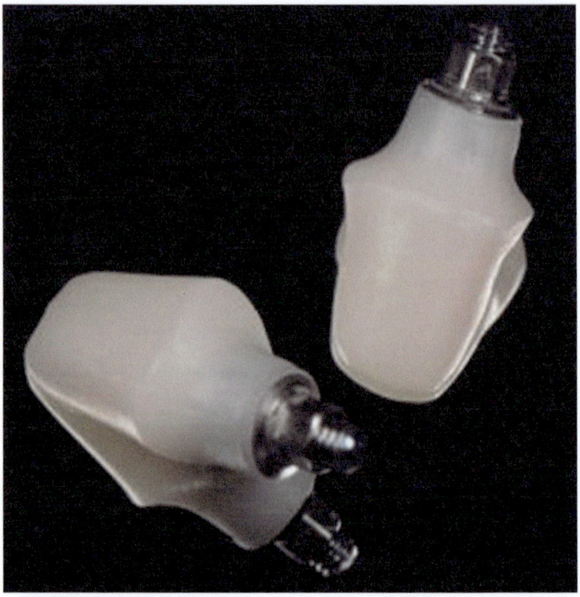

Fig. 11.123 The dentin-colored customized zirconia abutments create a good background for the lithium disilicate crowns

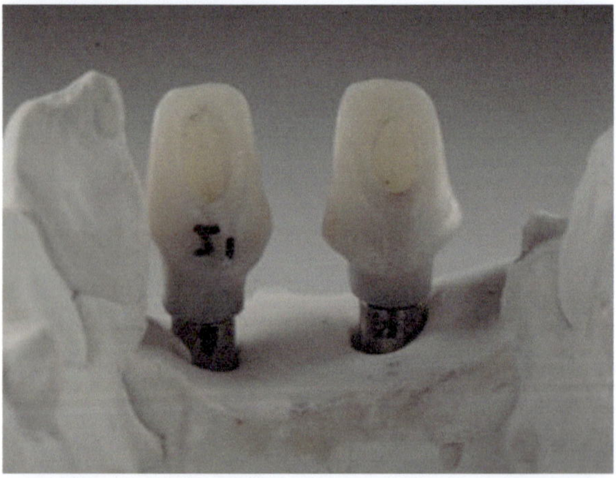

Fig. 11.124 Minimum cross-sectional thickness of at least 0.75 mm must be maintained for strength

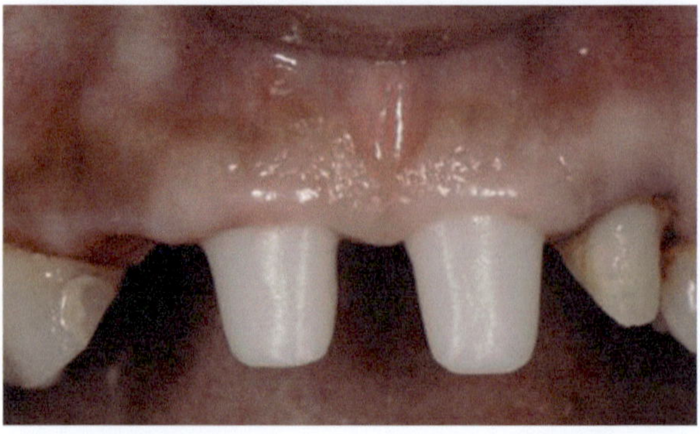

Fig. 11.125 The restorative margins on these abutments are placed <0.5 mm subgingival on the labial and proximal and equigingival on palatal areas to allow ease of access for cement cleaning

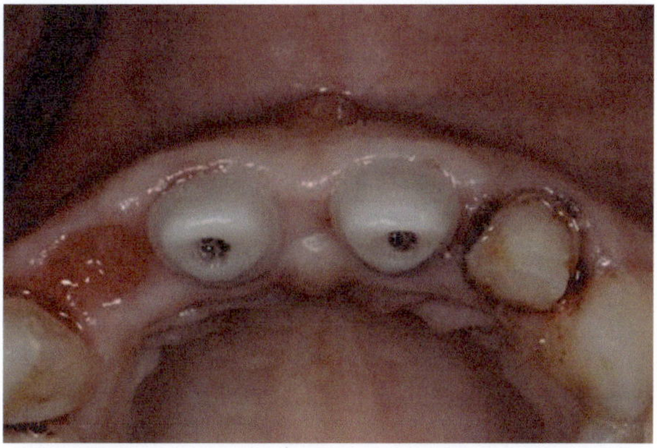

Fig. 11.126 The abutments torqued in and the tissue contour well maintained from beginning to end. The #12 area looks well maintained due to the root submergence

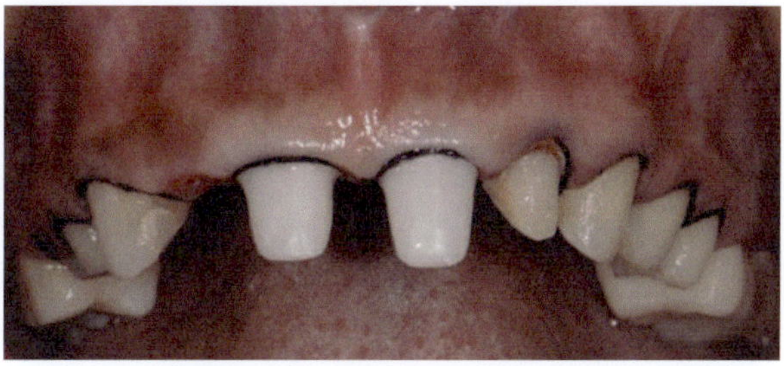

Fig. 11.127 The rest of the teeth visible in the smile have been prepared for aesthetic restorations and tissue management done to capture the abutments

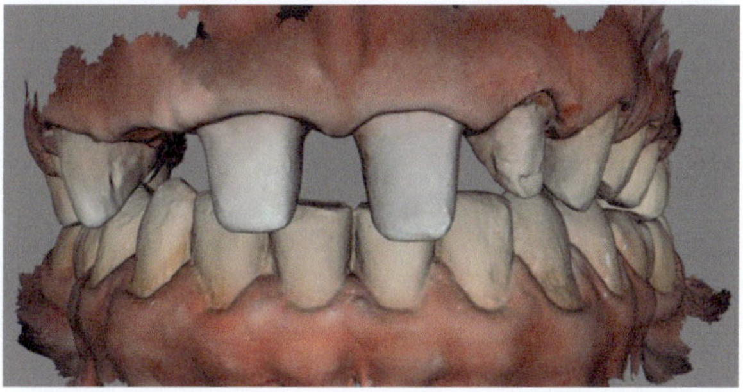

Fig. 11.128 The digital impression of all maxillary anterior teeth to receive the definitive aesthetic restorations

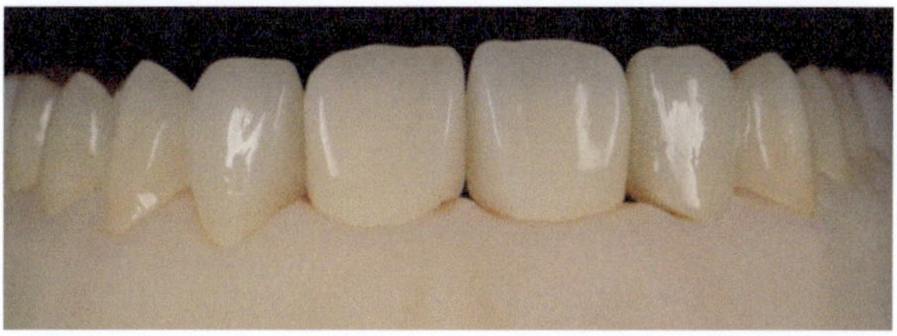

Fig. 11.129 The final layered lithium disilicate restorations

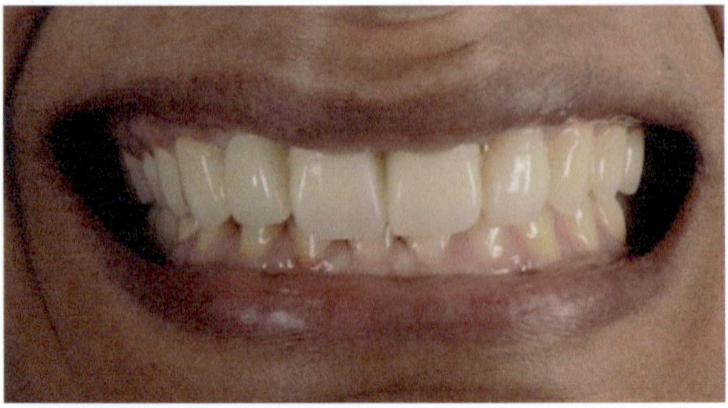

Fig. 11.130 The postoperative smile picture

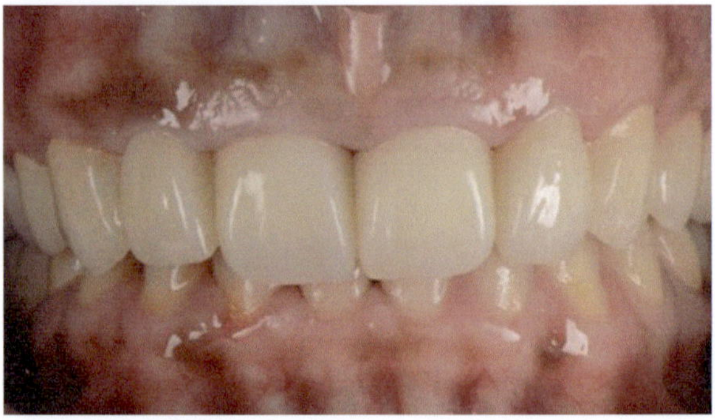

Fig. 11.131 The anterior final restorations

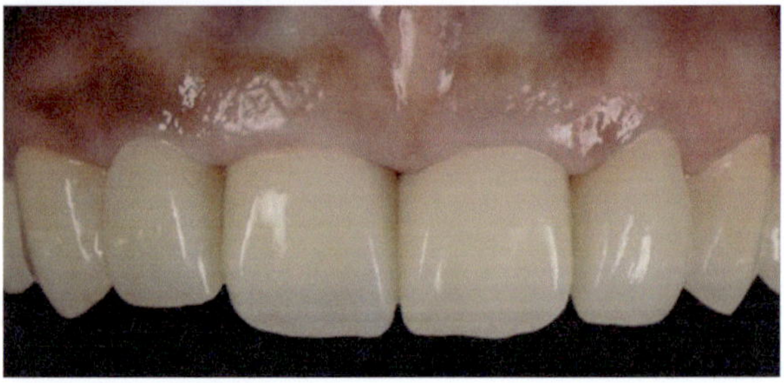

Fig. 11.132 The tissue quality and contour well maintained in #11, #21, and #12 region

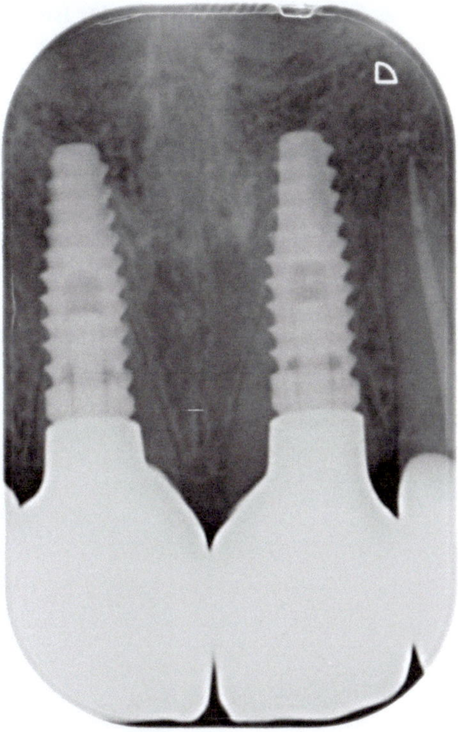

Fig. 11.133 The final postoperative radiograph showing maintenance of very good bone levels between these adjacent partial extraction therapy sites

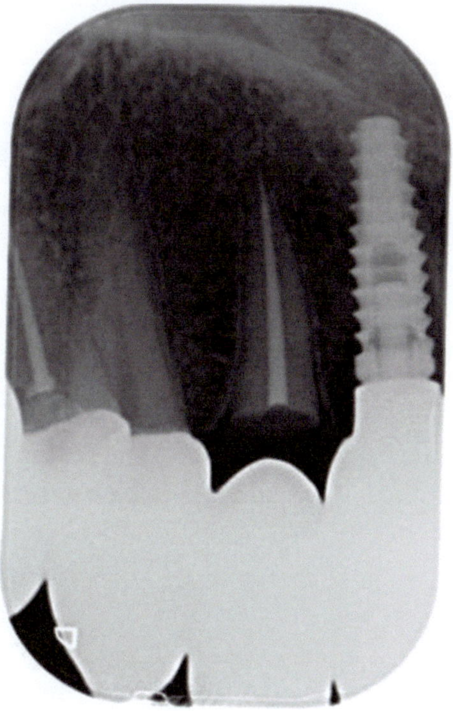

Fig. 11.134 Postoperative radiograph of #12 with root submergence

11.7.2 Case 7: Adjacent Lower Incisors

Surgical & Restorative Dentistry: Dr. Ali Tunkiwala.

Lab Credits: Danesh Vazifdar, Adaro Lab, Mumbai.

The challenge in regular cases in lower anterior region for adjacent implants lies in the fact that the mesio-distal space is less. Narrow, 3 mm platform implants can be done to maintain a minimum distance of 1.5 mm between implants. The possibility of getting a papilla in such cases with adjacent implants is slim, but since it is not visible in the smile, this can be considered a reasonable compromise between aesthetics and biomechanics (Figs. 11.135, 11.136, 11.137, 11.138, 11.139, 11.140, 11.141, 11.142, 11.143, 11.144, 11.145, 11.146, 11.147 and 11.148).

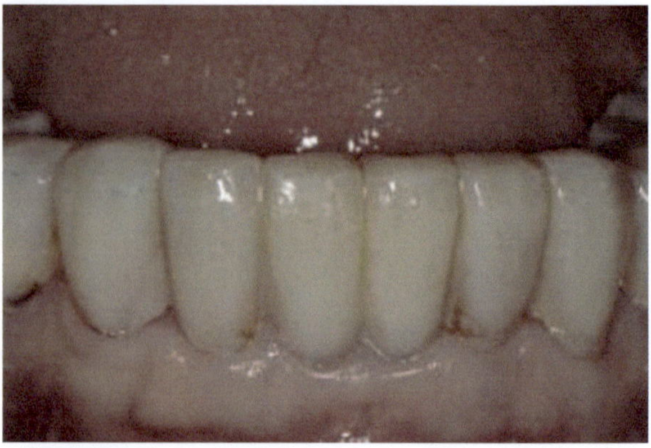

Fig. 11.135 Preoperative scenario with temporary teeth on failed #31 and #41

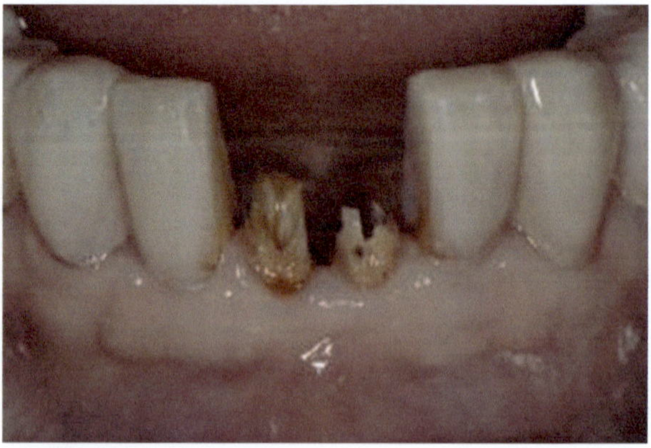

Fig. 11.136 #31 and #41 structurally unrestorable as there is no tooth structure on lingual side for a ferrule.

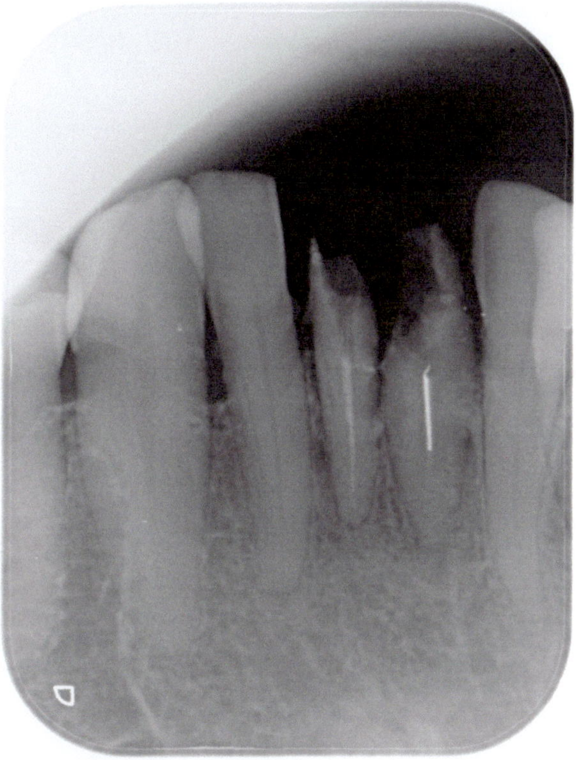

Fig. 11.137 Preoperative radiograph

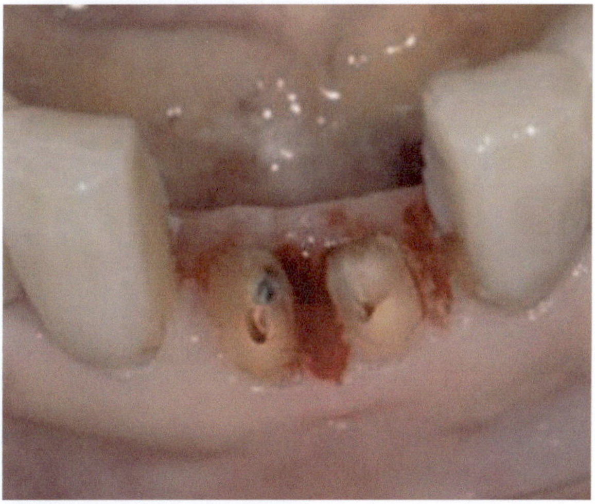

Fig. 11.138 Shield preparation initiated with decoronation

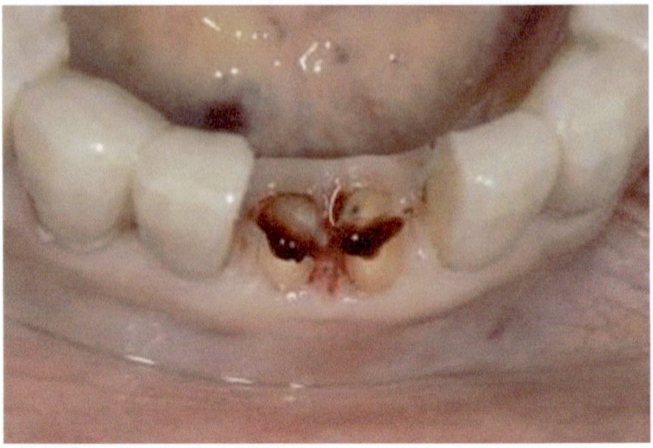

Fig. 11.139 The first horizontal cut to separate the lingual portion of the tooth from the labial

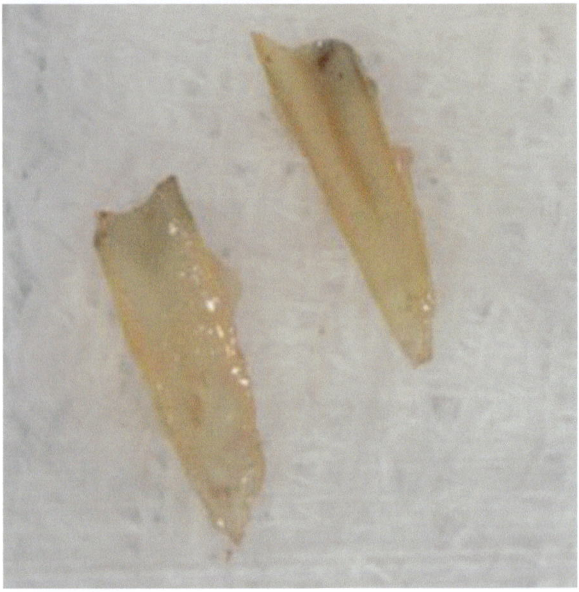

Fig. 11.140 Complete removal of lingual portion of the tooth with the apex

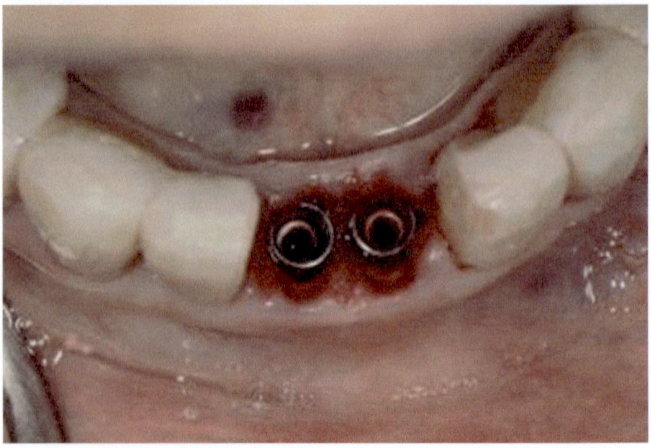

Fig. 11.141 3.0 mm by 12 mm implants placed in the sockets while maintaining minimum distance between them and the teeth and no contact with the shield

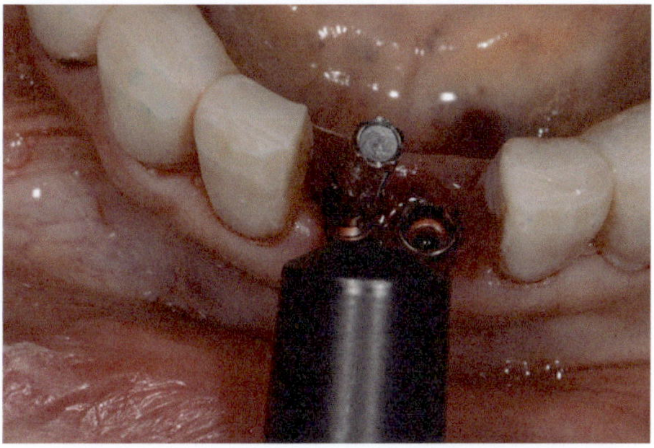

Fig. 11.142 ISQ values more than 70

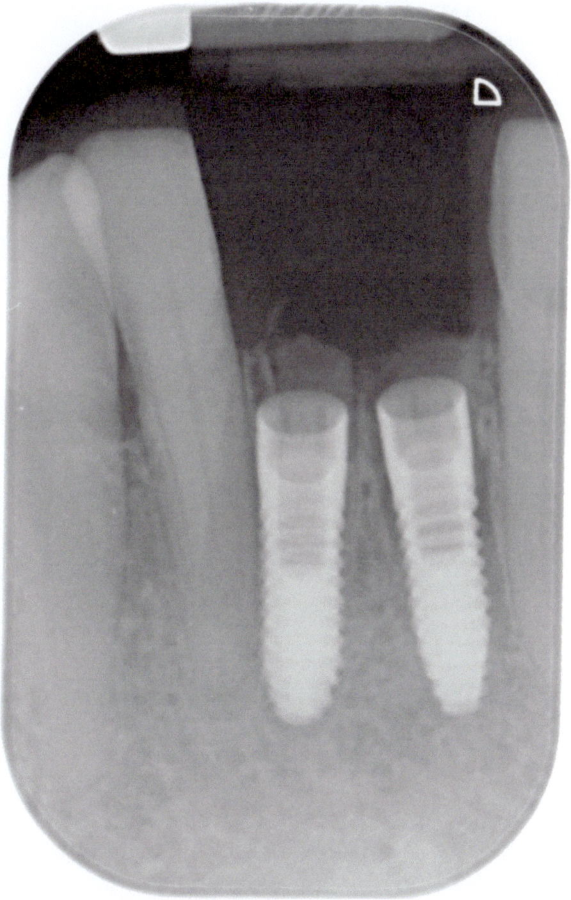

Fig. 11.143 Radiograph after implant placement

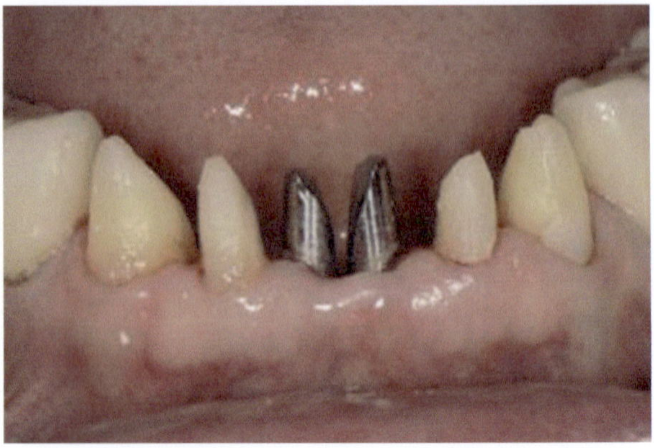

Fig. 11.144 At 3 months, final abutments in place with all lower anteriors ready to receive final restorations

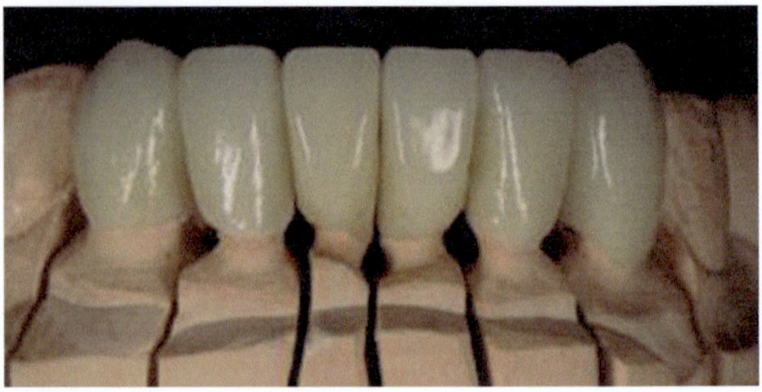

Fig. 11.145 The layered lithium disilicate crowns

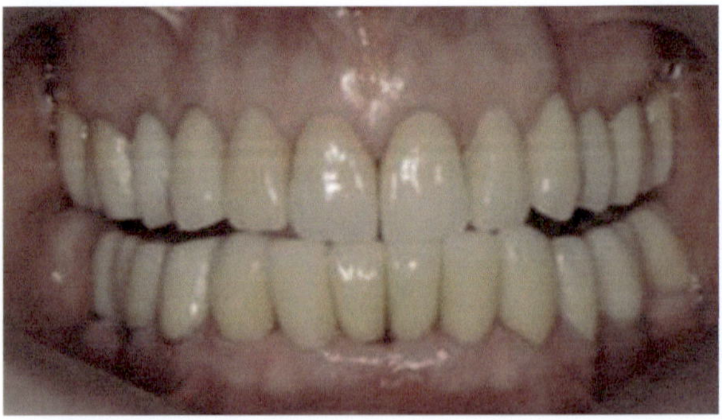

Fig. 11.146 Postoperative view of the final restorations

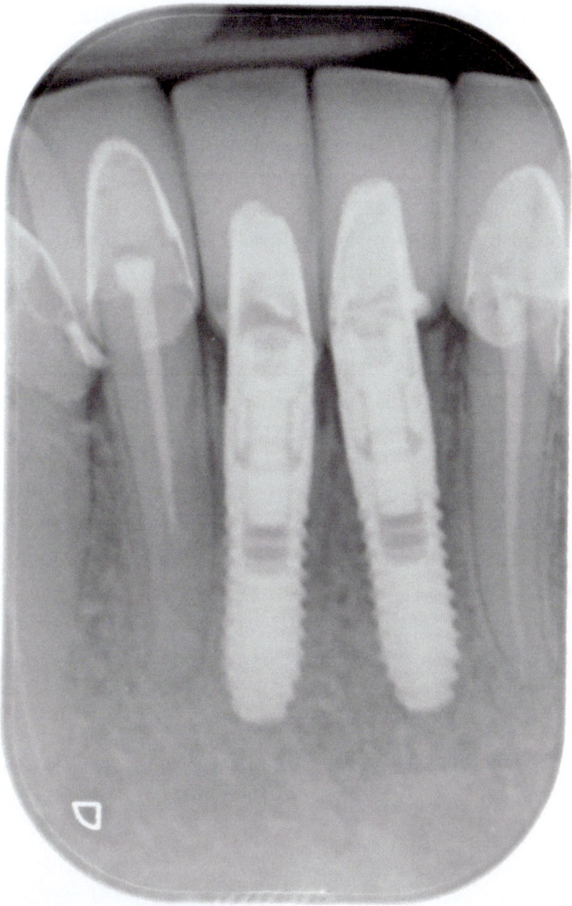

Fig. 11.147 Post-op X-ray

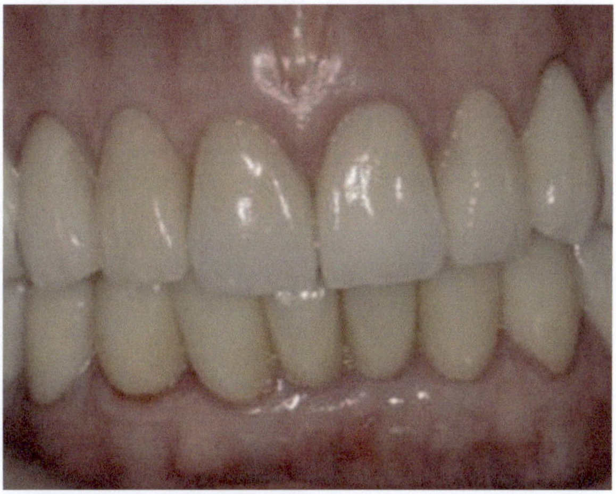

Fig. 11.148 2-year follow-up

11.7.3 Case 8: Adjacent Implants in Maxillary Anterior Region

Surgical Dentistry: Dr. Udatta Kher.

Restorative Dentistry: Dr. Ali Tunkiwala.

Lab Credits: Danesh Vazifdar, Adaro Lab, Mumbai.

A 25–year-old female patient reported with very unaesthetic anterior restorations. Upon removal of the faulty crowns, the underlying #12 and #11 teeth were found to be structurally poor. #21 and #22 were salvageable. Socket shield was performed for the right incisors. Once the implants were placed in the final position and good primary stability was ensured, a prefabricated Bio_HPP abutment was used to fabricate a cement-retained provisional restoration with due diligence to avoid any excess residual cement. The concept was to use this abutment as a final one-time abutment. At 4 months, the provisional restorations were removed and the final impressions were made using addition silicones; 4 individual lithium disilicate restorations were fabricated for these incisors (Figs. 11.149, 11.150, 11.151, 11.152, 11.153, 11.154, 11.155, 11.156, 11.157, 11.158, 11.159, 11.160, 11.161, 11.162, 11.163, 11.164, 11.165, 11.166, 11.167, 11.168, 11.169 and 11.170). The implants and prosthetic components in this case were sponsored by Bredent Medical, Germany.

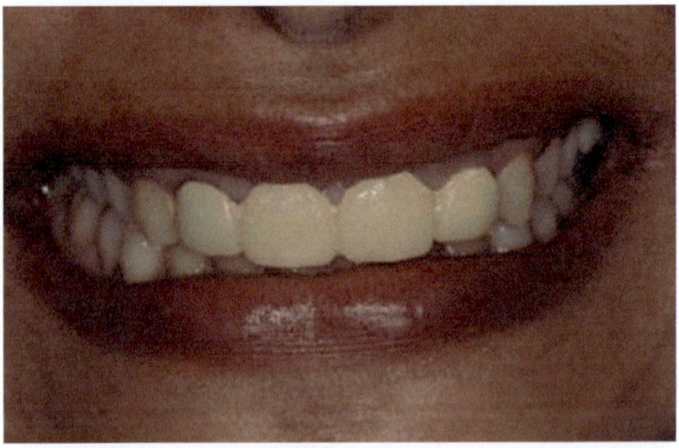

Fig. 11.149 Preoperative smile with unsightly incisors

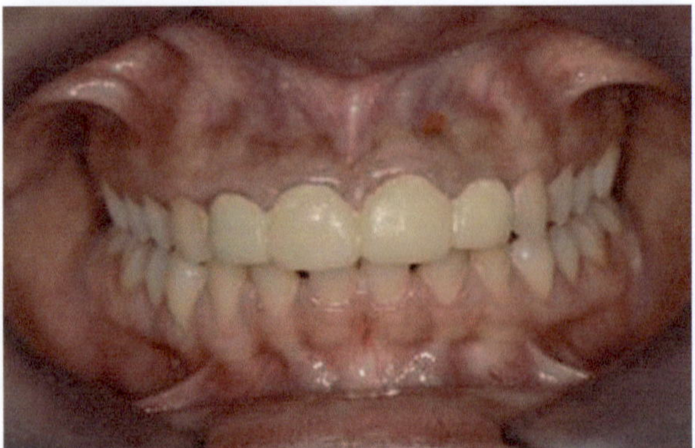

Fig. 11.150 Retracted intraoral view

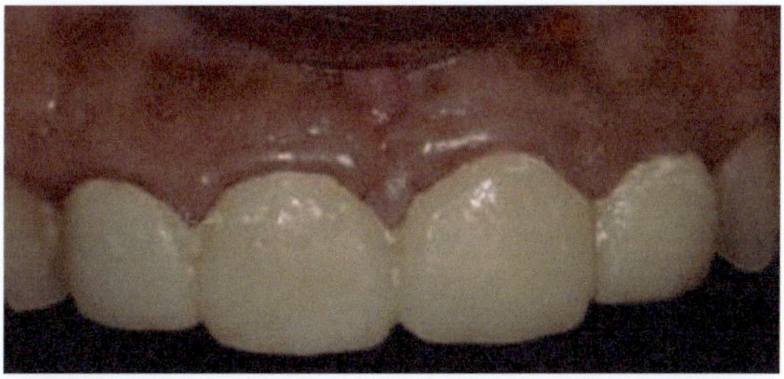

Fig. 11.151 Close-up view of existing restoration on incisors

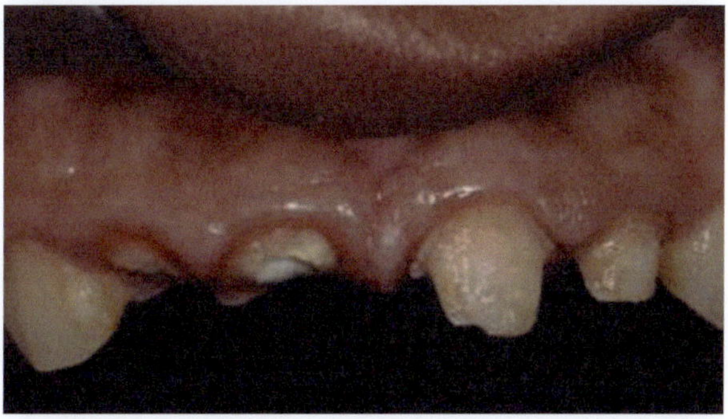

Fig. 11.152 #12 and #11 are structurally very poor. Partial extraction therapy planned for them. #21 and #22 were saved and restored with single crowns.

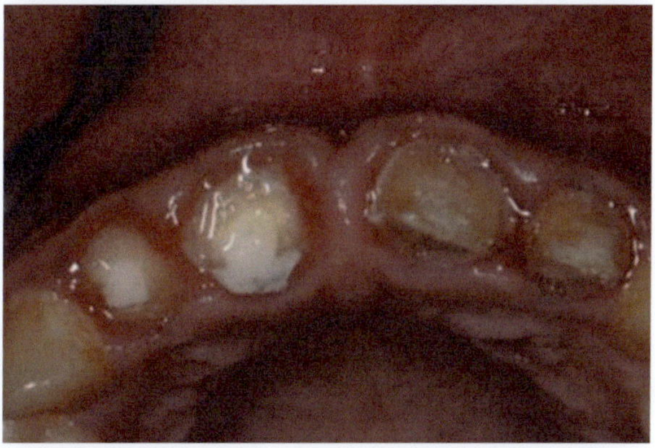

Fig. 11.153 Occlusal view of teeth showing good tissue contours to start with

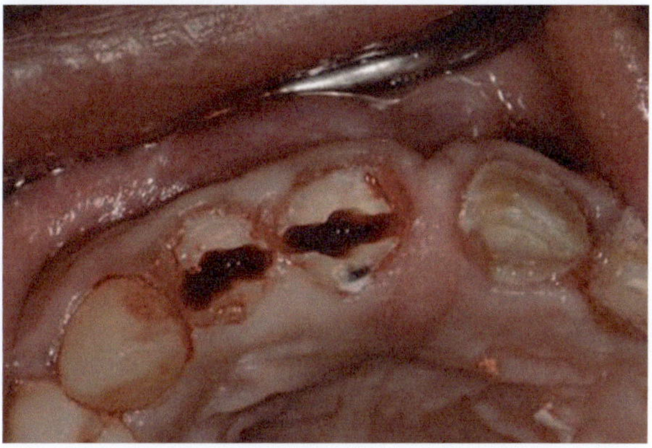

Fig. 11.154 Socket shield preparation initiated

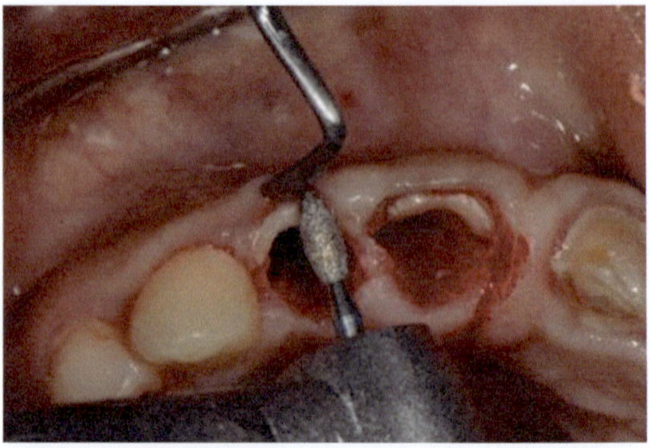

Fig. 11.155 Shield trimmed to bone with soft tissues protected

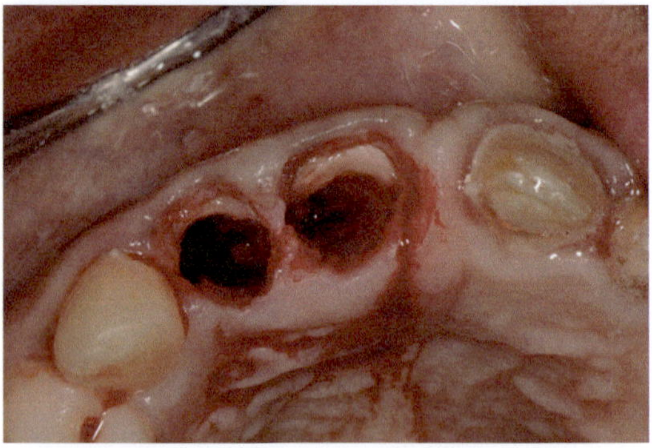

Fig. 11.156 Final shield preparation for #11 and #12

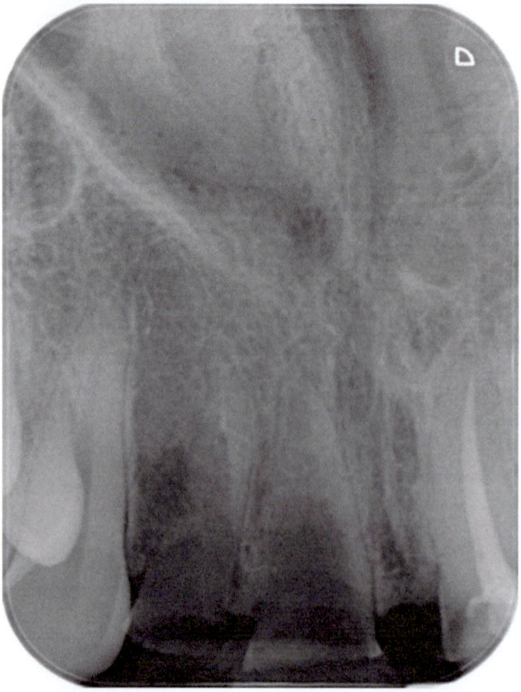

Fig. 11.157 Radiograph to confirm removal of all endodontic filling material

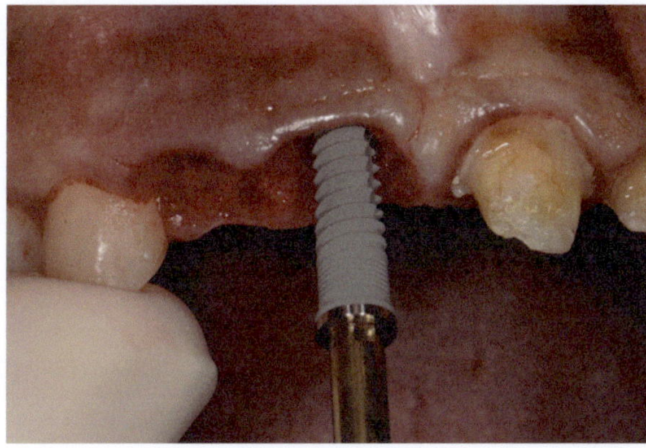

Fig. 11.158 Implant being placed in #11

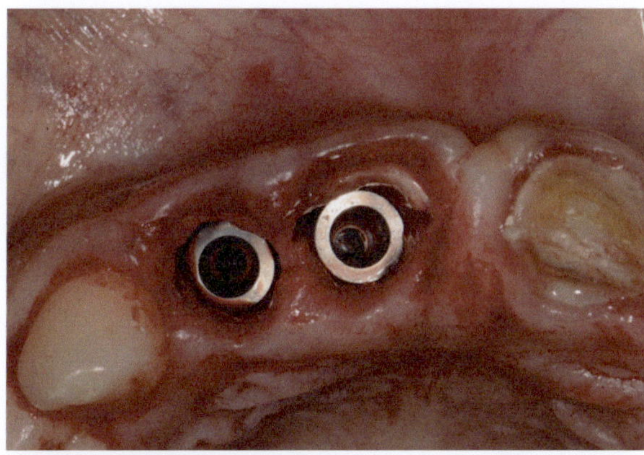

Fig. 11.159 Occlusal view showing both implants placed with socket shields

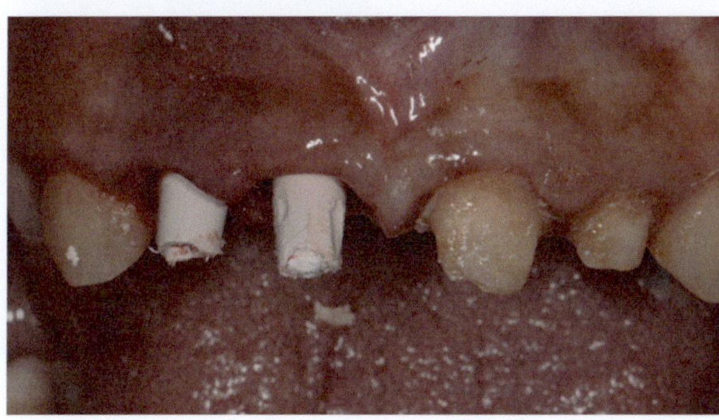

Fig. 11.160 Final Bio-HPP abutments fixated on the implants to receive a cement-retained provisional restoration

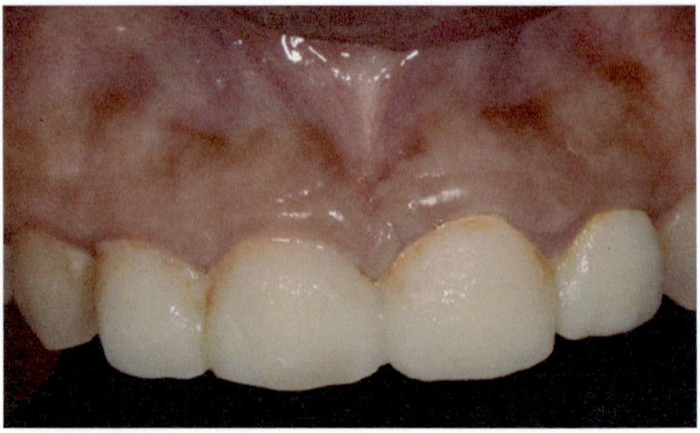

Fig. 11.161 Cement-retained provisional restorations placed

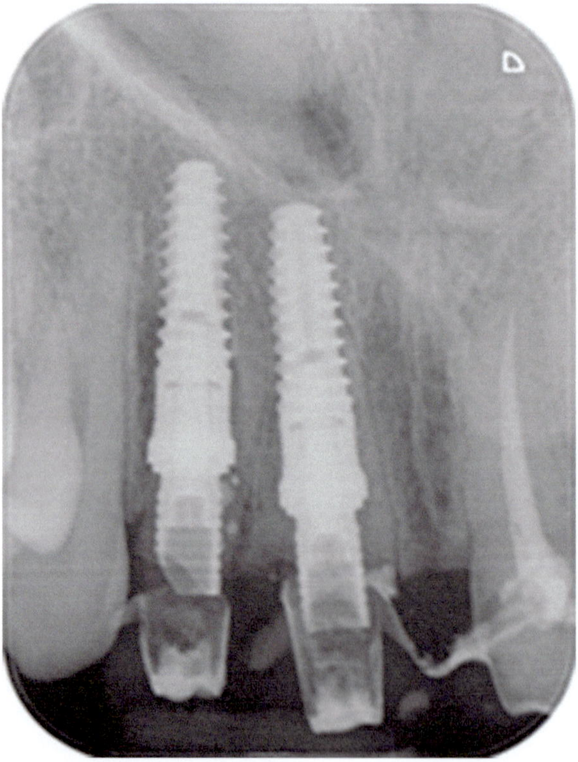

Fig. 11.162 Radiographs of implant placement

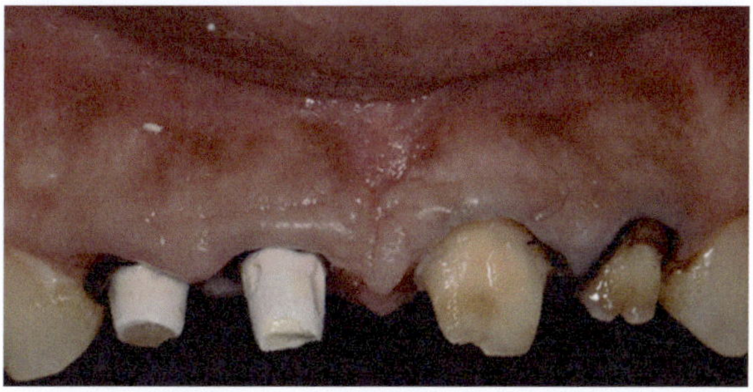

Fig. 11.163 At 4 months, the provisional restorations were removed and impressions made for all upper incisors

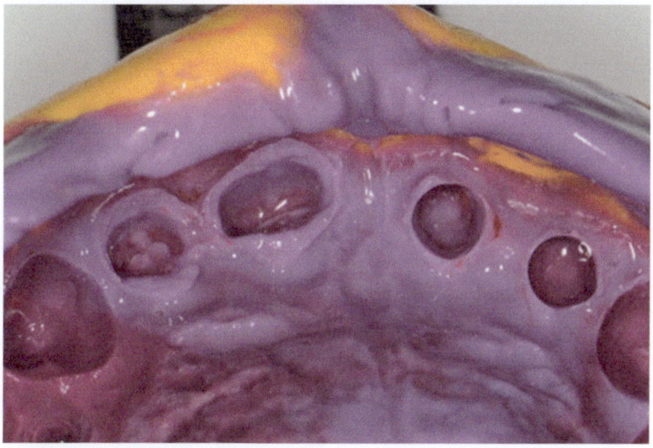

Fig. 11.164 Final impressions for final lithium disilicate restorations

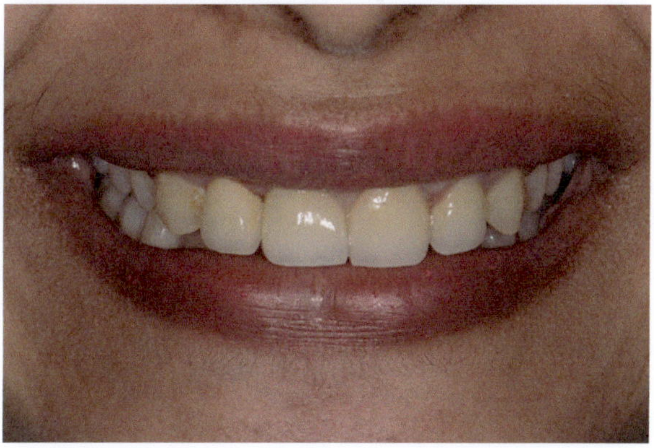

Fig. 11.165 Postoperative smile view

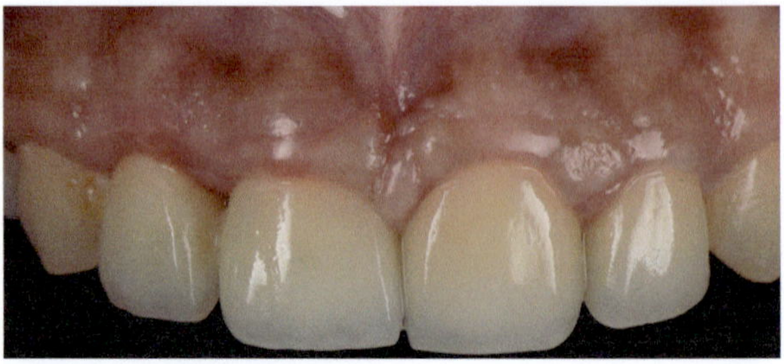

Fig. 11.166 Postoperative close-up view showing good tissue contours

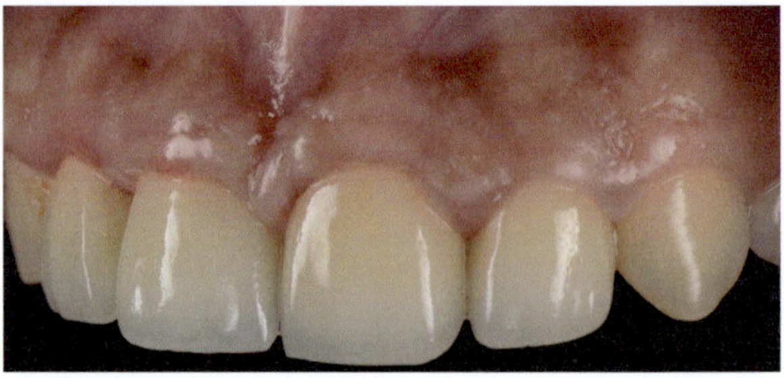

Fig. 11.167 Postoperative view depicting good emergence of site #11 and #12 in which implants with PET have been done

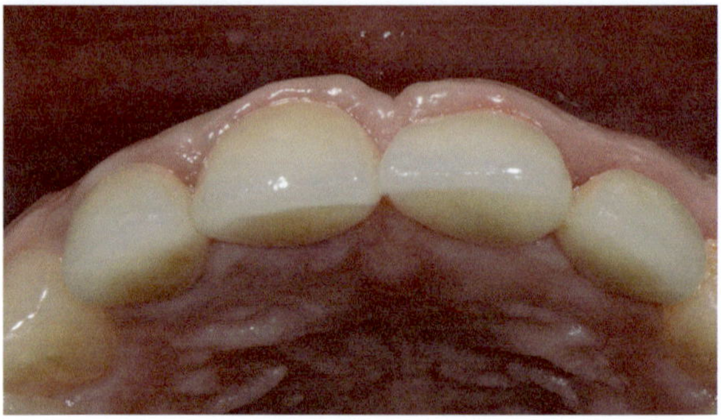

Fig. 11.168 Final occlusal view shows good tissue contours maintained due to the PET protocol

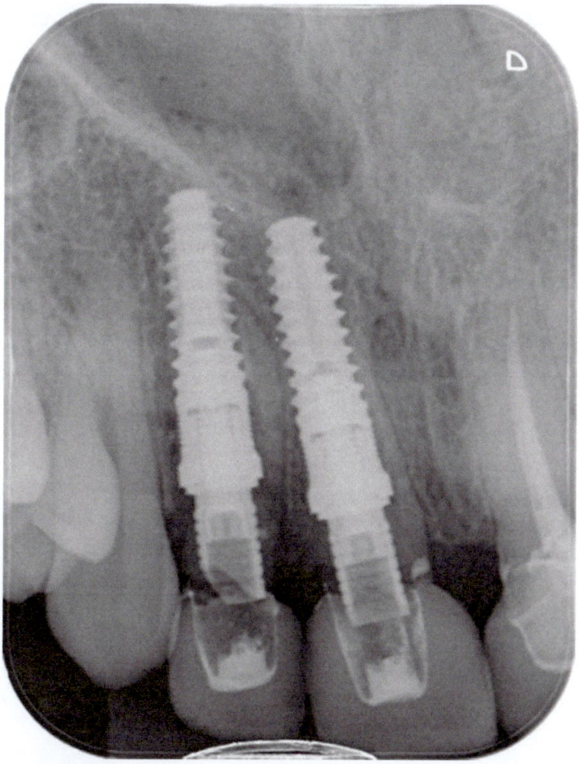

Fig. 11.169 Postoperative radiograph

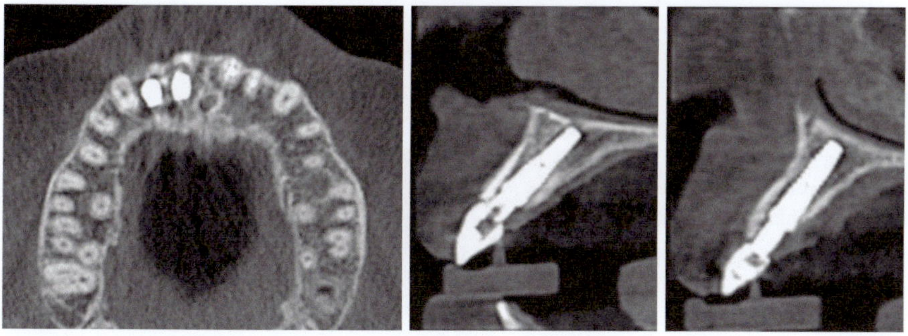

Fig. 11.170 Postoperative CBCT

11.7.4 Case 9: Multiple PET and Implants with Smile Design in Maxillary Anterior Region

Surgical & Restorative Dentistry: Dr. Ali Tunkiwala.

Lab Credits: Danesh Vazifdar, Adaro Lab, Mumbai.

A 35-year-old female patient reported with poor dental work in the aesthetic zone. The underlying teeth were compromised. Socket shield with implants was done in #12 and #22. Implant in healed site of 11 was done. The natural tooth #21 was saved and restored with a new full coverage restoration. Veneers/restorations were done on cuspids and first premolars to achieve a harmony in smile in the end result (Figs. 11.171, 11.172, 11.173, 11.174, 11.175, 11.176, 11.177, 11.178, 11.179, 11.180, 11.181, 11.182, 11.183, 11.184, 11.185, 11.186, 11.187, 11.188, 11.189, 11.190, 11.191, 11.192, 11.193 and 11.194).

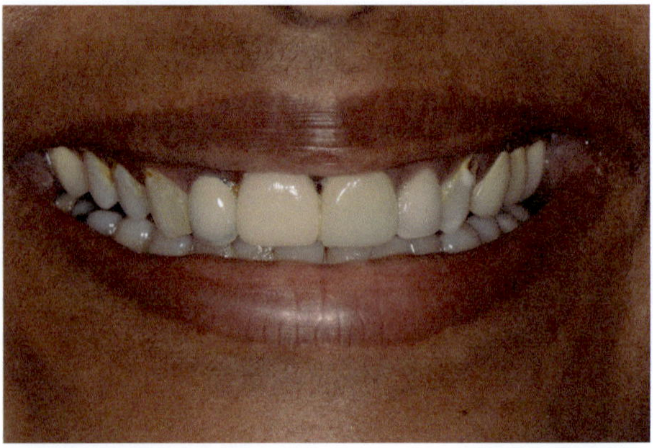

Fig. 11.171 Preoperative smile showing faulty restorations in anterior maxilla and carious lesion on left cuspid

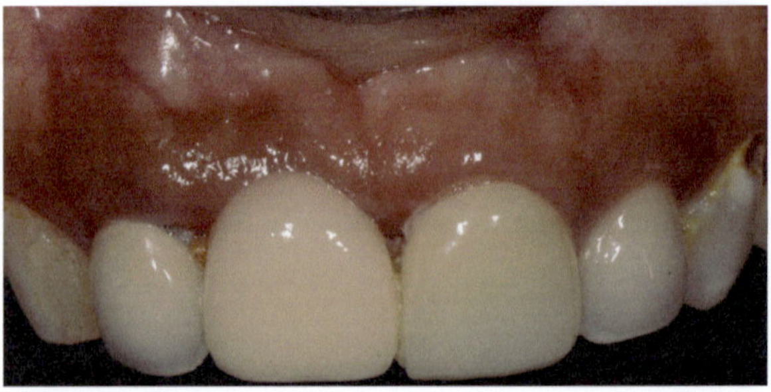

Fig. 11.172 The teeth proportions were unsightly and periodontal health was compromised

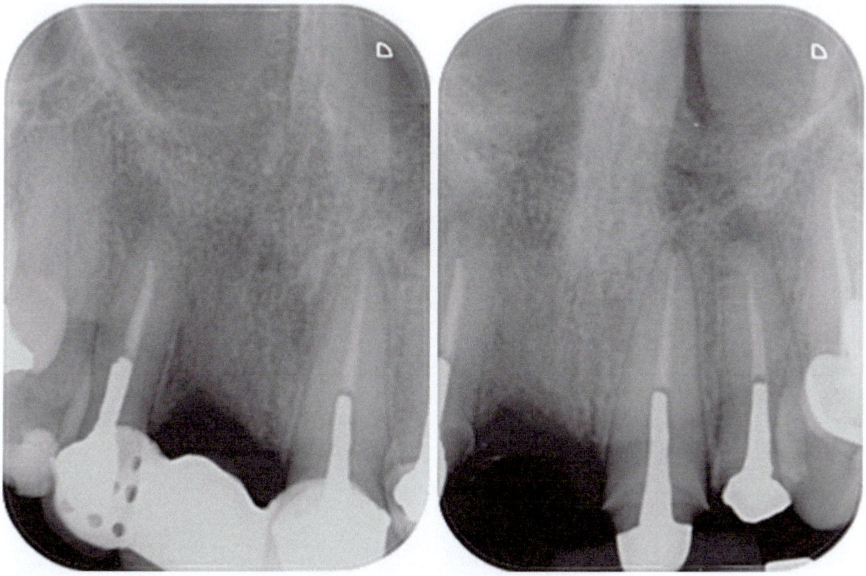

Fig. 11.173 Preoperative radiograph

Fig. 11.174 Teeth condition after removal of faulty restorations. Enough tooth structure on #21 to provide a ferrule. It was retained in the final plan

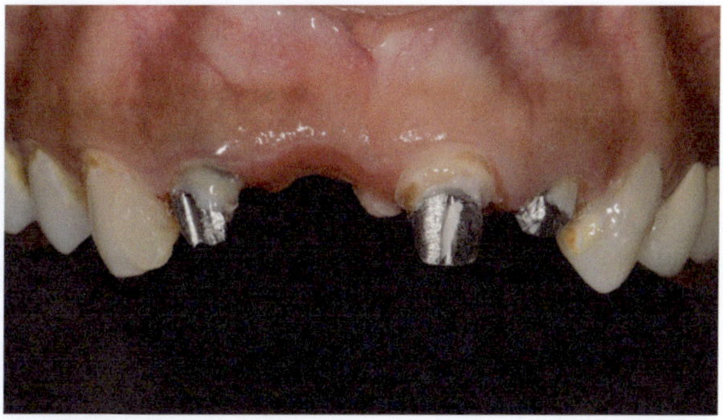

Fig. 11.175 #12 and #22 had no healthy tooth structure. Had to be extracted. Thus we decided to partially extract them.

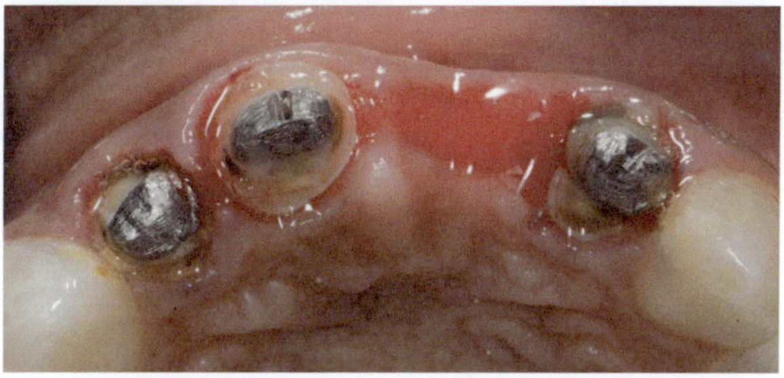

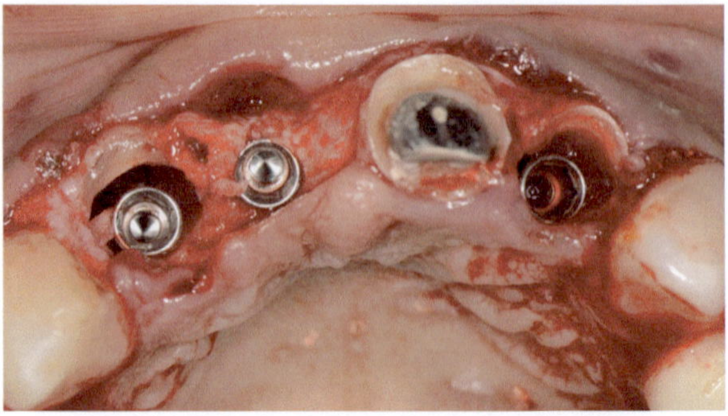

Fig. 11.176 Socket shield done for lateral incisors followed by implant placement. #11 was a delayed placement

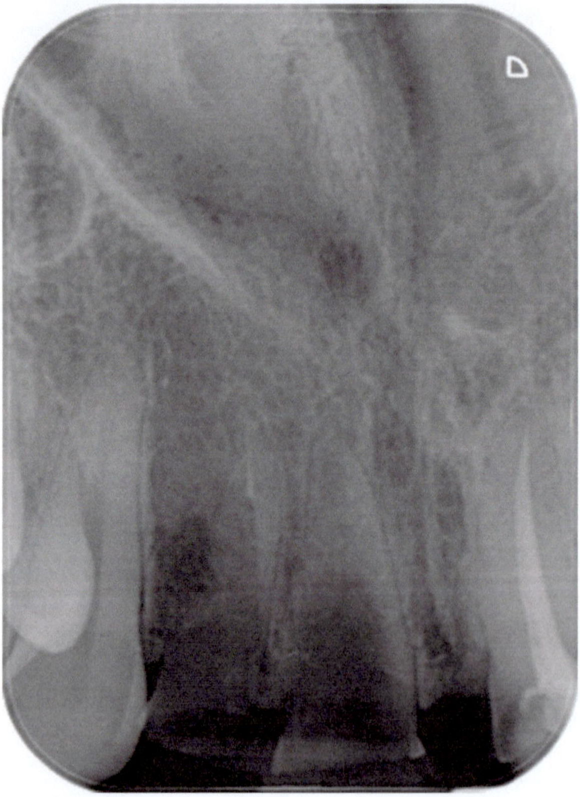

Fig. 11.177 Radiograph after shield preparation to confirm removal of all endodontic filling material

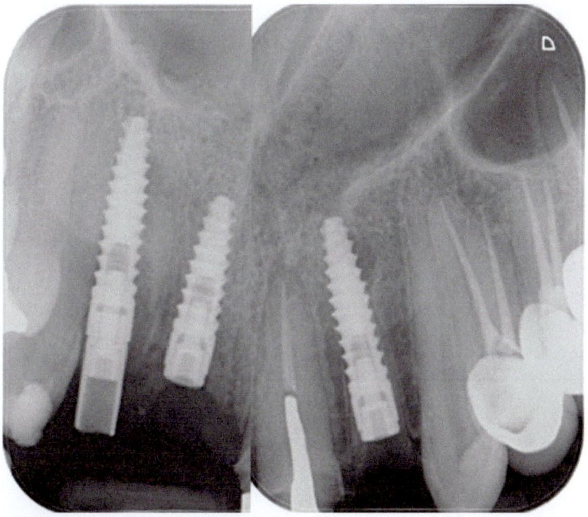

Fig. 11.178 Radiographs at implant placement

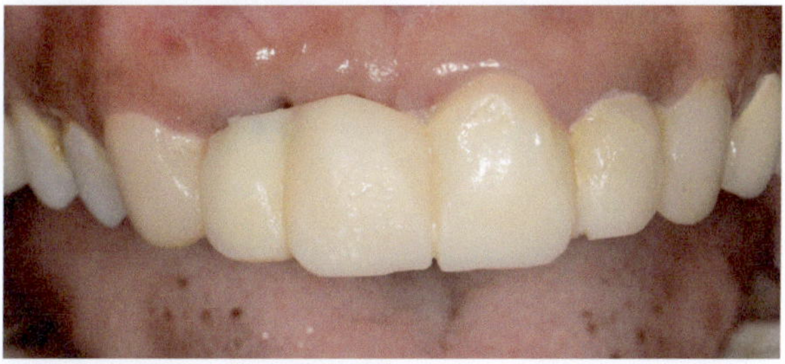

Fig. 11.179 A fixed provisional was fabricated using a cylinder on #12 and tooth #21

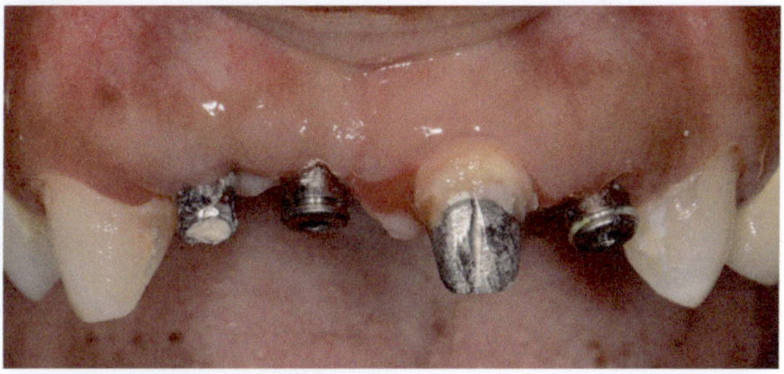

Fig. 11.180 Second stage surgery done for #11 at 4 months with a palatal roll technique to bulk

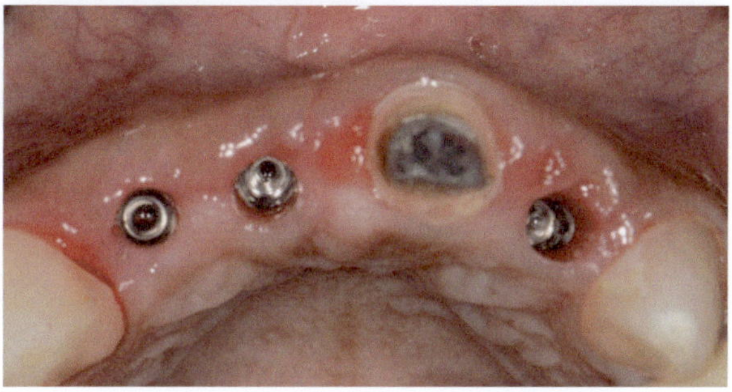

Fig. 11.181 Healed site after second stage surgery

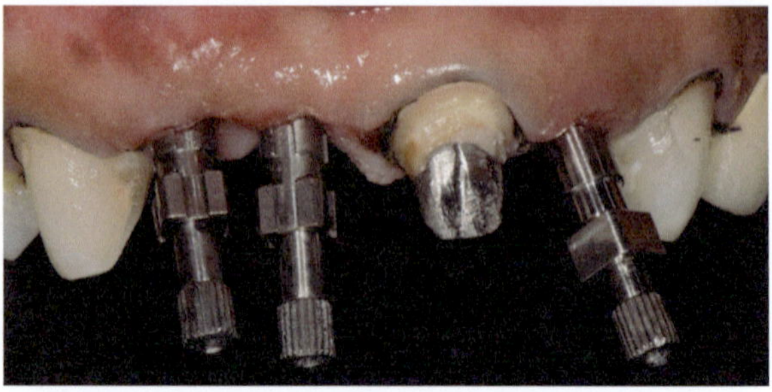

Fig. 11.182 Open tray impression copings to capture implant positions

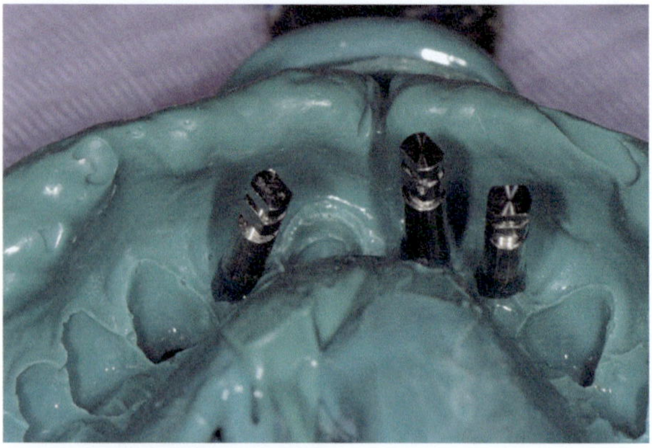

Fig. 11.183 Implant replica screwed in on the copings

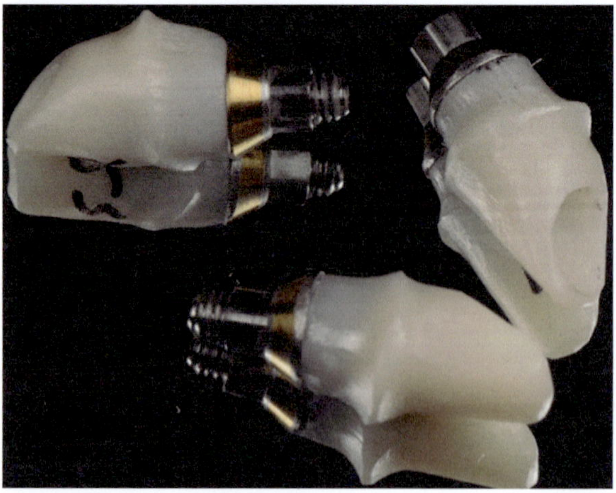

Fig. 11.184 Custom zirconia abutments fabricated on hybrid bases

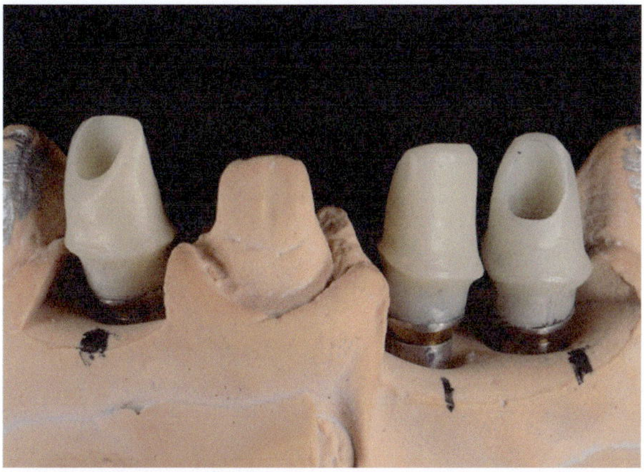

Fig. 11.185 The abutments have a concave subcritical contour to prevent any contact with the shield and maintain enough space for soft tissue

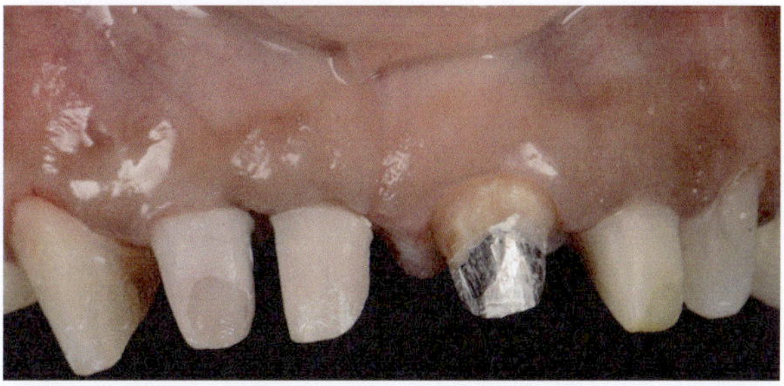

Fig. 11.186 The final zirconia custom abutments torqued in place

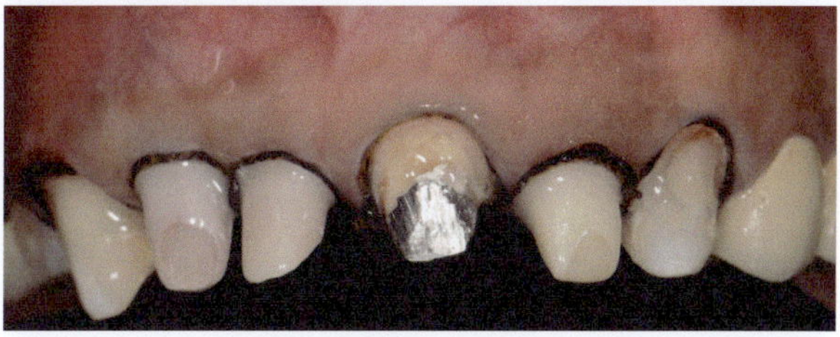

Fig. 11.187 Digital impressions of #15 to #24 made, to make final layered lithium disilicate restorations

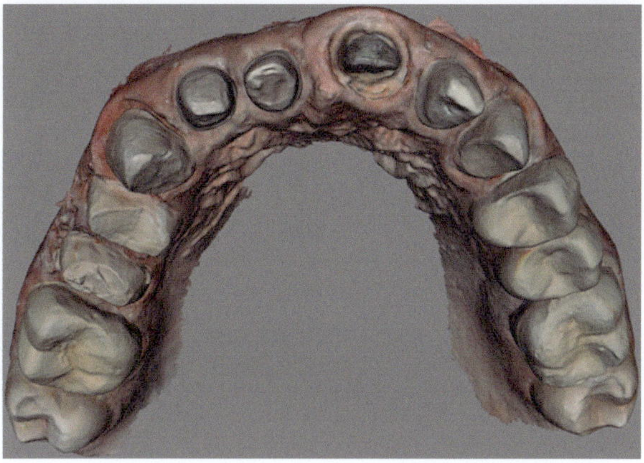

Fig. 11.188 Digital scans for final restorations

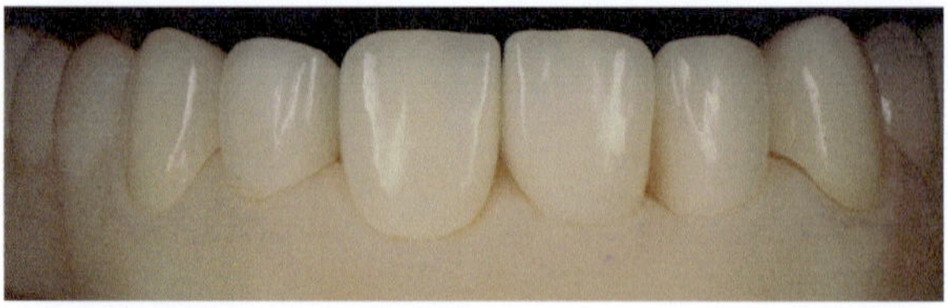

Fig. 11.189 Layered lithium disilicate restorations on 3D printed models

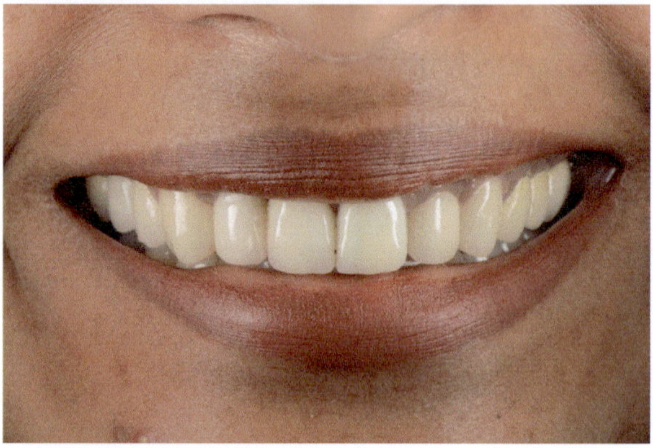

Fig. 11.190 Postoperative smile depicting a good dento-labial harmony

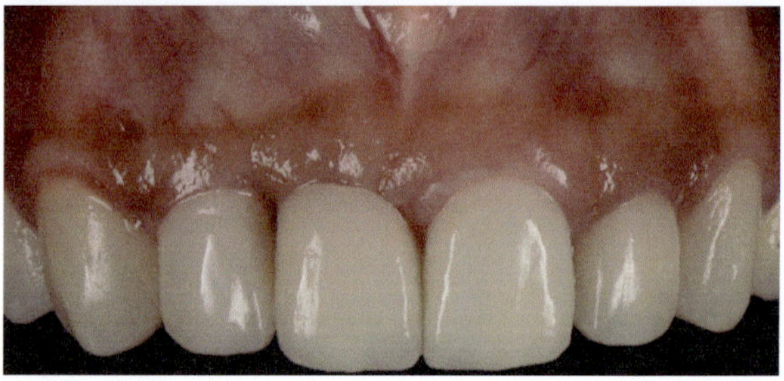

Fig. 11.191 Postoperative close-up view. The absence of papilla in between #12 and #11 was prosthetically managed with a long connector

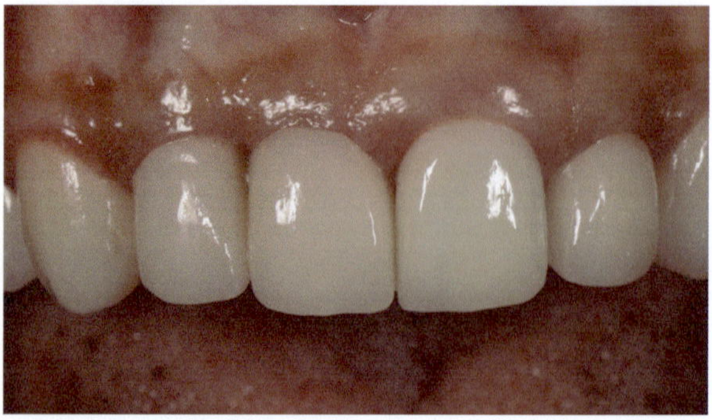

Fig. 11.192 One year Post-operative view. The convexity of tissue contours in areas on PET are well maintained

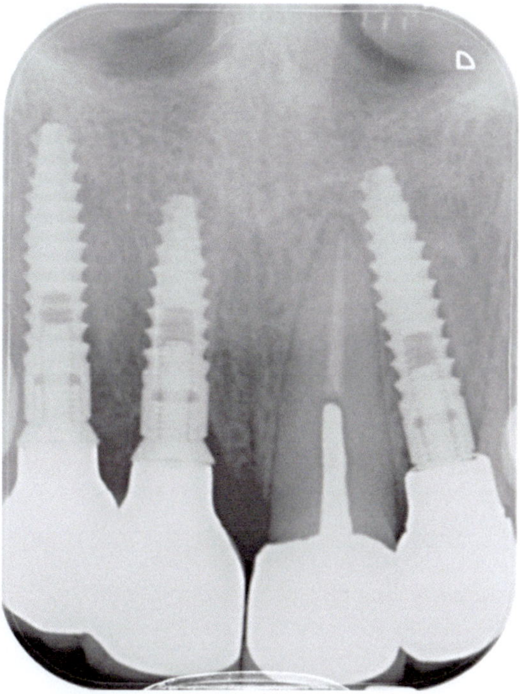

Fig. 11.193 Radiographs at 1 year showing stable interdental bone levels at this time

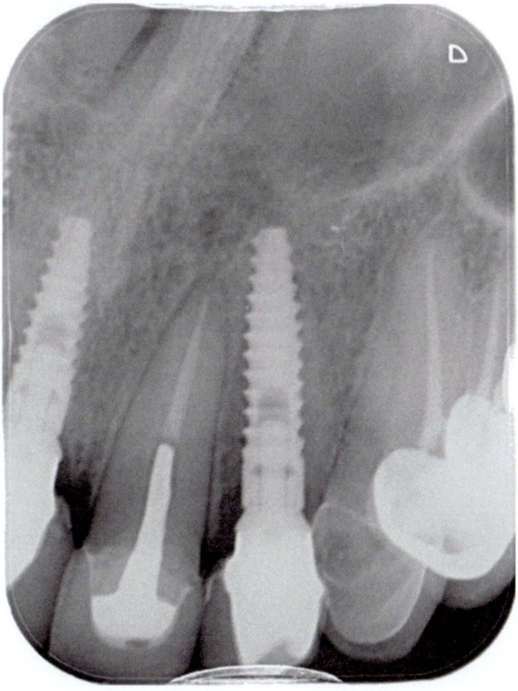

Fig. 11.194 Radiograph of 22 at 1 year

11.8 Socket Shield/Pontic Shield/Root Submergence in Maxillary Anterior Region

11.8.1 Case 10: Socket Shield in #12 and #21 and Pontic Shield in #11

Surgical & Restorative Dentistry: Dr. Ali Tunkiwala.

Lab Credits: Danesh Vazifdar, Adaro Lab, Mumbai:

A 62-year-old healthy male patient reported with unrestorable upper central incisors and right lateral incisor. Socket shield with one-time abutment placed in right lateral and left central positions and pontic shield used on right central to maintain tissue contour (Figs. 11.195, 11.196, 11.197, 11.198, 11.199, 11.200, 11.201, 11.202, 11.203, 11.204, 11.205, 11.206, 11.207, 11.208, 11.209, 11.210, 11.211, 11.212, 11.213, 11.214, 11.215, 11.216, 11.217, 11.218, 11.219, 11.220 and 11.221).

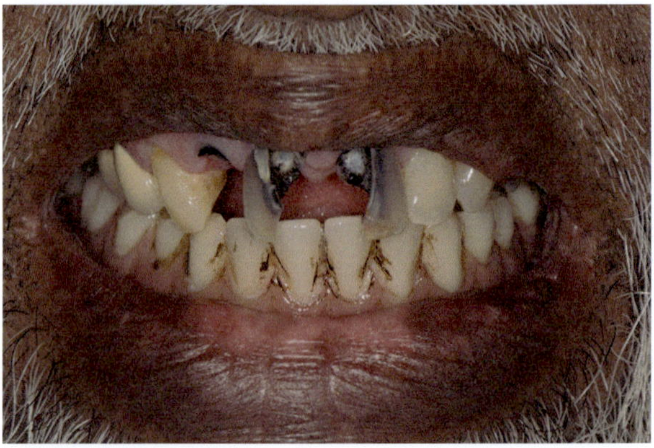

Fig. 11.195 Preoperative smile showing decayed, unrestorable incisors

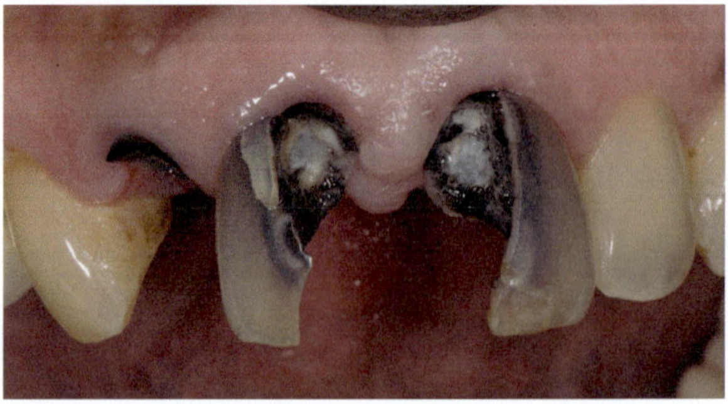

Fig. 11.196 #12 and #21 planned for socket shield and #11 for pontic shield.

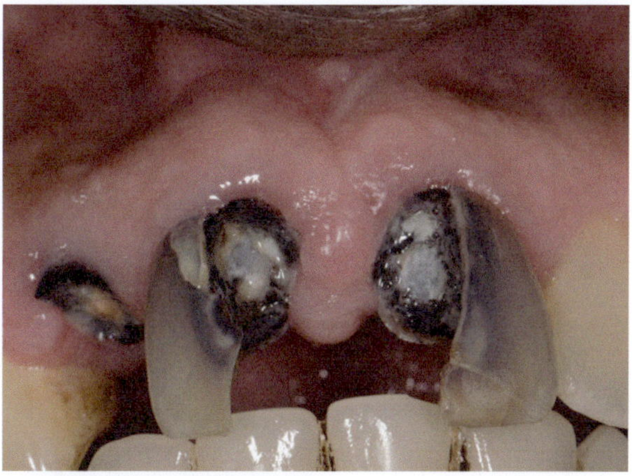

Fig. 11.197 The preoperative labial contour was pristine, our goal was to maintain that

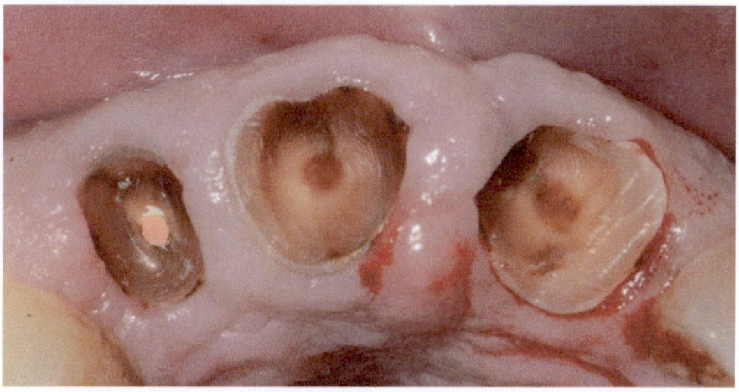

Fig. 11.198 The first step of decoronation

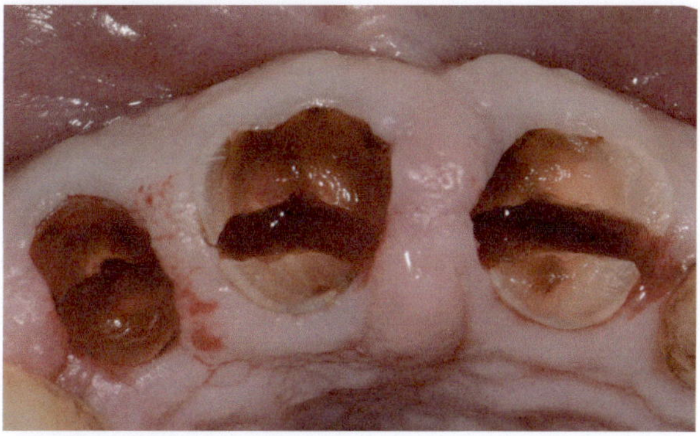

Fig. 11.199 The horizontal cuts

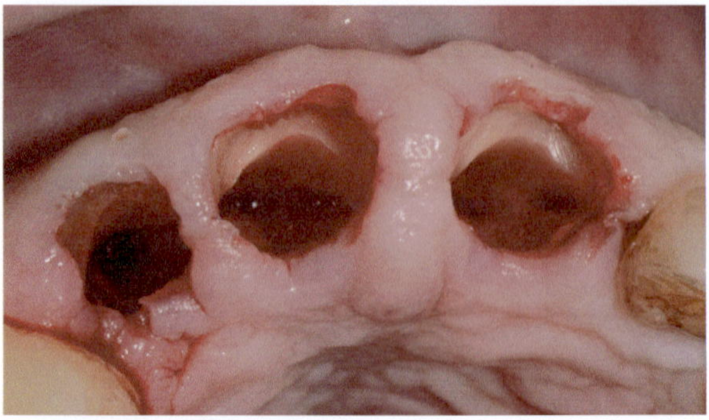

Fig. 11.200 The shields prepared. #11 had a periapical lesion, it was prepared as a pontic shield and not root submergence

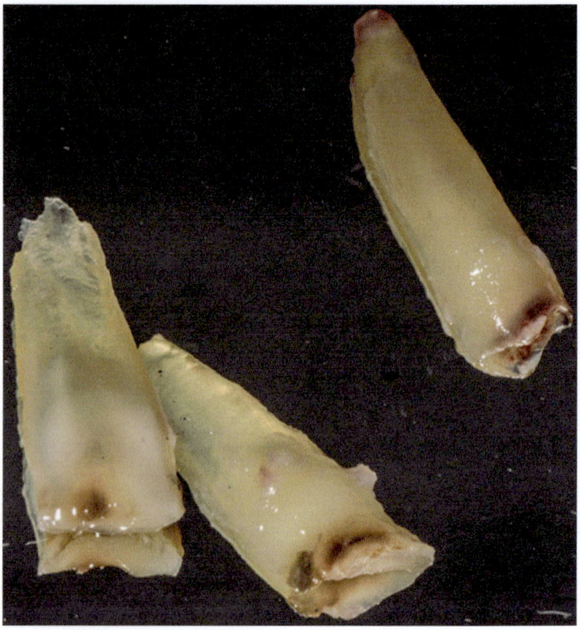

Fig. 11.201 The extracted palatal fragments and apices of teeth

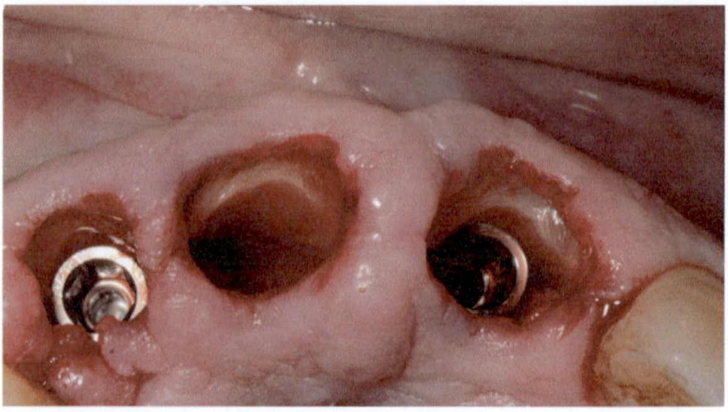

Fig. 11.202 Implants placed

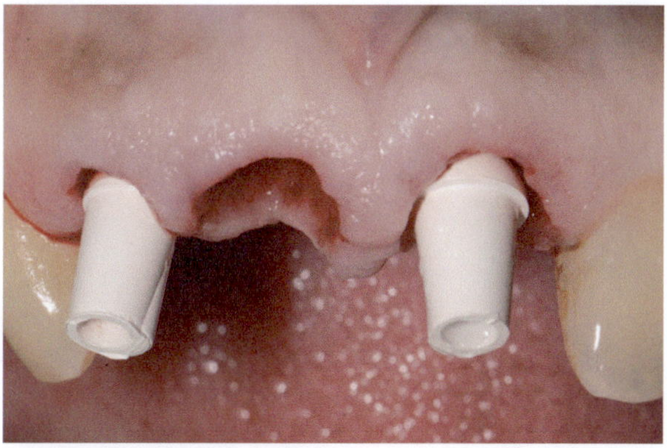

Fig. 11.203 BioHpp; Ceramic reinforced PEEK used as a one-time abutment option

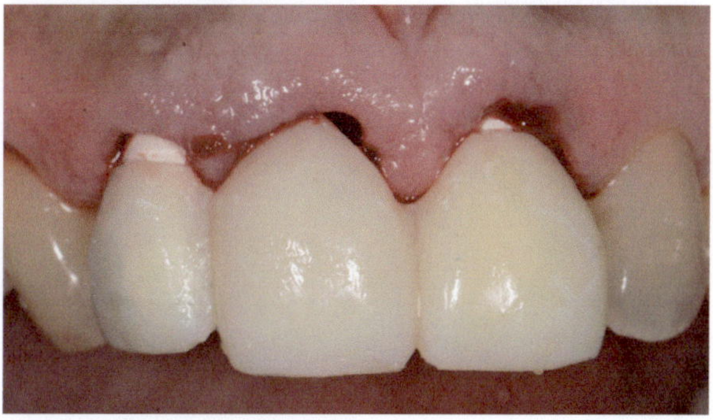

Fig. 11.204 The provisional restoration made from preoperative wax-up. Margins kept supragingival to allow gingival healing without interference from residual cement

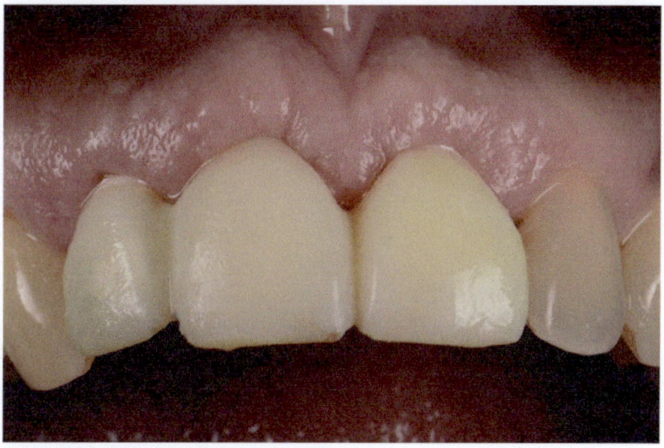

Fig. 11.205 The provisional restoration and surrounding peri-implant architecture at 4 months

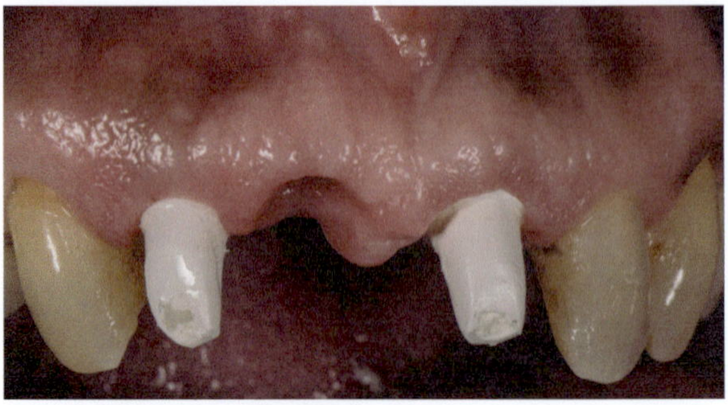

Fig. 11.206 Labial contour well maintained due to the partial extraction therapy with good soft tissue quality

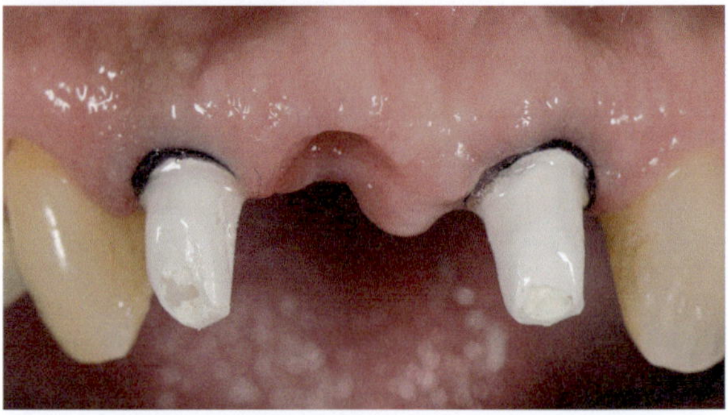

Fig. 11.207 Tissue contours on removal of the provisional restoration

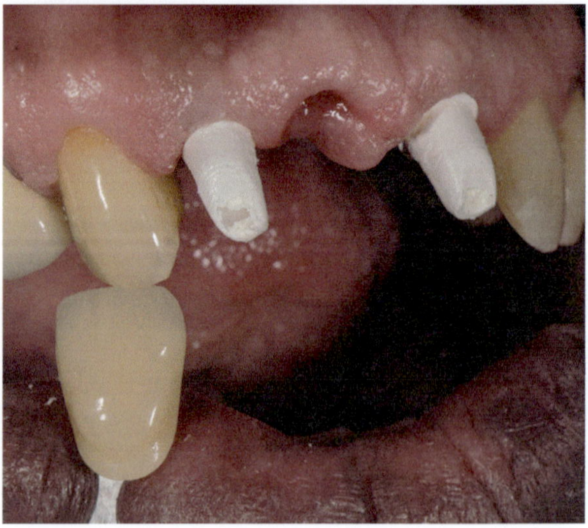

Fig. 11.208 Margins refined on the abutments and gingival retraction done to capture them

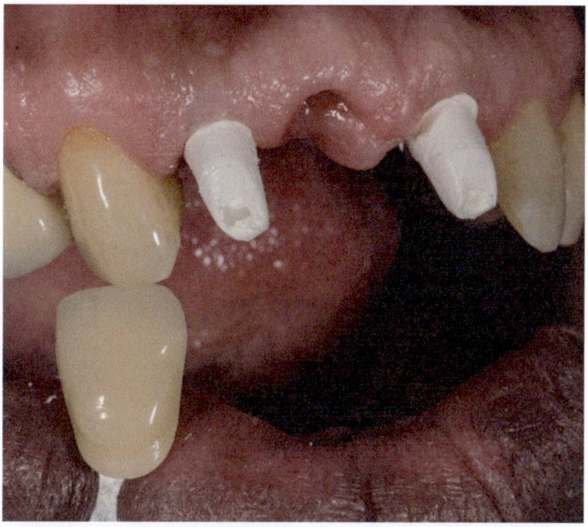

Fig. 11.209 Shade tab picture

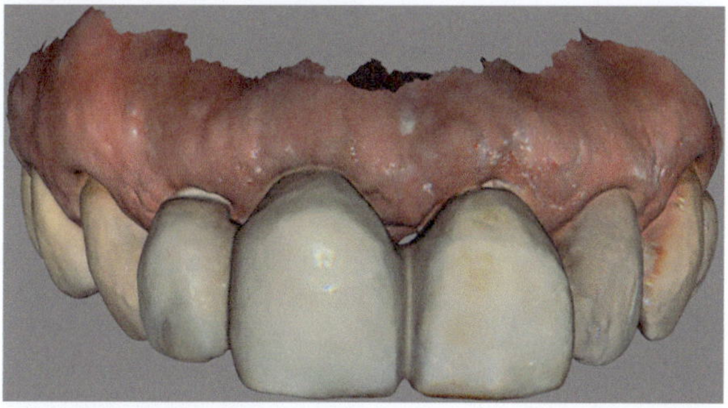

Fig. 11.210 Digital scan of approved provisional restoration to be used as guidance of length of final restorations

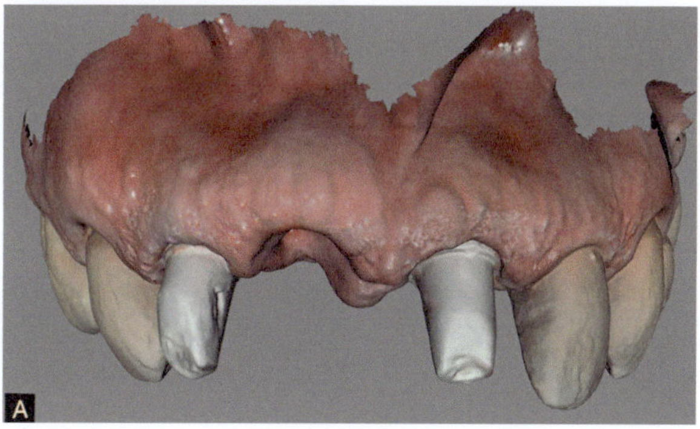

Fig. 11.211 Final digital impressions for fabricating a 3-unit implant bridge with an ovate pontic

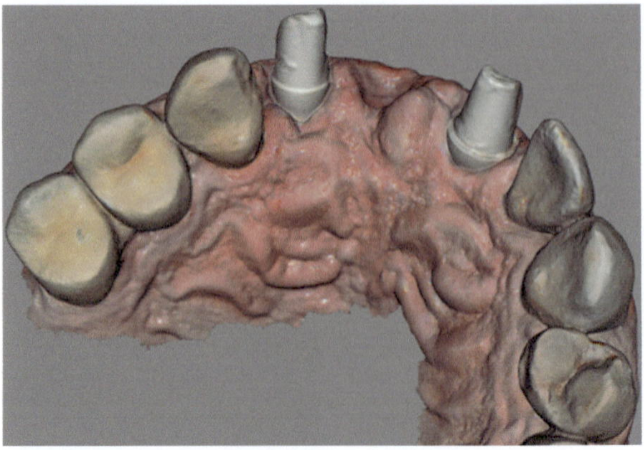

Fig. 11.212 Margins on palatal area kept 1 mm supragingival to allow easy clean-up of residual cement

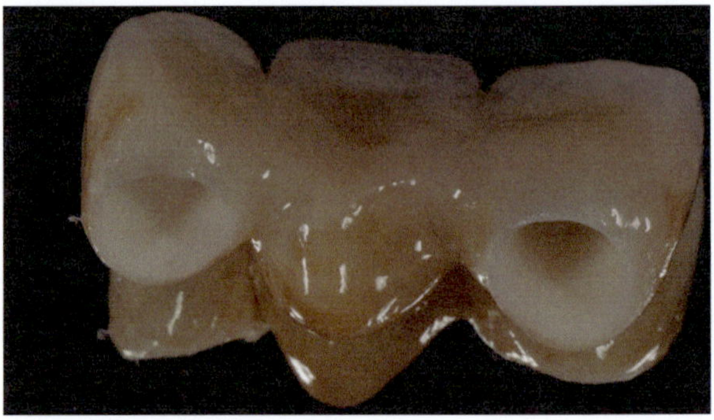

Fig. 11.213 Final lithium disilicate bridge with ovate pontic

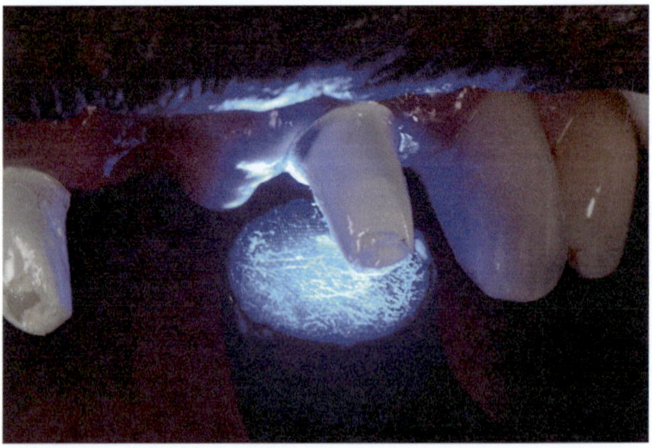

Fig. 11.214 Visio link bonding agent applied in thin layer on the abutments and light cured for 90 s

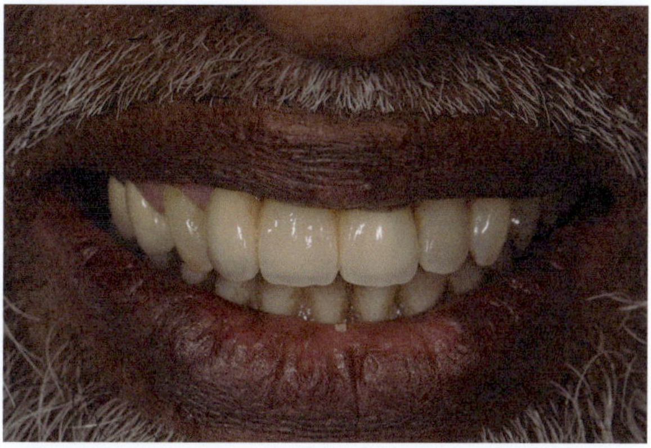

Fig. 11.215 Postoperative smile view

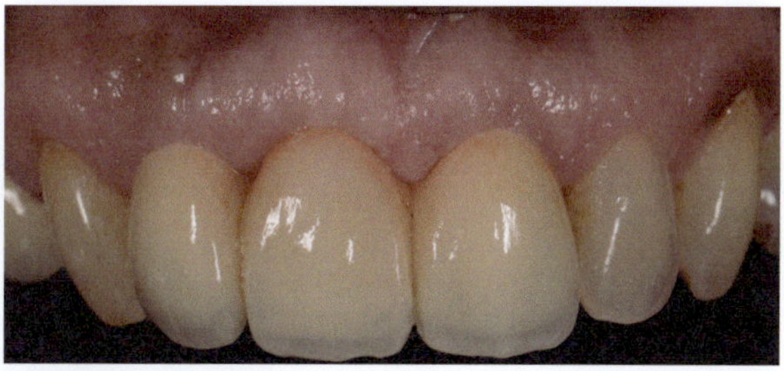

Fig. 11.216 Close-up view of final restorations. Good tissue contours evident. The partial extraction therapy allows good maintenance of gingival architecture

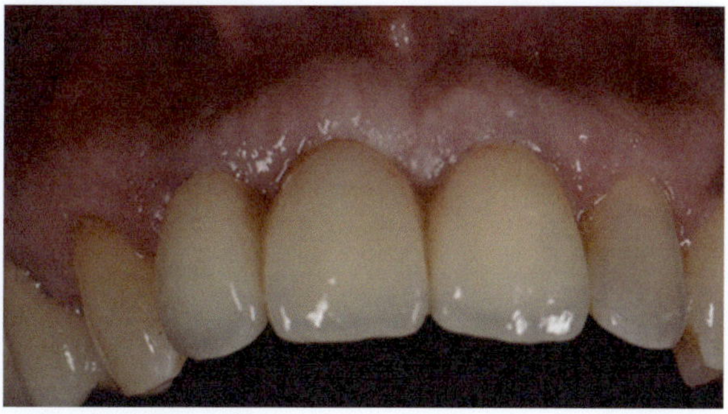

Fig. 11.217 Close-up view of final restorations. Good tissue contours evident. The partial extraction therapy allows good maintenance of gingival architecture

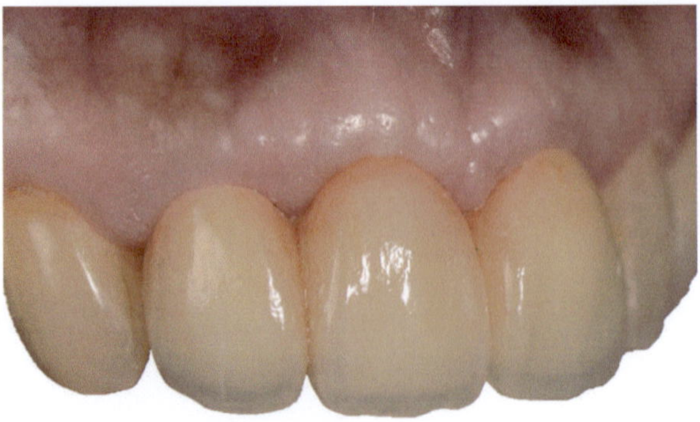

Fig. 11.218 The close-up profile allows better appreciation of tissue contours

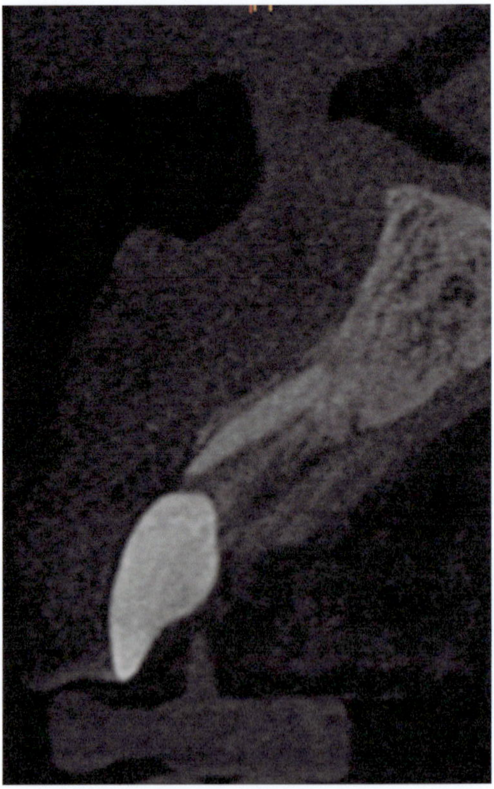

Fig. 11.219 Postoperative CBCT of tooth #11

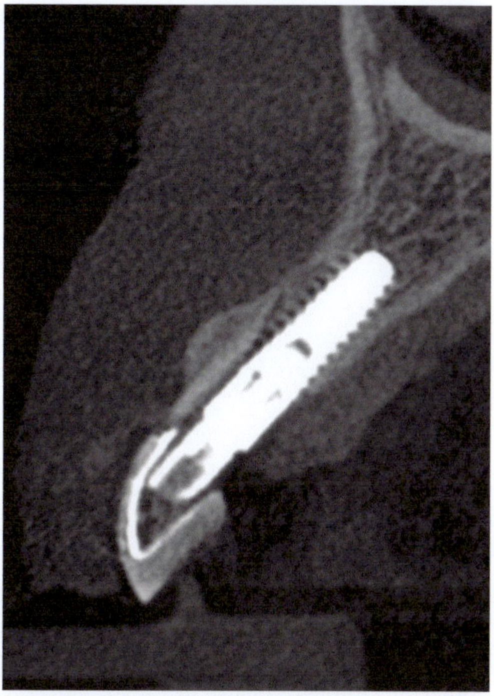

Fig. 11.220 Postoperative CBCT of tooth #12

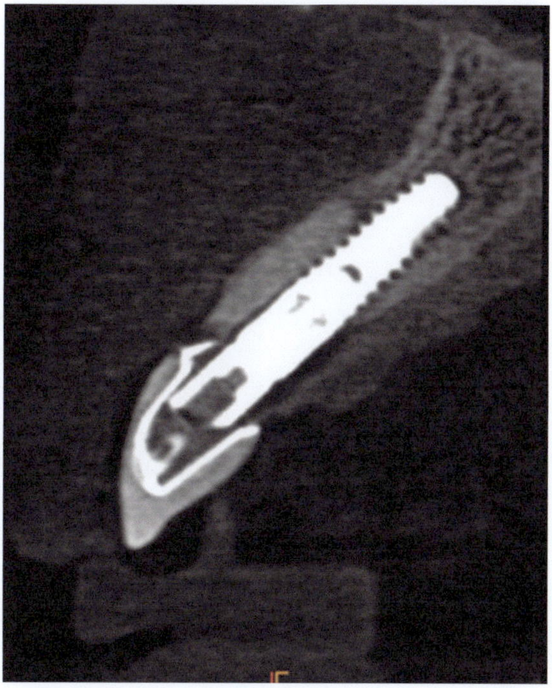

Fig. 11.221 Postoperative CBCT of tooth #21

11.8.2 Case 11: Socket Shield and Root Submergence in Maxillary Posterior Quadrant

Surgical and restorative dentistry: Dr. Udatta Kher.

Lab credits: Dentech Lab, Mumbai.

A 65-year-old female reported with a dislodged bridge from teeth 13, 14, 15, 16, 17. The 3 abutments on teeth 13 and 17 were broken down and were non-restorable. The abutment 15 was previously endodontically treated and in reasonable condition.

Challenges

1. Socket shield procedure for a maxillary second molar is a technically demanding procedure.

Partial extraction therapies done on teeth 18 and 15 were used to support an interim restoration during the surgical phase of treatment. Immediate loading or fixed provisional restorations were not made on the implants to minimize the risk of failure.

Whilst teeth 13 and 17 received a socket shield procedure; the tooth 15 was converted into a submerged root to provide a good emergence profile for the future pontic. A porcelain fused to metal cement retained restoration was fabricated supported on 3 implants placed in 13, 16, and 17 regions (Figs. 11.222, 11.223, 11.224, 11.225, 11.226, 11.227, 11.228, 11.229, 11.230, 11.231, 11.232, 11.233, 11.234 and 11.235).

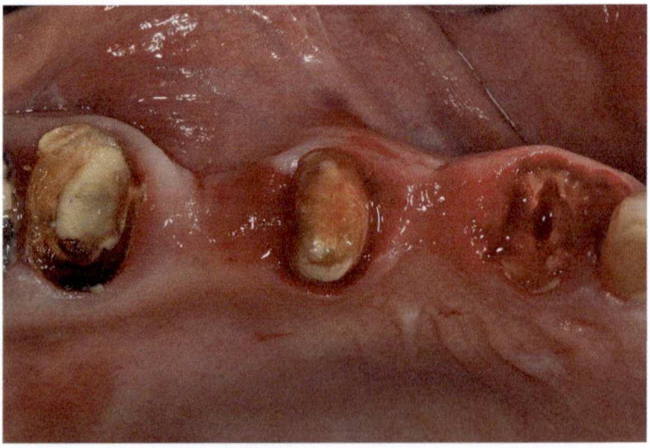

Fig. 11.222 Decayed and fractured teeth under a deboned old bridge

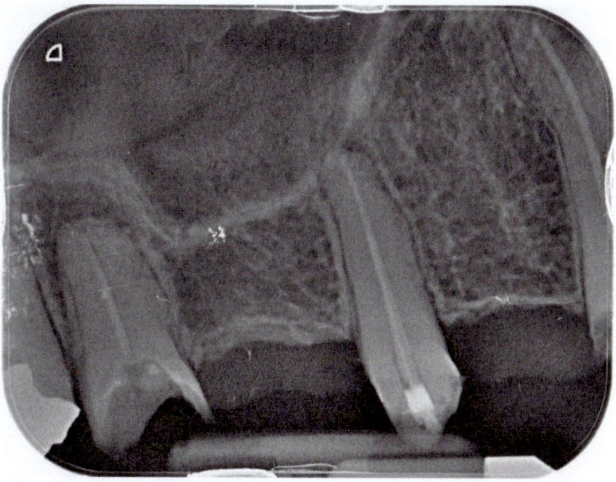

Fig. 11.223 Radiograph showing fractured and unrestorable bridge abutments

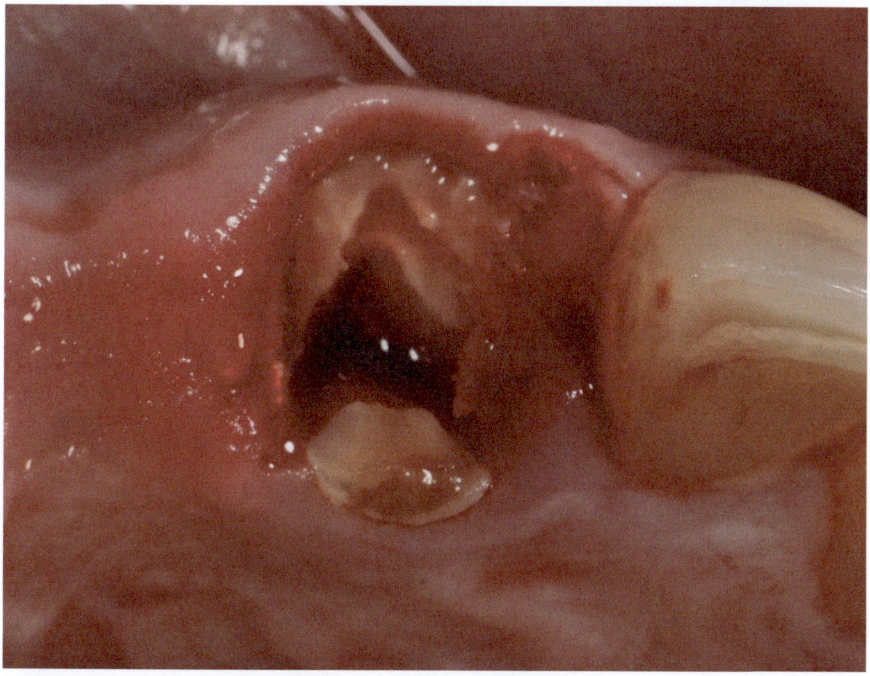

Fig. 11.224 Mesio-distal sectioning of tooth 13

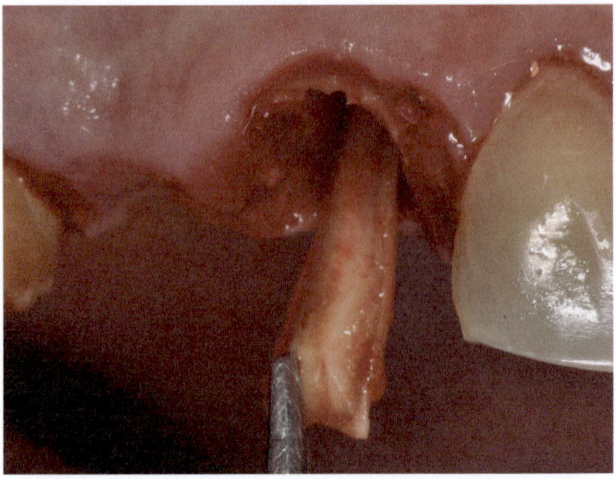

Fig. 11.225 Extraction of the palatal root fragment

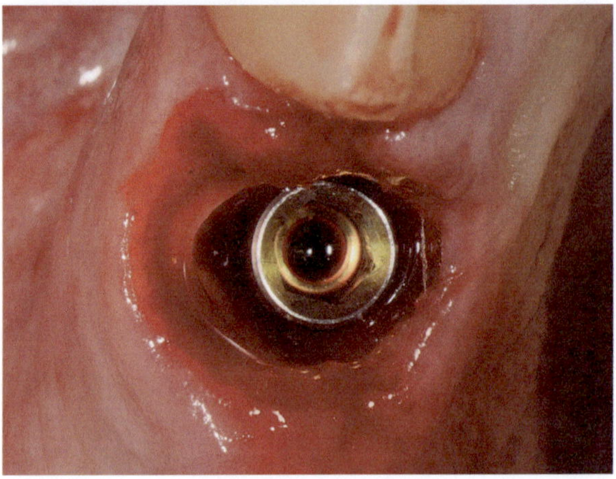

Fig. 11.226 Socket shield and implant placement for tooth 13

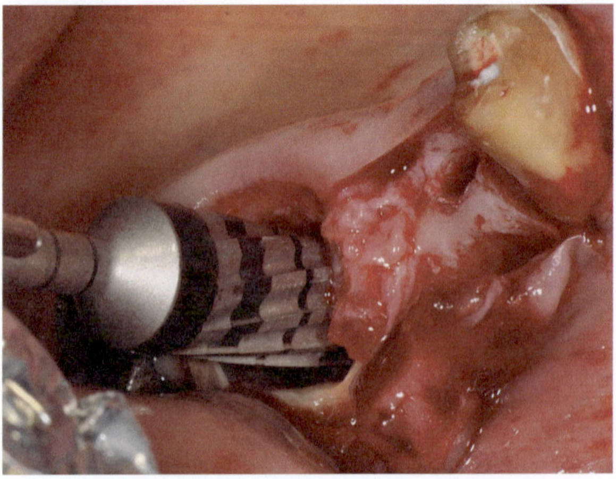

Fig. 11.227 Shield preparation followed by implant site preparation using Densah drill (Versah Inc., USA) in 17region

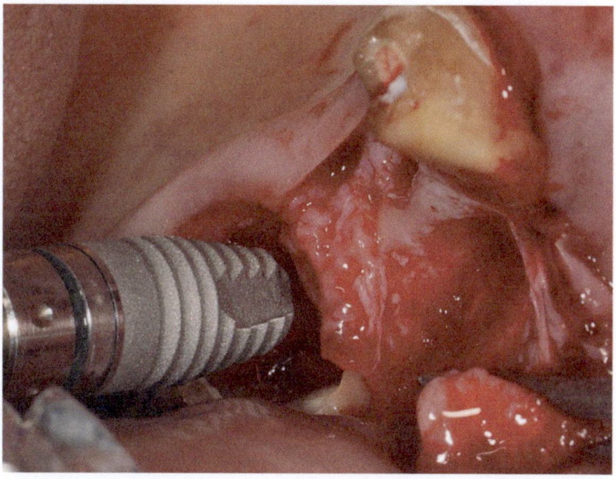

Fig. 11.228 Implant placement for tooth 17

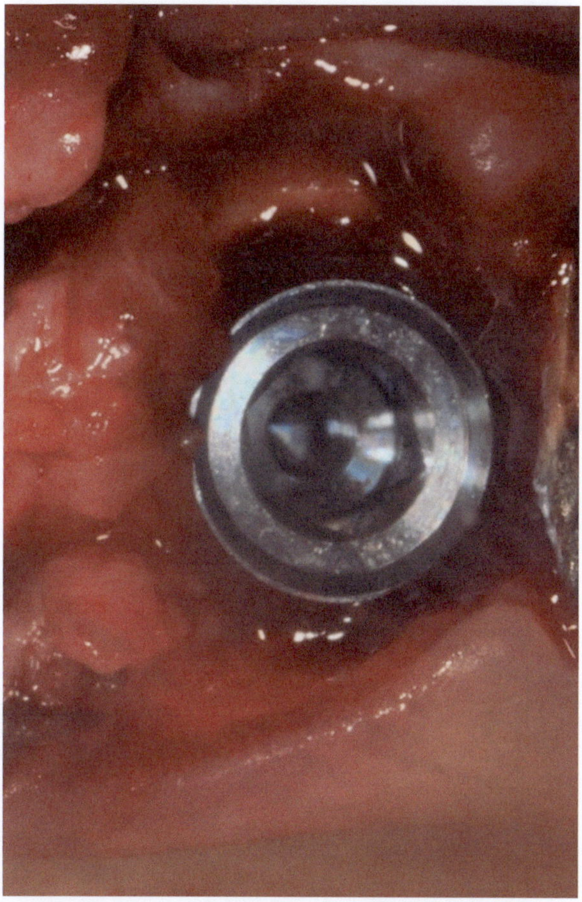

Fig. 11.229 Socket shield and implant placement for tooth #17

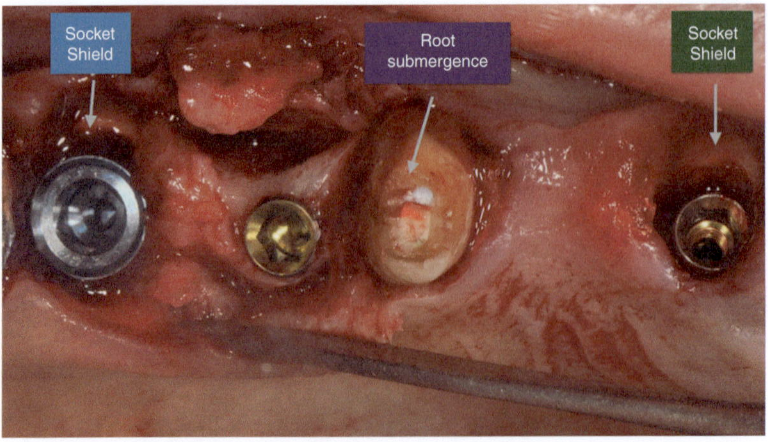

Fig. 11.230 Socket shields for teeth #13 and 17. Tooth #15 retained to support an interim restoration. To be submerged prior to final restoration

Fig. 11.231 Collagen sponge and sutures over the sockets

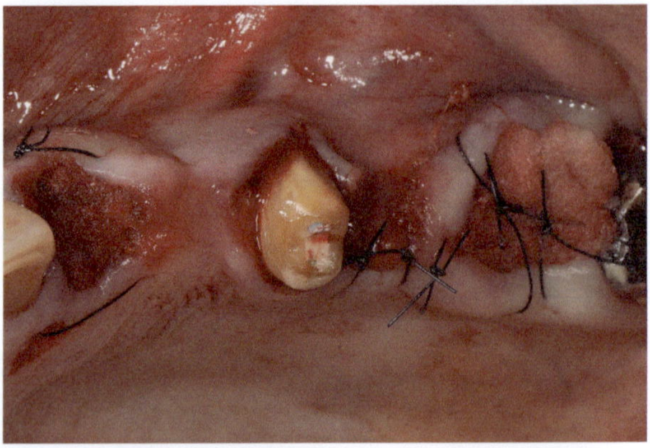

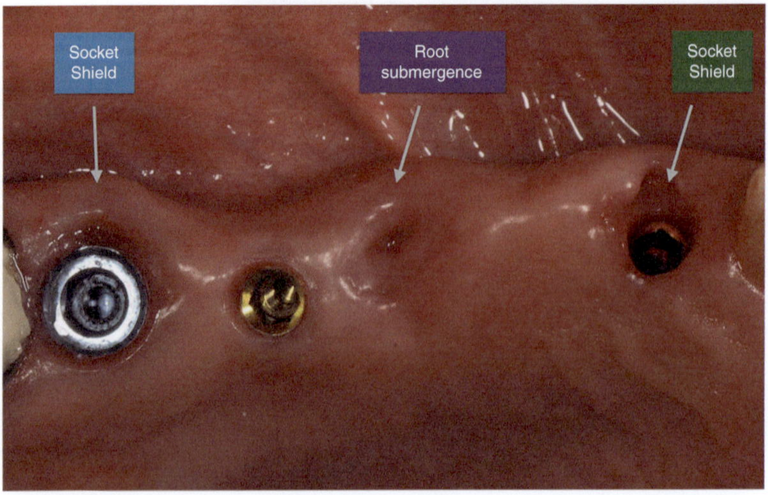

Fig. 11.232 Situation after complete healing. Root submergence done for tooth #15

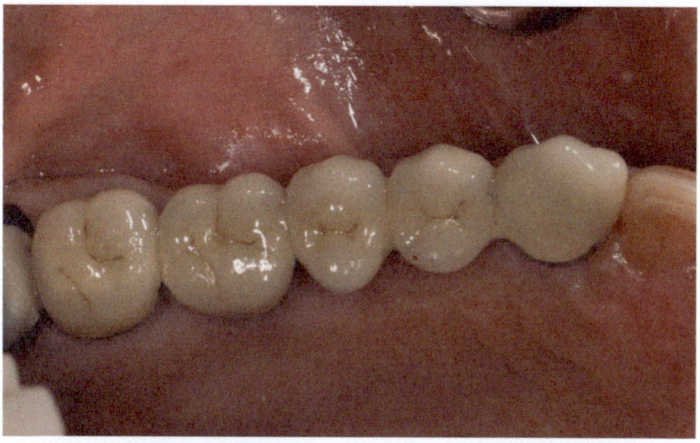

Fig. 11.233 Definitive porcelain fused to metal cement retained restoration

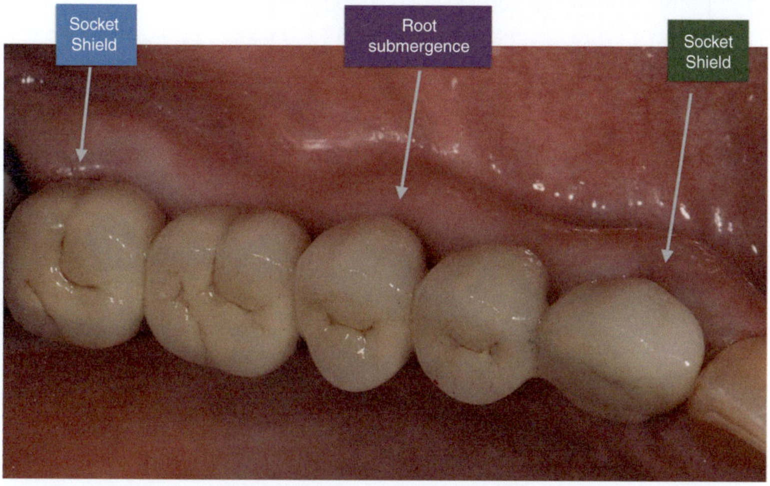

Fig. 11.234 Postoperative view displaying maintenance of tissue contours around the PET sites. Note ridge alteration in 14 and 16 regions

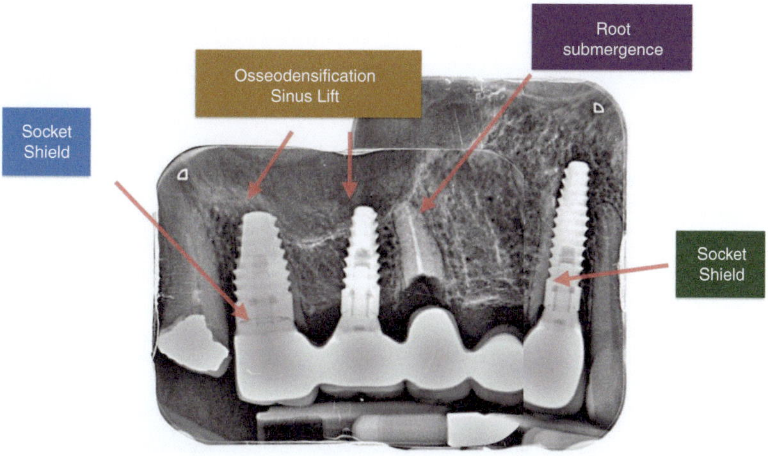

Fig. 11.235 Postoperative radiograph of the definitive restoration with submerged root

11.8.3 CASE 12: Pontic Shield with Multiple Adjacent Socket Shield in Aesthetic Zone

Surgical Dentistry: Dr. Udatta Kher.

Restorative Dentistry: Dr. Ali Tunkiwala.

Lab Credits: Adaro Dental Lab, Mumbai.

65 year old, male patient reported with faulty crowns on all upper anterior teeth with leaky margins. The underlying teeth were destroyed by decay and could not be saved. Tooth #13, 12, 11, 21 and 22 had to be extracted. Socket shield was performed for all teeth except #11 for which pontic shield was carried out. A one time abutment concept was used for immediate provisional restoration and then eventually after integration, lithium disilicate restorations were fabricated (Figs. 11.236, 11.237, 11.238, 11.239, 11.240, 11.241, 11.242, 11.243, 11.244, 11.245, 11.246, 11.247, 11.248, 11.249, 11.250, 11.251, 11.252, 11.253, 11.254, 11.255, 11.256, 11.257, 11.258, 11.259, 11.260, 11.261, 11.262, 11.263 and 11.264). The implants and prosthetic components in this case were sponsored by Bredent Medical, Germany

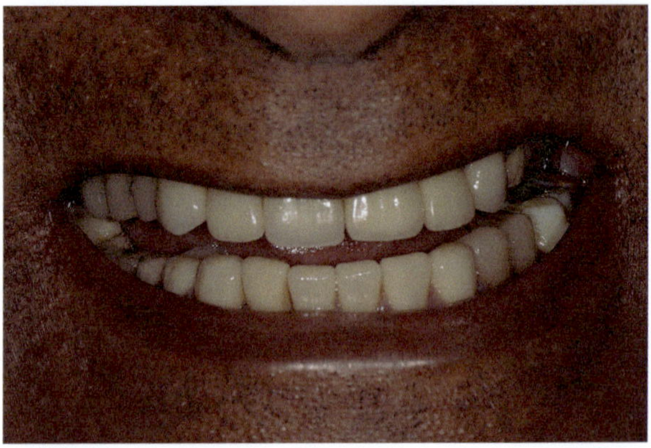

Fig. 11.236 Preoperative smile showing restorations on all upper and lower teeth

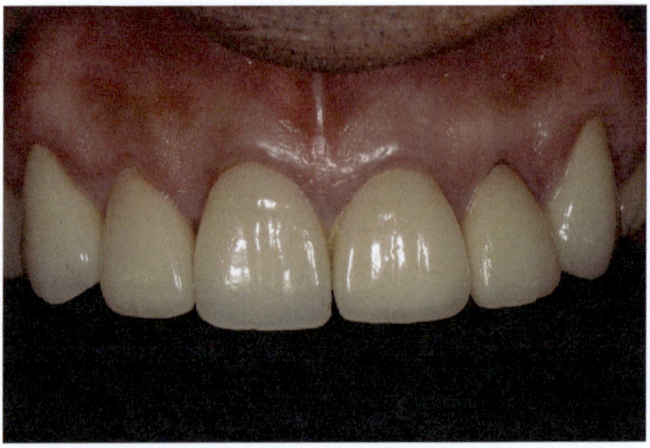

Fig. 11.237 13, 12, 11, 21, and 22 were structurally very poor and prone to fracture. #11 had a periapical lesion and was symptomatic

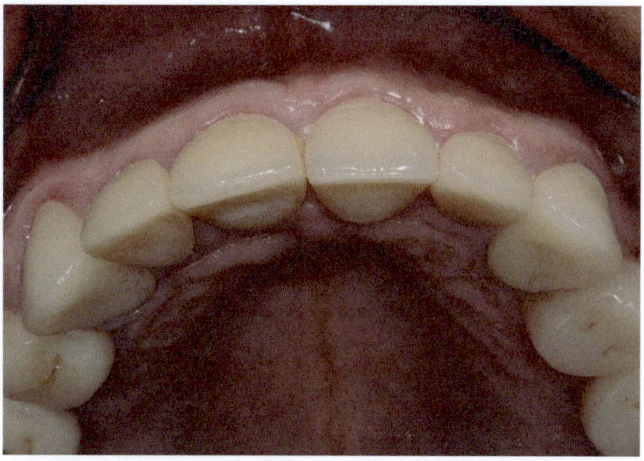

Fig. 11.238 Very good labial contours that needed to be preserved

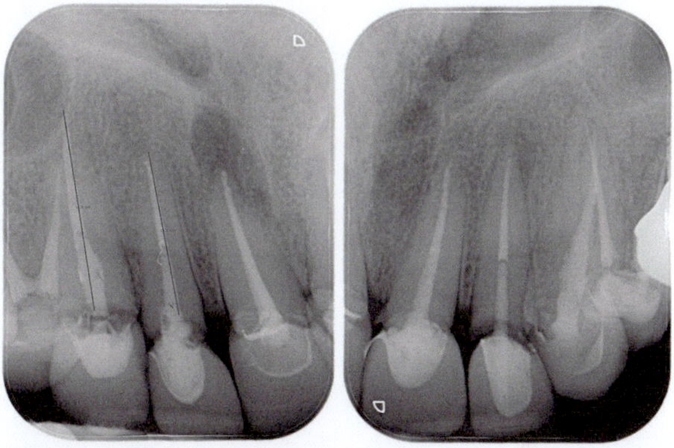

Fig. 11.239 Preoperative radiographs depicting the poor structure of teeth under the restorations and periapical lesions within bone

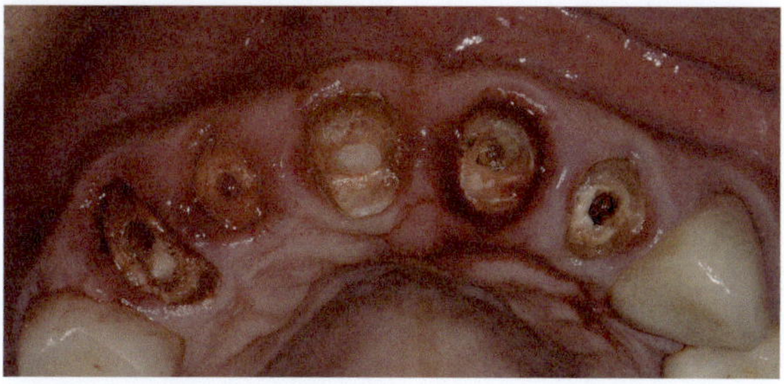

Fig. 11.240 Removal of all faulty restorations revealed the structurally poor teeth

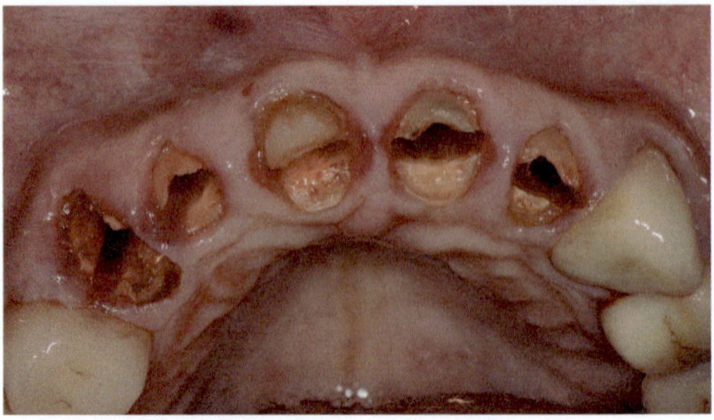

Fig. 11.241 Initiation of partial extraction therapies

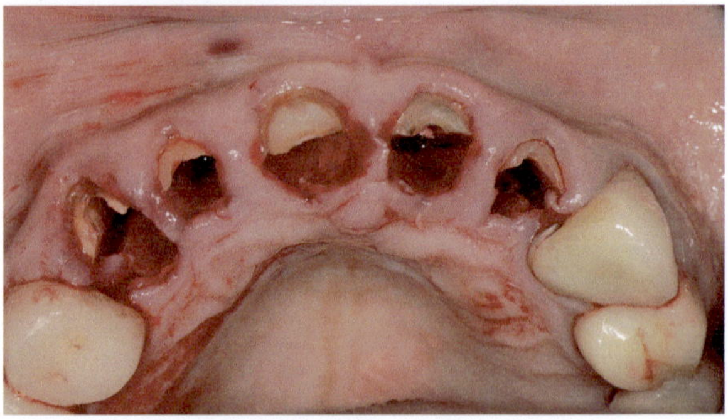

Fig. 11.242 Palatal portion of roots extracted with apices

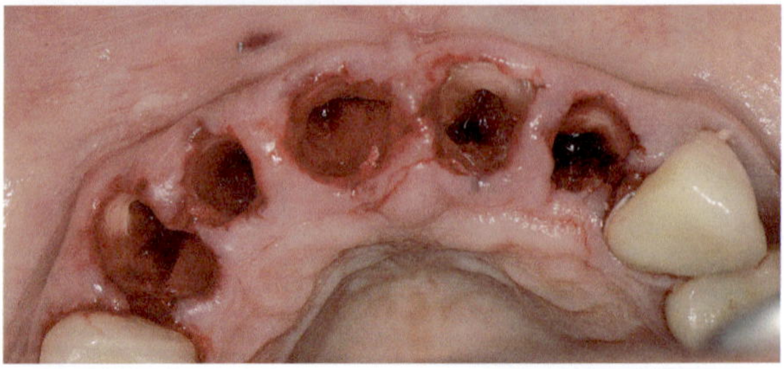

Fig. 11.243 Final shield preparations. #11 used as a pontic shield

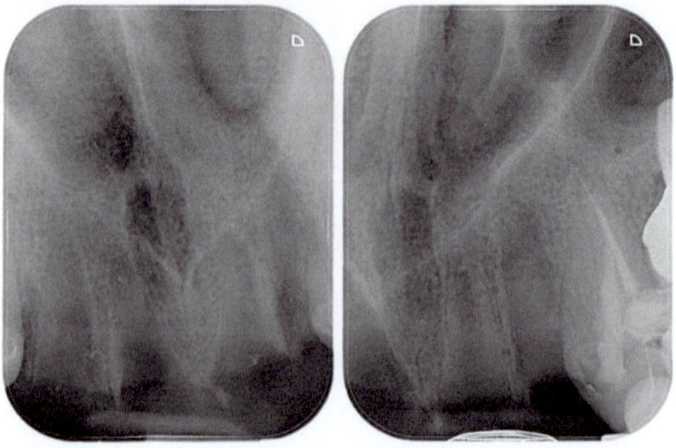

Fig. 11.244 Intra-surgical radiograph depicts no endodontic filling material after partial extractions and prior to implant placement

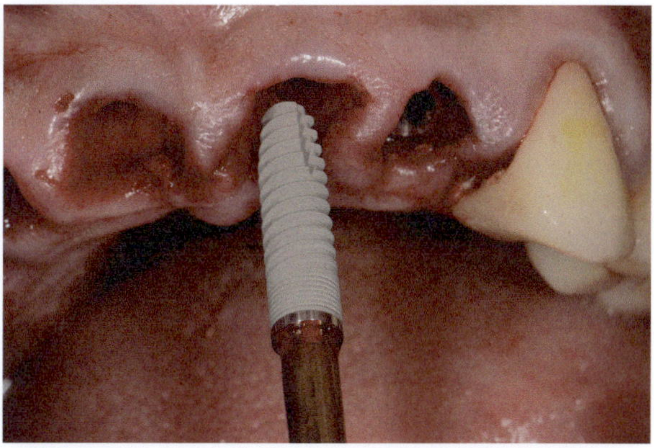

Fig. 11.245 Implants placed in the predetermined sites

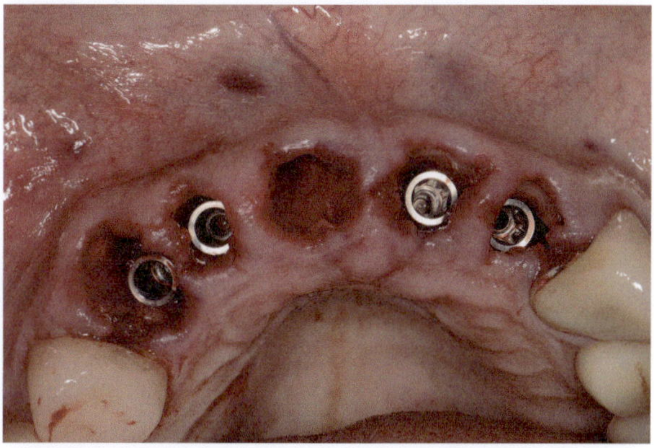

Fig. 11.246 #11 was a pontic shield. Rest all were socket shields with immediate placement

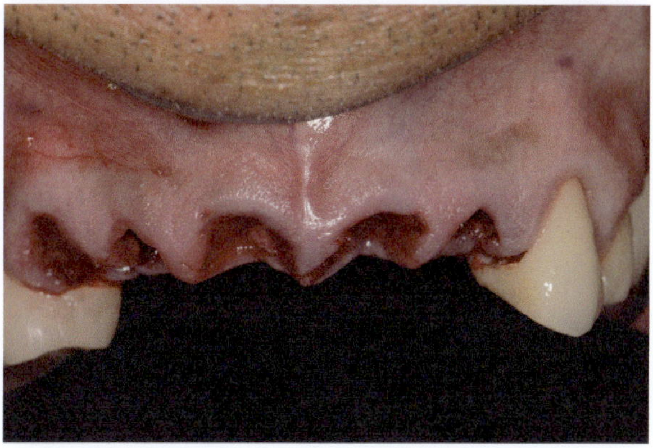

Fig. 11.247 Minimal trauma to tissues at the end of extractions, contours maintained

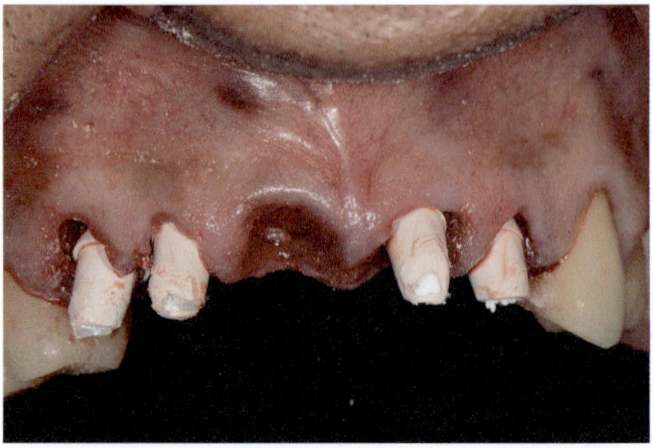

Fig. 11.248 Final Bio-HPP abutments placed as one-time abutment concept on 4 implants. The abutments were modified to achieve restorative clearance

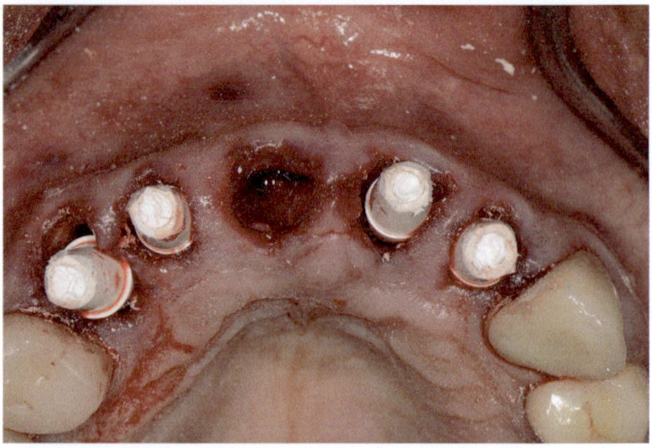

Fig. 11.249 The occlusal view showing the abutments in relation to implant sites with good tissue contours

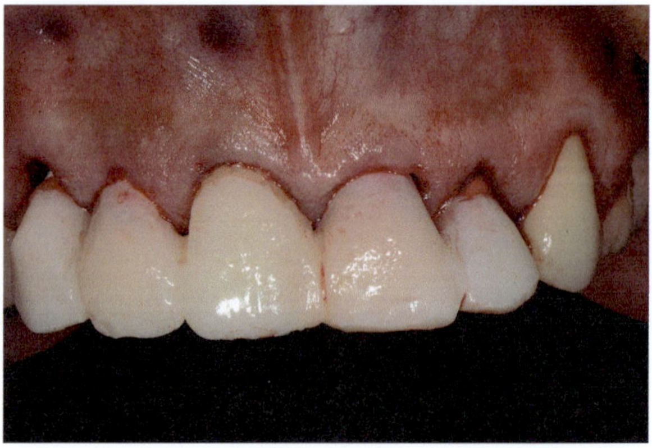

Fig. 11.250 Immediate chairside cement retained provisional restoration

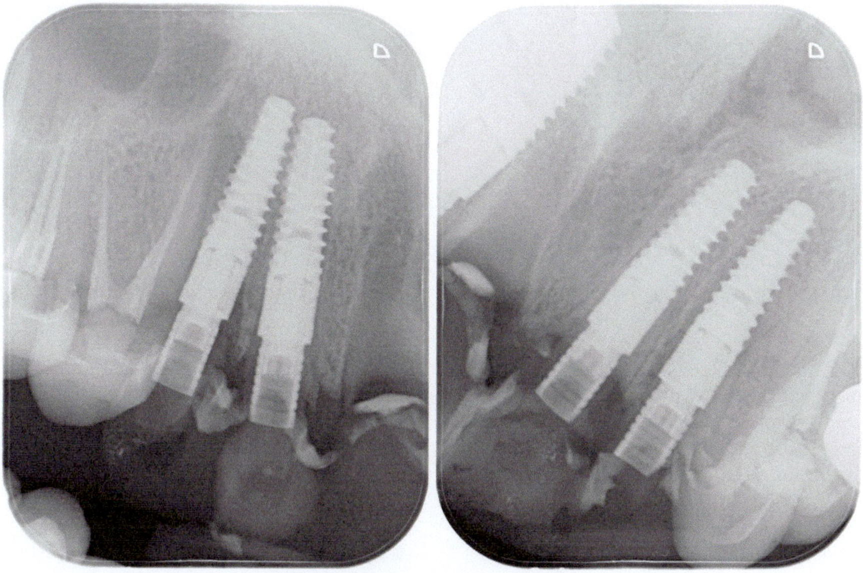

Fig. 11.251 Postsurgical radiographs

Fig. 11.252 Provisional restorations modified and well-integrated with surrounding peri-implant tissues at 72 h

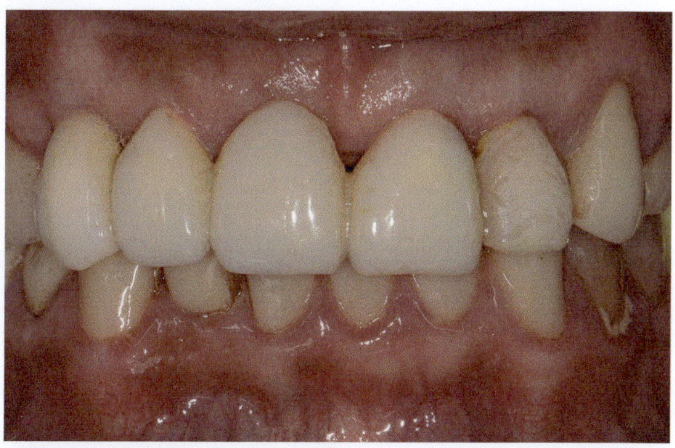

Fig. 11.253 Upon removal of provisional restorations at 4 months, the tissue levels looked good

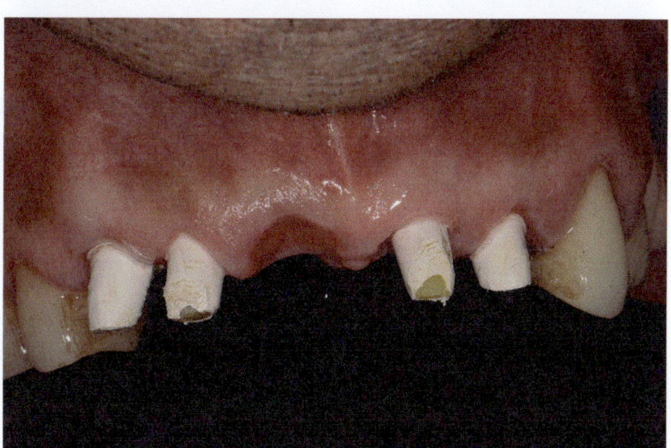

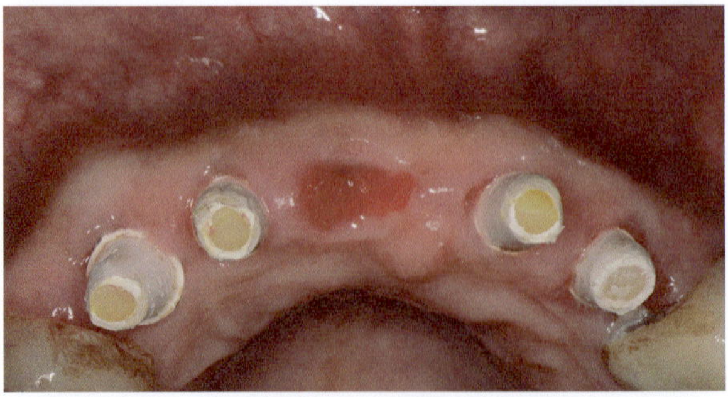

Fig. 11.254 Occlusal view at 4 months showing excellent labial tissue contours

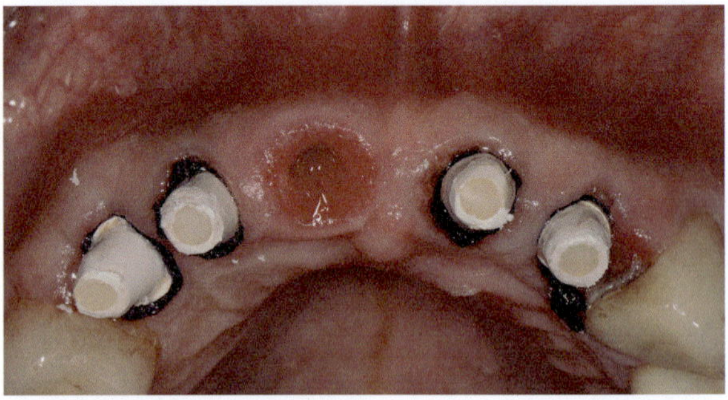

Fig. 11.255 Tissue management done with dry cord to capture the impression of the abutments on which final cement-retained restorations would be fabricated

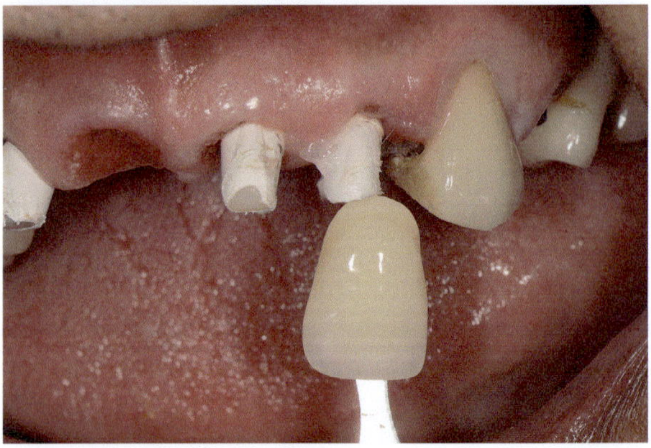

Fig. 11.256 Picture for shade matching

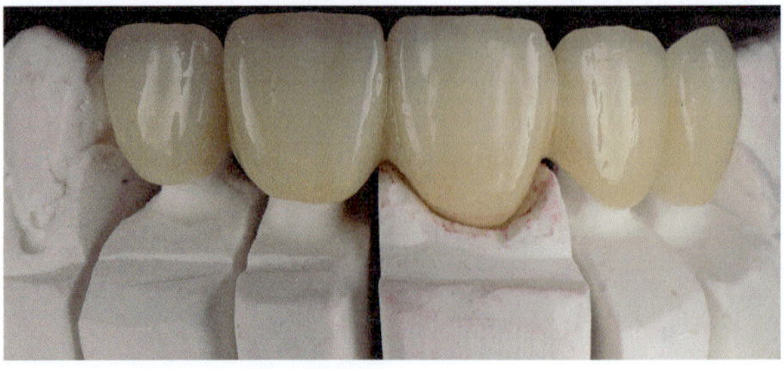

Fig. 11.257 Final lithium disilicate restorations

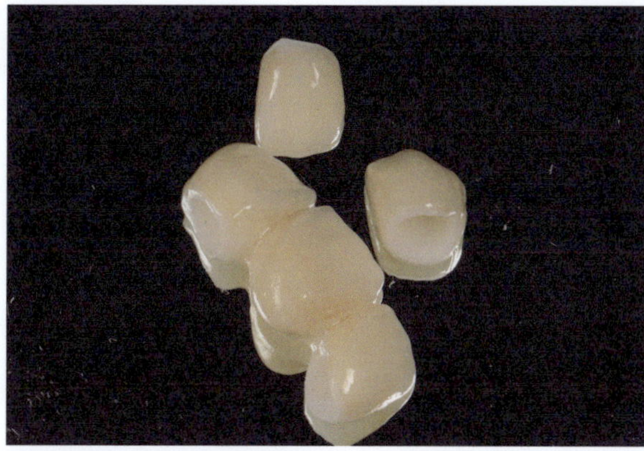

Fig. 11.258 #12, #11, and #21 was a 3-unit restoration and others were individual restorations

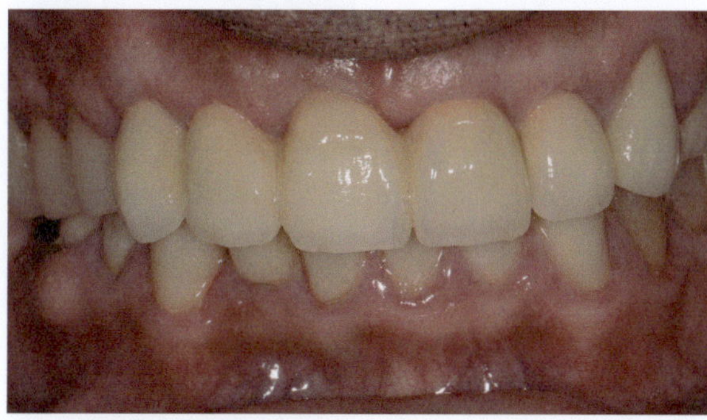

Fig. 11.259 Postoperative retracted view

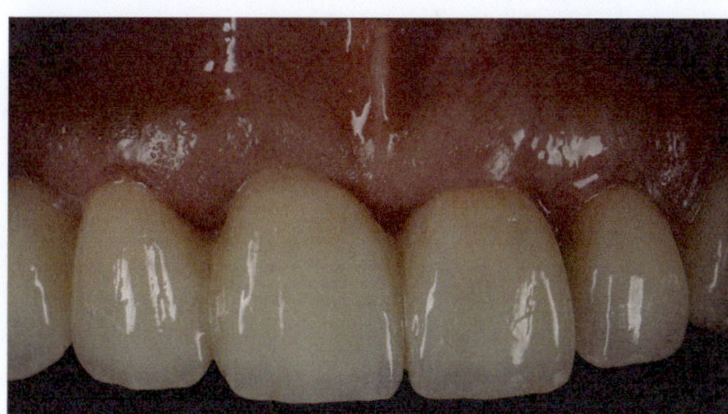

Fig. 11.260 Postoperative close-up view with excellent tissue levels and contours

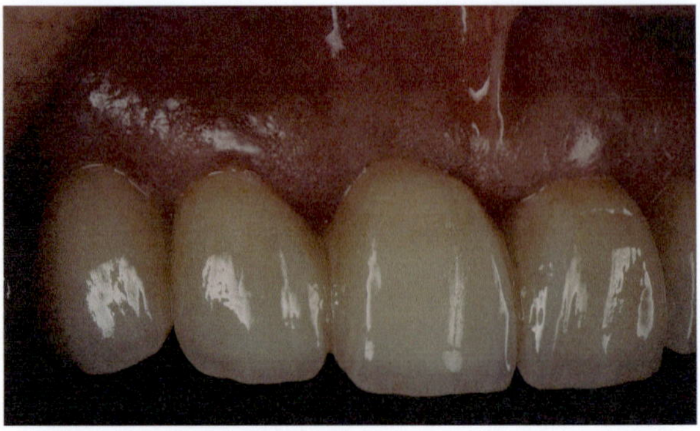

Fig. 11.261 Postoperative profile close up showing good tissue contours

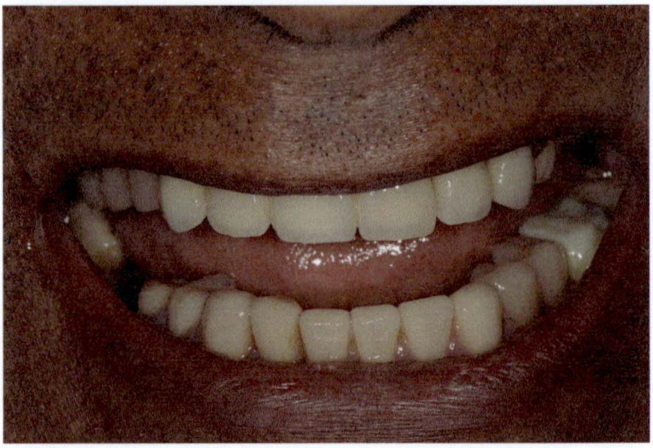

Fig. 11.262 Postoperative smile

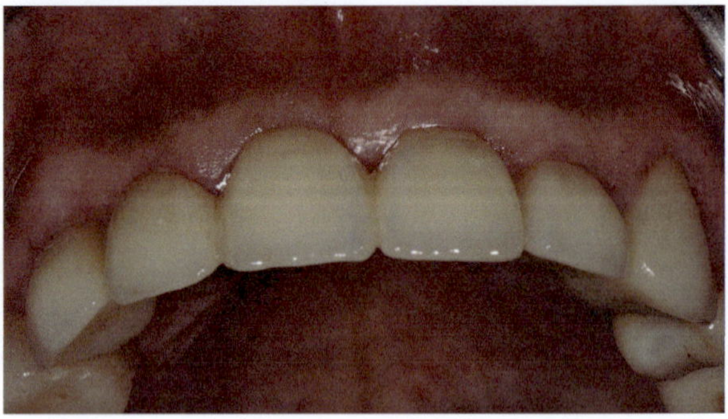

Fig. 11.263 Postoperative tissue contours showing a successful aesthetic outcome with PET

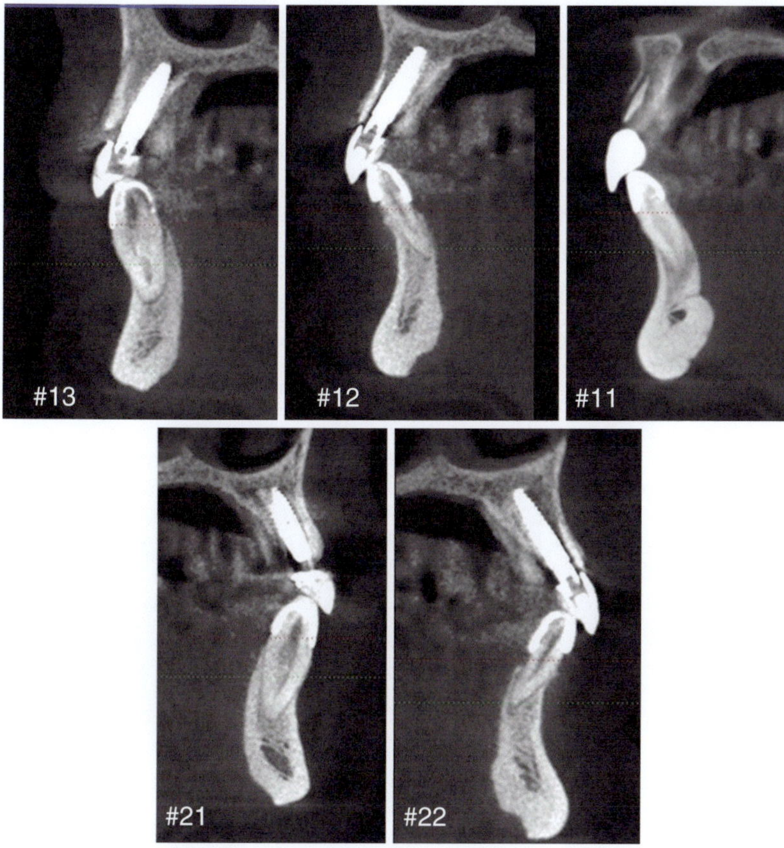

Fig. 11.264 Postoperative CBCT sections of each tooth with partial extraction therapy and implant with final restoration

11.8.4 CASE 13

Surgical and Restorative Dentistry: Udatta Kher

Lab credits: Katara Dental, Pune.

A 60-year-old lady reported with a failing anterior bridge. On removal of the bridge, it was observed that teeth 14, 22 and 23 were salvageable with post core and crown restorations. Teeth 11, 13 and 21 were non-salvageable due to lack of ferrule and subgingival caries.

Socket shield procedure with implant placement was done for teeth 13 and 21. Root of tooth 11 was submerged and a rotated palatal pedicled subepithelial connective tissue flap was used to cover it. Teeth 14, 22 and 23 were used to support a provisional restoration during the healing period.

Definitive porcelain fused to zirconia restoration was fabricated for the implant-supported restorations and for the crowns on teeth 14, 22 and 23 (Figs. 11.265, 11.266, 11.267, 11.268, 11.269, 11.270, 11.271, 11.272, 11.273, 11.274, 11.275, 11.276, 11.277, 11.278 and 11.279).

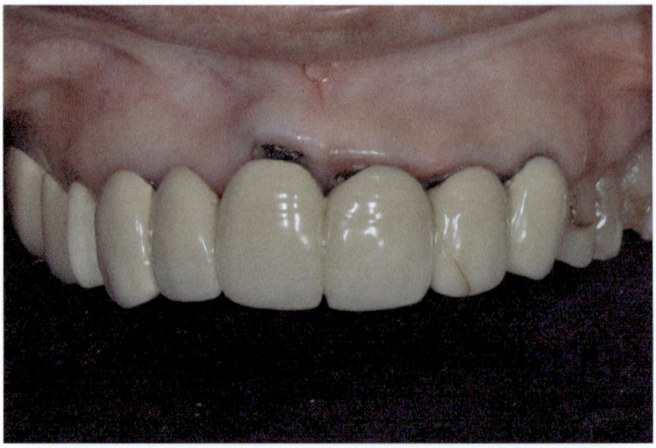

Fig. 11.265 Pre-operative situation. Failing anterior bridge

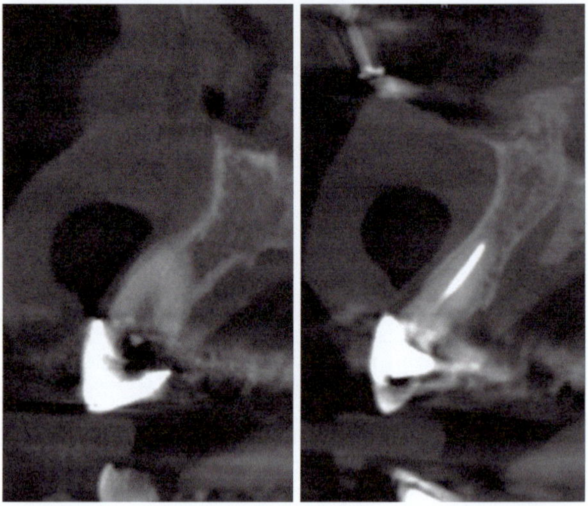

Fig. 11.266 Pre-operative scan for teeth 13 and 21, respectively

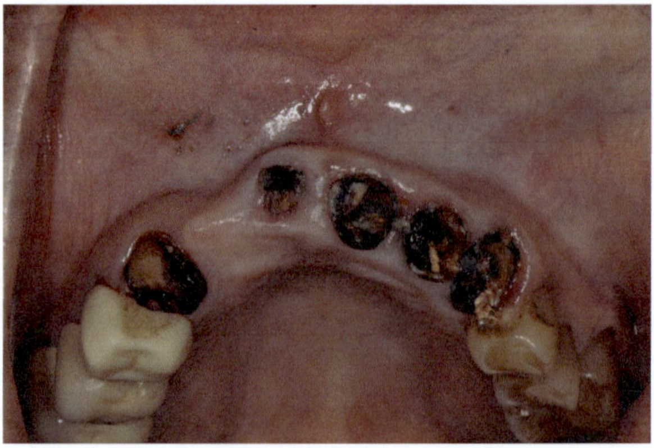

Fig. 11.267 Badly carious and broken down teeth. Teeth 13, 11 and 21 have subgingival caries and lack of ferrule for crowns

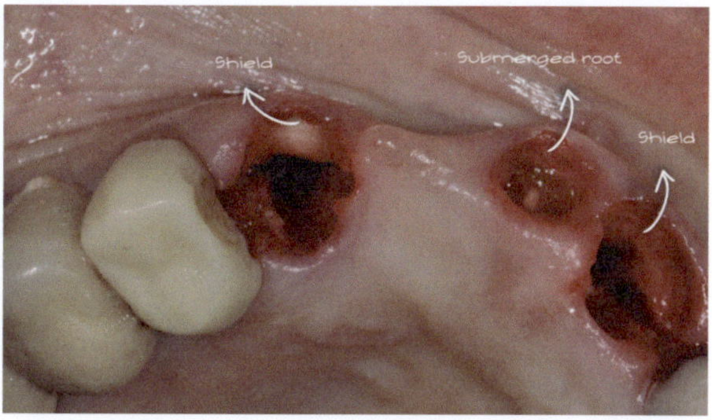

Fig. 11.268 Shield preparations done for teeth 13 and 21. Root submergence done for tooth 11

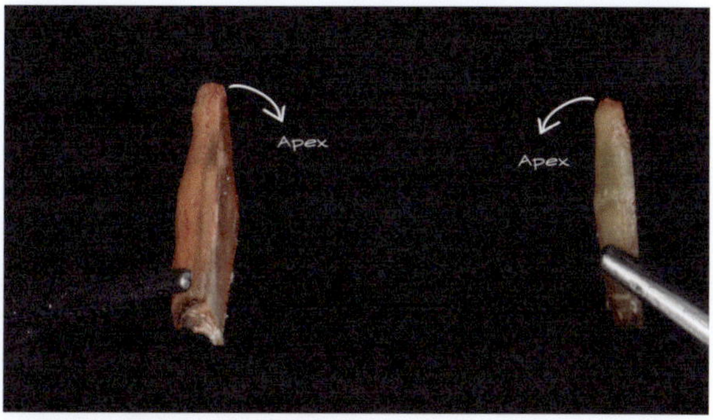

Fig. 11.269 Partial extractions of the roots displaying apices of the teeth

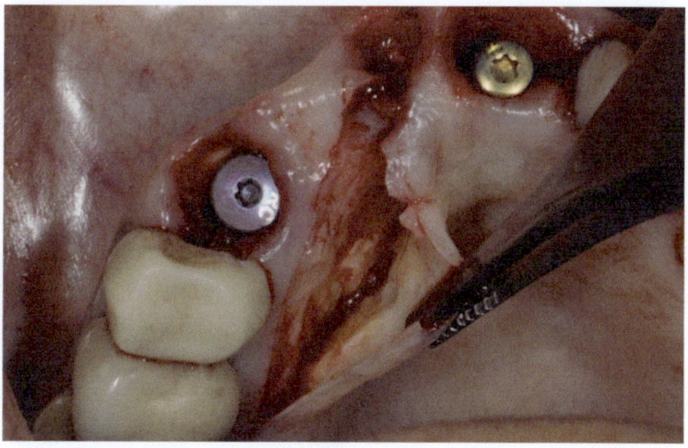

Fig. 11.270 Implant placements done in sockets of teeth 13 and 21. Partial thickness flap raised for harvesting connective tissue graft

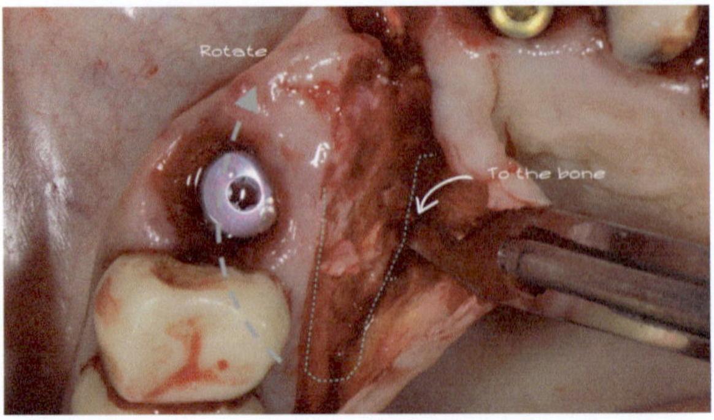

Fig. 11.271 Preparation for pedicled palatal connective tissue graft

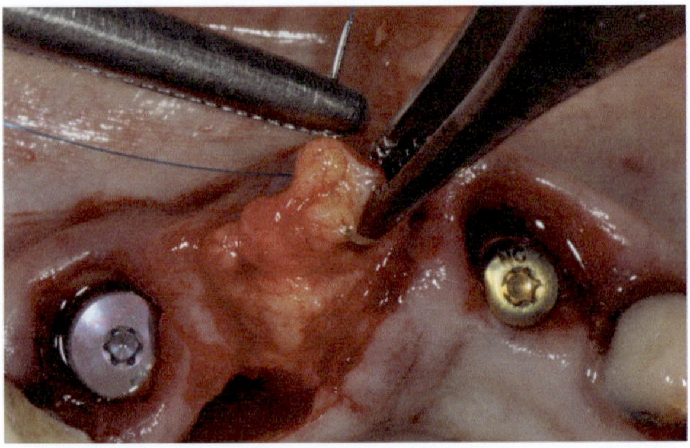

Fig. 11.272 The rotated pedicled graft

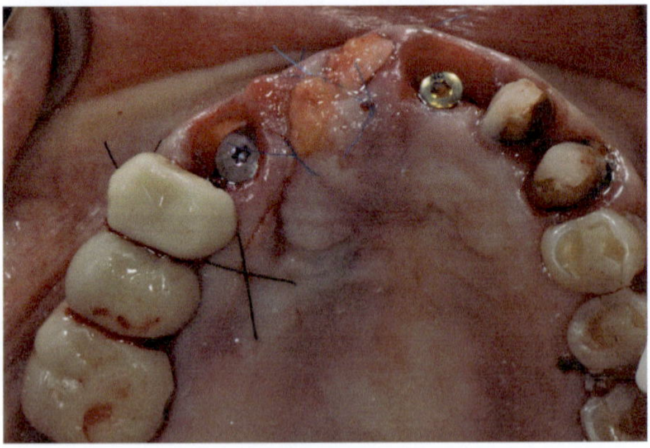

Fig. 11.273 Submerged root covered with the connective tissue graft. Recipient and donor site sutured

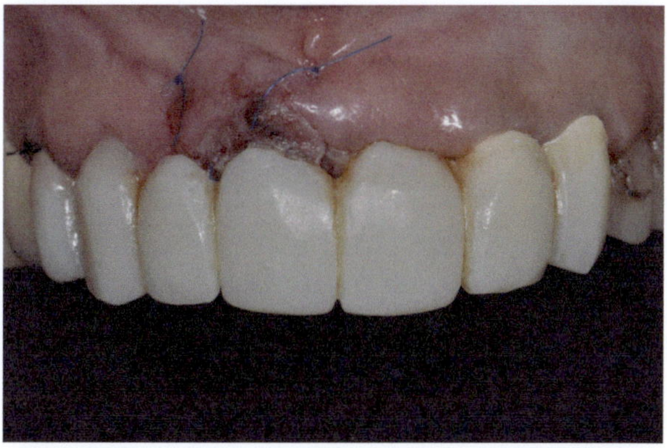

Fig. 11.274 Tooth supported provisional restoration

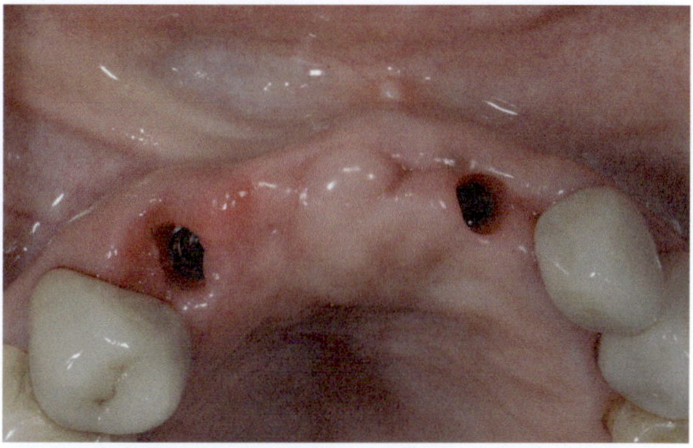

Fig. 11.275 Situation 4 months after surgery on removal of healing abutments

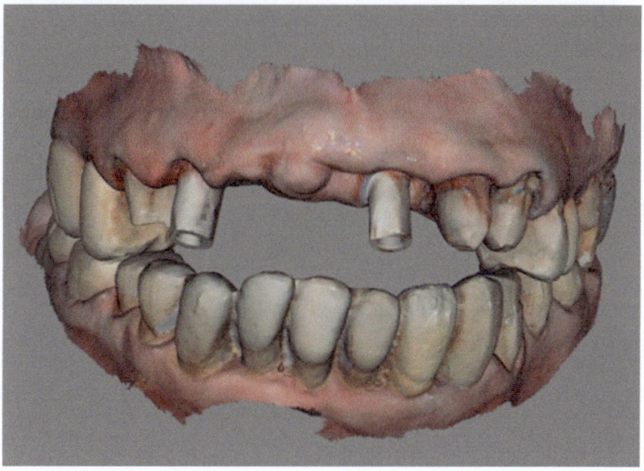

Fig. 11.276 Intraoral digital scan for final restorations

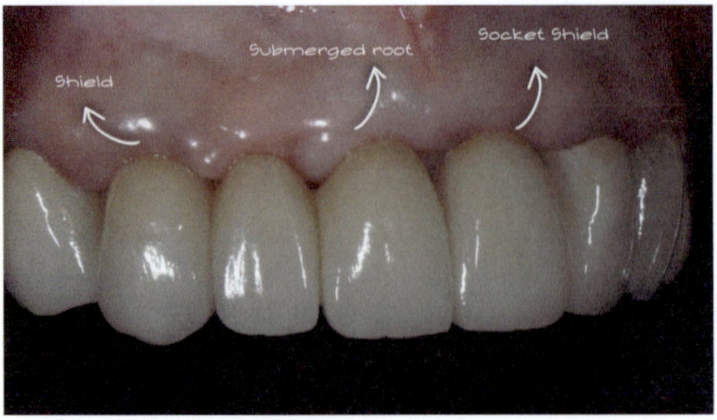

Fig. 11.277 Definitive implant-supported restoration

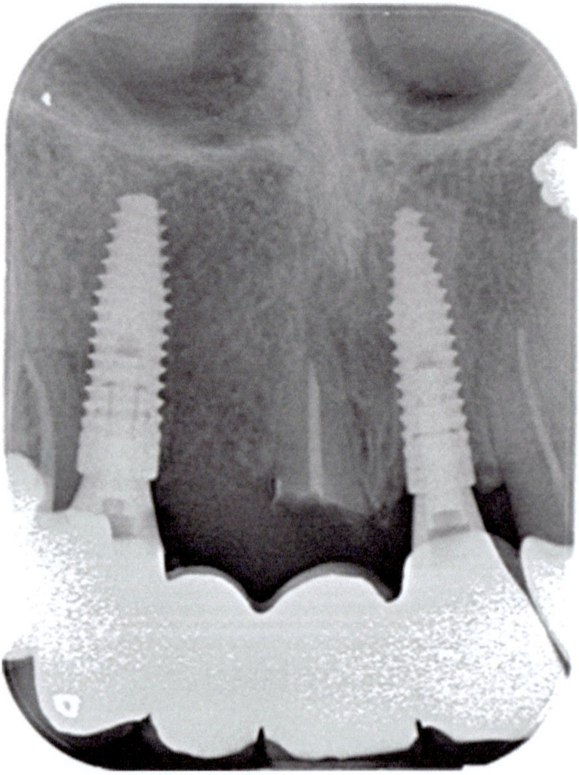

Fig. 11.278 Post-restoration radiograph

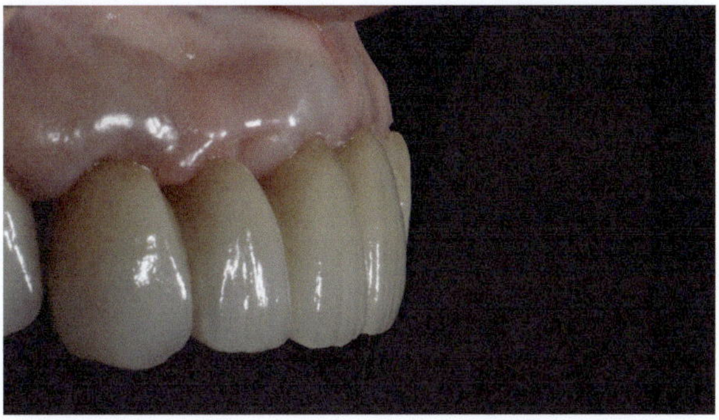

Fig. 11.279 Post-operative view displaying healthy peri-implant soft tissue contours and good emergence profile for the restoration

This compilation of work is a humble attempt by a group of wet-fingered clinicians who have been practicing and documenting PET cases over a 7-year period. The group has demonstrated high level of clinical success in performing these procedures by choosing appropriate cases for execution, meticulously following the technical guidelines and paying attention to details during the restorative phase. The group believes that PET procedures will become the preferred way of undertaking implant-supported restorations in the future.

Whilst these procedures have been published extensively over the past few years, there is scope to strengthen the level of evidence with well-designed clinical studies and long-term follow-ups.